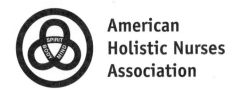
**American
Holistic Nurses
Association**

Core Curriculum
for HOLISTIC
NURSING

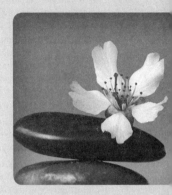

Edited by

Mary Helming, PhD, APRN, FNP-BC, AHN-BC
Track Coordinator for DNP and MSN Programs
Professor of Nursing
School of Nursing, Quinnipiac University
Hamden, Connecticut

Cynthia C. Barrere, PhD, RN, CNS, AHN-BC
Director of Faculty Development
Professor of Nursing
School of Nursing, Quinnipiac University
Hamden, Connecticut

Karen Avino, EdD, RN, AHN-BC, HWNC-BC
Coordinator, RN to BSN Program
Assistant Professor
School of Nursing, University of Delaware
Newark, Delaware

Deborah Shields, PhD, RN, CCRN, QTTT, AHN-BC
Associate Professor of Nursing
Capital University
Columbus, Ohio

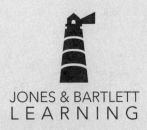
JONES & BARTLETT
LEARNING

World Headquarters
Jones & Bartlett Learning
5 Wall Street
Burlington, MA 01803
978-443-5000
info@jblearning.com
www.jblearning.com

Jones & Bartlett Learning books and products are available through most bookstores and online booksellers. To contact Jones & Bartlett Learning directly, call 800-832-0034, fax 978-443-8000, or visit our website, www.jblearning.com.

Substantial discounts on bulk quantities of Jones & Bartlett Learning publications are available to corporations, professional associations, and other qualified organizations. For details and specific discount information, contact the special sales department at Jones & Bartlett Learning via the above contact information or send an email to specialsales@jblearning.com.

Production Credits

Executive Publisher: William Brottmiller
Senior Acquisitions Editor: Nancy Anastasi Duffy
Editorial Assistant: Sara Bempkins
Associate Production Editor: Sara Fowles
Marketing Communications Manager: Katie Hennessy
VP, Manufacturing and Inventory Control: Therese Connell

Composition: Paw Print Media
Cover Design: Kristin E. Parker
Cover Image: © zimmytws/ShutterStock, Inc.
Printing and Binding: Edwards Brothers Malloy
Cover Printing: Edwards Brothers Malloy

To order this product, use ISBN: 978-1-284-03583-4

Library of Congress Cataloging-in-Publication Data
Core curriculum for holistic nursing / [edited by] Mary Helming ... [et al.].
-- 2nd ed.
p. ; cm.
Includes bibliographical references and index.
ISBN 978-1-284-03101-0 (pbk.)
I. Helming, Mary G.
[DNLM: 1. Holistic Nursing--Outlines. 2. Nurse's Role--Outlines. 3. Nursing Theory--Outlines. WY 18.2]
RT52
610.73076--dc23
                        2013010981
6048

Printed in the United States of America
17 16 15 14 13   10 9 8 7 6 5 4 3 2 1

Dedication

Visionaries are dreamers, people who see beyond the horizon and are able to illuminate the path for reaching goals never imagined. They believe in possibilities and, with humility and commitment, stand with us on our journey of discovery. Visionaries never give up the dream...nor do they give up on us! Barbara Montgomery Dossey, PhD, RN, AHN-BC, FAAN, HWNC-BC is among those we honor as a visionary and, to her, we dedicate the *Core Curriculum for Holistic Nursing, Second Edition.*

Dr. Dossey has, since the beginning of her career, worked tirelessly to create a healthcare system grounded in the core values of holism. Within her vision of caring/healing environments, clients and providers enter into partnerships in which both are able to grow in caring. Dr. Dossey clearly articulates the importance of an integrated model of holistic nursing where healing arts and technical competence are blended into a practice that supports the healing of self and other. Through her compassionate presence and commitment, Dr. Dossey shows us the way by living holistic nursing. She is an accomplished educator, researcher, theoretician, author and mentor who always, with grace and patience, teaches us to "stay the course," to dance with the possibilities and to have the courage to try new steps. Her gentle nudges move us on to the next step because they come from her belief in us...and ultimately, from her vision of a unified holistic discipline. Today, we are witnessing Dr. Dossey's vision blossoming throughout the world. We are blessed in her presence!

Contents

Prologue: Credentialing in Holistic Nursing

The American Holistic Nurses Credentialing Corporation (AHNCC) is pleased to share with readers information on national certification in Holistic Nursing. The *Core Curriculum for Holistic Nursing, Second Edition* is one reference for candidates to use as they prepare for the national examinations. A short overview of important information regarding AHNCC's history, work, and value is provided here.

HISTORY

AHNCC, incorporated in 1997 and governed by a board of directors, is responsible for the administration of certification examinations based on the precepts of holistic nursing. It currently certifies nurse coaches and holistic nurses at the basic (HN-BC and HNB-BC) and advanced levels (AHN-BC) as well as advanced practice registered nurses (APRNs) who seek to be credentialed as APHN-BC.

The American Nurses Association recognizes holistic nursing as an official nursing specialty. AHNCC certifies holistic nurses and nurses in other recognized specialties.

The American Holistic Nurses Association (AHNA) and AHNCC are autonomous organizations that collaborate to promote holistic nursing credentialing and practice. AHNCC is the credentialing body for AHNA and holistic nursing (HN).

CERTIFICATION EXAMINATIONS

The AHNCC certification examinations are based on nursing competencies specific to the standards of holistic nursing.[1] They are extrapolated from a review of the current literature including *Nursing: Scope and Standards of Practice*.[2] The competencies, reviewed by expert panels, are revised until approved and then used for a role delineation

(RDS) study. The results from the RDS are used to develop a blueprint, which guides the development of each exam.

A multiple-step process, overseen by Professional Testing Corporation of New York (PTC), is used to develop each examination including oversight and administration of the RDS, item writing to assess specific competencies, item reviews to assess content validity, and an examination development process to assess content and construct validity. An item bank is created from approved items, and certification examinations are drawn from these items. Items are consistently formatted and reviewed multiple times to ensure content and construct validity. An item analysis step, to assess for reliability, is conducted following the administration of each examination.

RECERTIFICATION

Certification is renewed every 5 years with submission of required documentation.

ASSISTANCE WITH PREPARING FOR CERTIFICATION EXAMINATIONS

Two documents, *Core Essentials for Basic Holistic Nursing* and *Core Essentials for the Practice of Advanced Holistic Nursing AHN-BC and APHN-BC*, provide important information for those who plan to sit for a certification examination.[3,4] Candidates should access these documents at www.ahncc.org. The Core Essentials documents are presented according to the standards of holistic nursing along with additional information to clarify each competency. Additional references can be found at the end of each Core Essentials document.

Candidates can also take a practice exam for the examination they plan to take. These exams consist of sample questions from the examination item bank and can be found on the PTC website: www.ptcny.com. Sample questions in the *Core Curriculum for Holistic Nursing, Second Edition* do not follow the rigorous development process followed by AHNCC. Although they help readers access basic knowledge and provide opportunities for personal exploration and evaluation, they are not to be viewed as predictive of success on AHNCC developed examinations.

■ NOTES

1. American Nurses Association. (2013). *Holistic nursing* (2nd ed.). Silver Spring, MD: Author.
2. American Nurses Association. (2010). *Nursing: Scope and standards of practice* (2nd ed.). Silver Spring, MD: Author.
3. American Holistic Nurses Credentialing Corporation. (2012). *Core essentials for basic holistic nursing.* Cedar Park, TX: Author.
4. American Holistic Nurses Credentialing Corporation. (2012). *Core essentials for the practice of advanced holistic nursing AHN-BC and APHN-BC.* Cedar Park, TX: Author.

Foreword

In the future, which I shall not see, for I am old, may a better way be opened! May the methods by which every infant, every human being will have the best chance at health—the methods by which every sick person will have the best chance at recovery, be learned and practiced. Hospitals are only an intermediate stage of civilization, never intended, at all events, to take in the whole sick population....

May we hope that, when we are all dead and gone, leaders will arise who have been personally experienced in the hard, practical work, the difficulties, and the joys of organizing nursing reforms, and who will lead far beyond anything we have done! May we hope that every nurse will be an atom in the hierarchy of ministers of the Highest! But she [or he] must be in her [or his] place in the hierarchy, not alone, not an atom in the indistinguishable mass of thousands of nurses. High hopes, which shall not be deceived!

—Florence Nightingale, *Sick-Nursing and Health-Nursing*

As I write this foreword in January 2013, I reflect back to January 17, 1981, the Woodlands, near Houston, Texas, and the thrilling founding meeting of the American Holistic Nurses Association (AHNA). With the AHNA founder, Charlotte "Charlie" McGuire, and 78 other nurses from eight states, we articulated the AHNA vision of caring and healing and uniting nurses in healing. We shared our stories about whole-person healing, human flourishing, and what it means to be a human being. We also explored how to create a fully integrated healing healthcare system and the leadership strategies needed for engaging in the restructuring and redesigning of healthcare delivery from an institutional curing paradigm to caring–healing practice.

As a founding AHNA member, and for more than 30 years, I have had the privilege to journey with holistic nursing colleagues to formalize our work and provide guidelines for our theoretical, empirical, caring–healing knowledge, competencies, and skills. Together, we have taken historical and bold steps to unite our voices, capacities, wisdom, and work of service—to create a healthy world—local to global. Our commitment to compassion, caring, and wholeness has shed light on the common quest and many possibilities for healing, health, and well-being for all humanity and planet Earth. This work has resulted in specialty status within the profession of nursing.

As the editor of the first edition of *AHNA Core Curriculum*, it brings me great joy to witness the

---

Note: The *AHNA Core Curriculum* (2nd edition) is adapted from B. M. Dossey and L. Keegan, *Holistic Nursing: A Handbook for Practice* (6th ed.). Burlington, MA: Jones & Bartlett Learning, 2013.

outstanding leadership of the editors of this second edition of *Core Curriculum for Holistic Nursing*, Mary Helming, Cynthia C. Barrere, Karen Avino, and Deborah Shields.[1] The second edition of *Core Curriculum for Holistic Nursing* is a guide for holistic nursing knowledge, competencies, and skills for transforming health care from a disease model of care to one that focuses on health and wellness.

This second edition of *Core Curriculum for Holistic Nursing* is published at an exciting time because it parallels the implementation of national strategies to stop disease before it starts and to create a healthy and fit nation. Holistic nurses recognize health prevention, healthy behaviors, and stress management as key factors in health, along with traditional healthcare screening and examinations. It is a "both/and" and not an "either/or."

The *Core Curriculum for Holistic Nursing, Second Edition* explores the complex nature of healing from many viewpoints and synthesizes holistic philosophy, theories, ethics, holistic caring process, holistic communication, healing environments, cultural diversity, holistic education and research, and holistic nurse self-care. It blends both the art and science of healing and spirituality and new, innovative, holistic ways of bringing balance and harmony into our chaotic times in health care and daily life.

Today, holistic nurses are challenged to carry forth Florence Nightingale's vision with a holistic, integrative, and integral philosophy.[2,3] The second edition of *Core Curriculum for Holistic Nursing* also assists us to bring our intention, intuition, compassion, and presence into all corners of health care, when technology tends to nudge them out—to recognize that patient care always requires "being with" rather than always "doing to." Intention is a volitional act of love and is consciously creating an image of a person's spiritual essence and wholeness that is experienced as a sacred space of inner calm.

Barbara Montgomery Dossey, PhD, RN, AHN-BC, FAAN, HWNC-BC

■ NOTES

1. Dossey, B. M. (1997). *American Holistic Nurses Association core curriculum for holistic nursing.* Gaithersburg, MD: Aspen.

2. Dossey, B. M. (2010). *Florence Nightingale: Mystic, visionary, healer* (Commemorative ed.). Philadelphia, PA: F. A. Davis.

3. Dossey. B. M. (2013). Nursing: Integral, integrative, holistic—local to global. In B. M. Dossey & L. Keegan (Eds.), *Holistic nursing: A handbook for practice* (pp. 3–57). Burlington, MA: Jones & Bartlett Learning.

Acknowledgments

The *Core Curriculum for Holistic Nursing, Second Edition* represents the work of many people. First and foremost is Barbara Montgomery Dossey who guided the creation and development of the first edition of the *AHNA Core Curriculum* in 1998. Although the first edition is still popular today, there have been many changes in healthcare and nursing practice. Barbara mentored the coeditors of *Core Curriculum for Holistic Nursing, Second Edition* through the process of designing and developing a resource that addresses these practice changes.

Deep appreciation is extended to the holistic nurse content experts who served as chapter contributors for this second edition of the *Core Curriculum for Holistic Nursing.* They generously shared their time and knowledge to provide this edition with the most current information about holistic nursing practice. The coeditors are grateful for their expertise and commitment to the development of this book.

The coeditors of the *Core Curriculum for Holistic Nursing, Second Edition* are also grateful to the American Holistic Nurses Association and the American Holistic Nurses Credentialing Center for their support of this work. The leadership, members and certificants of these associations are committed to the advancement of holistic nursing and the development of resources that are timely and helpful to nurses who wish to deepen their understanding of the core values and scope and standards foundational to the practice of holistic nursing.

And to each of you, the holistic nurses who are reading this resource to deepen your knowledge of holistic nursing or to utilize this as another resource in preparing for certification, the coeditors want to say thank you—thank you for, each and every moment, dedicating yourself to being in partnership with others as you cocreate paths of healing. You are the hearts and the voices of our envisioned future!

Editors' Note

A comprehensive table of common herbs and supplements is included within this text's supplemental resources, available exclusively online at http://go.jblearning.com/coreholistic.

Contributors

Veda Andrus, EdD, MSN, RN, HN-BC
Vice President, Education and
    Program Development
The BirchTree Center for Healthcare
    Transformation
Florence, Massachusetts

**Jeanne Anselmo, BSN, RN,
    BCIAC-SF, HNB-BC**
Holistic Nurse Educator/ Consultant
Sea Cliff, New York
Cofounder, Faculty
Contemplative Urban Law Program
City University of New York School of Law
Queens, New York
Faculty
Merton Contemplative Initiative, Iona College
New Rochelle, New York
Faculty
New York Open Center
New York, New York
Teacher, Order of Interbeing
Plum Village Tradition of Zen Master
    Thich Nhat Hanh
Philadelphia, Pennsylvania

**Karen Avino, EdD, RN, AHN-BC,
    HWNC-BC**
Coordinator, RN to BSN Program
Assistant Professor
School of Nursing, University of Delaware
Newark, Delaware

**Carol M. Baldwin, PhD, RN, CHTP,
    AHN-BC, FAAN**
Associate Professor and Southwest
    Borderlands Scholar
Director, Center for World Health Promotion
    and Disease Prevention
Affiliate Faculty, Southwest Interdisciplinary
    Research Center (SIRC) for Health Disparities

Affiliate Faculty, North American Center for
    Transborder Studies (NACTS)
Arizona State University College of Nursing
    and Health Innovation
Phoenix, Arizona

Linda A. Bark, PhD, RN, MCC, NC-BC
Founder and President, Bark Coaching Institute
Alameda, California
Adjunct Faculty, John F. Kennedy University
Pleasant Hill, California
Adjunct Faculty and Mentor, National Institute
    of Whole Health
Boston, Massachusetts
Author of *Wisdom of the Whole*--2012 Book of the
    Year by AJN for Professional Development
    and Issues
Coauthor of *The Art and Science of Nurse Coaching:
    The Providers Guide to Scope and Competencies*

Cynthia C. Barrere, PhD, RN, CNS, AHN-BC
Director of Faculty Development
Professor of Nursing
School of Nursing, Quinnipiac University
Hamden, Connecticut

**Megan McInnis Burt, MS, RN, CARN,
    PMH-BC, NC-BC**
Nurse Educator, North Shore LIJ Health System
Faculty, Huntington Meditation and
    Imagery Center
Faculty, International Nurse Coach Association
    (INCA)
Private Practice
Levittown, New York

Mary Ann Cordeau, PhD, RN
Nurse Historian
Assistant Professor of Nursing
Quinnipiac University
Hamden, Connecticut

Barbara Montgomery Dossey, PhD, RN, AHN-BC, FAAN, HWNC-BC
Codirector, International Nurse Coach Association (INCA)
Core Faculty, Integrative Nurse Coach Certificate Program (INCCP)
Miami, Florida
International Codirector, Nightingale Initiative for Global Health (NIGH)
Washington, DC and Neepawa, Manitoba, Canada
Director, Holistic Nursing Consultants
Santa Fe, New Mexico

Marty Downey, MSN, PhD, RN, AHN-BC, CHTIP, CNE
Associate Professor
School of Nursing
Boise State University
Boise, Idaho

Joan Engebretson, DrPH, AHN-BC, RN
Judy Fred Professor of Nursing
School of Nursing, Department of Family Nursing
University of Texas Health Science Center
Houston, Texas

Kimberley A. Evans, APRN, CNS-BC, AHN-BC, CNAT
Adjunct Faculty
Institute for Integrative Medicine
Bellarmine University Lansing School of Nursing
Louisville, Kentucky

Noreen Cavan Frisch, PhD, RN, ANC-BC, FAAN
Professor and Director, School of Nursing
University of Victoria
Victoria, British Columbia, Canada

Mary Helming, PhD, APRN, FNP-BC, AHN-BC
Track Coordinator for DNP and MSN Programs
Professor of Nursing
School of Nursing, Quinnipiac University
Hamden, Connecticut

Francie Halderman, RN, BSN, HN-BC
Integrative and Holistic Health Consultant
Strategic Planning and Culture Change for Resilient Organizations
Director, The Art of Universal Medicine
Philadelphia, Pennsylvania

Darlene R. Hess, PhD, RN, AHN-BC, PMHNP-BC, ACC, HWNC-BC
Brown Mountain Visions
Los Ranchos, New Mexico
Practitioner Faculty
University of Phoenix
Albuquerque, New Mexico
Faculty, RN to BSN Program
Northern New Mexico College
El Rito, New Mexico

Shannon S. Spies Ingersoll, DNP, CRNA
Independent Contractor
Anesthesia and KIND, LLC Home Care
Dover, Minnesota

Christina Bergh Jackson, PhD, APRN, PNP, AHN-BC, CNE
Professor, Nursing Curriculum Chair
Eastern University
St. Davids, Pennsylvania

Lynn Keegan, PhD, RN, AHN-BC, FAAN
Director, Holistic Nursing Consultants
Port Angeles, Washington
Partner, Absolutely: Business and Personal Strategic Consulting, LLC
Indianapolis, Indiana
Past President, American Holistic Nurses Association

Kamron Keep, RN, BSN
Primary Nurse, Radiation Oncology
St. Luke's Mountain States Tumor Institute
Boise, Idaho

Dorothy M. Larkin, PhD, RN
Associate Professor, The College of New Rochelle, School of Nursing
Coordinator and Faculty for the Clinical Specialist in Holistic Nursing Master's and Post-Master's Programs
New Rochelle, New York

Jackie D. Levin, RN, MS, AHN-BC, CHTP
Director, Leading Edge Nursing
Patient Advocate
Jefferson Healthcare
Port Townsend, Washington

Susan Luck, MA, RN, HNB-BC, CCN, HWNC-BC
Director, Integrative Nursing Institute (INI)
Codirector International Nurse Coach Association (INCA)

Core Faculty, Integrative Nurse Coach Certificate
  Association (INCCP)
Founder and Director, Earthrose Institute (ERI)
Miami, Florida

Carla Mariano, EdD, RN, AHN-BC, FAAIM
Adjunct Associate Professor
College of Nursing, New York University
New York, New York
Interim Nursing Program Director
Pacific College of Oriental Medicine
San Diego, California
Consultant, Holistic Nursing Education
Past President, American Holistic
  Nurses Association

**Deborah McElligott, DNP, AHN-BC,
  ANP-BC, HWNC-BC**
Nurse Practitioner, Southside Hospital
North Shore LIJ Health System
Bayshore, New York
Assistant Professor
Hofstra North Shore LIJ School of Medicine
Hofstra University
Hempstead, New York

Sharon S. Parker, MS, RN, CNS
Professor of Nursing
Capital University
Columbus, Ohio

Sue Popkess-Vawter, PhD, RN
Professor of Nursing
University of Kansas School of Nursing
Kansas City, Kansas

Pamela J. Potter, DNSc, RN, CNS
Assistant Professor, School of Nursing
University of Portland
Portland, Oregon

Janet F. Quinn, PhD, RN, FAAN
Director, HaelanWorks
www.HaelanWorks.com
Lyons, Colorado

Jennifer L. Reich, PhD, MA, RN
Assistant Professor
School of Nursing
College of Health and Human Services
Northern Arizona University
Flagstaff, Arizona

Ana Schaper, PhD, RN
Nurse Scientist
Gundersen Lutheran Health System
LaCrosse, Wisconsin

**Bonney Gulino Schaub, RN, MS,
  PMHCNS-BC, NC-BC**
Codirector, International Nurse
  Coach Association
Miami, Florida
Codirector, Huntington Meditation
  and Imagery Center
Huntington, NY

Marie Shanahan, MA, BSN, RN, HN-BC
President/CEO
The BirchTree Center for Healthcare
  Transformation
Florence, Massachusetts

David Shields, MSN, RN, QTTT
Assistant Professor of Nursing
Capital University
Staff Nurse, PACU
Doctors Hospital Ohio Health
Therapeutic Touch Therapist and Teacher
Columbus, Ohio

**Deborah Shields, PhD, RN, CCRN,
  QTTT, AHN-BC**
Associate Professor of Nursing
Capital University
Columbus, Ohio
Staff Nurse, PACU
Doctors Hospital Ohio Health
Therapeutic Touch Therapist and Teacher
Columbus, Ohio

**Victoria E. Slater, RN, PhD,
  AHN-BC, CHTP/I**
Holistic Nurse, Private Practice
Clarksville, Tennessee

**Mary Elaine Southard, RN, MSN,
  APHN-BC, HWNC-BC**
Director, Integrative Health Consulting and
  Coaching, LLC
Scranton, Pennsylvania

Lucia M. Thornton, RN, MSN, AHN-BC
President, Innovations in Healthcare
Fresno, California
Consultant and Educator, Whole Person Caring
Past President, American Holistic
  Nurses Association

**Rothlyn P. Zahourek, PhD, PMHCNS-BC,
  AHN-BC**
Adjunct Clinical Faculty
University of Massachusetts School of Nursing
Amherst, Massachusetts

Chapter 1

Nursing: Integral, Integrative, and Holistic: Local to Global

Barbara Montgomery Dossey

■ DEFINITIONS

Global health Exploration of the emerging value base and new relationships and innovations that occur when health becomes an essential component and expression of global citizenship; the increased awareness that health is a basic human right and a global good that needs to be promoted and protected by the global community.

Holistic nursing *See* the section "Nurses as Change Agents" that follows and Chapter 2 definitions in *Holistic Nursing: A Handbook for Practice, 6th ed.*

Integral *See* the following sections in this chapter: "Nurses as Change Agents" and "Theory of Integral Nursing."

Integrative *See* the section "Nurses as Change Agents" that follows.

Relationship-centered care A process model of caregiving that is based in a vision of community where the patient–practitioner, community–practitioner, and practitioner–practitioner relationships and the unique set of responsibilities of each are honored and valued.

■ NURSING: INTEGRAL, INTEGRATIVE, AND HOLISTIC: LOCAL TO GLOBAL

Nurses as Change Agents

1. Nurses are improving the health of the nation and are focused on increasing the "health span" of individuals by using an integral, integrative, and holistic approach rather than focusing on life span.

2. An *integral exploration* is an approach and a comprehensive way to organize multiple phenomena of human experience related to four perspectives of reality: (a) the individual interior (personal/intentional); (b) individual exterior (physiology/behavioral); (c) collective interior (shared/cultural); and (d) collective exterior (systems/structures).[1,2] See the section titled "Theory of Integral Nursing"[1,2] later in this chapter.

3. An integrative exploration is an approach that places the client at the center and addresses the whole person and full range of physical, emotional, mental, social, spiritual, and environmental influences that affect health; it includes the client's personalized action plan to maintain optimal health behaviors and human flourishing and to heal illness and disease. It makes use of all appropriate therapeutic approaches, healthcare professionals, and disciplines to achieve optimal health and healing.[3]

4. A holistic exploration is an approach that sees the patient as an interconnected unity and that includes physical, mental, social, and spiritual factors in any interventions. The whole is a system that is greater than the sum of its parts. It includes holistic communication that is a free flow of verbal and nonverbal interchange between and among people and significant beings such as pets, nature, and God/Life Force/Absolute/Transcendent. Holistic communication explores meaning and ideas leading to mutual understanding and growth.[4]

Global Nursing

1. Health and well-being of people everywhere can be seen as common ground to secure a sustainable, prosperous future for

everyone. Nurses engage in interdisciplinary and interprofessional collaboration and with concerned citizens to mobilize new approaches to education, healthcare delivery, and disease prevention.[5-8]

2. From an integral, integrative, and holistic nursing perspective, nurses are challenged to see global health imperatives as common concerns of humankind. These are not isolated problems in far-off countries. We must see prevention and prevention education as important to the health of humanity.

Global Health

1. Global health is the exploration of the emerging value base and new relationships and agendas that occur when health becomes an essential component and expression of global citizenship.[6] Global health encompasses an increased awareness that health is a basic human right and is "decent care"[8] that addresses the body, mind, and spirit. Health is a global good that needs to be promoted and protected by the global community.

2. The *Nightingale Declaration for a Healthy World* challenges nurses to act locally and think globally and to expand their awareness of integral, integrative, and holistic concepts and modalities in all ways of knowing, doing, and being. To expand our global consciousness and connect global nurses, interprofessionals, and concerned citizens to create healthy people living on a healthy planet by 2020, we can sign the Nightingale Declaration[9] at www.nightingaledeclaration.net.

3. United Nations Millennium Development Goals: In 2000, the 192 United Nations (UN) Member States adopted eight Millennium Development Goals (MDGs) to progress toward a sustainable quality of life for all of humanity by 2015.[10]

   a. Health is the common thread running through all eight UN MDGs. The UN MDGs are directly related to nurses as they work today to achieve global health at grassroots levels everywhere. Many nurses are engaged in sharing local solutions at the global level.

   b. Of these eight MDGs, three—MDG 4 Reduce child mortality, MDG 5 Improve maternal health, and MDG 6 Combat HIV/AIDS—are directly related to health and nursing. The other five goals—MDG 1 Eradicate extreme poverty and hunger, MDG 2 Achieve universal primary education, MDG 3 Promote gender equality and empower women, MDG 7 Ensure environmental sustainability, and MDG 8 Global partnerships for development—are factors that determine the health or lack of health of people. For each goal, one or more targets that use the 1990 data as benchmarks are set to be achieved by 2015.

Florence Nightingale's Legacy

1. Florence Nightingale overview

   a. Nightingale (1820–1910) is the philosophical founder of modern secular nursing and the first recognized nurse theorist. She also was an educator, administrator, communicator, statistician, and environmental activist.[11-13]

   b. Today we recognize Nightingale's work as global nursing. She envisioned what a healthy world might be with her integral, integrative, and holistic philosophy and expanded visionary capacities.

   c. Nightingale's major focus was worldwide service to humanity and communication of her knowledge.

2. Nightingale major accomplishments[11-13]

   a. Nightingale established the model for nursing schools throughout the world and created a prototype model of care for the sick and wounded soldiers during the Crimean War (1854–1856).

   b. She was an innovator in British Army medical reform. She reorganized the British Army Medical Department, created an Army Statistical Department, and collaborated on creating the first British Army medical school, including developing the curriculum and choosing the professors.

   c. She revolutionized hospital data collection and invented a statistical wedge diagram equivalent to today's circular histograms and circular statistical representation. In 1858, she became the first woman admitted to the Royal Statistical Society.

d. She wrote more than 100 combined books and official Army reports. Her 10,000 letters make up the largest private collection of letters at the British Library, with 4,000 family letters at the Wellcome Trust in London.[11-13] Nightingale addressed many themes in her *Notes on Hospitals* (1859),[14] *Notes on Nursing* (1860),[15] her formal letters to her nurses (1872–1900),[16] and her "Sick-Nursing and Health-Nursing" (1893).[17]

Eras of Medicine

Currently, three eras of medicine are operational in Western biomedicine.

1. Era I medicine: Era I medicine began to take shape in the 1860s, when medicine was striving to become more scientific. The underlying assumption of this era is that health and illness are completely physical in nature. The focus is on combining drugs, medical treatments, and technology to achieve health. A person's consciousness is considered a by-product of the chemical, anatomic, and physiologic aspects of the brain and is not considered a major factor in the origins of health or disease.

2. Era II medicine: In the 1950s, Era II therapies began to emerge. These therapies reflected the growing awareness that the actions of a person's mind or consciousness—thoughts, emotions, beliefs, meaning, and attitudes—influence the behavior of the person's physical body. In both Era I and Era II, a person's consciousness is said to be "local" in nature; that is, confined to a specific location in space (the body itself) and in time (the present moment and a single lifetime).

3. Era III medicine: This, the newest and most advanced era, originated in science. Consciousness is said to be nonlocal in that it is not bound to individual bodies. The minds of individuals are spread throughout space and time; they are infinite, immortal, omnipresent, and, ultimately, one. Era III therapies involve any therapy in which the effects of consciousness create bridges among different persons, as with distant healing, intercessory prayer, shamanic healing, so-called miracles, and certain emotions (e.g., love, empathy, compassion). Era

III approaches involve transpersonal experiences of being. They raise a person above control at a day-to-day material level to an experience outside his or her local self.

"Doing" and "Being" Therapies[18,19]

1. Holistic nurses use both "doing" and "being" therapies that are referred to as holistic nursing therapies, complementary and alternative therapies, or integrative and integral therapies.

   a. Doing therapies include almost all forms of modern medicine, such as medications, procedures, dietary manipulations, radiation, and acupuncture. In contrast, being therapies do not employ things, but instead use states of consciousness. These include imagery, prayer, meditation, and quiet contemplation, as well as the presence and intention of the nurse. These techniques are therapeutic because of the power of the psyche to affect the body.

   b. Doing therapies can be either directed or nondirected. A person who uses a directed mental strategy attaches a specific outcome to the imagery, such as the regression of disease or the normalization of the blood pressure. In a nondirected approach, the person images the best outcome for the situation but does not try to direct the situation or assign a specific outcome to the strategy. This reliance on the inherent intelligence within one's self to come forth is a way of acknowledging the intrinsic wisdom and self-correcting capacity within.

2. Doing and being therapies and eras of medicine:

   a. Era I medicine uses doing therapies that are highly directed in their approach. These therapies employ things, such as medications, for a specific goal.

   b. Era II medicine is a classic body–mind approach that usually does not require the use of things, with the exception of biofeedback instrumentation, music therapy, and use of CDs and videos to enhance learning and experience and increase awareness of body–mind connections. It employs being therapies that can be directed or nondirected, depending on the mental strategies selected (e.g., relaxation or meditation).

c. Era III medicine is similar to Era II medicine in that it requires a willingness to become aware, moment by moment, of what is true for our inner and outer experience. It is actually a "not doing" so that we can become conscious of releasing, emptying, trusting, and acknowledging that we have done our best, regardless of the outcome.

Rational Healing vs. Paradoxical Healing[18,19]

All healing experiences or activities can be arranged along a continuum from the rational healing domain to the paradoxical healing domain.

1. Rational healing and doing therapies
   a. These are therapies that make sense to our linear, intellectual thought processes and fall into the rational healing category.
   b. Based on science, these strategies conform to our worldview of commonsense notions. Often, the professional can follow an algorithm, which dictates a step-by-step approach. Examples of rational healing include surgery, irradiation, medications, exercise, and diet.
2. Paradoxical healing and being therapies
   a. Paradoxical healing experiences include healing events that might seem absurd or contradictory but are, in fact, true. They frequently happen without a scientific explanation.
   b. In psychological counseling, for example, a breakthrough is a paradox. When a patient has a psychological breakthrough, it is clear that the person has gained a new meaning. However, no clearly delineated steps lead to the breakthrough. Such an event is called a breakthrough for the very reason that it is unpredictable—hence, the paradox.
3. Exploring paradox[18,19]
   a. *Biofeedback* involves a paradox. When a person gives up trying to increase blood flow, induce relaxation, or shift brain wave activity and enters into a state of being, or passive volition, he or she allows these physiologic states changes to occur in the desired direction.

b. *Placebo* is a paradox. If the individual has just a little discomfort, a placebo does not work very well. The more pain a person has, however, the more dramatic the response to a placebo medication. A person who does not know that the medication is a placebo responds best. This is referred to as the "paradox of success through ignorance."

c. *Prayer* and *faith* fall into the domain of paradox because there is no rational scientific explanation for their effectiveness.[20]

d. *Miracle cures* also are paradoxical because no scientific mechanism can explain them. Every nurse has known, heard of, or read about a patient who had a severe illness confirmed by laboratory evidence that disappeared after the patient adopted a being approach.

■ RELATIONSHIP-CENTERED CARE

The Pew Health Professions Commission[21] describes three essential components of relationship care. Relationship-centered care is a model of caregiving based in a vision of community. The three types of relationships involve a unique set of tasks and responsibilities that address self-awareness, knowledge, values, and skills. Application of these components has been influential in relationship-centered care.[22-24]

1. Patient–practitioner relationship
   a. This includes expanding self-awareness, understanding the patient's experience of health and illness, developing and maintaining caring relationships with patients, and communicating clearly and effectively.
   b. Active collaboration includes the patient and family in the decision-making process, promotion of health, and prevention of stress and illness within the family.
   c. A successful relationship involves active listening and effective communication; integration of the elements of caring, healing, values, and ethics to enhance and preserve the dignity and integrity of the patient and family; and a reduction of the power inequalities in the relationship with regard to race, sex, education, occupation, and socioeconomic status.

2. Community–practitioner relationship
   a. The patient and his or her family simultaneously belong to many types of communities, such as the immediate family, relatives, friends, coworkers, neighborhoods, religious and community organizations, and the hospital community.
   b. The knowledge, skills, and values needed by practitioners include understanding the meaning of the community, recognizing the multiple contributors to health and illness within the community, developing and maintaining relationships with the community, and working collaboratively with other individuals and organizations to establish effective community-based care.
   c. Practitioners must be sensitive to the impact on patients of these various communities and foster the collaborative activities of these communities as they interact with the patient and family. Practitioners must identify and improve the restraints or barriers within each community that block the patient's healing to promote the patient's health and well-being.
3. Practitioner–practitioner relationship
   a. This involves many diverse practitioner–practitioner relationships and requires knowledge, skills, and values including developing self-awareness; understanding the diverse knowledge base and skills of different practitioners; developing teams and communities; and understanding the working dynamics of groups, teams, and organizations that can provide resources and services for the patient and family.
   b. Collaborative relationships require shared planning and action toward common goals. Responsibility for outcomes is shared with the interdisciplinary team in coordination with joint decision making, communication, and shared authority.
   c. All practitioners must understand and respect one another's roles and learn about the diversity of therapeutic and healing modalities that they each use (e.g., acupuncture, herbs, aromatherapy, touch therapies, music therapy, folk healers). This includes being open to

the potential benefits of different modalities and valuing cultural diversity. Ultimately, the effectiveness of collaboration among practitioners depends on their ability to share problem solving, goal setting, and decision making within a trusting, collegial, and caring environment.

■ CREATING OPTIMAL HEALING ENVIRONMENTS

1. Definition of optimal healing environments (OHEs): The Samueli Institute for Information Biology[25] (www.siib.org) defines optimal healing environments as "the social, psychological, spiritual, physical and behavioral components of health care [that] are oriented toward support and stimulation of healing and the achievement of wholeness."
   a. The OHE framework contains *four environmental domains*—internal, interpersonal, behavioral, and external. Under these four domains are *eight constructs*, each having several elements. These domains, components, and elements are integrated from the internal environments to the outer environments of the individual and the collective.
   b. Optimal healing environments always start with the individual, whether that is the practitioner, healer, healee (client/patient), a significant other, and/or the community as an entity. OHEs can lead to more cost-effective, efficient organizations where the environment truly facilitates healing and where practitioners are fully supported to connect to the "soul of healing" and the mission of caring.
2. Planetree International: This innovative patient-centered care model demonstrates that patient-centered care is not only an empowering philosophy, it is a viable, vital, and cost-effective model.[26]
   a. The Planetree model is implemented in acute and critical care departments, emergency departments, long-term care facilities, outpatient services, as well as ambulatory care and community health centers.
   b. The Planetree model of care is a patient-centered, holistic approach to health

care that promotes mental, emotional, spiritual, social, and physical healing. It empowers patients and families through the exchange of information and encourages healing partnerships with caregivers. It seeks to maximize positive healthcare outcomes by integrating optimal medical therapies and incorporating art and nature into the healing environment.

■ THEORY OF INTEGRAL NURSING

The Theory of Integral Nursing is presented in this chapter as its maps and expands nurses' capacities as 21st-century Nightingales, health diplomats, and integral health coaches who coach for integral health locally to globally. This one of many nursing theories used by holistic nurses is described in Chapter 5 of the sixth edition of the *Holistic Nursing Handbook*. For an in-depth discussion, see Dossey.[1,2] This is not a freestanding theory because it incorporates concepts and philosophies from various paradigms including holism, chaos, integral, multidimensionality, spiral dynamics, complexity, systems, and many others. Holistic nursing practice is included (embraced) and transcended (gone beyond).

Theory of Integral Nursing: Overview

1. The Theory of Integral Nursing is a grand theory that presents the science and art of nursing locally to globally. It includes an integral process, integral worldview, and integral dialogue that is praxis—theory in action. An integral understanding allows us to more fully comprehend the complexity of human nature and healing; it assists nurses to bring to health care and society their knowledge, skills, and compassion.[1,2]

2. Components: In the Theory of Integral Nursing, the subject matter and building blocks are as follows: (a) healing, (b) the metaparadigm of nursing theory, (c) patterns of knowing, (d) the four quadrants adapted from Wilber's integral theory (individual interior [subjective, personal/intentional], individual exterior [objective, behavioral], collective interior [intersubjective, cultural], and collective exterior [interobjective, systems/structures]), and (e) "all quadrants, all levels, all lines" that are adapted from Wilber.[27-29]

a. Healing: Healing embraces the individual as an energy field who is connected to the energy fields of all humanity and the world. Healing is transformed when we consider four perspectives of reality in any moment: (1) the individual interior (personal/intentional), (2) individual exterior (physiology/ behavioral), (3) collective interior (shared/cultural), and (4) collective exterior (systems/structures). Focusing our reflective integral lens on these four perspectives of reality assists us in experiencing a unitary grasp of the complexity that emerges in healing.

b. Metaparadigm of nursing theory: The metaparadigm in a nursing theory is nurse, person, health, and environment (society). Healing implies an interrelatedness, interdependence, and impact of these domains as each informs and influences the others; a change in one creates a degree of change in the others, thus affecting healing at many levels.

c. Patterns of knowing: The patterns of knowing in nursing (personal, empirical, aesthetic, ethical, not knowing, sociopolitical) assist nurses in bringing themselves into the full expression of being present in the moment, to integrate aesthetics with science, and to develop the flow of ethical experience with thinking and acting.

d. Quadrants: These four quadrants show the primary dimensions or perspectives of how we experience the world. They are represented graphically as the Upper-Left (UL), Upper-Right (UR), Lower-Left (LL), and Lower-Right (LR) quadrants. Each quadrant, which is intricately linked and bound to each other, carries its own truths and language. The specifics of the quadrants are as follows:

   ▪ Upper-Left (UL): In this "I" space (subjective; the inside of the individual) can be found the world of the individual's interior experiences. These are thoughts, emotions, memories, perceptions, immediate sensations, and states of mind (imagination, fears, feelings, beliefs, values, esteem, cognitive capacity, emotional maturity, moral development, and spiritual maturity). Integral nursing requires development of the I.

- Upper-Right (UR): In this "It" space (objective; the outside of the individual) can be found the world of the individual's exterior. This includes the material body (physiology [cells, molecules, neurotransmitters, limbic system], biochemistry, chemistry, physics), integral patient care plans, skill development (health, fitness, exercise, nutrition, etc.), behaviors, leadership skills, and integral life practices.

- Lower-Left (LL): In this "We" space (intersubjective; the inside of the collective) can be found the interior collective of how we can come together to share our cultural background, stories, values, meanings, vision, language, relationships and how to form partnerships to achieve a healing mission.

- Lower-Right (LR): In this "Its" space (interobjective; the outside of the collective) can be found the world of the collective, exterior things. These include social systems/structures, networks, organizational structures, systems (including financial and billing systems in health care), information technology, regulatory structures (environmental and governmental policies, etc.), and any aspect of the technological environment and the natural world.

- The left-hand quadrants (Upper Left, Lower Left) describe aspects of reality as interpretive and qualitative. In contrast, the right-hand quadrants (Upper Right, Lower Right) describe aspects of reality as measurable and quantitative.

e. All Quadrants, All Levels (AQAL): These levels, lines, states, and types are important elements of any comprehensive map of reality. The integral model simply assists us in further articulating and connecting all areas, awareness, and depth in these four quadrants. Briefly, these levels, lines, states, and types are as follows:[26]

- Levels: Levels of development become permanent with growth and maturity

(e.g., cognitive, relational, psychosocial, physical, mental, emotional, spiritual) and represent increased organization or complexity. These levels are also referred to as waves and stages of development. Each individual possesses the masculine and feminine voice or energy. Neither masculine nor feminine is higher or better; they are two equivalent types at each level of consciousness and development.

- Lines: Lines are developmental areas known as multiple intelligences: cognitive line (awareness of what is); interpersonal line (how I relate socially to others); emotional/affective line (the full spectrum of emotions); moral line (awareness of what should be); needs line (Maslow's hierarchy of needs); aesthetics line (self-expression of art, beauty, and full meaning); self-identity line (who am I?); spiritual line (where spirit is viewed as its own line of unfolding, and not just as ground and highest state); and values line (what a person considers most important).

- States: States are temporary changing forms of awareness: waking, dreaming, deep sleep, altered meditative states (resulting from meditation, yoga, contemplative prayer, etc.), altered states (resulting from mood swings, physiology, and pathophysiology shifts with disease, illness, seizures, cardiac arrest, low or high oxygen saturation, drugs), peak experiences (triggered by intense listening to music, walks in nature, love making, mystical experiences such as hearing the voice of God or the voice of a deceased person, etc.).

- Types: Types are differences in personality and masculine and feminine expressions and development (e.g., cultural creative types, personality types, enneagram).

f. Structure: The structure of the Theory of Integral Nursing illustrates that all content components are overlaid to create a mandala symbolizing wholeness. *Healing* is placed at the center, then the *metaparadigm of nursing* (integral nurse, person, integral health, integral environment), the *patterns of knowing* (personal, empirics, aesthetics, ethics, not knowing, sociopolitical), the *four quadrants* (subjective, objective, intersubjective, interobjective), and *all quadrants* and *all levels* of growth, development, and evolution. (Note: Although the patterns of knowing are superimposed as they are in the various quadrants, they can also fit into other quadrants.)

3. Four integral nursing principles
   a. Integral Nursing Principle 1: Nursing Requires Development of the "I": Integral Nursing Principle 1 recognizes the interior individual I (subjective) space. Each of us must value the importance of exploring our health and well-being starting with our own personal exploration and development on many levels.[1,2]
   b. Integral Nursing Principle 2: Nursing Is Built on "We": Integral Nursing Principle 2 recognizes the importance of the We (intersubjective) space where nurses come together and are conscious of sharing their worldviews, beliefs, priorities, and values related to enhancing integral self-care and integral health care.
   c. Integral Nursing Principle 3: "It" Is About Behavior and Skill Development: Integral Nursing Principle 3 recognizes the importance of the individual exterior "It" (objective) space. In this It space of the individual exterior, each person develops and integrates her or his integral self-care plan.
   d. Integral Nursing Principle 4: "Its" Is Systems and Structures: Integral Nursing Principle 4 recognizes the importance of the exterior collective "Its" (interobjective) space. In this Its space, integral nurses and the healthcare team come together to examine their work, their priorities, use of technologies, and any aspect of the technological environment.

■ NOTES

1. Dossey, B. M. (2013). Nursing: Integral, integrative, holistic—local to global. In B. M. Dossey & L. Keegan (Eds.), *Holistic nursing: A handbook for practice*. Burlington, MA: Jones & Bartlett Learning.

2. Dossey, B. M. (2013). Barbara Dossey's theory of integral nursing. In M. E. Parker & M. C. Smith (Eds.), *Nursing theories and nursing practice* (4th ed.). Philadelphia, PA: F. A. Davis.

3. Consortium of Academic Health Centers for Integrative Medicine. (2009, November). Definition of integrative medicine. Retrieved from http://www.imconsortium.org/about/home.html

4. American Holistic Nurses Association & American Nurses Association. (2013). *Holistic nursing: Scope and standards of practice* (2nd ed.). Silver Spring, MD: Nursebooks.org.

5. Beck, D. M., Dossey, B. M., & Rushton, C. H. (2011). Integral nursing and the Nightingale Initiative for Global Health (NIGH): Florence Nightingale's integral legacy for the 21st century—local to global. *Journal of Integral Theory and Practice, 6*(4), 71–92.

6. Gostin, L. O. (2007). Meeting the survival needs of the world's least healthy people. *Journal of American Medical Association, 298*(2), 225–227.

7. Interprofessional Education Collaborative Expert Panel. (2011). *Core competencies for interprofessional collaborative practice: Report of an expert panel.* Washington, DC: Interprofessional Education Collaborative.

8. Karph, T., Ferguson, J. T., & Swift, R. Y. (2010). Light still shines in the darkness: Decent care for all. *Journal of Holistic Nursing, 28*(4), 266–274.

9. Nightingale Initiative for Global Health. *Nightingale Declaration.* Retrieved from http://www.nightingaledeclaration.net

10. United Nations. (2000). *United Nations Millennium Development Goals.* Retrieved from http://www.un.org/millenniumgoals/

11. Dossey, B. M. (2010). *Florence Nightingale: Mystic, visionary, healer.* (Commemorative ed.). Philadelphia, PA: F. A. Davis.

12. Dossey, B. M., Beck, D.-M., Selanders, L. C., & Attewell, A. (2005). *Florence Nightingale today: Healing, leadership, global action.* Silver Spring, MD: Nursesbooks.org.

13. McDonald, L. (2001–2012). *The collected works of Florence Nightingale* (Vols. 1–16). Waterloo, Ontario: Wilfrid Laurier Press.

14. Nightingale, F. (1859). *Notes on hospitals.* London, England: Parker & Son.

15. Nightingale, F. (1860). *Notes on nursing.* London, England: Harrison.

16. Nightingale, F. Letters to her nurses (1872–1900). In B. M. Dossey, D.-M. Beck, L. C. Selanders, & A. Attewell (Eds.), *Florence Nightingale today: Healing, leadership, global action* (pp. 203–285). Silver Spring, MD: Nursesbooks.org.

17. Nightingale, F. (2005). Sick-nursing and health-nursing. In B. M. Dossey, D.-M. Beck, L. C. Selanders, & A. Attewell (Eds.), *Florence Nightingale today:*

Healing, leadership, global action (pp. 288–303). Silver Spring, MD: Nursesbooks.org. (Original work published 1893)

18. Dossey, L. (1999). *Reinventing medicine: Beyond mindbody to a new era of healing.* San Francisco, CA: HarperSanFrancisco.

19. Dossey, L. (1991). *Meaning and medicine: A doctor's tales of breakthrough and healing.* New York, NY: Bantam Books.

20. L. Dossey, *Healing Words: The Power of Prayer and the Practice of Medicine* (San Francisco: Harper SanFrancisco, 1993).

21. Tresoli, C. (1994). *Pew-Fetzer Task Force on Advancing Psychosocial Health Education: Health professions education and relationship-centered care.* San Francisco, CA: Commission at the Center for the Health Professions, University of California.

22. Belack, J. P., & O'Neill, E. H. (2000). Recreating nursing practice for a new century: Recommendations and implications of the Pew Health Professions Commission's final report. *Nursing Health Care Perspective, 21*(1), 14–21.

23. Suchman, A. L., Sluyter, D. J., & Williamson, P. R. (2011). *Leading change in healthcare: Transforming organizations using complexity, positive psychology, and relationship-centered care.* London, England: Radcliffe Publishing.

24. Frankel, R. M., Eddins-Folensbee, F., & Irui, T. S. (2011). Crossing the patient-centered divide: Transforming health care quality through enhanced faculty development. *Academy of Medicine, 86*(4), 445–452.

25. Samueli Institute of Information Biology. (2012). Optimal healing environments. Retrieved from http://www.siib.org/research/research-home/optimal-healing.html

26. Planetree International. About us. Retrieved from http://planetree.org/?page_id=510

27. Wilber, K. (2000). *Integral psychology.* Boston, MA: Shambhala.

28. Wilber, K. (2005). *Integral operating system.* Louisville, CO: Sounds True.

29. Wilber, K. (2005). *Integral life practice.* Denver, CO: Integral Institute.

■ STUDY QUESTIONS

Basic Level

1. To improve the health of the nation on which of the following do nurses primarily focus?
   a. Commitment to community health care and shelters for the homeless
   b. Increasing the health span of individuals using an integral, integrative, and holistic approach rather than focusing on life span
   c. Preparing more nurses to become nurse practitioners and DNPs
   d. Increasing enrollment in schools of nursing and graduate internships

2. What was Florence Nightingale's major focus?
   a. The Nightingale School of Nursing
   b. Legislative resolutions to improve workhouses
   c. Applied statistics in medical reform and hospitals
   d. Worldwide service to humanity and communication of her knowledge

3. What overall goal do the United Nations Millennium Development Goals established in 2000 progress toward?
   a. Safer child birth in the world
   b. Decreased hunger and poverty in the world
   c. Increased literacy in the world
   d. A sustainable quality of life for all humanity

4. Eras of medicine are relevant because they focus on which of the following?
   a. Combination of medical treatments and technology
   b. Three distinct medical eras that consider local and nonlocal data
   c. Consciousness as a brain-bound mind state
   d. Mind–body therapies and outcomes

5. What are the three components of relationship-centered care?
   a. Patient–practitioner, community–practitioner, practitioner–practitioner
   b. Caring, values, and ethics
   c. Decision making, effective communication, and prevention of stress and illness
   d. Reduction of power inequalities, socioeconomic status, practitioner knowledge base

Advanced Level

6. Optimal healing environments include which four environmental domains?
   a. Leadership, lifestyle, technology, social support
   b. Internal, interpersonal, behavioral, external

c. Healing organizations, mission, purpose, and strategies

d. Integrative medicine, sustainability, technology, protocols

7. An integral worldview is a way to organize multiple phenomena of human experience related to which of the following?
   a. Two perspectives: (1) traditional medicine, and (2) complementary therapies
   b. Three perspectives: (1) traditional medicine, (2) Chinese medicine, and (3) Ayurvedic medicine
   c. Four perspectives of reality: (1) the individual interior, (2) individual exterior, (3) collective interior, and (4) collective exterior
   d. Five perspectives of reality: (1) spiritual, (2) moral, (3) psychosocial, (4) interpersonal, and (5) emotional

8. What are the Theory of Integral Nursing building blocks?
   a. Rational and paradoxical healing, complexity science
   b. Whole-person care, psychological counseling, positive psychology

c. Nonlocality of consciousness, miracles, chaos theory

d. Healing, metaparadigm of nursing theory, patterns of knowing, quadrants

9. Which of the following choices accurately describes the Theory of Integral Nursing?
   a. Midrange theory that focuses on healing the healthcare system
   b. Free-standing theory that incorporates complexity science
   c. Grand theory that maps nurses' capacities—local to global
   d. Midrange theory that focuses on human nature and emotions

10. What does the Theory of Integral Nursing show?
    a. Values are interpretive, and qualitative data are preferred over measurable, quantitative data.
    b. Each quadrant has its own truth and language and is intricately linked and bound to all other quadrants.
    c. Right-hand quadrants focus on the individual and exterior quantitative data.
    d. Left-hand quadrants focus on the individual and interior qualitative data.

Chapter 2

Holistic Nursing: Scope and Standards of Practice

Carla Mariano

■ SCOPE AND STANDARDS OF HOLISTIC NURSING PRACTICE

The second edition of *Holistic Nursing: Scope and Standards of Practice*[1] articulates the scope and standards of the specialty practice of holistic nursing and informs holistic nurses, the nursing profession, other healthcare providers and disciplines, employers, third-party payers, legislators, and the public about the unique scope of knowledge and the standards of practice and professional performance of a holistic nurse.

Holistic Nursing: Scope and Standards of Practice is the foundational document and resource for holistic nursing education at all levels (undergraduate, graduate, continuing education) and for holistic nursing practice, research, advocacy, and certification.

1. Function of the scope of practice statement of holistic nursing
   a. Describes the *who, what, where, when, why*, and *how* of the practice of holistic nursing
   b. Builds on a foundation provided by *Nursing: Scope and Standards of Practice*, 2nd edition (2010),[2] the *Guide to the Code of Ethics for Nurses: Interpretation and Application* (2010),[3] and *Nursing's Social Policy Statement: The Essence of the Profession* (2010)[4]
2. Function of the standards of holistic nursing
   a. Standards of professional nursing practice are authoritative statements of the

duties that all registered nurses, regardless of role, population, or specialty, are expected to perform competently.
   b. Standards reflect the values and priorities of the profession.
   c. The standards of holistic nursing practice are specific to this specialty but build on the standards of practice expected of all registered nurses.
   d. Standards provide guidance in professional activities, knowledge, and performance that is relevant to basic and advanced levels of holistic nursing.[5]
3. Function of competencies accompanying standards of holistic nursing
   a. A *competency* is an expected and measurable level of nursing performance that integrates knowledge, skills, abilities, and judgment, based on established scientific knowledge and expectations for nursing practice.

Holistic Nursing Scope of Practice

1. Definition and overview of holistic nursing
   a. Defined as "all nursing practice that has healing the whole person as its goal"[6]
   b. Honors the interconnectedness of self, others, nature, and spirituality
   c. Draws on nursing knowledge, holistic theories, other theories, expertise, and intuition
   d. Focuses on protecting, promoting, and optimizing health and wellness;

This chapter is derived from *Holistic Nursing: Scope and Standards of Practice,* 2nd ed. (2013), Carla Mariano, primary contributor. Printed with permission of the American Holistic Nurses Association (AHNA) and American Nurses Association (ANA).

assisting healing; preventing illness and injury; alleviating suffering; and supporting people to find peace, comfort, harmony, and balance through the diagnosis and treatment of human response

e. Identifies a nurse as an instrument of healing and facilitator in the healing process

f. Is healing oriented and centered on the relationship with the person in contrast to an orientation toward diseases and their cures

g. Emphasizes practices of self-care, intentionality, presence, mindfulness, and therapeutic use of self

h. Incorporates conventional nursing and complementary/alternative/integrative modalities (CAM) and interventions into practice

i. Creates environments conducive to healing, using techniques that promote empowerment, peace, comfort, and a subjective sense of harmony and well-being for the person

j. Acts in partnership with the individual or family in providing options and alternatives regarding health and treatment

k. Assists the person to find meaning in the health and illness experience

2. Philosophical principles of holistic nursing
   a. Person: Unity, totality, and connectedness of everyone and everything. Human beings are unique, diverse, and inherently good.
   b. Healing/health: Health is balance, integration, harmony, right relationship, and the betterment of well-being, not just the absence of disease.
   c. Practice: Practice is a science and an art. The values and ethic of holism, caring, moral insight, dignity, integrity, competence, responsibility, accountability, and legality underlie holistic nursing.
   d. Nursing roles: Using warmth, compassion, caring, authenticity, respect, trust, and relationship as instruments of healing.
   e. Self-reflection and self-care: Self-reflection, self-assessment, self-care, healing, and personal development are necessary for service to others, growth/change in the nurse's own well-being,

and understanding of the nurse's own personal journey.

3. Integrating the art and science of nursing: Core values
   a. Core Value 1: Holistic Philosophy, Theories, and Ethics
      - Recognize the human health experience as a complicated, dynamic relationship of health, illness, and wellness, and value healing as the desired outcome of the practice of nursing.
      - Recognize the holistic philosophy is grounded in nursing knowledge and skill and guided by holistic nursing and other theories.
      - Recognize and honor the person as the authority on his or her own health experience.
      - Believe that people heal themselves; the holistic nurse acts as a guide and facilitator of the individual's own healing.
      - Embrace a professional ethic of caring and healing that seeks to preserve the wholeness and dignity of self and others.
   b. Core Value 2: Holistic Caring Process
      - Provide care that recognizes the totality of the human being (the interconnectedness of body, mind, emotion, spirit, social/cultural, relationships, context, environment, and energy).
      - Incorporate a number of complementary/alternative/integrative modalities along with conventional nursing interventions.
      - Use an iterative process that involves six steps, which often occur simultaneously: assessment, diagnosis (identification of pattern/problem/need/issue), outcomes identification, therapeutic plan of care, implementation, and evaluation.
      - Strongly emphasize partnership with individuals in the healing process.
   c. Core Value 3: Holistic Communication, Therapeutic Healing Environment, and Cultural Diversity
      - Ensure that each individual experiences the presence of the nurse as

authentic, caring, compassionate, and sincere.

- Provide deep listening, with conscious intention and without preconceptions, busy-ness, distractions, or analysis.
- Recognize the nurse is not "the expert" regarding another's health and illness experience but is a "learner."
- Encourage and support others in the use of prayer, meditation, and other spiritual and symbolic practices for healing purposes.
- Assist individuals to find meaning in their experience.
- Possess knowledge and understanding of numerous cultural traditions and healthcare practices and use these understandings to provide culturally competent care.
- Participate in building an ecosystem that sustains the well-being of all life.

d. Core Value 4: Holistic Education and Research
- Provide information on health promotion and disease prevention and opportunities to enhance well-being through comprehensive health counseling, motivational interviewing, and coaching.
- Value all the ways of knowing and learning including empiric, ethical, aesthetic, personal, narrative, transpersonal, embedded, sociopolitical, and unknowing.
- Assess health literacy and individualize learning and teaching.
- Assist others to know themselves and access their own inner wisdom to enhance growth, wholeness, and well-being.
- Disseminate advancements in holistic nursing knowledge.
- Conduct and evaluate research in diverse areas such as outcome measures of various holistic therapies and instrument development to measure holistic phenomena.

e. Core Value 5: Holistic Nurse Self-Reflection and Self-Care
- Self-reflection and self-care, as well as personal awareness of and continuous focus on being an instrument of healing, are significant requirements for holistic nurses.
- Value self and mobilize the necessary resources to care for themselves.
- Strive to achieve harmony/balance in their own lives and to assist others to do the same.

Standards of Holistic Nursing Practice

The complete and comprehensive statement of standards of holistic nursing practice is contained in *Holistic Nursing: Scope and Standards of Practice*, 2nd ed. (2013), which can be obtained from the American Holistic Nurses Association (1-800-278-2462; www.ahna.org or info@ahna.org).

Holistic nurses express, contribute to, and promote an understanding of the following: a philosophy of nursing that values healing as the desired outcome; the human health experience as a complex, dynamic relationship of health, illness, disease, wellness, and well-being; the scientific foundations of nursing practice; and nursing as an art. The philosophical principles of holistic nursing (see pp. 12–13 in this chapter) are embedded in every standard of practice and standard of professional performance.

There are 16 standards in the *Holistic Nursing: Scope and Standards of Practice* (2013), 6 for practice and 10 for professional performance.[1] Each standard addresses measurement criteria/competencies for both the registered nurse and the graduate-level or advanced practice registered nurse. Included here is one example of measurement criteria for each standard.

1. Standards of practice for holistic nursing
   a. Standard 1. Assessment: The holistic registered nurse collects comprehensive data pertinent to the person's health and/or the situation.
      - The holistic registered nurse: Collects comprehensive data including but not limited to physical, functional, psychosocial, emotional, mental, sexual, cultural, age-related, environmental, spiritual/transpersonal, economic, and energy field assessments in a systematic and ongoing process

while honoring the uniqueness of the person.

- The graduate-level-prepared holistic nurse or the advanced practice registered nurse: Explores the meanings of the symbolic language expressing itself in areas such as dreams, images, symbols, narratives, sensations, and prayers that are a part of the individual's health experience.

b. Standard 2. Diagnosis: The holistic registered nurse analyzes the assessment data to determine the diagnosis or issues expressed as actual or potential patterns/problems/needs.

- The holistic registered nurse: Assists the person to explore the meaning of the health/disease experience.
- The graduate-level-prepared holistic nurse or the advanced practice registered nurse: Utilizes complex data and information obtained during interview, examination, and diagnostic procedures in identifying diagnoses.

c. Standard 3. Outcomes Identification: The holistic registered nurse identifies expected outcomes for a plan individualized to the person or the situation. The holistic nurse values the evolution and the process of healing as it unfolds. This implies that specific unfolding outcomes might not be immediately evident because of the nonlinear nature of the healing process. Both expected/anticipated and evolving/emerging outcomes are considered.

- The holistic registered nurse: Partners with the person to identify realistic goals based on the person's present and potential capabilities and quality of life.
- The graduate-level-prepared holistic nurse or the advanced practice registered nurse: Identifies expected outcomes that incorporate scientific evidence and are achievable through implementation of evidence-based practices.

d. Standard 4. Planning: The holistic registered nurse develops a plan that prescribes strategies and alternatives to attain expected outcomes.

- The holistic registered nurse: In partnership with the person, family, and others develops an individualized plan that considers the person's characteristics or situation, including, but not limited to, values, beliefs, knowledge and understanding, spiritual and health practices, preferences, choices, developmental level, coping style, culture and environment, and available technology.
- The graduate-level-prepared holistic nurse or the advanced practice registered nurse: Identifies assessment strategies, diagnostic strategies, therapeutic interventions, therapeutic effects, and side effects that reflect current evidence, including data, research, literature, expert clinical knowledge, and the person's experiences.

e. Standard 5. Implementation: The holistic registered nurse implements the identified plan in partnership with the person.

- The holistic registered nurse: Partners with the person, family, significant others, and caregivers as appropriate to implement the plan in a safe, realistic, and timely manner.
- The graduate-level-prepared holistic nurse or the advanced practice registered nurse: Incorporates new knowledge and strategies to initiate change in nursing care practices if desired outcomes are not achieved.

f. Standard 5A. Coordination of Care: The holistic registered nurse coordinates care delivery.

- The holistic registered nurse: Manages the person's care so as to maximize independence and quality of life.
- The graduate-level-prepared holistic nurse or the advanced practice registered nurse: Provides leadership in the coordination of interprofessional health care for integrated delivery of person-care services across continuums, settings, and over time.

g. Standard 5B. Health Teaching and Health Promotion: The holistic registered nurse employs strategies to promote health/wellness and a safe environment.

- The holistic registered nurse: Provides health teaching to individuals, families, and significant others or caregivers that enhances the body-mind-emotion-spirit-environment connection by addressing such topics as healthy lifestyles, risk-reducing behaviors, developmental needs, activities of daily living, and preventive self-care.

- The graduate-level-prepared holistic nurse or the advanced practice registered nurse: Synthesizes empirical evidence on risk behaviors, decision making about life choices, learning theories, behavioral change theories, motivational theories, epidemiology, and other related theories and frameworks when designing holistic health education information and programs.

h. Standard 5C. Consultation: The graduate-level-prepared holistic nurse or advanced practice registered nurse provides consultation to influence the identified plan, enhance the abilities of others, and effect change. The graduate-level-prepared holistic nurse or the holistic advanced practice registered nurse:

- Synthesizes clinical data, theoretical frameworks, belief/value systems, and evidence when providing consultation.

- Facilitates the effectiveness of a consultation by involving all stakeholders, including the individual, in decision making and negotiating role responsibilities.

i. Standard 5D. Prescriptive Authority and Treatment: The advanced practice registered nurse uses prescriptive authority, procedures, referrals, treatments, and therapies in accordance with state and federal laws and regulations.

- The graduate-level-prepared holistic nurse or the advanced practice registered nurse: Prescribes evidence-based treatments, therapies, and procedures considering the person's comprehensive healthcare needs and holistic choices.

j. Standard 6. Evaluation: The holistic registered nurse evaluates progress toward attainment of outcomes while recognizing and honoring the continuing holistic nature of the healing process.

- The holistic registered nurse: Evaluates, in partnership with the person, the effectiveness of the planned strategies in relation to the person's responses and the attainment of the expected and unfolding outcomes.

- The graduate-level-prepared holistic nurse or the advanced practice registered nurse: Uses the results of the evaluation analyses to make or recommend process or structural changes, including policy, procedure, and/or protocol revision, as appropriate to improve holistic care.

2. Standards of professional performance

a. Standard 7. Ethics: The holistic registered nurse practices ethically.

- The holistic registered nurse: Uses *Code of Ethics for Nurses with Interpretative Statements*[7] and *Position Statement on Holistic Nursing Ethics*[8] to guide practice and articulate the moral foundation of holistic nursing.

- The graduate-level-prepared holistic nurse or the advanced practice registered nurse: Engages others to incorporate a holistic perspective of ethical situations and decision making.

b. Standard 8. Education: The holistic registered nurse attains knowledge and competence that reflect current nursing practice.

- The holistic registered nurse: Demonstrates a commitment to lifelong learning through self-reflection and inquiry to identify learning and personal growth needs.

- The graduate-level-prepared holistic nurse or the advanced practice registered nurse: Uses current healthcare research findings and other evidence to expand clinical knowledge, skills, abilities, and judgment; to enhance holistic role performance; and to increase knowledge of professional issues and changes in national standards for practice and trends in holistic care.

c. Standard 9. Evidence-Based Practice and Research: The holistic registered nurse integrates evidence and research findings into practice.
- The holistic registered nurse: Utilizes the best available evidence, including current evidence-based nursing knowledge, theories, and research findings, to guide practice.
- The graduate-level-prepared holistic nurse or the advanced practice registered nurse: Contributes to nursing knowledge by conducting or synthesizing research that discovers, examines, and evaluates current practice, knowledge, theories, philosophies, context, criteria, and creative approaches to improve holistic healthcare outcomes.

d. Standard 10. Quality of Practice: The holistic registered nurse contributes to quality nursing practice.
- The holistic registered nurse: Participates in quality improvement activities for holistic nursing practice.
- The graduate-level-prepared holistic nurse or the advanced practice registered nurse: Designs innovations to effect change in practice and improve holistic health outcomes.

e. Standard 11. Communication: The holistic registered nurse communicates effectively in a variety of formats in all areas of practice.
- The holistic registered nurse: Uses intention, centering, presence, caring, intuition, and deep listening in creating and maintaining healing and person-centered communication.
- The graduate-level-prepared holistic nurse or the advanced practice registered nurse: Establishes practice environments that recognize and value holistic communication as fundamental to holistic care.

f. Standard 12. Leadership: The holistic registered nurse demonstrates leadership in the professional practice setting and the profession.
- The holistic registered nurse: Oversees the nursing care given by others while retaining accountability for the quality of care given to the healthcare consumer.
- The graduate-level-prepared holistic nurse or the advanced practice registered nurse: Influences decision-making bodies to improve holistic integrative care, the professional practice environment, and holistic healthcare consumer outcomes.

g. Standard 13. Collaboration: The holistic registered nurse collaborates with the healthcare consumer, family, and others in the conduct of holistic nursing practice.
- The holistic registered nurse: Partners with others to effect change, enhance holistic care, and produce positive outcomes through the sharing of knowledge of the person and/or the situation.
- The graduate-level-prepared holistic nurse or the advanced practice registered nurse: Partners with other disciplines to enhance holistic care and outcomes through interprofessional activities such as education, consultation, referral management, technological development, or research opportunities.

h. Standard 14. Professional Practice Evaluation: The holistic registered nurse evaluates her or his own nursing practice in relation to professional practice standards and guidelines, relevant statutes, rules, and regulations.
- The holistic registered nurse: Reflects on his or her practice and how personal, cultural, and/or spiritual beliefs, experiences, biases, education, and values can affect care given to individuals, families, and communities.
- The graduate-level-prepared holistic nurse or the advanced practice registered nurse: Engages in a formal process of seeking feedback regarding his or her own practice from individuals receiving care, peers, professional colleagues, and others.

i. Standard 15. Resource Utilization: The holistic registered nurse utilizes appropriate resources to plan and provide nursing services that are holistic, safe, effective, and financially responsible.

- The holistic registered nurse: Assists the person, family, significant others, and caregivers, as appropriate, in identifying and securing appropriate and available services to address needs across the healthcare continuum.
- The graduate-level-prepared holistic nurse or the advanced practice registered nurse: Formulates innovative solutions for healthcare consumer care problems that utilize resources effectively and maintain quality.

j. Standard 16. Environmental Health: The holistic registered nurse practices in an environmentally safe and healthy manner.

- The holistic registered nurse: Assesses the practice environment for factors that threaten health, such as sound, odor, noise, and light.
- The graduate-level-prepared holistic nurse or the advanced practice registered nurse: Acts as a leader, collaborator, consultant, and change agent in evaluating global health issues and environmental safety; anticipating the potential effect of environmental hazards on the health or welfare of individuals, groups, and communities; and assisting in reducing or eliminating environmental hazards.

Settings for Holistic Nursing Practice

1. Because holistic nursing is a worldview—a way of "being" in the world and not just a modality—holistic nurses can practice in any setting, anywhere, and with individuals throughout the life span.
2. Holistic nursing takes place wherever healing occurs.[9]

Educational Preparation for Holistic Nursing Practice

1. Holistic nurses are registered nurses who are educationally prepared for practice from an approved school of nursing and are licensed to practice in their individual state, commonwealth, or territory.

2. *Holistic Nursing: Scope and Standards of Practice* identifies the scope of practice of holistic nursing and the specific standards and associated measurement criteria of holistic nurses at both the basic and advanced levels.[1]
3. Basic practice level:
   a. The educational focus of most basic nursing programs is on specialties often emanating from the biomedical disease model and cure orientation.
   b. In holistic nursing programs, the individual across the life span is viewed in context as an integrated totality of body, mind, emotion, environment, society, energy, and spirit, with the emphasis on wholeness, well-being, health promotion, and healing using both conventional and complementary/alternative practices.
4. Advanced practice level:
   a. Holistic nurses at advanced level are expected to hold a master's or doctoral degree and demonstrate a greater depth and scope of knowledge, a greater integration of information, increased complexity of skills and interventions, and notable role autonomy.
   b. They provide leadership in practice, teaching, research, consultation, advocacy, and policy formation in advancing holistic nursing to improve the holistic health of people.

Certification in Holistic Nursing

Competency mechanisms for evaluating holistic nursing practice as a specialty exist through a national certification/recertification process overseen by the American Holistic Nurses Certification Corporation (AHNCC).

■ NOTES

1. American Holistic Nurses Association & American Nurses Association. (2013). *Holistic Nursing: Scope and Standards of Practice* (2nd ed.). Silver Spring, MD: Nursebooks.org.
2. American Nurses Association. (2010). *Nursing: Scope and Standards of Practice* (2nd ed.). Silver Spring, MD: Nursebooks.org.
3. American Nurses Association. (2010). *Guide to the Code of Ethics for Nurses: Interpretation and Application.* Silver Spring, MD: Nursebooks.org.

4. American Nurses Association. (2010). *Nursing's Social Policy Statement: The Essence of the Profession.* Silver Spring, MD: Nursebooks.org.

5. Mariano, C. (2006). *Proposal for Recognition of Holistic Nursing as a Nursing Specialty.* Unpublished document submitted to ANA.

6. American Holistic Nurses Association. (1998). *Description of Holistic Nursing.* Flagstaff, AZ: Author.

7. American Nurses Association. (2001). *Code of Ethics for Nurses with Interpretative Statements.* Silver Spring, MD: Nursebooks.org.

8. American Holistic Nurses Association. (2012). *Position Statement on Holistic Nursing Ethics.* Retrieved from http://www.ahna.org/Resources /Publications/PositionStatements/tabid/1926 /Default.aspx#P2

9. Mariano, C. (2009). Holistic nursing: Every nurse's specialty. *Beginnings, 29*(4), 4–7.

■ STUDY QUESTIONS

Basic Level

1. The second edition of *Holistic Nursing: Scope and Standards of Practice* is the foundational document and resource for which of the following four areas of holistic nursing?
   1. Education
   2. Reimbursement
   3. Research
   4. Certification
      a. 1, 2, 4
      b. 1, 3, 4
      c. 2, 3, 4
      d. All of the above

2. Which of the following best describes standards of holistic nursing practice?
   a. Expected and measurable levels of holistic nursing performance
   b. The who, what, where of holistic nursing
   c. Reflection of the values and priorities of holistic nursing
   d. Principles including person, healing/health, practice, roles

3. Which of the following best describes the function of the scope of practice statement of holistic nursing?
   a. Expected and measurable levels of holistic nursing performance
   b. The who, what, where, when, why, and how of holistic nursing

   c. Reflection of the values and priorities of holistic nursing
   d. Principles including person, healing/health, practice, roles

4. A holistic nursing competency is best defined as which of the following?
   a. An expected and measurable level of nursing performance
   b. An outcomes measure of patient care
   c. The knowledge level of the holistic nurse
   d. The knowledge level of the patient and his or her ability to understand instructions provided by the holistic nurse.

5. According to the core values, which of the following statements is accurate?
   a. Self-reflection and self-care are significant requirements for holistic nurses.
   b. Only advanced level holistic nurses are required to practice self-care.
   c. As long as the holistic nurse practices self-care, patients do not need to do so.
   d. Self-reflection is a needless activity for a holistic nurse.

Advanced Level

6. The core values of holistic nursing focus on which of the following?
   1. Holistic philosophy and ethics
   2. Providing care that recognizes the totality of the human being
   3. Pathology and relief of symptoms
   4. Education and research
      a. 1, 3, 4
      b. 2, 3, 4
      c. 1, 2, 4
      d. All of the above

7. Which of the following statements describe the scope of holistic nursing practice?
   1. It is the foundational document for holistic nursing education and research.
   2. It builds on the *Nursing Social Policy Statement.*
   3. It defines expected and measurable levels of holistic nursing performance.
   4. It describes the when, where, and how of holistic nursing practice.
      a. 1 and 3
      b. 2 and 4
      c. 2 and 3
      d. 1 and 4

8. The philosophical principles of holistic nursing include all of the following ideas except which one?
   a. Holistic nurses use primarily complementary and alternative modalities in practice.
   b. People find meaning and purpose in their own life, experiences, and illness.
   c. Holistic nurses assist other nurses to nurture and heal themselves.
   d. Practice is a science and an art.

9. A holistic nurse practitioner notices that end-of-life patients who are visited each day by the pet therapy dog at the extended care facility where she practices have lower pain ratings; however, few nurses at the facility initiate pet therapy. She conducts a quality improvement project to collect data, which validate her observations. Upon sharing the data with the unit nurses and manager, pet therapy visit requests significantly increase, resulting in an increase in end-of-life patient comfort levels. But the patients need to wait too long for the pet therapy visit. The nurse practitioner then meets with nursing administration and influences the hiring of an additional pet therapist to ensure an adequate numbers of pets are available for the increase in daily visits. Which holistic nursing standard does the holistic nurse practitioner in this scenario best exemplify?
   a. Collaboration
   b. Resource utilization
   c. Environmental health
   d. Leadership

10. Holistic nurses contribute to and promote which of the following ideas?
    1. The scientific foundations of nursing practice
    2. The human health experience as a complex, dynamic relationship
    3. Cure as the desired outcome
    4. Nursing as a top 10 career choice
       a. 1 and 2
       b. 1 and 3
       c. 3 and 4
       d. All of the above

Chapter 3

Current Trends and Issues in Holistic Nursing

Carla Mariano

■ HEALTH CARE IN THE UNITED STATES

1. The American public increasingly demands health care that is compassionate and respectful, provides options, is economically feasible, and is grounded in holistic ideals. A shift is occurring in health care where people desire to be more actively involved in health decision making. They have expressed their dissatisfaction with conventional (Western allopathic) medicine and are calling for a care system that encompasses health, quality of life, and a relationship with their providers.

2. The National Center for Complementary and Alternative Medicine's *Strategic Plan for 2011–2015*[1] and the U.S. Department of Health And Human Services initiative *Healthy People 2020*[2] prioritize enhancing physical and mental health and wellness, preventing disease, and empowering the public to take responsibility for their health.

3. Chronic diseases—such as heart disease, cancer, hypertension, diabetes, depression—are the leading causes of death and disability in the United States, accounting for 70% of all deaths in the United States, which is 1.7 million deaths each year.[3]

4. Stress accounts for 80% of all healthcare issues in the United States.

5. Healthcare costs have been rising for several years.
   a. Costs surpassed $2.3 trillion in 2008 and are projected to be $2.7 trillion in 2011 and $4.3 trillion by 2017.[4]
   b. Accounts for 16.2% of the nation's gross domestic product (GDP); this is among the highest of all industrialized countries. Total healthcare expenditures continue to outpace inflation and the growth in national income.[5] The U.S. healthcare system is the most expensive in the world.
   c. Employees pay a much larger share of the rising expense. The total cost of health care for a typical family of four is $19,393.[6]

6. Health coverage:
   a. There is an increased number of uninsured Americans at 50.7 million, or 16.7% of the population.[7]
   b. The number of underinsured has grown 60% to 25 million over the past 4 years.[8]
   c. Reasons for the rise in uninsured and underinsured include workers losing their jobs in the recession, companies dropping employee health insurance benefits, and families going without coverage to cut costs—primarily as a result of the high costs of health care.

7. Forces driving healthcare costs:[5]
   a. Technology and prescription drugs
   b. Chronic disease
   c. Aging of the population
   d. Administrative costs

8. Containing healthcare costs:[5]
   a. Invest in information technology (IT).
   b. Improve quality and efficiency.
   c. Adjust provider compensation and increase comparative effectiveness research (CER).
   d. Increase government regulation in controlling per capita spending.
   e. Increase prevention efforts.
   f. Increase consumer involvement in purchasing.

9. Need for focus on quality-based medicine (health care) with disease prevention, health promotion, and wellness, not just evidence-based medicine.

■ USE OF CAM IN THE UNITED STATES

1. The American public has pursued alternative and complementary care at an ever-increasing rate.
   a. In 1993, 33% or 61 million Americans were using some form of alternative or complementary medicine.[9]
   b. In 1998, 42% or 83 million Americans were using some form of alternative or complementary medicine. The out-of-pocket dollars the American public spent on CAM was $12.2 billion.[10]
   c. The most recent survey, the 2007 National Health Interview Survey,[11] indicates that 38.3% of adults in the United States aged 18 years and older (almost 4 of 10 adults) and nearly 12% of children aged 17 years and younger (1 in 9 children) used some form of CAM. Americans spent $33.9 billion out-of-pocket on CAM, accounting for approximately 1.5% of total U.S. healthcare expenditures and 11.2% of total out-of-pocket expenditures.[12]
   d. CAM therapies most commonly used by U.S. adults are natural products, deep breathing exercises, meditation, chiropractic or osteopathic manipulation, massage, and yoga.
   e. People who use CAM approaches:
      - Seek ways to improve their health and well-being.
      - Attempt to relieve symptoms associated with chronic or even terminal illnesses or the side effects of conventional treatments.
      - Have a holistic health philosophy or desire a transformational experience that changes their worldview.
      - Want greater control over their health.
      - Do so to complement conventional care rather than as an alternative to conventional care.

2. People 50 years and older tend to be high users of CAM.[13]
   a. Fifty-three percent of people 50 years and older reported using CAM at some point in their lives, and 47% reported using it in the past 12 months.
   b. Herbal products or dietary supplements were most commonly used, followed by massage therapy, chiropractic manipulation, and other bodywork mind–body practices, and naturopathy, acupuncture, and homeopathy.
   c. Women were more likely than men to report using any form of CAM.
   d. The most common reasons for using CAM were to prevent illness, for overall wellness to reduce pain or treat painful conditions, to treat a specific health condition, and to supplement conventional medicine.
   e. Patients receive information about CAM from a variety of sources: family or friends, the Internet, their healthcare provider, publications including magazines, newspapers, and books, and radio or television.

3. There is great interest in CAM practices among those who are chronically ill, those with life-threatening conditions, and those at the end of their lives.

4. There is a lack of discussion of CAM use with healthcare providers.[13]
   a. Two-thirds (67%) of patients/clients had not discussed CAM with any healthcare provider.
   b. Use of CAM was brought up by the patient 55% of the time, by the healthcare provider 26% of the time, or by a relative/friend 14% of the time.
   c. Reasons for nondiscussion: The provider never asks patients/clients, patients/clients did not know that they should bring up the topic, there is not enough time during a visit, the healthcare practitioner (HCP) would have been dismissive or told the respondent not to do it, or the respondent did not feel comfortable discussing the topic with the HCP.
   d. Nondisclosure raises important safety issues, such as the potential interactions

of medications with herbs used as part of a CAM therapy and incorrect use of CAM products and procedures.

e. Healthcare providers and clients, patients, and families need to have an open dialogue to ensure safe and appropriate integrated medical care.

■ HEALTHCARE REFORM AND INTEGRATIVE HEALTH CARE

1. The comprehensive health reform, the *Patient Protection and Affordable Healthcare Act*, was signed into law in 2010 to expand health coverage, control health costs, and improve the healthcare delivery system. It incorporates the following:[14]

    a. Inclusion of licensed practitioners insurance coverage, allowing participation of any healthcare provider within the scope of that provider's license or certification in insurance plans and coverage

    b. Inclusion of licensed complementary and alternative medicine practitioners in medical homes, establishing community-based interdisciplinary, interprofessional teams to support primary care practices

    c. Use of integrative health care and integrative practitioners in prevention strategies

    d. Use of demonstration projects concerning individualized wellness plans

    e. Inclusion of licensed complementary and alternative providers and integrative practitioners in workforce planning

    f. Use of experts in Integrative health and state-licensed integrative health practitioners in comparative effectiveness research or patient-centered outcomes research

■ TRENDS IN HEALTH CARE

1. Workplace clinics[15]

    a. Employers offering clinics that provide a full range of wellness, health promotion, and primary care services.

    b. Tool to contain medical costs, such as specialist visits, nongeneric prescriptions, emergency department visits, and avoidable hospitalizations; boost productivity; reduce absenteeism; prevent disability claims and work-related injuries.

c. Nation's largest employers are focusing on prevention and disease management by adopting an integrative medicine approach.

2. Primary care: The Institute for Alternative Futures forecasts the following aspects of the future of primary care in 2025:[16]

    a. Focus on primary prevention.

    b. Health will be continually assessed and worked on along multiple dimensions such as physical, medical, nutritional, behavioral, psychological, social, spiritual, and environmental.

    c. Trusting relationships between providers and patients will be the basis of primary care's capacity for promoting health and managing disease.

    d. Primary care team members will include the patient, nurse practitioners, physicians, a psychologist, a pharmacist, a health information technician, and community health workers.

    e. Focus on behavioral change.

    f. Focus on quality and safety.

    g. Use of genome and epigenetic data.

    h. Broadened vital signs including personal and community vital signs.

    i. Person-centered care where the whole person is the focus of care.

    j. The knowledge of conventional, unconventional, complementary, alternative, traditional, and integrative medicine disciplines will be used.

    k. Health care will be available anytime and everywhere.

3. Healthcare issues[17]

    a. Industry-wide, intense efforts to reduce healthcare costs

    b. Increased oversight, tax changes, coverage, and consumer demand

    c. Adoption of healthcare IT

    d. Technology and telecommunications sectors playing leading roles in health care

    e. Pharmaceutical and life sciences companies promoting wellness and prevention and patient outcomes

    f. Physician groups joining health systems, with more and more hospitals employing physicians

    g. Alternative care delivery models emerging as traditional care delivery gives way

to alternative models outside of physicians' offices and hospitals; for example, services in work sites, health clinics, home health services, and technology-enabled delivery such as email, tele-health, and remote monitoring
h. Community health becoming a new social reality
4. Health workforce: Job growth will continue in the healthcare sector.
5. Holistic health
   a. Eight transitions that will bring light and balance to health care:[18]
      - From health care being a science to also being an art
      - From health care being a business to also being a calling
      - From the Dominator Model ("what is good for me?") to the Partnership Model ("what is good for all of us?")
      - From focus on individual health only to focus on community health also
      - From type II medical malpractice (doing the wrong thing the right way) to no malpractice or only type I medical malpractice (doing the right thing the wrong way)
      - From unrealistic expectations of the medical system to more realistic expectations
      - From living in fear of illness and death to acceptance of illness and death as normal parts of life
      - From single-causality mentality to an understanding and acceptance of the multiple causalities of disease
   b. Holistic nurses have knowledge of a wide range of complementary, alternative, and integrative modalities; health promotion and restoration and disease prevention strategies; and relationship-centered, caring ways of healing and are in a prime position to provide leadership in national trends.

RECOMMENDATIONS FOR HEALTH CARE IN THE UNITED STATES

1. White House Commission on CAM Policy (WHCCAMP) *Final Report*:[19]
   a. Include more evidence-based teaching about CAM approaches in the conventional health professions schools.

b. Emphasize approaches to prevent disease and promote wellness for the long-term health of the American people.
c. Teach the principles and practices of self-care and provide lifestyle counseling in professional schools so that health professionals can provide this guidance to their patients as well as improve their own health.
d. Provide those in the greatest need access to the most accurate, up-to-date information about which therapies and products can help and which can harm.
e. Design the education and training of all practitioners to increase the availability of practitioners knowledgeable in both CAM and conventional practices.
2. Institute of Medicine report *Complementary and Alternative Medicine in the United States*:[20]
   a. Health professionals take into account a patient's individuality, emotional needs, values, and life issues and implementation strategies to enhance prevention and health promotion.
   b. Health professions schools (e.g., medicine, nursing, pharmacy, allied health) incorporate sufficient information about CAM into the standard curriculum at the undergraduate, graduate, and postgraduate levels.
   c. National professional organizations of all CAM disciplines ensure the presence of training standards and develop practice guidelines.
   d. Healthcare professional licensing boards and crediting and certifying agencies (for both CAM and conventional medicine) should set competency standards in the appropriate use of both conventional medicine and CAM therapies.
   e. Needed is a moral commitment of openness to diverse interpretations of health and healing, a commitment to finding innovative ways of obtaining evidence, and an expansion of the knowledge base relevant and appropriate to medical practice.
   f. Research aimed at answering questions about outcomes of care is crucial so that healthcare professionals provide evidence-based, comprehensive care that encourages a focus on healing, recognizes the importance of compassion

and caring, emphasizes the centrality of relationship-based care, encourages patients to share in decision making about therapeutic options, and promotes choices in care that can include complementary and alternative medical therapies when appropriate.

g. The National Institutes of Health (NIH) and other public and private agencies sponsor research to compare the outcomes and costs of combinations of CAM and conventional medical treatments and develop models that deliver such care.

3. Wellness Initiative for the Nation (WIN):[21]

a. Created to prevent disease and illness proactively, promote health and productivity, and create well-being and flourishing of the people of the United States

b. Addresses preventable chronic illness and creating a productive, self-care society

c. Establishes a network of Systems Wellness Advancements Teams (SWAT) with national and local leaders in health promotion and integrative practices; establishes educational and practice standards for effective, comprehensive lifestyle and integrative healthcare delivery; creates an advanced information tracking and feedback system for personalized wellness education; and creates economic incentives for individuals, communities, and public and private sectors to create and deliver self-care training, wellness products, and preventive health practices

4. *National Prevention Strategy*[22] convened by the Surgeon General:

a. Vision: Working together (state, local, and territorial governments, businesses, health care, education, and community faith-based organizations) to improve the health and quality of life for individuals, families, and communities by moving the nation from a focus on sickness and disease to one based on wellness and prevention

b. Goals: Create community environments that make the healthy choice the easy and affordable choice, to implement effective preventive practices by creating and recognizing communities that support prevention and wellness, to connect

prevention-focused health care and community efforts to increase preventive services, to empower and educate individuals to make healthy choices, and to eliminate disparities in traditionally underserved populations

c. Priorities: Active lifestyles, countering alcohol/substance misuse, healthy eating, healthy physical and social environment, injury- and violence-free living, reproductive and sexual health, mental and emotional well-being

5. Summit on Integrative Medicine and the Health of the Public[23] convened by Institute of Medicine (IOM) and the Bravewell Collaborative:

a. The progression of many chronic diseases can be reversed and sometimes even completely healed through lifestyle modifications.

b. Genetics is not destiny. Recent research shows that gene expression can be turned on or off by nutritional choices, levels of social support, stress reduction activities such as meditation, and exercise.

c. The environment influences health.

d. Improving the primary care and chronic disease care systems is paramount.

e. The reimbursement system must be changed. The current reimbursement system rewards procedures rather than outcomes, and changes are needed that incentivize healthcare providers to focus on the health outcomes of their patients/clients.

f. Changes in education will fuel changes in practice. All healthcare practitioners should be educated in team approaches and the importance of compassionate care that addresses the biopsychosocial dimensions of health, prevention, and well-being.

g. Evidence-based medicine/health care is the only acceptable standard. Research must better accommodate multifaceted and interacting factors.

ISSUES IN HOLISTIC NURSING

In December 2006, holistic nursing was officially recognized by the American Nurses Association (ANA) as a distinct nursing specialty with a defined scope and standards of practice, acknowledging holistic nursing's unique contribution to the health and healing of people and society. This recognition provides holistic nurses with clarity and a foundation for their practice and gives holistic nursing legitimacy and voice within the nursing profession and credibility in the eyes of the healthcare world and the public.

1. Education
   a. Educational challenges in holistic nursing:
      - Both students and faculty need knowledge of and skill in the use of complementary/alternative/integrative therapies.
      - Holistic, relationship-centered philosophies and integrative modalities (both content and practical experiences) need to be integrated into nursing curricula at the basic and advanced levels.
      - Faculty development programs also are necessary to support faculty in understanding and integrating holistic philosophy, content, and practices into curriculums.
   b. *Essentials of Baccalaureate Education for Professional Nursing Practice*:[24]
      - Includes language on preparing the baccalaureate generalist graduate to practice from a holistic, caring framework; engage in self-care; develop an understanding of complementary and alternative modalities; and incorporate patient teaching and health promotion, spirituality, and caring, healing techniques into practice.
      - Holistic nurses will need to continue to work with the accrediting bodies of academic degree programs to ensure that this content is included in educational programs.
   c. *Educating Nurses: A Call for Radical Transformation*[25] recommendations:
      - Broadening clinical experiences to community health care
      - Promoting and supporting students learning the skills of inquiry and research
      - Teaching the ethics of care and responsibility, the ethos of self-care in

the profession, skills of involvement and clinical reasoning and reflection
      - Teaching strategies for organizational change, organizational development, policy making, leadership, and improvement of healthcare systems
      - Incorporating evidence-based practice and critical reflection
      - Assisting students to better understand the patient's context and how they can help patients improve their access and continuity of care
      - Teaching relational skills of involvement and caring practices
      - Teaching collegial and collaborative skills
   d. The National Educational Dialogue, an outgrowth of the Integrated Healthcare Policy Consortium (IHPC),[26] sought to identify a set of core values, knowledge, skills, and attitudes necessary for all healthcare professional students.
      - Wholeness and healing—interconnectedness of all people and things with healing as an innate capacity of every individual
      - Clients/patients/families as the center of practice
      - Practice as a combined art and science
      - Self-care of the practitioner and commitment to self-reflection, personal growth, and healing
      - Interdisciplinary collaboration and integration embracing the breadth and depth of diverse healthcare systems and collaboration with all disciplines, clients, and families
      - Responsibility to contribute to the improvement of the community, the environment, health promotion, healthcare access, and the betterment of public health
      - Attitudes and behaviors of all participants in health care demonstrating respect for self and others, humility, and authentic, open, courageous communication
   e. *The Future of Nursing: Leading Change, Advancing Health*:[27]
      - Nurses should achieve higher levels of education and training through

improved educational systems, by increasing the proportion of nurses with a baccalaureate degree to 80% by 2020, and by ensuring that nurses engage in lifelong learning.

- Nurses need more education and preparation to adopt new roles to respond to a rapidly changing and evolving healthcare system.
- Competencies are needed in community, geriatrics, leadership, health policy, system improvement and change, research and evidence-based practice, and teamwork and collaboration.

f. Continuing education programs at national and regional specialty organizations and conferences needed for holistic and CAM education.

2. Research
   a. Research in holistic nursing is increasingly important in the future especially in whole systems research, exploration of healing relationships, and outcomes of healing interventions, particularly in the areas of health promotion and prevention.
   b. Need for an evidence base to establish the effectiveness and efficacy of complementary/alternative/integrative therapies and development of instruments to measure these outcomes.
   c. The IOM report on CAM in the United States recommends qualitative and quantitative research to examine the following:[20]
      - The social and cultural dimensions of illness experiences, the processes and preferences of seeking health care, and practitioner–patient interactions
      - How often users of CAM, including patients and providers, adhere to treatment instructions and guidelines
      - The effects of CAM on wellness and disease prevention
      - How the American public accesses and evaluates information about CAM modalities
      - Adverse events associated with CAM therapies and interactions between CAM and conventional treatments
      - Accessing information about CAM

d. *NCCAM Third Strategic Plan Exploring the Science of Complementary and Alternative Medicine: 2011–2015:*[1]
   - Advance research on mind and body interventions, practices, and disciplines.
   - Advance research on natural products.
   - Increase understanding of "real-world" patterns and outcomes of CAM use and its integration into health care and health promotion.
   - Improve the capacity of the field to carry out rigorous research.
   - Develop and disseminate objective, evidence-based information on CAM interventions.

e. Patient-Centered Outcomes Research Institute (PCORI), created by the Patient Protection and Affordable Care Act:[28]
   - Assists patients, clinicians, purchasers, and policymakers in making informed health decisions by carrying out research projects that provide high-quality, relevant evidence on how diseases, disorders, and other health conditions can effectively and appropriately be prevented, diagnosed, treated, monitored, and managed
   - Helps people make informed healthcare decisions and allows their voice to be heard in assessing the value of healthcare options

f. Research methodologies need to be expanded to capture the wholeness of the individual's experience because the philosophy of these therapies rests on a paradigm of wholeness.

g. Whole practices, whole systems, and related research that takes into consideration the *interactive* nature of the body-mind-emotion-spirit-environment need professional and organizational attention.[29]

h. Investigations into the concept and nature of the placebo effect also are needed because one-third of all medical healings are the result of the placebo effect.[30]

i. Nurses need to address how to secure funding for their holistic research and to be represented in study sections and review panels to educate and convince the biomedical and NIH community about the value of nursing research; the need for models of research focusing on health promotion and disease prevention, wellness, and self-care instead of only the disease model; and the importance of a variety of designs and research methodologies including qualitative studies rather than sole reliance on randomized controlled trials.

j. Advanced practice holistic nurses must disseminate their research findings to various media sources (e.g., television, newsprint) and at nonnursing, interdisciplinary conferences. Publishing in nonnursing journals and serving on editorial boards of nonnursing journals also broaden the appreciation in other disciplines for nursing's role in setting the agenda and conducting research in the area of holism and CAM.

3. Clinical practice
   a. Clinical care models reflecting holistic assessment, treatment, health, healing, and caring are important in the development of holistic nursing practice. Implementing holistic and humanistic models in today's healthcare environment will require a paradigm shift.
   b. Licensure and credentialing:
      - IOM report *The Future of Nursing*[27] notes that regulations defining scope-of-practice limitations vary widely by state. Some states have kept pace with the evolution of the healthcare system, but the majority of state laws have not. The IOM recommends that *nurses should practice to the full extent of their education and training* and that *scope-of-practice barriers should be removed*.
      - In 2010, the American Holistic Nurses Association (AHNA) conducted a preliminary survey to ascertain the number of state boards of nursing that accepted and recognized holistic nursing and/or permitted holistic practices with their regulations and/or the state's nurse practice act. Eight states include holistic nursing in their nurse practice act. Forty-seven of 51 states/territories have some statements or positions

that include holistic wording such as *self-care*, *spirituality*, *natural therapies*, and/or specific complementary/alternative therapies under the scope of practice.
      - It will be important in the future to monitor state boards of nursing for evidence of their recognition and support of holistic, integrative nursing practice and requirements that include CAM. It will also be important to work with the state boards to incorporate this content into the National Council Licensure Examination to ensure the credibility of this practice knowledge.
   c. Nursing shortage:
      - Addressing the nursing shortage in this country is crucial to the health of our nation. Multiple surveys and studies confirm that the shortage of RNs influences the delivery of health care in the United States and negatively affects patient outcomes. According to the American Hospital Association, the United States is in the midst of a significant shortage of registered nurses that is projected to last well into the future. Nationally, there is an average vacancy rate of approximately 8.1%.[31]
      - Demand for RNs will increase as large numbers of RNs retire. A large and prolonged shortage of nurses is expected to hit the United States in the latter half of the next decade.[32]
      - The American Association of Colleges of Nursing report *2010–2011 Enrollment and Graduations in Baccalaureate and Graduate Programs in Nursing* found that in 2010 U.S. nursing schools turned away 67,563 qualified applicants because of insufficient number of faculty, clinical sites, classroom space, clinical preceptors, and budget constraints. Almost two-thirds of the nursing schools pointed to faculty shortages as a reason for not accepting all qualified applicants into their programs.[31]
      - Forty-one percent of nurses are dissatisfied with their present job. Nationally, nurses give themselves burnout

scores of 30–40%, and 17% of nurses are not working in nursing. Thirteen percent of newly licensed RNs had changed principal jobs after 1 year, and 37% reported that they felt ready to change jobs.

- Nurses often change jobs or leave the profession because of unhumanistic and chaotic work environments and professional and personal burnout. Reduction of perceived stress is related to job satisfaction. Holistic nurses, through their knowledge of self-care, resilience, caring cultures, healing environments, and stress management techniques, can influence and improve the healthcare milieu, both for healthcare providers and for clients and patients.[33]

4. Policy

   a. Four major policy issues face holistic nursing in the future: leadership, reimbursement, regulation, and access.

   b. *The Future of Nursing*[27] recommends that *nurses should be full partners with physicians and other health professionals in redesigning health care in the United States.* Nurses should be prepared and enabled to lead change in all roles and should have a voice in health policy decision making and be engaged in implementation efforts related to healthcare reform. Nurses must see policy as something they can shape rather than something that happens to them.

   c. Public or private policies regarding coverage and reimbursement for healthcare services play a crucial role in shaping the healthcare system and will play a crucial role in deciding the future of wellness, health promotion, and CAM in the nation's healthcare system.

   d. Holistic nurses will need to work with Medicare and other third-party payers, insurance groups, boards of nursing, healthcare policymakers, legislators, and other professional nursing organizations to ensure that holistic nurses are appropriately reimbursed for services rendered.

   e. Reimbursement must be included for the process of holistic and integrative care, not just for providing a specific modality.

   f. There are many barriers to the use of holistic therapies by potential users, including lack of awareness of the therapies and their benefits, uncertainty about their effectiveness, inability to pay for them, and limited availability of qualified providers.

   g. Holistic nurses have a responsibility to educate the public more fully about health promotion, complementary/alternative modalities, and qualified practitioners and to assist people in making informed choices among the array of healthcare alternatives and individual providers.

   h. Holistic nurses also must actively participate in the political arena as leaders in this movement to ensure quality, an increased focus on wellness, and access and affordability for all.

■ NOTES

1. National Center for Complementary and Alternative Medicine. (2011). *Exploring the science of complementary and alternative medicine: Third strategic plan 2011–2015.* Washington, DC: U.S. Department of Health and Human Services, National Institutes of Health.

2. U.S. Department of Health and Human Services. (2010). *Healthy People 2020.* Washington, DC: Author. Retrieved from http://www.healthypeople.gov

3. Centers for Disease Control and Prevention. (2011, May 11). Chronic disease prevention and health promotion. Retrieved from http://www.cdc.gov/chronicdisease/index.htm

4. Centers for Medicare and Medicaid Services. (2012, April 11). National health expenditure data. Retrieved from http://www.cms.hhs.gov/NationalHealthExpendData

5. KaiserEdu.org. (2010, March). U.S. health care costs: Background brief. Retrieved from http://www.kaiseredu.org/Issue-Modules/US-Health-Care-Costs

6. Milliman, L. M. (2011, May 11). Milliman Medical Index indicates healthcare costs for typical American family of four have doubled in fewer than nine years. [Press release]. Retrieved from http://www.milliman.com/news-events/press/pdfs/milliman-medical-index-indicates.pdf

7. Wolf, R. (2010, September 10). Number of uninsured Americans rises to 50.7 million. *USA Today.*

8. HealthCareProblems.org. (2011, September). Health care statistics. Retrieved from http://www.healthcareproblems.org/health-care-statistics.htm

9. Eisenberg, D., Kessler, R. C., Foster, C., Norlock, F. E., Calkins, D. R., & Delbanco, T. L. (1993). Unconventional medicine in the United States: Prevalence, costs and patterns of use. *New England Journal of Medicine, 328*(4), 246–252.

10. Eisenberg, D., Davis, R. B., Ettner, S. L., Appel, S., Wilkey, S., Van Rompay, M., Kessler, R. C. (1998). Trends in alternative medicine use in the United States, 1990-1997. *Journal of the American Medical Association, 280*, 1569–1575.

11. Barnes, P. M., Bloom, B., & Nahin, B. R. (2008, December). Complementary and alternative medicine use among adults and children: United States, 2007. *CDC National Health Statistics Reports, 10*(12), 1–23.

12. National Center for Complementary and Alternative Medicine. (2009, July 30). Americans spent $33.9 billion out-of-pocket on complementary and alternative medicine. Retrieved from http://nccam.nih.gov/news/2009/073009.htm

13. AARP & National Center for Complementary and Alternative Medicine. (2011, April). *Complementary and alternative medicine: What people aged 50 and older discuss with their health care providers.* Washington, DC: U.S. Department of Health and Human Services.

14. Weeks, J. (2010, May 10). Reference guide: Language and sections on CAM and integrative practice in HR 3590/Healthcare Overhaul. Integrator Blog. Retrieved from http://theintegratorblog.com/site/index.php?option=com_content&task=view&id=658&Itemid=2

15. Tu, H., Boukus, E., & Cohen, G. (2010). Workplace clinics: A sign of growing employer interest in wellness (HSC Research Brief no. 17). Retrieved from http://www.hschange.com/CONTENT/1166/

16. Bezold, C. (2011, April 25). Alert: Major study on future of primary care seeks input on IM therapies and CAM practitioners. Integrator Blog. Retrieved from http://theintegratorblog.com/index.php?option=com_content&task=view&id=744&Itemid=189

17. Manos, D. (2009, December 17). Healthcare IT among PricewaterhouseCoopers's (PWC) list of top 10 healthcare issues for 2010. HealthcareITNews.com. Retrieved from http://www.healthcareitnews.com/news/healthcare-it-among-pwcs-list-top-10-healthcare-issues-2010

18. Manahan, B. (2009, January 14). Revisioning healthcare in 2009: Eight transitions that will help bring light and balance to healthcare. Integrator Blog. Retrieved from http://theintegratorblog.com/site/index.php?option=com_content&task=view&id=519&Itemid=189

19. White House Commission on Complementary and Alternative Medicine Policy. (2002). *Final report.* Washington, DC: U.S. Government Printing Office.

20. Institute of Medicine. (2005). *Complementary and alternative medicine in the United States.* Washington, DC: National Academies Press.

21. Samueli Institute. (2009). *A wellness initiative for the nation (WIN).* Retrieved from http://www.lifesciencefoundation.org/WellnessInitiative11feb09.pdf

22. U.S. Office of the Surgeon General. (2011). *The national prevention and health promotion strategy (national prevention strategy).* Washington, DC: U.S. Department of Health and Human Services.

23. Institute of Medicine. (2009). *Summit on integrative medicine and the health of the public.* Washington, DC: National Academy of Sciences.

24. American Association of Colleges of Nursing. (2008). *The essentials of baccalaureate education for professional nursing practice.* Washington, DC: Author.

25. Benner, P., Sutphen, M., Leonard, V., & Day, L. (2010). *Educating nurses: A call for radical transformation.* San Francisco, CA: Jossey-Bass.

26. Goldblatt, E., Snider, P., Quinn, S., & Weeks, J. (2009). *Clinicians' and educators' desk reference on the licensed complementary and alternative healthcare professions.* Seattle, WA: Academic Consortium for Complementary and Alternative Health Care.

27. Institute of Medicine. *The future of nursing: Leading change, advancing health.* Washington, DC: National Academies Press. Retrieved from http://www.iom.edu/nursing

28. Weeks, J. (2011, September 26). Culture change: Patient-centered outcomes at the center of new $600-million/year quasi-governmental research institute (PCORI). Integrator Blog. Retrieved from http://theintegratorblog.com/index.php?option=com_content&task=view&id=781&Itemid=1

29. Mariano, C. (2008). Contributions to holism through critique of theory and research. *Beginnings, 28*(2), 26.

30. Mariano, C. (2011, March). *Research in holism: A nursing perspective* [Keynote presentation]. Lexington, KY.

31. American Association of Colleges of Nursing. (2011, April). Nursing shortage [Fact sheet]. Retrieved from http://www.aacn.nche.edu/media-relations/fact-sheets/nursing-shortage

32. Buerhaus, P., Auerbach, D. I., & Staiger, D. O. (2009). The recent surge in nurse employment: Causes and implications. *Health Affairs, 28*(4), w657–w668.

33. Mariano, C. (2007). The nursing shortages: Is stress management the answer? *Beginnings, 27*(1), 3.

■ STUDY QUESTIONS

Basic Level

1. Which of the following are forces driving healthcare costs?
   1. Technology
   2. Aging of the population
   3. Chronic disease
   4. Administrative costs
      a. 1 and 3
      b. 2 and 4
      c. 4
      d. All of the above

2. People who use complementary and alternative medicine (CAM) modalities do so for all of the following reasons except which one?
   a. They desire greater control over their own health.
   b. CAM is less costly than most conventional treatments.
   c. They are seeking ways to improve their health and well-being.
   d. CAM can relieve symptoms associated with side-effects of conventional treatments.

3. Clients often do not discuss alternative treatments and CAM use with their healthcare providers because of which of the following reasons?
   1. The provider is a specialist.
   2. The provider does not ask about use of CAM.
   3. The patient does not feel comfortable bringing up the topic of CAM use.
   4. Insurance does not cover the CAM treatment.
      a. 1 and 2
      b. 2 and 3
      c. 1 and 4
      d. 2 and 4

4. Which of the following major policy issues face holistic nursing in the future?
   1. Reimbursement
   2. The nursing shortage
   3. Access to holistic care
   4. Research dissemination
      a. 1 and 2
      b. 1 and 3
      c. 2 and 4
      d. 3 and 4

Advanced Level

5. Healthcare costs in the United States can be contained by which of the following methods?
   a. Increasing employees' share of healthcare coverage.
   b. Having consumers pay more for health insurance.
   c. Increasing prevention efforts.
   d. Using less information technology (IT).

6. Which answer best describes the consequences of a patient's nondisclosure of alternative or complementary treatments to his or her healthcare provider?
   a. It raises important safety issues such as potential interactions of medications and herbs.
   b. It negates the effects of conventional treatments.
   c. It compromises the relationship between patient and health provider.
   d. It empowers the patient in healthcare decision making.

7. The Institute of Medicine report *The Future of Nursing: Leading Change, Advancing Health* recommends which of the following ideas?
   1. More nurses are needed in acute care facilities.
   2. Nurses should achieve higher levels of education.
   3. Nurses need preparation and competency in geriatrics, health policy, and evidence-based practice.
   4. Nurses need to adopt to new roles.
      a. 1, 2, 4
      b. 1, 3
      c. 2, 3, 4
      d. All of the above

8. Research in holistic nursing is particularly important in all of the following areas except which one?
   a. Whole systems research
   b. Biomedical randomized controlled clinical trials
   c. Exploration of healing relationships
   d. Outcomes of healing interventions

Chapter 4

Transpersonal Human Caring and Healing

Janet F. Quinn

■ DEFINITIONS

Habitats for healing Healthcare practice environments that provide a context of caring, for the purpose of healing, which can include curing.[1]

Healing The emergence of right relationship at one or more levels of the body-mind-spirit system.[2]

Healing system A true healthcare system in which people can receive adequate, nontoxic, and noninvasive assistance in maintaining wellness and in healing the body, mind, and spirit, together with the most sophisticated, aggressive curing technologies available.

Human caring The ideal of nursing in which the nurse brings his or her whole self into relationship with the whole self of the patient or client to protect the vulnerability and preserve the humanity and dignity of the one caring and the one cared for.[3]

Right relationship A process of connection among or between parts of the whole that increases energy, coherence, and creativity in the bodymindspirit system.

Transpersonal That which transcends the limits and boundaries of individual ego identities and possibilities to include acknowledgment and appreciation of something greater. *Transpersonal* can refer to consciousness, intrapersonal dynamics, interpersonal relationships, and lived experiences of connection, unity, and oneness with the larger environment, cosmos, or Spirit.

■ TRANSPERSONAL HUMAN CARING AND HEALING: CONCEPTS AND THEORY

1. Within the discipline of nursing, there is widespread acceptance of the concept of caring as central to practice.[4,5]
2. When we enter into caring–healing relationships with patients, bringing with us an acknowledgment and appreciation of the body, mind, and spirit dimensions of our own and their human existence, we are engaged in a transpersonal human caring process.
3. In this type of relationship, we feel ourselves to be interconnected with the patient and with the larger environment and cosmos. We know that we are walking on sacred ground when we walk this path with our patients, and we recognize that neither of us will be the same afterward. Watson calls these healing encounters "caring occasions,"[3p59] which actually transcend the bounds of space and time.
4. The field of consciousness created in and through the caring–healing relationship has the potential to continue healing the patient long after the physical separation of nurse and patient.
5. When nurses are able to engage their full, caring selves in the art of nursing, it is both energizing and satisfying. It is often assumed that nurses burn out as a result of caring too much. However, today's nurses are far more likely to burn out for a different reason: the difficulty in finding the time to care for patients with their whole selves within healthcare systems that do not value caring.[6]

Healing: Emergence of Right Relationship as the Goal of Holistic Nursing

1. The origin of the word *heal* is the Anglo-Saxon word *haelan*, which means to be or to become whole.
2. *Wholeness* is frequently understood to mean harmony of body, mind, and spirit, whereas *harmony* is defined as "an esthetically pleasing set of relationships among the elements of the whole."
3. These terms begin to suggest that wholeness is not just about structure and function of the physical body, and neither is it a state of being in perfect balance at every level. Rather, wholeness is fundamentally about relationship.
4. Healing is a process rather than a state. It is the emergence of "right relationship" at any one or more levels of the human body-mind-spirit system.
5. Human beings as living systems are self-organizing systems, capable of—indeed, striving toward—order, self-transcendence, and transformation.[7]
6. The healing process itself is inherent within the person. This urge toward healing, toward right relationship, when manifested, can be thought of as the *"haelan* effect."[8]
7. *Right relationship*, in the whole systems context, refers to a process in which energy in the body-mind-spirit system is maximized to do the work of the system. Right relationship increases coherence and decreases chaos in the system, thus gaining for the system maximum freedom, choice, and capacity to creatively unfold. [9–12]
8. For this reason, true healing is always a process of emergence into something new, rather than a simple returning to prior states of being.[13]
9. Some examples of healing at different levels are the following:
   a. Body: The bonding together, the new relationship, of cells and tissues as wounds close or fractures knit.
   b. Mind/emotion: One's relationship to an event in the past shifts from resentment to forgiveness, releasing energy for new growth and an expanded consciousness.
   c. Spirit: One suddenly has the experience of being loved unconditionally and for all time, allowing her to transcend her sense of separateness and feel at one with God and all of creation.

Healing vs. Curing

1. Curing is the elimination of the signs and symptoms of disease, which might or might not correspond to an end to the patient's disease or distress.
2. Curing can occur in the complete absence of healing, for example, in the patient who undergoes bypass surgery and returns to exactly the same lifestyle as he/she had before the surgery. More dramatically, imagine the transplant patient whose body rejects the new organ. Cure, the elimination of the diseased organ, was complete, but the new relationship did not emerge. This patient might die, cured.
3. Healing can occur in the complete absence of curing, for example, in the person who is living with AIDS, or someone who is dying of cancer. Relationship to long hidden or rejected parts of the self, estranged family members, or one's God might all shift during the dying process, which can be thought of in this context as a healing process of its own.
4. Healing is always possible, whereas curing is not. Healing, the emergence of *right relationship*, can occur up to and including the moment of death. In fact, some spiritual traditions call death "the ultimate healing." In this context, a healing model is always optimistic, always hopeful.

The Healer

1. There is no way to predict how any individual's healing process will look or how long it will take or what new relationship will emerge. Healing is completely unique and cannot be coerced, manipulated, or controlled by the one healing or by anyone else. The nurse healer is a facilitator of this process, a sort of midwife, but is not the one doing the healing. Neither is the locus of the healing an isolated part of the patient, the "mind" or the "spirit."
2. All healing emerges from within the unique body-mind-spirit of the patient, sometimes with the assistance of therapeutic interventions, but not because of them. Therapeutics

(drugs, surgery, complementary therapies) might be necessary for the patient to be cured or healed, but they are not sufficient. Think about all the patients you have had who "should have" gotten better but didn't, as well as the ones who "should have" died, but went on to live long, healthy lives.

3. The assumption that all healing and curing are accomplished by the patient does not mean that all healing and curing are controlled by the patient. The causes of illness and cure are so complex and multifaceted that no simple statement of cause and effect is appropriate to describe either.

4. One can participate knowledgeably in the healing process, formulating a healing intention and doing what he or she believes is best in this situation, but the outcome of that process is a mystery even to the one healing. If we accept the premise that we are indeed body-mind-spirit, we must also accept that at least part of our healing process will always be mystery unfolding. Suggesting otherwise to patients can contribute to their sense of failure when they are unable to cure themselves of disease. Remember that caring is a moral commitment to protect the vulnerability of another, not add to it.

A True Healing Healthcare System

1. The current healthcare system continues to focus almost exclusively on the curing process, thus making it more akin to a sickness–cure system, despite 2010 reforms, which were primarily about access rather than approach.

2. Although necessary and excellent in its own right, this system is incomplete. The use of new tools of care, including alternative, holistic, or complementary therapies, without a fundamental shift in the philosophy of care with which they are used will not transform the sickness–cure system into a true, healing healthcare system.

3. The way in which practitioners use the tools available, whether the tools are conventional or complementary, and their willingness to become a midwife to nature rather than the hero of success stories make the care holistic or integrative.

4. Holistic nurses have a key role to play in facilitating this level of change in the existing systems[14-21] and in revisioning/re-creating hospitals and clinics, wellness centers and hospices, as Habitats for Healing, optimal healing environments in which nurses thrive and patients heal.

5. Habitats for Healing are characterized by autonomy of the nursing staff, a holistic, caring/healing/relationship-centered framework that guides practice, and the integration of complementary and alternative healing modalities into regular nursing care.[1]

Integration of the Masculine and the Feminine

1. The Western sickness–cure/medical system is characterized almost exclusively by attributes usually ascribed to the masculine principle and usually carried by men. These attributes include an emphasis on decisive intervention, curing, fixing, precision, "power over," and goal-/outcome-oriented approaches. These attributes are part of a way of being that might be thought of as "getting the job done."

2. These attributes may be extremely useful in the treatment of acute injury and disease, but without the attributes usually ascribed to the feminine principle, they provide an incomplete foundation for a true, integrative healing healthcare system.

3. To facilitate true healing in another the holistic nurse must learn to become comfortable with walking in the unknown, using all ways of knowing, and following the lead of the patient. These qualities, which can be thought of as holding sacred space rather than getting the job done, are usually associated with the feminine principle of receptivity and are typically carried by women.

4. "Getting the job done" includes these characteristics:
   a. Authority vested in the external "expert"
   b. Source of healing: what the expert provides
   c. Gathering, collecting, taking in information
   d. Problem solving/fixing
   e. Making "something" happen, where something is
      - Defined by the external expert
      - Defined ahead of time
      - Meeting the goal

f. Directing/taking over to make it happen

g. Doing to or for

h. Leading

i. Power over

j. Expert is accountable and responsible for outcome

k. Failure is the nonachievement of predetermined outcome

5. "Holding sacred space" includes these characteristics:

a. Authority vested in the individual client(s)

b. Source of healing: the body-mind-spirit of the client(s)

c. Receiving information

d. Life unfolding/facilitating

e. Allowing "something" to happen, where something is
   - Defined mutually
   - Defined in the moment
   - Emergence of mystery

f. Guiding/helping to allow it to happen

g. Being with

h. Walking with

i. Power with

j. Facilitator is accountable and responsible for competent practice

k. Failure is giving up on the unfolding process

6. The true healthcare system will finally emerge when both sets of attributes, masculine and feminine, are equally valued and available to guide the work of all men and women. This shift, not the mere introduction of new tools, alternative medicines, or complementary therapies, will create the world's finest healing healthcare system.

The Nurse as Healing Environment

1. One of the most powerful tools for healing that we possess is our presence as "the nurse" in the patient's environment. Of all the elements in the patient's environment, when the nurse is there, the nurse is the most impacting element. Simply by virtue of the role, a nurse has all the ritual power of the shaman of other cultures. The nurse is guardian of the patient's journey through illness and healing. He or she is the keeper and bestower of information, medicines, and treatments. He or she mediates the system and the comings and goings of others in the system.

2. In a model of the universe that includes the nonlocal nature of consciousness[22p43] or the possibility for the existence of a human energy field[23] that extends beyond the skin, the nurse is not simply part of the patient's environment, but rather, the nurse is the patient's environment. The healing environment of the patient can be maximized when the nurse intentionally shifts consciousness into a centered or meditative state. Through the interconnectedness of the energy fields of the nurse and the patient, this can facilitate relaxation, rest, and/or healing in the patient.[24]

3. When the nurse is centered in the present moment and has the intention to be a healing environment, this intention can be carried in the energy field and manifested in the voice, the eyes, and the quality of touching the nurse administers.[25]

4. Consider how the use of your voice, as a vibrational correlate of your state of consciousness, can affect your patient. The voice of a relaxed and centered person carries a different vibration than does the voice of someone who is stressed, hurried, or angry. Do patients hear in your voice that you care? That you have time for them? That they are safe with you?

5. Consider the impact of how you look at your patient. What is the quality of your facial expression? Of your eyes? Do they communicate your care and compassion, or are they perfunctory and distant? Does the patient feel seen by you or overlooked? If the eyes are the windows of the soul, what is your soul saying to the soul of your patient? What is the patient's soul saying to you?

6. Consider how you use your touch. Are you focused on the task at hand and simply touching the patient to get the job done? Or does your touch convey care, support, nurturance, and competence? (See chapter on touch for more information.)

7. Learning how to shift consciousness into a healing state is a basic skill for the holistic nurse. We are not simply separate selves "doing to" the patient, but an integral part of the patient's environment, "being

with" the patient on the healing journey. The quality of the energy with which the patient is interacting is part of what we attend to, and this means attending to our own state of consciousness and well-being before, during, and after our interactions with patients.

8. Taking time for ourselves, to learn and practice relaxation, meditation, centering, or other self-care strategies, becomes essential in this model. We are not being selfish by taking this time. We are recognizing that unless we are energized, relaxed, and centered, we are trying to give what we don't have to give. This results in less than optimal care for our patients and burnout for us.[26-28]

■ NOTES

1. Quinn, J. F. (2010). Habitats for healing: Healthy environments for health care's endangered species. *Beginnings, 30*(2), 10-11.

2. Quinn, J. F. (1997). Healing: A model for an integrative health care system. *Advanced Practice Nursing Quarterly, 3*(1), 1-7.

3. Watson, J. (1988). *Nursing: Human science and human care.* New York, NY: National League for Nursing.

4. Covington, H. (2003). Caring presence. Delineation of a concept for holistic nursing. *Journal of Holistic Nursing, 21*(3), 301-317.

5. Cowling, W. R., & Taliaferro, D. (2004). Emergence of a caring-healing perspective: Contemporary conceptual and theoretical directions. *Journal of Theory Construction and Testing, 8*(2), 54-59.

6. Quinn, J. F. (2002). Revisioning the nursing shortage: A call to caring for healing the healthcare system. *Frontiers of Health Services Management, 19*(2), 3-21.

7. Holden, L. M. (2005). Complex adaptive systems: Concept analysis. *Journal of Advanced Nursing, 52*(6), 651-657.

8. Quinn, J. (1989). On healing, wholeness and the haelan effect. *Nursing and Health Care, 10*(10), 553-556.

9. Skyttner, L. (2002). *General systems theory.* River Edge, NJ: World Scientific Publishing Company.

10. Morin, E. (2008). *On complexity: Advances in systems theory, complexity, and the human sciences.* New York: Hampton Press.

11. Lindberg, C., Nash, S., & Lindberg, C. (2008). *On the edge: Nursing in the age of complexity.* Bordentown, NJ: Plexus Press.

12. Davidson, A. W., Ray, M. A., & Turkel, M. C. (2011). *Nursing, caring and complexity science.* New York, NY: Springer.

13. McElligott, D. (2010). Healing: The journey from concept to nursing practice. *Journal of Holistic Nursing, 28*(4), 251-259.

14. Tonuma, M., & Winbolt, M. (2000). From rituals to reason: Creating an environment that allows nurses to nurse. *International Journal of Nursing, 6*(4), 214-218.

15. Taylor, M., & Keighron, K. (2004). Healing is who we are...and who are we? *Nursing Administration Quarterly, 28*(4), 241-248.

16. Watson, J. (2006). Caring theory as an ethical guide to administrative and clinical practices. *Nursing Administration Quarterly, 30*(1), 48-55.

17. McDonough-Means, S. I., Kreitzer, M. J., & Bell, I. R. (2004). Fostering a healing presence and investigating its mediators. *Journal of Alternative and Complementary Medicine, 10*(Suppl. 1), S25-S41.

18. Bernick, L. (2004). Caring for older adults: Practice guided by Watson's caring–healing model. *Nursing Science Quarterly, 17*(2), 128-134.

19. Stichler, J. F. (2001). Creating healing environments in critical care units. *Critical Care Nursing Quarterly, 24*(3), 1-20.

20. Stickley, T., & Freshwater, D. (2002). The art of loving and the therapeutic relationship. *Nursing Inquiry, 9*(4), 250-256.

21. Watson, J., & Foster, R. (2003). The attending nurse caring model: Integrating theory, evidence and advanced caring–healing therapeutics for transforming professional practice. *Journal of Clinical Nursing, 12*(3), 360-365.

22. Dossey, L. (1993). *Healing words.* San Francisco, CA: Harper San Francisco.

23. Rogers, M. (1990). Nursing: Science of unitary, irreducible, human beings: Update 1990. In E. A. M. Barrett (Ed.), *Visions of Rogers science-based nursing.* New York, NY: National League for Nursing.

24. Quinn, J. F. (1992). Holding sacred space: The nurse as healing environment. *Holistic Nursing Practice, 6*(4), 26-36.

25. Quinn, J. F. (2013). Transpersonal human caring and healing. In B. Dossey & L. Keegan (Eds.), *Holistic nursing: A handbook for practice* (6th ed., pp. 107-114). Burlington, MA: Jones & Bartlett Learning.

26. Turkel, M. C., & Ray, M. A. (2004). Creating a caring practice environment through self-renewal. *Nursing Administration Quarterly, 28*(4), 249-254.

27. Christianson, J. D., Finch, M. D., Findlay, B., Jonas, W. B., & Choate, C. G. (2007). *Reinventing the patient experience.* Chicago, IL: Health Administration Press.

28. Vitale, A. (2009). Nurses' lived experience of Reiki for self-care. *Holistic Nursing Practice, 23*(3), 129-145.

■ STUDY QUESTIONS

Basic Level

1. Which statement best describes the relationship between healing and curing?
   a. Healing and curing are unrelated processes.
   b. Curing is required for healing to begin.
   c. Healing can occur with or without curing.
   d. Once healing has begun, curing will follow.

2. Which way of being is usually attributed to the "feminine principle"?
   a. A focus on the outcome rather than the process
   b. Decisive intervention designed to fix the problem
   c. An attitude of precise action
   d. Allowing space for the unfolding mystery

3. Which of the following statements characterizes healing?
   a. Healing is another way of talking about curing.
   b. Healing is an outcome of treatment given by the medical staff.
   c. Healing is measurable by standard tests and empirical observations.
   d. Healing is the emergence of right relationship at one or more levels.

4. Which of the following most accurately reflects the holistic nurse's understanding of the healing process?
   a. Healing emerges from within the body-mind-spirit of the patient but cannot be manipulated or controlled.
   b. Healing is the result of what we do as healthcare providers.
   c. The outcome of a healing process can be determined at the outset by the patient and/or the healthcare team.
   d. Patients are in control of the healing process and we must help them to achieve their goals.

5. Which of the following statements about transpersonal human caring best explains how it can be applied in patient care?
   a. It is first and foremost a process of relationship.
   b. It is a set of intervention strategies anyone can use.

   c. It requires nurses to take more time with patients.
   d. It cannot happen if the patient cannot communicate.

Advanced Level

6. Before you enter a patient's room to provide his treatments you take a moment to center yourself in the present moment, letting go of any of the tensions you are carrying from an unpleasant encounter just prior to this. This action is the application of which principle related to transpersonal caring and healing?
   a. The nurse should be quiet when entering the patient's environment.
   b. The nurse is the patient's environment.
   c. The nurse needs to maintain healthy boundaries with the patient.
   d. The nurse needs to be undistracted to provide the treatment.

7. You are the nurse educator charged with helping unit nurses to create a more healing environment. As you prepare your in-service presentation on this topic, which of the following is the *main idea* that you will emphasize?
   a. The unit nurses need to become skillful in using a variety of alternative therapies.
   b. Nurses need to remember that they are the healers in the healing environment.
   c. When the nurse is present, he or she is the healing environment for the patient.
   d. Healing is sometimes possible even when curing isn't.

8. Which of the following answer choices correctly completes the statement "Right relationship in the context of healing _____"?
   a. Maximizes free energy to do the work of the system
   b. Decreases order and coherence in the system
   c. Minimizes freedom for creativity and change
   d. Increases feelings of power and control

9. When you come in to see him, Paul has just gotten the results of his latest CT scan, which shows widespread metastasis

of his cancer. He explains that his doctors have told him there is nothing else that the healthcare system can do for him and that he should get his affairs in order. In responding to Paul, which of the following would be *least* consistent with the transpersonal caring–healing framework?

a. Following Paul's lead in where and how his sharing unfolds, remembering that it is his process and you are only the midwife

b. Expressing your condolences and asking if there is someone that he might like you to call to help him begin getting his affairs in order

c. Letting Paul know that, although there might be no further medical options open to him for treatment of his cancer, that doesn't mean there is nothing that can be done to support his healing

d. Maintaining a safe, loving space for Paul to talk about his responses to the news

10. Maureen is a 51-year-old woman who was recently diagnosed with hypertension. She wants to treat her hypertension holistically, so she is not taking the medications that were prescribed for her. She wants to work with you, a holistic nurse, using alternative medicine. She has already begun using meditation because she believes it can help contribute to her healing process. Which of the following assumptions that appear to be influencing Maureen's course of action is erroneous?

a. All healing emerges from within the unique body-mind-spirit of the patient.

b. Healing might or might not include the elimination of the signs and symptoms of disease.

c. Healing is a process rather than an event or state.

d. Holistic care requires the use of alternative therapies instead of standard, allopathic treatments.

Chapter 5

Nursing Theory in Holistic Nursing Practice

Noreen Cavan Frisch and Pamela J. Potter

■ DEFINITIONS

Concept An abstract idea or notion.

Conceptual model A group of interrelated concepts described to suggest relationships among them.

Framework A basic structure; the context in which theory is developed; the structure that permits theory to be understood.

Grand theory A theory that covers a broad area of the discipline's concerns.

Metaparadigm Concepts that identify the domain of a discipline.

Metatheory Theory about theory development; theory about theory.

Midrange theory A focused theory for nursing that deals with a portion of a nurse's concerns, or one that is oriented to patient outcomes.

Model A representation of interactions between and among concepts.

Nursing theory A framework; a set of interrelated concepts that are testable; a way of seeing the factors that contribute to nursing practice and nursing thought.

Worldview A perspective; a way of viewing, perceiving, and interpreting one's experience.

■ NURSING THEORY

1. Nursing theory: A framework from which professional nurses can think about their work. Theory is a means of interpreting one's observations of the world and is an abstraction of reality.

2. Domain of nursing: Each discipline has a set of concepts or ideas that represent the core content of the discipline. These core concepts are called the *metaparadigm* of the discipline. For nursing, the core concepts are person, health, nursing, and environment. These concepts have been thought to represent the domain of nursing.

3. Expanded domain of nursing: Some current nursing scholars suggest that, as the discipline has matured, other concepts might well be as central to the core content as the four original concepts.[1] These other concepts include caring, healing, energy fields, development, adaptation, consciousness, and nurse–client relationships.

■ THEORY AND RESEARCH

Nursing theory is grounded in research and can help to provide a scientific basis for care. There are two kinds of research approaches to theory development.

1. Theory-building research: Research that examines the relationships between and among core concepts of nursing and that uses the results of these examinations to develop models or frameworks for the discipline. For example, a researcher might examine the relationship of a caring environment to healing and develop a theoretical model of how the two could be associated.

2. Theory-validating research: Research that applies a defined theory to practice and evaluates outcomes.

■ USE OF NURSING THEORY

1. Schools of nursing: Almost all schools of nursing develop curriculums based on nursing theories so that students learn a way of thinking about nursing and approaching nursing care based on theory. Sometimes nursing theory concepts are taught as assumptions (i.e., *This* is what nursing is), and other times the concepts are presented explicitly as part of an identified theory.

2. Holistic nursing practice: The American Holistic Nursing Association (AHNA) description of holistic nursing practice indicates that there are five elements for nursing practice: knowledge, theory, expertise, intuition, and creativity.[2] Theory is included because use of theory requires the nurse to reflect on practice, bring practice behaviors in line with beliefs and values, and consider alternatives of care before selecting from care options.

3. AHNA Core Value 1: AHNA's *Holistic Nursing: Scope and Standards of Practice* incorporates theory into its first core value that includes holistic philosophy, theory, and ethics. Use of theory helps the nurse articulate his or her fundamental philosophical beliefs about the discipline and provides the framework for self-reflection required of professional holistic practice.

4. Theory in an era of evidence-based/evidence-informed practice: Theory provides the nurse with a framework from which to understand and make meaning out of complex experiences and a framework from which to study the actual complexities of the human health condition. At a time where there is an increasing need to practice on the basis of evidence, theory helps us examine evidence and the assumptions behind evidence.

■ SELECTED HOLISTIC NURSING THEORIES

1. The Theory of Environmental Adaptation: This is the current name given to Florence Nightingale's work. Nightingale first presented views on concepts important to nursing and directed nurses in the provision of care. To Nightingale, the overarching goal of nursing care is putting patients in the best condition for nature to act upon them.[3] According to this theory:
   a. The focus of nursing care is the creation of an environment so that natural healing may take place.
   b. Cleanliness, fresh air, and order are emphasized, as are the patient's needs for nutrition.
   c. The theory has been studied and modernized by nurse scholars who have described it in terms of theory development used today. Selanders has written about the principle of environmental alteration, and how Nightingale's work has formed a basis for current nursing research.[4,5]
   d. A definitive statement on Nightingale's life and work is available in a biography prepared by Dossey.[6]

2. The Modeling and Role-Modeling Theory (M-RM): M-RM draws on work from many theoretical perspectives, including Maslow's Basic Needs, Erickson's Stages of Development, Piaget's Theory of Cognitive Development, and Selye's Stress Theory. First published by Helen Erickson and her colleagues in 1983,[7] this theory emphasizes nursing as a process that demands an interpersonal and interactive relationship with the client. According to this theory:
   a. Facilitation, nurturance, and unconditional acceptance must characterize the nurse's caregiving; the human person is viewed as a holistic being with interacting subsystems (biologic, psychologic, social, and cognitive) and with an inherent genetic base and spiritual drive; the whole is greater than the sum of its parts; health is a dynamic equilibrium between subsystems; and the environment is viewed as both internal and external.
   b. The client is viewed as an individual with strengths that can and should be used to mobilize resources to adapt to stress. *Adaptive potential* is a theory-specific term used to describe conditions of adaptation–equilibrium (which can be adaptive or maladaptive), arousal, and impoverishment.
   c. The theory presents five aims of all nursing interventions: (1) to build trust, (2) to promote positive orientation, (3) to promote perceived control, (4) to promote

strengths, and (5) to set mutual goals that are health directed.

d. The nurse uses this theory by creating a model of the client's world (modeling) and using that model to plan interventions and to demonstrate and support health-producing behaviors from within the client's worldview (role modeling).

e. In her most recent text on the theory, Erickson writes that nurses who practice holistically need to discover that their gift to clients is the gift of themselves.[8] She provides a foundation for self-nurturance, self-discovery, and self-growth as conditions of holistic nursing that becomes a way of living and provides meaning in life.

3. The Theory of Transpersonal Caring and Caring Science: First presented as a philosophy and science of caring,[9] Jean Watson's theory emphasizes the humanist aspects of nursing combined with scientific knowledge.

a. In using the Theory of Transpersonal Caring, the foremost role of the nurse is to establish an intimate, caring relationship with the client. The nurse must be able to understand the client's subjective experiences and interact with the client in a meaningful relationship.

b. Person is seen holistically with the knowledge that the whole is greater than, and different from, the sum of the parts; every person is a valued individual to be cared for, cared about, and understood; health is a subjective state that has to do with unity and harmony; illness can be understood as disharmony. Caring is achieved through the environment because the environment provides social, cultural, and spiritual influences that can be perceived as caring.

c. The "caring occasion" or the "caring moment" are important concepts within this theory and represent situations when nurses and clients come together in unique ways such that there is a truly transformational encounter, leaving both the nurse and the client changed.

d. The strength of the theory relies on the nurse's ability to provide quality, caring interactions with the client while simultaneously promoting health through nursing knowledge and interventions.

e. Watson has advocated for a postmodern view of nursing, and of science, that comprises multiple truths, physical and nonphysical realities, and the relativity of time and space.[10,11]

4. The Science of Unitary Human Beings: Martha Rogers was the first theorist to describe nursing in relation to the view that a person is an energy field. In addition, she believed that nursing is a "humanistic science dedicated to compassionate concern for maintaining and promoting health, preventing illness, and caring for and rehabilitating the sick and disabled."[12] Rogers's theory, which is an abstract system, is the basis for the Science of Unitary Human Beings. According to this theory:

a. Nursing is the scientific study of human and environmental energy fields.

b. A person is a unified whole, defined as a human energy field; human beings evolve irreversibly and unidirectionally in space and time. Health is understood in terms of culture and, according to Rogers, is individually defined by the subjective values of each person. The environment is the environmental energy field that is in constant interaction with the human energy field. There are no boundaries to the environmental or human energy fields.

c. Over the years many studies have tested concepts of this theory, and several authors have suggested research methodologies specifically appropriate to the Science of Unitary Human Beings. These include the Unitary Field Pattern Portrait Research Method described by Butcher,[13] rational hermeneutics described by Alligood and Fawcett,[14] and case study approaches described by Cowling.[15]

d. Current development of the theory is being carried out by a number of Rogerian scholars and perhaps most notably Howard Butcher, who reminds us that Rogers understood that knowledge and practice were inseparable—thus, at the theory's core is the praxis of nursing thought and action.

5. The Theory of Expanding Consciousness: Margaret Newman included Rogers's concepts of energy patterns and unitary

human beings in the development of her theory. Newman viewed nursing as a profession that is moving to an integrated role; nursing is caring, and caring is a moral imperative for nursing.[16] Within this theory:

a. The person is viewed as a dynamic energy field; humans are identified by their field patterns. Health is expanding consciousness that includes an individual's total pattern; pathologic conditions are manifestations of the individual's total pattern. Environment is the wholeness of the universe; there are no boundaries.

b. For Newman, people are not separate entities but instead are "open energy systems constantly interacting and evolving with each other."[17]

c. Health and illness are paired as a unitary process of complementary forces of order and disorder that are essential in each person's continuing development.

d. Newman notes that experiencing a significant illness often results in a turning point (a choice point) for a person where the person sees himself or herself differently. Thus, a person can expand consciousness after transcending limitations of disease and other life events.

6. The Theory of Human Becoming: Rosemarie Rizzo Parse further developed the idea of the person as a unitary whole and suggested that the person can be viewed only as a unity.[18] Nursing is viewed as a scientific discipline, but the practice of nursing is an art in which nurses serve as guides to assist others in making choices affecting health. Within this theory:

a. Person is a unified, whole being. Health is a process of becoming; it is a personal commitment, an unfolding, a process related to lived experiences. Environment is the universe. The human universe is inseparable and evolving as one.

b. Research on the theory of human becoming documented the importance of intersubjective dialogue in assisting clients to move toward different meanings and choices in their lives and has described the sense of caring that clients perceive from nurses guided by the theory.

c. The concept of presence is critically important for this theory because the nurse offers authentic presence to each client in the process of becoming and living experiences.

7. The Theory of Integral Nursing (TIN): In 2008, Barbara Dossey presented her work on the development of a grand theory of nursing that incorporated work from two other prominent theorists: Wilber's Integral Theory and Carper's theory on Ways of Knowing.[19] As a grand theory, this theory is abstract and is meant to address very broad areas of the discipline's concerns. For some, this theory can be considered a metatheory, or a theory of theories.

a. TIN has three intentions: to embrace the unitary whole person and the complexity of nursing and health care; to explore the application of an integral process and worldview; and to expand nurses' capacities for current and future demands.[19]

b. The concept of healing is central to the TIN and within this theory, healing includes knowing, doing, and being and becomes a lifelong journey.

c. TIN recognizes the metaparadigm of nursing and views the four concepts of person, health/healing, nurse, and environment from within the four quadrants of Wilber's theory: individual interior (intentional personal), individual exterior (behavioral/biological), collective interior (cultural/shared), and collective exterior (systems/structures).

d. TIN also embraces the concept of development and, again, based on Wilber's Integral Theory, development occurs through levels of growth/maturity and through areas such as cognitive, interpersonal, moral, needs, identity, and spirituality.

e. TIN is applied within an environmental context that both understands and accepts the environment as interior and exterior and that which has meaning to the individual.

f. As a new theory, TIN might be shifting our paradigm in nursing to expand our notions of who and what we are.

■ MIDRANGE THEORY

1. Definition: Over the years, many nurses have been interested in focused or midrange theories that deal with only a portion

of a nurse's concerns and that are very often oriented to patient outcomes.

2. Need for midrange theories: Midrange theories originated from an emphasis on providing nurse-sensitive outcomes as part of our professional accountability. Thus, some of these midrange theories have been useful to practicing holistic nurses dealing with specific issues such as pain alleviation, postpartum depression, and maternal role attachment.

3. Kolcaba's Theory of Comfort: This theory is an example of a midrange theory that is based on holistic philosophies and values.[20]
   a. According to the theory, comfort is not simply the absence of pain or distress; it is a positive subjective feeling reflecting a sense of holistic well-being. Comfort is understood as a holistic phenomenon such that comfort is manifested as feelings of relief, ease, and transcendence occurring "all at once."
   b. The theory has been applied to nurses' work with many populations across the life span and across care environments. Also, several comfort measures have been identified to make every effort to determine the client's response to nursing actions as a perceived state of comfort or a feeling of being comforted.

4. Use of midrange theories: Attention to midrange theories can provide helpful and immediate applications of theory to current work settings and assist holistic nurses to begin documenting nurse-sensitive outcomes of their practices.

■ THEORY AND THE HOLISTIC CARING PROCESS

1. A nurse who uses a theory in practice takes on the worldview of that theory and "sees" the world from the lens of that theory. Thus, our theoretical perspective influences how we assess, analyze, select outcomes, plan nursing actions, and evaluate our care.

2. Important points in relation to the holistic caring process are as follows:
   a. The language of the nursing process and nursing diagnoses are atheoretical; thus, the standardized words used to record assessments, diagnoses, and outcomes (for example, words contained in the NANDA-NIC-NOC taxonomies/classifications) name a condition or state and can be used with any theory.
      ▪ The written nursing diagnostic statements that includes a "related to" clause frequently use the language of the theoretical perspective in the "related to" description of the nursing phenomena of concern. Example: NDX: Fatigue r/t state of impoverishment. (M-RM)
   b. When the nurse evaluates outcomes of care, the nurse should consider and record how the theoretical perspective affected the diagnoses and influenced the options for nursing interventions.
      ▪ The interventions and care outcomes might also be recorded based on the theory. Example: For a client demonstrating anxiety and sleep disturbance, the intervention of *therapeutic presence* can have an impact on restored sleep.
   c. Use of theory can also have an impact on the nurse as a person and on the practice environments at the unit/system level.
      ▪ A nurse might use holistic theory and its values to consider the task of handwashing between patient encounters as a symbolic cleansing of herself as a tool of healing—rinsing away that which is not healthful and making ready for each new patient encounter.
      ▪ An organization committed to patient-centered care might embrace the practice of nurturing the caregivers through support for collaborative and mutually enriching and energizing actions among nursing staff.

■ NOTES

1. Parker, M. E. (2006). *Nursing theories and nursing practice* (2nd ed.). Philadelphia, PA: F. A. Davis.
2. American Holistic Nurses Association & American Nurses Association. (2007). *Holistic nursing: Scope and standards of practice*. Silver Spring, MD: Nursesbooks.org.
3. Nightingale, F. (1860). *Notes on nursing*. London, England: Harrison.
4. Selanders, L. C. (1998). The power of environmental adaptation: Florence Nightingale's original theory for nursing practice. *Journal of Holistic Nursing, 16*, 247–263.

5. Selanders, L. C. (2010). The power of environmental adaption. *Journal of Holistic Nursing, 28,* 81–88.

6. Dossey, B. M. (2000). *Florence Nightingale, Mystic, visionary, healer.* Springhouse, PA: Springhouse.

7. Erickson, H., Tomlin, E. M., & Swain, M. A. P. (1983). *Modeling and role-modeling: A theory and paradigm for nursing.* Lexington, KY: Pine Press.

8. Erickson, H. L. (2006). *Modeling and role-modeling: A view from the client's world.* Cedar Park, TX: Unicorns Unlimited.

9. Watson, J. (1988). *Human science and human care.* New York, NY: National League for Nursing.

10. Watson, J. (1999). *Postmodern nursing.* London, England: Churchill Livingstone.

11. Watson, J. (2006). *Caring science as sacred science.* Philadelphia, PA: F. A. Davis.

12. Rogers, M. (1970). *The theoretical basis for nursing.* Philadelphia, PA: F. A. Davis.

13. Butcher, H. K. (1998). Crystallizing the process of the unitary field pattern portrait research method. *Visions: The Journal of Rogerian Nursing Science, 6,* 13–26.

14. Alligood, M. E., & Fawcett, J. (1999). Acceptance of the invitation to dialogue: Examination of an interpretive approach for the science of unitary human beings. *Visions: The Journal of Rogerian Nursing Science, 8,* 5–13.

15. Cowling, W. R. (1998). Unitary case inquiry. *Nursing Science Quarterly, 12,* 139–141.

16. Newman, M. (1994). *Health as expanding consciousness* (2nd ed.). New York, NY: National League for Nursing.

17. Newman, M. (1999). *Health as expanding consciousness.* (3rd ed.). Sudbury, MA: Jones and Bartlett.

18. Parse, R. R. (1992). Human becoming: Parse's theory of nursing. *Nursing Science Quarterly, 5,* 35–42.

19. Dossey, B. M. (2008). Theory of integral nursing. *Advances in Nursing Science, 31*(1), e52–e73.

20. Kolcaba, K. (2003). *Comfort theory and practice.* New York, NY: Springer.

■ STUDY QUESTIONS
Basic Level

1. Which of the following best describes a nursing theory?
   a. A framework for thinking about one's work
   b. A basis for evidence-informed practice
   c. A precondition for professionalism
   d. A tool for making complete client assessments

2. Florence Nightingale's original work has been updated by Selanders. What is it called?
   a. The Theory of Adaptive Potential
   b. The Theory of Unitary Human Beings
   c. The Theory of Environmental Adaptation
   d. The Theory of Caring

3. Which of the following is a core concept of Watson's theory for nursing?
   a. Human development
   b. Energy fields
   c. The four quadrants
   d. Human caring

4. According to Newman's Theory of Expanding Consciousness, illness and wellness are related in what way?
   a. There is a continuum from wellness to illness.
   b. Illness and wellness are opposites.
   c. Illness is an inevitable condition of living.
   d. Wellness can occur at the time of illness.

5. Holistic nurse Marion is using the Theory of Unitary Human Beings in her practice. When completing her initial nursing assessment, which of the following actions will Marion take?
   a. Evaluate the integrity of her client's energy field.
   b. Assess her client's current level of environmental stress.
   c. Complete a thorough neurological assessment.
   d. Evaluate her client's need for social interaction.

Advanced Level

6. Susan, a patient in a hospital, awaits surgery tomorrow morning. Susan's physical state is stable. Susan talks with the nurse about feeling worried and expresses discomfort with the idea of surgery because she has never had surgery before. In enacting the values of Parse's Theory of Human Becoming, what will Susan's nurse, Debra, do?
   a. Reassure Susan that her surgery is needed and that the hospital staff will do everything possible to make her feel safe and comfortable.

b. Complete a physical assessment and share her findings with Susan.

c. Provide a sleep protocol as a nursing intervention to support restful sleep.

d. Engage Susan in dialogue about Susan's feelings and subjective experiences.

7. In making a home visit to a postpartum family with their first child, the nurse assesses that the mother is doing well with establishing breastfeeding, yet she expresses worry about her ability to breast-feed the baby. Using Erickson's Modeling Role-Modeling theory, what will the nurse do?

a. Identify the mother's strengths as a new mother and emphasize these in her interactions with the mother.

b. Provide health promotion teaching on breastfeeding and maternal nutrition.

c. Assist the mother to create an uncluttered and nurturing environment in the home.

d. Evaluate the mother's developmental state and create support for the mother to move into her new role.

8. Bob is a nurse working in a cardiac critical care unit. He frequently sits at the bedside of his patients and talks to them about how they are feeling and what they are experiencing in the unit. He tells the other nurses that he is a student of Watson's theory and wants to provide a presence of caring and support for patients, and he encourages other nurses to do the same. How could the nursing unit best approach Bob's suggestions?

a. Ask for more nursing time from administration to enact this theory.

b. Write their nursing care plans to include stress-reduction interventions.

c. Identify probable patient outcomes from such interactions and evaluate whether they occur.

d. Develop their own theory of human interaction and explain how interaction and healing might be related.

9. Nurse Mary is caring for her client, Nora, who is undergoing outpatient chemotherapy for a lymphoma. Nora has every expectation of a successful recovery from this condition. Mary notes that her client is physically stable and, although nausea after chemotherapy has been a concern, it is being controlled reasonably well through medication. During her current visit with Nora, Mary notes that Nora expresses feelings questioning why she is undergoing this illness and tries to understand the full impact of this cancer on her life. Using Newman's theory, which of the following does Mary assess?

a. Nora is undergoing an expected period of anxiety resulting from the uncertain outcome of her treatment.

b. Nora is searching for additional social interactions and activities that will help her to regain a sense of balance and normalcy in her life.

c. Nora is at risk for depression and needs additional nursing and social service supports that put her in touch with others who have had the same illness.

d. Nora is facing a choice point in her life and could benefit from nursing interventions that focus on exploring personal meanings.

10. Elizabeth is the chief nursing officer of a large medical center. Daily, she is faces issues of how to provide quality care within available resources, how to maintain a supportive working environment for nurses, and how to articulate the need for professional nursing to members of an interdisciplinary team. Elizabeth believes that nurses' knowledge and use of nursing theories can help her hospital simultaneously meet the mandates for patient satisfaction and nurse retention. If this idea is correct, what could she provide as an explanation to others?

a. Nursing theories offer a way to initiate care planning that connects nursing activities with nurse-sensitive outcomes.

b. Nursing theories provide for client-centeredness.

c. Nursing theories result in cost-effective practice.

d. Nursing theories define the role of professional nursing.

Chapter 6

Holistic Ethics

Mary Ann Cordeau

Original Authors: Margaret A. Burkhardt
and Lynn Keegan

■ DEFINITIONS

Being The state of existing or living.

Consciousness A state of knowing or awareness.

Earth ethics A code of behavior that incorporates the understanding that the Earth community has core value in and of itself and includes ethical treatment of the non-human world and the Earth as a whole. This code influences the way that we individually and collectively interact with the environment and all beings of the Earth.

Ethical code A written list of a profession's values and standards of conduct.

Ethics The study or discipline concerned with judgments of approval and disapproval, right and wrong, good and bad, virtue and vice, and desirability and wisdom of actions, as well as dispositions, ends, objects, and states of affairs; disciplined reflection on the moral choices that people make.

Holistic Concerned with the interrelationship of body, mind, and spirit in an ever-changing environment.

Holistic ethics The basic underlying concept of the unity and integral wholeness of all people and of all nature, which is identified and pursued by finding unity and wholeness within one's self and within humanity. In this framework, acts are not performed for the sake of law, precedent, or social norms, but rather from a desire to do good freely, to witness, identify, and contribute to unity.

Informed consent A process by which patients or participants in research studies are informed of the purpose, possible outcomes, alternatives, risks, and benefits of treatment or the research protocol; individuals are required to freely give their consent for the treatment or participation in the study.

Morals Standards of right and wrong that are learned through socialization.

Nursing ethics A code of values and behavior that influences the way nurses work with those in their care, with one another, and with society.

Personal ethics An individual code of thought, values, and behavior that governs each person's actions.

Values Concepts or ideals that give meaning to life and provide a framework for decisions and actions.

■ THE NATURE OF ETHICAL PROBLEMS

1. Ethical issues reflect diverse values and perspectives and are extremely complex.
2. Many factors affect ethical decision making such as the following:
   a. Life-sustaining technology
   b. Advances in medical technology
   c. Genetic engineering
   d. Allocation of increasingly scarce resources
   e. Greater recognition of patients' rights
   f. Malpractice cases

g. Court-ordered treatment
h. End-of-life decisions
i. Relationship between ethical treatment of the Earth and human health
3. Ethical dilemmas occur when there are two or more unsatisfactory answers or conflicting responses.
4. Technological sources of ethical dilemmas include the following:
   a. Changes in knowledge that forms the basis of our values and advances in health care are leading to new sources of ethical dilemmas.
   b. Computers and confidentiality affect ethical dilemmas.
   c. Life support might prolong living but might also increase suffering and delay the dying process, thus causing a potential ethical dilemma.

■ MORALS AND PRINCIPLES

1. Ethical principles serve as a guide for ethical decision making.
2. Major ethical principles:
   a. Autonomy: To respect wishes of a competent person
   b. Beneficence: To take actions that benefit others
   c. Nonmaleficence: To not harm others
   d. Veracity: To be truthful, to disclose information
   e. Confidentiality: To respect privacy and protect confidential information
   f. Justice: To distribute benefits and harms fairly
   g. Fidelity: To keep promises and contracts
3. Principle of double effect: Many actions have untoward consequences.
4. Four conditions that must be met before a double principle act can be justified:
   a. The act itself must be morally good, or at least indifferent.
   b. The good effect must not be achieved by means of the bad effect.
   c. Only the good effect must be intended, even though the bad effect is foreseen and known.
   d. The good effect intended must be equal to or greater than the bad effect.[1]
5. Moral problems
   a. Incorporate a mix of values, risks, benefits, and harms
   b. Include elements of uncertainty and conflict, and defy easy solutions
   c. Ethics addresses different types of moral problems:
      ■ Moral uncertainty (i.e., unsureness about moral principles or rules that may apply, or the nature of the ethical problem itself)
      ■ Moral distress (i.e., inability to take the action known to be right because of external constraints)
6. Practical dilemmas: Situations in which moral claims compete with nonmoral claims.[1] Ethical debate helps to relieve moral uncertainty by clarifying questions and illuminating the ethical features of a situation. A holistic approach to ethical problems incorporates both thinking and feeling as credible ways of knowing and recognizes a legitimate role for both in ethical decision making. Heart and mind, reason and emotion need to be attended to when making ethical decisions, appreciating that what one feels in relation to the circumstances of the situation is as important as what one thinks is right or wrong.
   Many factors contribute to the complexity of ethical problems:
   a. Context (i.e., a person's unique life circumstances)
   b. Uncertainty (i.e., a lack of predictability of the outcome of a given act)
   c. Multiple stakeholders with potentially strong and diverse preferences
   d. Power imbalance within the healthcare institution
   e. Variables outside of the direct patient care setting, such as institutional policies
   f. Urgency (i.e., situations in which a decision must be made before one has a chance to deliberate as much as one would like)[2]

■ TRADITIONAL ETHICAL THEORIES

1. A number of ethical theories have played a role in Western civilization and have laid the foundation for the development of modern ethics.
   a. Aristotelian theory is based on the individual manifesting specific virtues and developing his or her own character. Aristotle (384–322 B.C.E.) believed that

an individual who practices the virtues of courage, temperance, integrity, justice, honesty, and truthfulness will know almost intuitively what to do in a particular situation or conflict.[3]

b. Immanuel Kant (1724–1804) formulated the historical Christian idea of the Golden Rule: "So act in such a way as your act becomes a universal for all mankind."[3p273] Kant was very much concerned with the "personhood" of human beings and persons as moral agents.

c. Jeremy Bentham (1748–1832) and John Stuart Mill (1806–1873) proposed Utilitarianism: The consequences of our actions are the primary concern, the means justify the ends, and every human being has a personal concept of good and bad.

d. Natural Rights Theory of John Locke (1632–1714), and the Contractarian Theory of Thomas Hobbes (1588–1679): Briefly stated, the consequentialist, or the Contractarian Theory of Hobbes, contends that morality involves a social contract indicating what individuals can and cannot do.[3pp163-169]

e. Traditional ethical styles:
   - Deontologic style: *Deontologic* derives from a Greek root meaning knowledge of that which is binding and proper. Duty or obligation is based on the intrinsic aspects of an act rather than its outcome, meaning that action is morally defensible on the basis of its intrinsic nature.
   - Teleologic style: *Teleologic* derives from a Greek root meaning knowledge of the ends. Duty or obligation is based on the consequences of the act, meaning that action is morally defensible on the basis of its extrinsic value or outcome.

■ THE DEVELOPMENT OF HOLISTIC ETHICS

1. Holistic ethics is a philosophy that couples both reemerging and rapidly evolving concepts of holism and ethics. It involves a basic underlying concept of the unity and integral wholeness of all people, and of all nature, which is identified and pursued by finding unity and wholeness within one's self, within humanity, and within the larger Earth community.

   a. Framework of holistic ethics: Acts are not performed solely for the sake of law, precedent, or social norms; they are performed from a desire to do good freely, to witness, identify, and contribute to unity of the self and of the universe, of which the individual is a part.
      - Encompassing traditional ethical views, the holistic view is characterized by the balance and integration evident in the Eastern monad of the yin-yang mode and in the Western concept of masculine-feminine.
      - Holistic ethics originates in the individual's own character and in the individual's relationship to the universe. In some ways, the universe is present totally in each individual; paradoxically, the person is just a small part of that same universe.
      - Holistic ethics is grounded or judged not so much in the act performed or in the distant consequences of the act as in the conscious evolution of an enlightened individual who performs the act.
      - By understanding that all things are connected, the primary concern is the effect of the act on the individual and his or her larger self (i.e., that unity of which the individual is a part).
      - Holistic ethics embraces and strives for the fusion between self and others. In the process, it becomes a cosmic ecology, a flowing with the universal tide of events, and a cocreator of celestial harmony.
      - All events and ethical decisions become part of the unfolding of a harmonious order and a realization of potentials.
      - Even tragic events can be analyzed within this harmonious spectrum with full realization of the fusion of relationships.
      - One's own actions can become courageous, full of truth, full of being and beauty, assured, detached, virtuous.

2. Unethical acts are those that degrade or brutalize the individual who performs the

act and that detract from his or her conscious evolution, which, in turn, degrades the whole.

  a. The effect of an unethical act is to make us aware of the deprivation of divinity within humanity and of humanity itself.
  b. The unethical act dissolves the unity of matter and takes away wholeness.
  c. Acts must be judged in this setting to determine whether they promote wholeness and integration of either an individual or the collective whole.

3. Moral acts can be judged not solely in terms of their intrinsic nature nor solely in terms of their ends, but in both ways. The act can affect the nature of the person performing the act (the "I") and his or her relationships, as well as affect the object of the act and the object's relationships.

  a. Holistic ethics is both deontologic and teleologic.
  b. Holistic ethics is specifically teleologic in questioning the meaning and quality of life.

4. Code of ethics for holistic nurses: The American Holistic Nurses Association has written a position statement on holistic nursing ethics.[4] The fundamental responsibilities of the nurse are to promote health, facilitate healing, and alleviate suffering. Inherent in nursing is the respect for life, dignity, and right of all persons.

  a. Nurses and self: The nurse has a responsibility to model health behaviors. Holistic nurses strive to achieve harmony in their own lives and assist others striving to do the same.
  b. Nurses and the client: The nurse's primary responsibility is to the client needing nursing care. The nurse strives to see the client as a whole and provides care that is professionally appropriate and culturally consonant. The nurse holds in confidence all information obtained in professional practice and uses professional judgment in disclosing such information. The nurse enters into a relationship with the client that is guided by mutual respect and a desire for growth and development.
  c. Nurses and coworkers: The nurse maintains cooperative relationships with coworkers in nursing and other fields.

Nurses have a responsibility to nurture each other and to assist nurses to work as a team in the interest of client care. If a client's care is endangered by a coworker, the nurse must take appropriate action on behalf of the client.

  d. Nurses and nursing practice: The nurse carries personal responsibility for practice and for maintaining continued competence. Nurses have the right to utilize all appropriate nursing interventions and have the obligation to determine the efficacy and safety of all nursing actions. Wherever applicable, nurses utilize research findings in directing practice.
  e. Nurses and the profession: The nurse plays a role in determining and implementing desirable standards of nursing practice and education. Holistic nurses may assume a leadership position to guide the profession toward holism. Nurses support nursing research and the development of holistically oriented nursing theories. The nurse participates in establishing and maintaining equitable social and economic working conditions in nursing.
  f. Nurses and society: The nurse, along with other citizens, has responsibility for initiating and supporting actions to meet the health and social needs of the public.
  g. Nurses and the environment: The nurse strives to manipulate the client's environment to become one of peace, harmony, and nurturance so that healing can take place. The nurse considers the health of the ecosystem in relation to the need for health, safety, and peace of all persons.

5. Earth ethics: A sense that the human experience is separate from and in opposition to nature has engendered and permitted a destructive attitude toward Earth and a belief that all species and resources of the Earth have been put here primarily for human use. This attitude promotes little sense of ethical responsibility toward the nonhuman world.

  a. There is an urgent need for holistic nurses and all of humanity to move beyond a human-centered focus in ethical concerns and begin to relate to all parts of the Earth community as having core value.

b. We need to incorporate Earth ethics into our understanding and practice of holistic ethics.

c. As humans, we are only one part of the interconnected Earth community, and we recognize the interdependence and unity of all in the natural world, we appreciate that all species have an intrinsic right to exist.

d. The moral imperative of holistic ethics directs us to apply principles of beneficence, nonmaleficence, and justice to our treatment of the whole Earth community, not only to its human members.

■ DEVELOPMENT OF PRINCIPLED BEHAVIOR

Holistic nurses need to be aware of personal values and know how these values influence relationships with themselves, others, and the Earth community.

1. Values clarification: A process of illuminating and understanding values and beliefs that enables individuals and groups to participate in ethical decision making.

   a. Values develop over time and have cultural, familial, environmental, and educational components.

   b. Values clarification is a never-ending process in which an individual becomes increasingly aware of what is important and just—and why.

   c. Understanding and openly discussing different views in a given situation helps us to appreciate the truth inherent in the various perspectives.

   d. Values clarification within groups and organizations requires conscious identification of spoken and written (i.e., overt) values as well as those values that are unspoken or unwritten (i.e., covert) values.

   e. Patients must clarify their values to participate fully in ethical decision making. Holistic nurses can assist patients in this process in a variety of ways.

      ▪ Reflection: Listen carefully and reflect back what nurses hear patients say is personally important to them.

      ▪ Rank order: List several health behaviors or values such as happiness, good relationships with family, health, and independence, and ask patients to rank them or to identify how they incorporate them into their lives.

2. Legal aspects and holistic ethics: Healthcare providers must adhere to the law. Whatever an individual nurse's personal ethic, he or she must still adhere to the standards of practice and to the law.

   a. All nurses are responsible and accountable to comply with the Nursing Practice Act as well as the rules and regulations of the board of nurse examiners in the state where they are licensed and work.

   b. Standards of professional nursing practice require that each nurse practice to the level of his or her knowledge and skills.

   c. Holistic nurses need to be familiar with and adhere to the standards of practice for holistic nurses.[5]

■ ETHICAL DECISION MAKING

1. Frameworks for ethical decision making: To make decisions appropriately, holistic nurses need to be grounded in an understanding of the integral wholeness of all beings and do their best to articulate and examine their core values and their relationship to nursing and institutional standards. It is necessary that nurses operate from a set of principles and have facility with processes that help sort out and classify the elements of the problem.

2. The five-step ethical decision-making process of Burkhardt and Nathaniel: A framework of a decision-making process that is spiral in nature.[2] This process requires an ongoing evaluation and assimilation of information, with each step being revisited as often as is required and molded by the dynamics of changing facts, evolving beliefs, unexpected consequences, and participants who move in and out of the process.

   a. Articulate the problem: Clearly articulate and identify the problem and goal.

   b. Gather data and identify conflicting moral claims:

      ▪ Clarify the issues by gathering information that provides evidence of conflicting goals, obligations, principles, duties, rights, loyalties, values, or beliefs.

- Include information about facts as well as feelings that seem important, such as expectations, preferences, quality-of-life issues, understanding of the situation, relationships and supports, and projected outcomes of available options.
- Identify gaps in information.
- Identify key participants (which include healthcare providers), including who is affected and how; who is legitimately empowered to make the decision; issues of conflict and agreement among participants and what is most important to each; the level of competence of the person most affected; and the rights, duties, authority, and capabilities of all participants.

c. Explore strategies:
- Consider legal and other consequences to determine which alternatives best meet the identified goals and fit participant basic beliefs, lifestyles, and values.
- Review options with both head and heart, eliminate unacceptable alternatives and begin the process of listing, weighing, prioritizing, and sensing the energy of those that are considered acceptable, recognizing that there is rarely a perfect solution.
- Once an option is chosen, the decision makers must be willing to act on the choice.

d. Implement the strategy:
- This can be one of the most difficult parts of the process.
- Emotions laced with both certainty and doubt about the rightness of the decision often emerge.
- Empowering patients and families to make difficult decisions requires special attention to the emotions that often manifest at this point of the process.

e. Evaluate outcomes of action:
- Determine whether the original ethical problem has been effectively resolved and whether other problems have emerged related to the action.

- As new data emerge and the situation changes, participants might identify subsequent moral problems that require adjusting the course of action based on both new information and responses to the previous decision.

3. The four-component process of Jonsen and colleagues:[6]
   a. Medical indications:
   - The underlying ethical principles in considering medical indications are beneficence—be of benefit—and do no harm.
   - Discussion should focus on discerning the relationship among the pathophysiology and the diagnostic and therapeutic interventions (both conventional and integrative) available to remedy the patient's pathologic condition.
   - Questions regarding the overall goal of the care are important considerations in this component.

   b. Patient preferences:
   - In all interventions, the preferences of the patient are relevant.
   - Whenever possible, it is essential to ensure the patient's right to self-determination based on his or her personal values and evaluation of risks and benefits is honored.
   - It is necessary to be clear about what is realistically feasible in relation to the patient's wishes.
   - In the case of a child, nurses must ask the questions: Do the parents understand the situation? Do the parents appear to have the best interests of the child at heart? Are the parents in agreement or discord?

   c. Quality of life: This component can be a difficult part of the analysis of clinical problems, but it is indispensable.
   - The objective of healthcare interventions is to improve quality of life.
   - What does quality of life mean, in general? In particular?
   - How are others responding to their perceptions of it?
   - How do particular levels of quality impose obligations, if any, on providers?

   d. Contextual issues: Every case has a patient at its center.

- The patient exists in a social, psychological, spiritual, economic, and relational environment.
- All decisions must be considered in the light of this expanded conceptual and holistic view of personhood and personality.
- The major factors affected are psychological, emotional, financial, legal, scientific, educational, and spiritual.

e. Holistic approach: The holistic approach adds relationship questions to the four-component process of Jonsen and colleagues.[6]
- Who am I?
- What is my relationship to others and to the whole?
- What other factors are contributing to my decisions?
- Am I wise and courageous enough to perceive and respect others' differences and honor them as I would honor my own beliefs?

■ ADVANCE DIRECTIVES

1. Many ethical dilemmas arise surrounding end-of-life care options and choices. Supporting a patient's right and ability to make choices is an essential element of holistic nursing practice and holistic ethics.

   a. The Patient Self-Determination Act, effective December 1, 1991, requires that all individuals receiving medical care also receive written information about their right to accept or refuse medical or surgical treatment and their right to initiate advance directives.

   b. Advance directives are instructions that indicate healthcare interventions to initiate or withhold or that designate someone who will act as a surrogate in making such decisions in the event that decision-making capacity is lost.

   c. Advance directives support people in making decisions on their own behalf and help to ensure that patients have the kind of end-of-life care they want.

   d. Advance medical directives are of two types: treatment directives (often referred to as living wills), and appointment directives (often referred to as powers of attorney or health proxies).

- A living will specifies the medical treatment that a patient wishes to refuse in the event that he or she is terminally ill and cannot make those decisions.
- A durable power of attorney for health care appoints a proxy or surrogate, usually a relative or trusted friend, to make medical decisions on behalf of the patient if he or she can no longer make such decisions. It has broader applications than a living will and can apply to any illness or injury that causes the patient to lose decision-making capacity temporarily or long term.

   e. The authority of the surrogate is effective only for the duration of the loss of decision-making capacity.

   f. An advance directive applies only if a patient is incapacitated. It might not apply if, in the opinion of two physicians, the patient can make decisions.

   g. Individuals can cancel advance directives at any time.

   h. Individuals should give a copy of the advance directive to their family members and physician and should carry a copy if and when hospital admission is necessary.

Ethical Considerations in Practice and Research

1. Informed consent

   a. Ensures legal and ethical protection of a patient's right to personal autonomy

   b. Necessary for medical and other treatments and for participation in research studies

   c. Provides the opportunity for the patient to choose a course of action regarding plans for health care, including the right to refuse medical recommendations and to choose from available therapeutic alternatives

   d. An informed consent must include the following:
   - The nature of the health concern and prognosis if nothing is done
   - Description of all treatment options, even those that the healthcare provider does not favor or cannot provide

- The benefits, risks, and consequences of the various treatment alternatives, including nonintervention

2. Informed consent and complementary/ alternative modalities (CAM)
   a. Listing alternative treatments is one of the elements of an informed consent; nurses must consider whether it is an ethical duty for practitioners of bioscientific medicine to include discussion of CAM in discussion of therapeutic alternatives.
   b. Nurses also need to ask whether practitioners of other healing modalities should ensure that their clients are aware of biomedical alternatives.
   c. Holistic nurses who offer CAM therapies should explain the intervention and discuss risks, expected effects and benefits, and treatment options prior to initiating therapy.
   d. Because CAM therapies can affect conventional interventions in varying ways, it is important to inform other health team members of the use of these therapies.

3. Informed consent and research: Research expands the unique body of knowledge of nursing and provides an organizing framework for nursing practice.
   a. Informed consent in research refers to freely choosing to participate in a research study after the research purpose, expected commitment, risks and benefits, any invasion of privacy, and ways that anonymity and confidentiality will be addressed have been explained.
   b. The principles that underlie the ethical conduct of research include the following:
      - Respect for human dignity (i.e., the rights to full disclosure and self-determination or autonomy)
      - Beneficence (i.e., the right to protection from harm and discomfort, as in balancing between the benefits and risks of a study)
      - Justice (i.e., the rights of fair treatment and privacy, including anonymity and confidentiality)[7]
   c. Nurses who assist with research or who work on units where research is being conducted need to be familiar with elements of informed consent and be attentive to ensuring informed consent is obtained from research participants.
   d. A particular area of concern is protection of human rights in research studies focused on vulnerable populations such as children; persons with disabilities; persons who are challenged, institutionalized, or incarcerated; older adults; pregnant women; and those who are dying.
   e. Nurses who are involved in research are accountable to professional standards for reporting research findings.
   f. An important consideration in this regard is the ethical treatment of data, which demonstrates the integrity of research protocols and honesty in reporting data.

Cultural Diversity Considerations

1. Cultural values and beliefs: Cultural values and beliefs guide our way of being in the world and our reaction to life experiences in patterned ways.
   a. Patterns influenced by culture that are significant in providing holistic health care include beliefs about health and practices related to health and healing.
   b. The increasing cultural diversity in modern society can present challenges in transcultural ethical decision making for healthcare workers.
   c. Transcultural issues arise when nurses, patients, and families are guided by different moral paradigms and hold differing views of what is important or necessary regarding health, recovery, illness, or the dying process.

2. Ethical or legal dilemmas can arise from lack of understanding of language, procedures, expectations, and other elements of the culture that lead to miscommunication, unclear decisions, and a sense of powerlessness or lack of control.

3. Becoming sensitive to the culture of another is to understand one's own culture and its influence on personal perceptions and behaviors.

4. When considering definitions of health and values such as autonomy, beneficence, justice, or the right to self-determination, it is important to ask from whose perspective these values are understood—that of the nurse or that of the patient.

5. Flowing from the concept of the unity and integral wholeness of all people, holistic ethics must encompass a global perspective. This perspective includes cultural competence and cultural humility that enable the nurse to acknowledge and respect multiple ethical paradigms.

6. Broad principles and concepts that can guide holistic nursing practice and research with cultures other than one's own include:
   a. Respect for persons and for communities
   b. Honoring the unity and wholeness of all beings
   c. Beneficence
   d. Justice
   e. Respect for human rights
   f. Contextual caring
   g. Fidelity to one's professional code of ethics

■ NOTES

1. McIntyre, A. (2011). Doctrine of double effect. In E. N. Zalta (Ed.), *Stanford encyclopedia of philosophy*. Retrieved from http://plato.stanford.edu/entries/double-effect

2. Burkhardt, M. A., & Nathaniel, A. K. (2008). *Ethics and issues in contemporary nursing* (3rd ed.). Albany, NY: Delmar.

3. Sidgwick, H. (1960). *Ethics*. Boston, MA: Beacon Press.

4. American Holistic Nurses Association. (2012). *Position Statement on Holistic Nursing Ethics*. Retrieved from http://www.ahna.org/Resources/Publications/PositionStatements/tabid/1926/Default.aspx#P2

5. American Holistic Nurses Association & American Nurses Association. (2007). *Holistic nursing: Scope and standards of practice*. Silver Spring, MD: Nursebooks.org.

6. Jonsen, A. R., Siegler, M., & Winslade, W. (2010). *Clinical ethics: A practical approach to ethical decisions in clinical medicine* (7th ed.). New York, NY: McGraw-Hill/Appleton Lange.

7. U.S. Department of Health and Human Services. (n.d.). Office for Human Research Protections. Retrieved from http://www.hhs.gov/ohrp

■ STUDY QUESTIONS

Basic Level

1. Which of the following statements defines ethics?

   a. Acts reflecting values and beliefs

   b. The study or discipline concerned with judgments of approval and disapproval, right and wrong, good and bad, virtue and vice, and desirability and wisdom of actions, as well as dispositions, ends, objects, and states of affairs; disciplined reflection on the moral choices that people make

   c. Behavior that reflects personal, cultural, and political beliefs of individuals and groups

   d. A code of behaviors of a particular discipline

2. Which of the following is a difference between ethics and holistic ethics?

   a. Holistic ethics is based on a holistic ethical theory whereas ethics is not.

   b. Holistic ethics focuses on identifying the underlying ethical issues rather than application of ethical theories.

   c. Holistic ethics focuses on wholeness and the unity and integral wholeness of all people and of all nature.

   d. Holistic ethics examines free will in relation to individual behavior.

3. Which of the following best describes an ethical dilemma?

   a. A situation when there are two or more unsatisfactory answers or conflicting responses

   b. A situation when an individual's behavior is not considered to be moral

   c. A situation when only one ethical theory can be applied

   d. A situation when more than one ethical theory can be applied

4. A holistic approach to ethical problems incorporates which of the following?
   a. A single ethical theory and ethical principle that applies to the dilemma
   b. Multiple ethical theories that apply to the dilemma
   c. Thinking and feeling as credible ways of knowing for examining ethical dilemmas
   d. Cognition and spirituality as they apply to the dilemma

5. Holistic ethics is both deontologic and teleologic. Which of the following represents a teleologic perspective?
   a. A hospital offers free flu vaccines to employees and encourages all employees to receive the flu vaccine because it decreases the number of hospital-associated flu cases.
   b. A hospital mandates that all employees receive a yearly flu vaccination if they wish to continue employment even though it is known that a small percentage of the employees will suffer adverse effects of the vaccine.
   c. A hospital offers free flu vaccines to employees with the belief that everyone will be vaccinated voluntarily based on the Golden Rule.
   d. A hospital mandates that all employees receive a yearly flu vaccination if they wish to continue employment based on their moral responsibility to society.

Advanced Level

6. A holistic nurse holds a leadership position on a newly formed statewide committee that will examine the environmental impact of medical waste. At the first meeting, the nurse states, "It is important for this committee to include a statement regarding the ethical treatment of the nonhuman world and the earth itself." This statement is based on which of the following principles?
   a. Autonomy
   b. Moral uncertainty
   c. Consciousness
   d. Earth ethics

7. The parents of a young adult patient who is brain dead and on life support following a motor vehicle accident have been approached by the transplant team. The son's driver's license indicates that he is an organ donor. The father wishes to donate his son's organs, but the mother is very reluctant, stating that she does not want to "kill her son by taking him off of the breathing machine." The holistic nurse helps the family engage in values clarification by using which of the following methods?
   a. Listening to the parents, reflecting back what is being said, and helping them to rank positive and negative outcomes of the organ donation
   b. Listening to the mother and encouraging her to seek professional help with this dilemma
   c. Helping the father convince the mother that organ donation is their son's wish
   d. Listening to the mother and helping her to understand that she is not killing her son

8. The ethics committee is using Burkhardt and Nathaniel's ethical decision-making process to make a decision about a patient. The committee is exploring strategies for resolving an ethical dilemma. This step involves which of the following?
   a. Determining whether the original ethical problem has been effectively resolved and whether other problems have emerged related to the action
   b. Identifying patient preferences
   c. Considering legal and other consequences to determine which alternatives best meet the identified goals and fit participant basic beliefs, lifestyles, and values
   d. Identifying key participants (which include healthcare providers), including who is affected and how, and who is legitimately empowered to make the decision

9. A holistic nurse is planning to use thera-peutic touch as a part of a comprehensive pain management strategy for a patient with chronic lower back pain. Before implementing the therapeutic touch, the nurse should do which of the following?

    a. Give the patient literature on therapeu-tic touch to read at home when she has time to understand the effects.

    b. Use therapeutic touch informally with this patient to determine how she reacts before discussing its use with her.

    c. Inform the patient that therapeutic touch is very effective for treating pain.

    d. Discuss the risks, expected effects, and benefits of therapeutic touch prior to implementation.

10. A nurse wishes to examine the effects of foot massage on behavioral symptoms in nursing home residents with dementia. Prior to beginning the study, which of the following steps does the nurse take?

    a. Obtains informed consent from patients to determine their desire to participate in the study

    b. Obtains approval for the study from the agency and obtains informed consent from individuals who have power of at-torney or serve as a healthcare proxies for the patients

    c. Discusses the benefits of foot massage with the patients but does not mention the research study with this population because that can confound the results

    d. Skips obtaining informed consent be-cause foot massage is a nursing interven-tion that does not need prior consent

Chapter 7

Holistic Leadership

Veda Andrus and Marie Shanahan

To manage is to control; to lead is to liberate.

Harrison Owen, *The Spirit of Leadership:*
Liberating the Leader in Each of Us, p. 53

■ DEFINITIONS

Appreciative inquiry An asset-based approach based on the assumption that every organization has things that work well and these strengths can be the starting point for positive change.

Cultural change agent An individual who holds the vision for and works to actualize a plan to transform the culture of an organization to become a caring–healing environment.

Influential leadership Understanding why people are doing what they are doing and whether that behavior can be made more effective to drive performance. Three domains of influential leadership are self-awareness, collaboration, connectivity.

Intention Attention directed toward an object or idea. The energy and the spark that transform the plan to action.

Moral distress Inability to act upon ethically appropriate action and/or acting in a manner contrary to personal/professional values.

Nurse empowerment A state in which nurses assume control over their practice, enabling successful fulfillment of professional nursing responsibilities.[1]

Nurse engagement A positive state of fulfillment and dedication experienced by nurses at work. When nurses are engaged they feel energetic and dedicated to their work and become immersed in work activities.

Servant leadership A philosophy and set of practices that enrich the lives of individuals, build better organizations, and ultimately create a more just and caring world. A servant leader focuses primarily on the growth and well-being of people and the communities to which they belong. The servant leader shares power, puts the needs of others first, and helps people develop and perform as highly as possible.

Structural empowerment Solid structures and processes developed by influential leadership provide an innovative environment where strong professional practice flourishes and where the mission, vision, and values come to life to achieve the outcomes believed to be important for the organization.

Transformational leadership Style of leadership in which the individual identifies the needed change and (co)creates a clearly articulated vision to guide the change through inspiration, integrity, and mutual respect. The change is accomplished with the commitment of the members of the group and through maximizing human potential and mentorship.

Transparency An intentional, ethical choice to be clear, plain, forthright, and above board.

Visionary Having or marked by foresight and imagination.[2]

Vision statement An inspiring, compelling, clear, direct statement of intention that guides the fulfillment of the purpose of an individual or organization.

■ THEORETICAL FRAMEWORKS AND MODELS IN HOLISTIC NURSING PRACTICE

Leadership Theories

1. Leadership *theories* incorporate conceptual perspectives such as the following:
   a. Leader philosophy, values, and world-view.
   b. Leader relationships with self, others, and organization.
   c. Leader ability to facilitate group process and goal achievement.
   d. Leader (personal) traits and (professional) characteristics.
   e. Leader acquired skills, behaviors, and experience.
   f. Leader influence and ability to manifest change.
   g. Leader competencies and outcomes.
2. Integral Leadership Theory[3]
   a. Developed from Ken Wilber's *Integral Philosophy*.
   b. A framework for examining and applying several leadership perspectives through Wilber's four-quadrant model
   c. Major concepts:
      ▪ Focuses on creating communities of collective wisdom.
      ▪ Intersects multiple approaches of leadership to arrive at/derive good leadership practice.
      ▪ Increases levels of leadership awareness and influence through an integrated approach.
3. Theory U[4]
   a. Developed by Otto Scharmer.
   b. Process of leading from a vision of one's highest future possibility.
   c. Major concepts:
      ▪ Leaders are all who engage in creating change or shaping their future, regardless of position in organization.
      ▪ Requires awareness of blind spot and willingness to let go of the past.

▪ Highest future possibility exists in the future field.
▪ "Presencing" is connecting with the source of the highest possible future and bringing it into the present moment.
▪ The U: One process, five movements
▪ For more information on Theory U: http://www.ottoscharmer.com/publications/summaries.php

4. Leadership and the New Science
   a. Developed by Margaret Wheatley.
   b. Application of quantum physics principles in the practice of leadership.
   c. Major concepts:
      ▪ Organizations are self-organizing fields exhibiting complexity, chaos, and natural order.
      ▪ Chaos is necessary for change.
      ▪ Natural order is inherent in chaos and eventually emerges.
      ▪ Leaders have low reliance on task, more ability to facilitate process and participation.
      ▪ Leaders foster ownership before implementation.
      ▪ Leaders work to increase organizational flexibility and adaptability.
5. Transformational Leadership
   a. Introduced by Robert MacGregor Burns (1978) as *transforming* leadership, and later expanded as *transformational* leadership by Bernard Bass (1985).
   b. Leadership style in which leader influences followers' high performance through attention to moral ideals, respect, trust, personal motivation, and compelling vision.
   c. Major concepts:
      ▪ Intellectual stimulation: Leader respects follower's creativity and encourages new ways of doing things (challenges the status quo) and new solutions.
      ▪ Individualized consideration: Leader maintains open communication, offers support and recognition, and fosters supportive relationships with individual followers.
      ▪ Inspirational motivation: Leader articulates and models a compelling

vision that inspires followers to pas-
sionately execute the vision.
- Idealized influence: Leader acts as a
role model for followers; followers
emulate leader.
6. Servant Leadership[5]
a. Developed by Robert Greenleaf.
b. Values-based style of leadership in which
leaders must place the needs of followers,
customers, and the community ahead of
their own interests to be effective.
c. Major concepts:
- Servant leader has a natural drive to
serve first; the leader emerges as a result of that inherent desire.
- Servant leader's primary focus is on
the growth, development, and well-
being of people, leading to greater
performance.
- Shares power with others, does not
attempt to accumulate powers.
- Leader adopts Ten Principles of Servant Leadership.
- Equated with high employee satisfaction.

Leadership Models

1. Leadership *models* provide leaders with a
course of action to operationalize theoretical components.
2. Nyberg's Caring in Nursing Administration
Model
a. Developed by Jan Nyberg.
b. Model for identifying the practices,
effects, domains, and outcomes of
caring in nursing administration, demonstrated through leadership actions.
c. Major concepts: Leader actions:
- Understanding and communicating
caring as a philosophy and ethic for
the organization through process,
structure, and relationships.
- Developing skills of caring relationships and caring presence in formal
and informal relationships with individuals and groups.
- Being alert for opportunities for
modeling and articulating caring ethics with staff and colleagues.
- Providing leadership in implementing and evaluating experimental
models of caring based on theoretical-
philosophical values.

- Implementing theoretical models
of caring to critique and transform
nursing practice.
- Promoting and supporting research
on caring and healing.
- Pursuing relationships and data that
document relationship between and
among caring practice models and
nurse retention, nurse–patient satisfaction, healing outcomes, and cost.
- Becoming stewards of caring economics by incorporating caring as a
valuable economic resource and as a
foundational ethical variable in cost-
benefit ratios.
- Experimenting with new demonstration projects that showcase models
of caring–healing excellence, new
professional practice models.
3. Quality-Caring Model
a. Developed by Joann Duffy.
b. Integrates caring processes with quality
concepts to promote excellence in nursing practice.
c. Major concepts:
- The development of caring nurse-
patient relationships assists nurses
in anticipating needs, planning care,
and evaluating outcomes.
- Nurses form caring relationships
with patients/families and collaborative relationships with other care
team members.
- Nurse caring has been linked to improved clinical and service outcomes,
higher patient satisfaction, and cost
containment.
- Caring values, attitudes, and behaviors influence the structure, process,
and outcomes of the nurse–person
relationship, nurse–(other) care provider relationship, and nurse–organization relationship.
- Leaders must value caring relationships and create opportunities for
nurses to "be with" patient and others.
4. Renaissance Caring Model (See Figure 7-1)
a. Developed by Marie Shanahan and Veda
Andrus.
b. An integrative interdisciplinary progressive model of personal and professional transformation that promotes

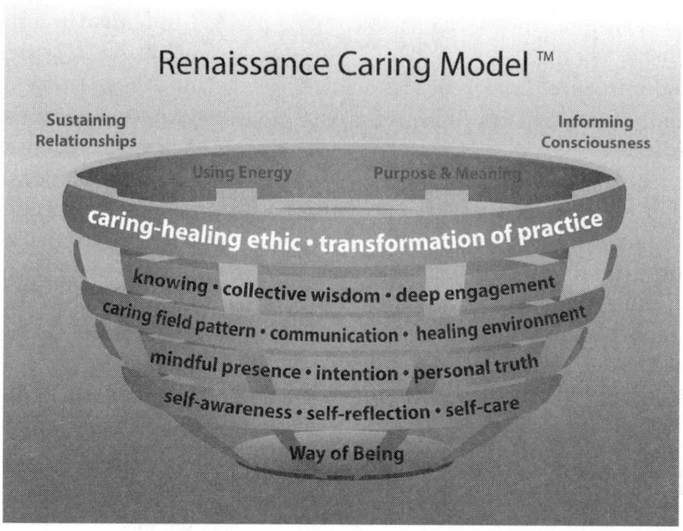

FIGURE 7–1 Renaissance Caring Model.

consistent and sustainable holistic practice in health care, supportive processes,
and stages of unfolding. Individual
builds capacity for personal transformation; organizations build capacity for
cultural transformation.

c. Major concepts:
- An individual's way of being has a direct impact on the development of a
caring–healing ethic and the transformation of practice.
- An individual's way of being is revealed and transformed through self-
awareness, self-reflection, self-care,
renewal, and restorative practices
(Self-3RRP) (*Informing Consciousness*).
- Self-3RRP builds personal field pattern for mindful presence, intentionality, and personal truth in practice
(*Using Energy*).
- Expanded personal-professional field
pattern (mindful intention) expresses
caring-collaborative communication
and generates therapeutic healing environments (*Sustaining Relationships*).
- Field pattern manifests personal
knowing, collective wisdom, and deep
engagement with self, others, practice,
and workplace (*Meaning and Purpose*).
- Development of caring–healing ethic
and transformation of practice.

5. Synergy Model for Patient Care[6]
a. Created by the American Association
of Critical-Care Nurses (AACN) in response to the need for a conceptual
framework for critical-care nurse certification that shifts the paradigm from
task and pathology orientation to person and nurse as interrelated entities.
b. Developed into a model for nursing
practice that identifies synergy as the
ideal match of nurse competencies with
patient/family needs necessary to produce optimal patient outcomes.
- Needs or characteristics of patients
and families influence and drive the
characteristics or competencies of
nurses.
- System includes:
  - Eight characteristics of patients,
  clinical units, and systems of concern to nurses.
  - Eight nurse competencies of concern for patients, clinical units,
  and systems.
- Assessment of patient needs, unit
characteristics, and nurse competencies provides nurse leaders with a
decision-making process of matching
patients to nurses.
- Links clinical practice with patient
outcomes.

▣ RESEARCH MODELS

1. Quantitative research methods
   a. Objective, systematic form of research.
   b. Reductionist approach used to measure nursing *science*.
2. Qualitative research methods
   a. Subjective form of research that describes life experiences and provides meaning.
   b. Measures both the *art and the science* of holistic inquiry.
3. Appreciative inquiry
   a. Shift from a deficit-based approach to group engagement in studying what does work and building solutions from this knowledge base—yields greater creativity.
   b. Fosters excitement, enthusiasm, and commitment in the nursing staff through inclusivity of those who might have the best insights into solutions.
   c. Enhances nurse engagement in studying what does work rather than focusing on what has not worked.
   d. Focus:
      ▪ Optimal performance.
      ▪ System strengths and resources.
      ▪ What the organization does best.
   e. Introduces opportunity for creative and innovative solutions.
   f. Is evidence-based (based on people's experiences).
   g. 5-D cycle of appreciative inquiry:
      ▪ Definition: Reframe focus of the inquiry in the affirmative and on topics valuable to the people involved.
      ▪ Discovery: A collaborative search for the best of what is that already provides optimal performance. Discovery involves meaningful conversations.
      ▪ Dream: Dialogue, reflection, envisioning. Explore what might be where people collectively explore their hopes and dreams.
      ▪ Design: Coconstruct the vision created in the dream phase into specific changes to create a preferred future.
      ▪ Destiny: Focus on personal commitments and implementation of innovation.
   h. Appreciative inquiry is a cycle: When *destiny* is implemented, the cycle starts again with *definition*.

▣ CHARACTERISTICS OF A HOLISTIC LEADER

Holistic Leader as *Visionary*

Inspired leadership is the ability to work from intention so that your very being brings forth visionary thinking in your colleagues.

Gay Hendricks and Kate Ludeman,
The Corporate Mystic

1. Visionary leaders
   a. Catalyst for innovation (thought leader), working with imagination, insight, and boldness.
   b. Care for the souls of individuals and the soul of the organization.
   c. Recognize everyone is a leader and draws forth each person's creative potential.
   d. Understand the deeper spiritual needs of people: the need for fulfillment of purpose and meaning.
   e. Call forth the best in people and brings them together around a shared sense of purpose.
   f. Work with the power of intention and alignment with a higher purpose.
   g. Architects of change (change agents), seeing the big picture, utilizing out-of-the-box thinking, bringing words into innovative strategic actions.
   h. Know how to listen and learn from other points of view and have fine-tuned communications skills.
   i. Promote a partnership approach with coparticipative strategies.
   j. Recognize the need for and actively engage in succession planning.
2. Vision statement
   a. A statement of intention cocreated by a group to serve as an energetic directive of shared purpose.
   b. Vision is a field that brings energy into form.
   c. Must be inspiring, compelling, clear, and direct.
   d. Developed through an inclusive, collaborative, and shared process.
      ▪ Creative approach must be identified and utilized to include everyone in the development process.

- Vision statement is *not* developed only by a small select group of individuals.
  e. Four steps of vision statement development:
  - Record each individual's vision for nursing practice.
  - Identify challenges or concerns with manifesting the vision.
  - Revisit visions and allow the core elements to emerge.
  - Develop the vision statement (one to four sentences in length).
  f. Broadcast/communicate the vision to create a strong field that then brings the vision into reality.
  g. Revisit the vision statement annually to ensure that it continues to align with purpose and meaning.
3. Servant leadership
  a. "The servant-leader is *servant* first... it begins with the natural feeling that one wants to serve, to serve *first*. Then conscious choice brings one to aspire to lead. That person is sharply different from one who is *leader* first."[5]
  b. Servant leader serves those who serve others.
  c. Outcome of servant leadership in nursing:
  - Improves nursing satisfaction.
  - Enhances quality of care.
  - Assists nurses in finding meaning in their work.
  - Integrates business ethics with spirituality in the workplace.
  d. Ten principles of servant leadership:[7]
  - Listening: Commitment to deep listening through the practice of full presence.
  - Empathy: Understands circumstances of others. Recognizes and accepts others for their unique contributions.
  - Healing: Healing relationships with self and others become a transformative process within an organization.
  - Awareness: Being awake to strengths and growing edges. Servant leaders have a strong sense of what is going on around them, looking for input to enhance the quality of relationships and develop meaningful solutions to challenges.
  - Persuasion: Through awareness, the servant leader coparticipates in shared decision making and is effective at building consensus within groups.
  - Conceptualization: Sees big picture and supports creative process for fulfillment while seeking a delicate balance between conceptualization and a day-to-day focus.
  - Foresight: Understands lessons from the past, present reality, and anticipates how decisions made in the present can influence the future.
  - Stewardship: Responsibility for preparing an organization to fulfill its mission and contribute to the betterment of society.
  - Growth: Servant leaders have a strong commitment to the growth of people and actively work to help them reach their true potential, as nurses and as human beings.
  - Building community: Fosters connection among the people within the organization by being inclusive rather than competitive. This is accomplished by identifying shared values and a common sense of purpose.
4. Influential leadership
  a. Understands why people are doing what they are doing and whether that behavior can be made more effective to drive performance.
  b. Three domains of influential leadership are self-awareness, collaboration, and connectivity: Self-aware, influential leaders are in a better position to collaborate and connect with others and to lead the organization to success.[8]

Holistic Leader as *Inspirational Presence*

Leaders cannot demand inspiration from others; they must create the environment that encourages such inspiration.

L. Secretan, *Inspirational Leadership: Destiny, Calling and Cause*

1. Motivates and inspires
  a. Motivation: "A means for altering the behavior of others, determined by an external force."[9p50]

b. Inspiration: "Emotions and behaviors are determined by powers from within. Inspired people arouse the hearts of others."[9p51]

2. Creates the environment to *inspire* people to be their best selves through respect, recognition, acknowledgment, and inclusion.

3. Embodies a sense of personal integrity and radiates a sense of energy and vitality.

4. Incorporates an understanding of emotional intelligence (EI):
   a. Ability to perceive and moderate own emotions and bring that awareness to others to positively influence communication and teamwork.
   b. Self-mastery (self-awareness and self-regulation) plus social intelligence (empathy and social awareness) are essential.
   c. Recognition that you have to lead yourself before you can lead others.
   d. Understands that an expression of positive energy has an affirming correlation with productivity and job performance.

5. Gathers stories as exemplars of compassionate care and professional excellence to inspire others within the organization and community.

Holistic Leader as *Role Model*

Be the change you want
to see in the world.

Gandhi

1. Core principles of a holistic leader role model:
   a. Integrity: Adheres to superior moral and ethical principles; not willing to trade integrity for personal advancement.
   b. Ethical: Models a professional code of holistic nursing ethics (caring and healing).
   c. Courageous: Stands in own truth and knowing; takes risks to advance nursing excellence.
   d. Visible-approachable-accessible: For example, presents vision statement at nursing orientation; practices unit-based and safety rounding.

2. Demonstrates a passion for nursing and a love of the profession.

3. Models respectful holistic communication style:
   a. Makes no assumptions.

b. Compassionate and sincere.
c. Nonjudgmental.
d. Inquisitive; draws information from a broad range of sources.
e. Engages in deep listening (heart-mind) through full presence.
f. Reflective and responsive, rather than reactive.
g. Models transparency through open and honest dialogue.

4. Models self-reflection and self-care
   a. Engages in self-reflective and self-care activities on a regular/consistent basis.
      - Personal: Rest/sleep, nutritious meals, movement/exercise, contemplative reflection, spiritual practice.
      - Professional: Takes lunch breaks, utilizes reflective time for decision making, and departs workplace in a timely manner at end of day.
   b. Practices grounding and centering techniques.
      - Uses breath prior to meetings, during all interactions, in transitions.
      - Practices techniques to cope with workplace stressors.
      - Practices lovingkindness toward self, others, organization, community.

Holistic Leader as *Mentor*

1. Commits to lifelong learning.
   a. Fosters commitment to professional growth and continued career advancement in nursing leadership.
   b. Strengthens competence and confidence.
   c. Enhances nurse engagement.
   d. Increases nursing satisfaction.

2. Develops a mentorship environment and culture.
   a. Identifies projects for skill development.
   b. Sponsors leadership development workshops.

3. Views mentorship as a mutually beneficial process.
   a. Mentorship is an "individualized, tailor-made, one-on-one environment for giving and receiving the gift of wisdom."[10]
   b. A shared, rather than hierarchical, process where both people learn and grow from each other's experience, insights, and wisdom.

Holistic Leader as *Champion for Clinical Excellence*

1. Promotes education and learning at every level where staff values themselves, values each other, values the patient/family, and values the organization.
2. Elevates the professionalism of the nursing staff by encouraging and supporting ongoing professional development and clinical competence through advanced degrees and certifications.
3. Promotes membership in professional organizations.
4. Participates in the National Database of Nursing Quality Indicators (NDNQI) Program of the American Nurses Association National Center for Nursing Quality.[11]
   a. Providing national comparative data to participating hospitals.
   b. Conducting research on the relationship of nursing care and patient outcomes.
5. Implements innovative care delivery models to engage nurses.
   a. Applying principles/processes of Transforming Care at the Bedside (TCAB).[12]
      ▪ Safe and reliable care.
      ▪ Vitality and teamwork.
      ▪ Patient-centered care.
      ▪ Value-added care processes.
   b. Renaissance Caring Model.
6. Utilizes research and publications for evidence-based best practices.
7. Strives for highest level of nurse recognition.

Holistic Leader as *Courageous Advocate*

1. For the *advancement of holistic nursing and the nursing profession.*
   a. Visible and vocal advocate for holistic nursing.
   b. Active in professional organizations (e.g., American Holistic Nurses Association, American Organization of Nurse Executives, Sigma Theta Tau International).
   c. Informed on healthcare policy and healthcare financing.
   d. Enhances practice through research and publication.
   e. Builds business *and* caring case for nursing.

2. For *nurses*
   a. Views caring for nurses as foundational as a holistic leader.
      ▪ Regards nurse self-care as a nursing competency.
      ▪ Endorses nurses taking their breaks.
      ▪ Supports creation of workplace renewal spaces for nurses.
      ▪ Encourages unit-based self-care activities (e.g., tea time, hand/foot massage).
   b. Promotes economic value of nurses.
   c. Upholds the four key messages of the Institute of Medicine *Future of Nursing* report:[13]
      ▪ Nurses should practice to the full extent of their education and training.
      ▪ Nurses should achieve higher levels of education and training through an improved education system that promotes seamless academic progression.
      ▪ Nurses should be full partners, with physicians and other healthcare professionals, in redesigning health care in the United States.
      ▪ Effective workforce planning and policymaking require better data collection and an improved information infrastructure.
3. For *patients*
   a. Creates an innovative culture and workplace environment that enhances the patient experience.
      ▪ Providing Relationship-Centered Holistic Care.
      ▪ Creating a healing healthcare environment (e.g., quiet time, compassionate and loving care).
      ▪ Delivering integrative therapies at the bedside (e.g., healing touch, aromatherapy, reflexology).
   b. Upholds a culture of safety and nursing competence.
   c. Strives for excellent patient perception/satisfaction scores on the Hospital Consumer Assessment of Healthcare Providers and Systems (HCAHPS) survey.
4. For *community* (local, regional, national, international).
   a. Builds collaborative relationships/partnerships with community organizations.

b. Networks with other organizational leaders to promote community-based health and wellness educational programs.

c. Is an articulate and influential nurse-spokesperson on social issues (e.g., gun violence, domestic violence).

5. For the *Earth*
    a. Fosters environmental education and resources for nurses.
    b. Encourages awareness regarding environmental factors (e.g., noise, lights, use of toxic cleaning materials).
    c. Implements organizational programs for the care of the Earth (e.g., recycling programs, double-sided copying set as default in printers).

Holistic Leader as *Cultural Transformational Agent*

Moving from a "chain of command" to a "web of influence."

Andrus, V. (2011). *Transformational Leadership for Organizational Change.* The Integrative Healing Arts Program Training Manual: Session One. Florence, MA: BirchTree Center Press. p. 55.

1. Facilitates people becoming their best selves through (co)creating an inspiring and engaging work environment that:
    a. Supports genuine human fulfillment.
    b. Provides purpose and meaning.
    c. Nurtures creative use of self.
2. Cultivates a *therapeutic healing environment* for nurses and patients.
    a. Builds a learning community where everyone is viewed as a teacher/learner.
    b. Fosters healthy relationships.
    c. Creates avenues and opportunities for *nurse empowerment.*
        ▪ Shifts language from *follower* to *partner.*
        ▪ Promotes mutual respect, empathy, and dignity.
        ▪ Engages nurses in shared governance.
    d. Upholds a culture of safety.
        ▪ Reduces interruptions and noisy, distracting work environments.
3. Develops an organizational culture that supports *nurse engagement.*
    a. Works to close the engagement gap through:

▪ Catalyzing a passion for nursing.
▪ Being an advocate for nurses.
▪ Encouraging autonomy.
▪ Promoting participatory management by fostering a culture of shared decision making.
▪ Supporting professional growth.
▪ Encouraging involvement in professional associations.
▪ Recognizing nurses for providing excellent care.
    b. Proactively resolves performance issues.
4. Provides *structural empowerment*
    a. Creates an infrastructure for an innovative, collaborative practice environment.[14]
        ▪ Organizational structure.
        ▪ Personnel policies and programs.
        ▪ Image of nursing.
        ▪ Professional development.
5. Encourages/supports policy and procedure development for clinical use of integrative modalities.
6. Endorses evidence-based best practices.
7. Promotes *moral courage* within the work environment.
    a. Recognizes the complexity of the healthcare environment and its relationship with potential moral and ethical conflicts.
    b. Creates a culture that supports acts of moral courage in nursing practice.
    c. Utilizes the *AACN 4As to Rise Above Moral Distress:*[15]
        ▪ Ask, affirm, assess, act.
    d. Anticipates potential moral residue from unresolved moral distress and is proactive in interrupting the repetitive cycle leading to moral residue.
8. Endorses *just* culture[16]
    a. Creates an environment of disclosure and transparency that promotes blame-free error reporting.
    b. Views errors as educational opportunities for improvement and learning.
9. Upholds *zero tolerance* policy[17]
    a. Zero tolerance policy: Opposed to intimidating and disruptive behaviors that undermine a culture of safety.
    b. Develops appropriate avenues for addressing and reporting disruptive behaviors in the workplace.

■ HOLISTIC NURSING PROCESS

Holistic Assessment

1. Engage in collaborative assessment with colleagues.
   a. Role model inclusivity.
   b. Cocreate empowering community.
   c. Inspire colleagues to view challenge as an opportunity for change.
      ▪ Set intention together.
   d. Explore meaning and purpose—why is this challenge occurring now?
   e. Gather information—look at the integral picture.
2. Apply *definition* step of 5-D cycle of *appreciative inquiry*.
   a. Frame challenge in the affirmative.
3. Align with care model and theory to provide framework for assessing challenge.
4. Assess elements of structural empowerment.
   a. Review policies, programs, organizational structure.

Identification of Patterns/ Challenges/Needs

1. Apply *discovery* step of 5-D cycle of *appreciative inquiry*.
   a. Collaborative search for what already provides optimal performance.
   b. Look for strengths.
2. Identify resources (people, services, technology).
3. Listen to experience, contribution, and insight from each person.

Outcome Identification

1. Apply *dream* step of 5-D cycle of *appreciative inquiry*.
   a. Reflection, dialogue, envisioning.
   b. *Responsive* rather than *reactive*.
2. Utilize out-of-the-box creative and critical thinking.
3. Compare to NDNQI.
   a. Gain information from national comparative data of participating hospitals.
4. Implement evidence-based best practices.
5. Coparticipate in shared decision making.

Therapeutic Care Plan

1. Apply *design* step of 5-D cycle of *appreciative inquiry*.
   a. Coconstruct specific changes to create a preferred future.
2. Partnership approach with coparticipative strategies.
3. Present to Professional Holistic Nurse Practice Council for insight and feedback.
4. Align with nursing vision statement.

Implementation

1. Apply *destiny* step of 5-D cycle of *appreciative inquiry*.
   a. Implementation of innovation.
2. Implement with enthusiasm, confidence, and commitment.

Evaluation

1. Reflect on process, remaining open to revision as needed.
2. Celebrate process and outcome.
   a. Recognize each person for their valuable contribution.
3. Include as exemplar in mentorship program.
4. Consider possibility for research and publication.
5. Apply *definition* step of 5-D cycle of *appreciative inquiry*.
   a. Begin cycle again....

■ NURSING INTERVENTIONS

1. Vision statement development.
2. Identifies and shares best practices.
3. Participates in and facilitates shared governance model.
   a. Professional Holistic Nurse Practice Council.
4. Institutes holistic practitioner position.
5. Establishes mentorship programs.
6. Participates in leadership development programs—institutes/academies.

■ NOTES

1. Rao, A. (2012). The contemporary construction of nurse empowerment. *Journal of Nursing Scholarship, 44*(4), 396–402.
2. Free Dictionary. (n.d.). Visionary. Retrieved from http://www.thefreedictionary.com/visionary
3. Reams, J. (2005). What's integral about leadership? A reflection on leadership and integral theory. Retrieved from http://integral-review.org/documents/Whats%20Integral%20About%20Leadership%201,%202005.pdf
4. Scharmer, O. C. (2009). *Theory U: Leading from the future as it emerges*. San Francisco, CA: Berrett-Koehler.

5. Accessed December 20, 2012. https://www .greenleaf.org/what-is-servant-leadership/

6. American Association of Critical-Care Nurses. (2013). Assumptions guiding the AACN synergy model for patient care. Retrieved from http ://www.aacn.org/wd/certifications/content /synmodel.pcms?menu=#Assumptions.

7. Neill, M., & Saunders, N. (2008). Servant leadership: Enhancing quality care and staff satisfaction. *JONA, 28*(9), 395–400.

8. Accessed December 22, 2012. http://nebraska ruralhealth.org/wp-content/uploads/2011/05 /Frisina.pdf

9. Secretan, L. (1999). *Inspirational leadership: Destiny, calling and cause.* Toronto, Ontario: MacMillan Canada.

10. Huang, C. A., & Lynch, J. (1999). *Tao mentoring.* New York, NY: Marlowe and Company.

11. National Database of Nursing Quality Indicators. (n.d.). About us. Retrieved from https://www .nursingquality.org/discover.aspx

12. Institute for Healthcare Improvement. (2013). Transforming care at the bedside. Retrieved from http://www.ihi.org/offerings/initiatives/past strategicinitiatives/tcab/pages/default.aspx

13. Institute of Medicine. (2010, October). *The future of nursing: Leading change, advancing health.* Washington, DC: Author. Retrieved from http://www.iom.edu/~/media/Files/Report%20 Files/2010/The-Future-of-Nursing/Future%20 of%20Nursing%202010%20Report%20Brief.pdf

14. American Nurses Credentialing Center. (2013). Magnet Recognition Program model: Structural empowerment. Retrieved from http://www.nurse credentialing.org/Magnet/ProgramOverview /New-Magnet-Model#StructuralEmpowerment

15. Retrieved from http://www.aacn.org/WD/Practice /Docs/4As_to_Rise_Above_Moral_Distress.pdf

16. Accessed December 24, 2012. http://www .americannursetoday.com/article.aspx?id=8242 &fid=8172

17. The Joint Commission, 2009. Accessed December 27, 2012. http://www.jointcommission.org /assets/1/18/SEA_40.PDF

■ STUDY QUESTIONS

Basic

1. When in non-emergency chaos, a holistic leader:
   a. Rushes in to fix the problem
   b. Steps back to see the big picture
   c. Tells staff what the solution is so they can solve the problem themselves
   d. Initiates a Quality Improvement process

2. Building a healthy work environment for nurses leads to:
   a. Higher staff job satisfaction
   b. Lower turnover and vacancy rates
   c. Increased patient safety
   d. Improved quality of care
   e. All of the above

3. Visionary nurse leaders:
   a. Facilitate the potential of those they lead to become future managers
   b. Unite people around a shared sense of purpose
   c. Listen carefully to all points of view before deciding what is best for a group
   d. Respect timeframes when conducting staff meetings

4. As a new unit manager, Amy is attempting to learn many new things to feel competent in her role. After a stressful staff meeting to introduce a new staffing model the hospital will be adopting, she realizes the nursing staff is divided on their opinions about the new model. Amy knows this may affect the successful implementation of the model. Should she:
   a. Poll the staff to determine how many nurses support the new model
   b. Avoid controversial topics in future staff meetings
   c. Appoint a committee to decide how to implement the model
   d. Seek support and guidance from her mentor to strengthen her skills as a holistic leader

5. Gerard leads the Professional Practice Council in his rural acute care hospital. The nurses in the Critical Care Unit want to integrate aromatherapy into clinical practice. They have proposed the use of Lavender Angustifolia to promote relaxation for patients in the unit. Gerard is reviewing their proposal and is pleased to see they have included all but **one** of the following steps:
   a. Reviewing the literature on the use of aromatherapy with critically ill patients
   b. Creating a committee to research and recommend best practices
   c. Requiring all critical care nurses implement the practice after attendance at an

in-service on the use of aromatherapy in critical care settings

d. Evaluating the results of a two week clinical trial

Advanced

6. Kim submits data to the National Database of Nurse Quality Indicators from her organization. She has been following the results of a 6 month course for nurse interns that includes self-care instruction and has noted positive outcomes. When presenting this data to the nurse executive team at her hospital she references this theoretical framework
   a. Synergy Model for Patient Care
   b. Duffy's Quality-Caring Model
   c. Relationship Based Care Model
   d. Health Belief Model

7. Maryann believes she is a visionary holistic leader and has been evaluating her resume in preparation for submission to a search team seeking a new Chief Nursing Officer. She believes it is important for the search team to know her philosophy of leadership in her cover letter. Which statement best conveys that philosophy:
   a. I believe nurse satisfaction is the key to patient satisfaction.
   b. I believe holistic nurses should always place patient's needs first.
   c. I believe families should be included in the patient care plan to facilitate the patient's highest level of healing.
   d. I believe every nurse is a leader and it is my role to draw forth their potential.

8. Vickie leads an 8 person staff development department that is training nurses to use the Renaissance Caring Model in practice. Her educators are busy developing curriculum for the training program. They are also incorporating the model into their Magnet application. She reviews their final draft of the curriculum. Which of the following statements is NOT congruent with the Renaissance Care Model?
   a. Patients are biological, psychological, social and spiritual entities who present at a particular developmental stage.

   b. It is an integrative, interdisciplinary progressive model of personal and professional transformation.
   c. An individual's way of being is transformed through self-awareness, self-reflection and self-care.
   d. As the person relates purpose and meaning to their work their field pattern manifests deep engagement with self, others and the workplace.

9. Gayle is known as a thoughtful, innovative leader who models holistic leadership. Recently she was asked to lead a task force to discover why a particular unit was having trouble adopting the use of the Rapid Response Teams. She gathered nurses in small groups to hear their concerns. While listening to them list several issues she realized they had developed workarounds rather than confront the central issues. After analyzing the issues Gayle called the small groups together again and asked them to identify what was working well on their teams. Once they identified their strong points and their success, she asked them how they might build on those areas. Quickly this generated several excellent solutions from the groups. Gayle method of working with the nursing staff employed the principles of:
   a. The 8 Competencies of the Synergy Model of Patient Care
   b. The 10 Clinical Caritas
   c. The 5-D Cycle of Appreciative Inquiry
   d. The Four Stages of Group Dynamics

10. Mary has had a passion for holistic nursing since the start of her career. She has been instrumental in developing holistic nursing in her oncology unit. Now she has the opportunity to spearhead holistic nurse certification at her organization. Which of the following actions will assist Mary in realizing her goal:
    a. Starting a study group for nurses interested in board certification.
    b. Becoming active in the American Holistic Nurses Association.
    c. Encouraging evidence-based introduction of modalities at her facility
    d. All of the above

Chapter 8

The Holistic Caring Process

Pamela J. Potter and Noreen Cavan Frisch

■ DEFINITIONS

Electronic health record (EHR) A patient care record in digital format.

Holistic caring process (HCP) A circular process that involves six steps that may occur simultaneously. These steps are assessment, patterns/challenges/needs, outcomes, therapeutic care plan, implementation, and evaluation.

Holistic nursing All nursing practice that has healing the whole person as its goal.

Intuition The perceived knowing of things and events without the conscious use of rational processes; using all of the senses to receive information.

NANDA-I diagnosis A multiaxial classification schema for the organization of nursing diagnoses based on functional domains and classes.[1]

Nursing diagnosis (NDx) "A clinical judgment about the individual, family, or community responses to actual and potential health problems or life processes. A nursing diagnosis is the basis for the selection of nursing interventions to achieve outcomes for which the nurse is accountable."[2p332]

Nursing Interventions Classification (NIC) A standardized comprehensive classification or taxonomy of treatments that nurses perform, including both independent and collaborative, as well as direct and indirect.[3]

Nursing Outcomes Classification (NOC) A standardized comprehensive taxonomy of frequently identified Goals: measurable responses to nursing interventions.[4]

Nursing process The original model describing the "work" of nursing, defined as steps used to fulfill the purposes of nursing, such as assessment, diagnosis, client outcomes, plans, intervention, and evaluation.

Paradigm A model for conceptualizing information.

Patterns/challenges/needs A person's actual and potential life processes related to health, wellness, disease, or illness, which might or might not facilitate well-being.

Perso An individual, client, patient, family member, support person, or community member who has the opportunity to engage in interaction with a holistic nurse.

Standards of practice A group of statements describing the expected level of care by a holistic nurse.

Taxonomy of nursing practice (NDx/NIC/NOC [NNN]) An atheoretical taxonomic framework that describes nursing practice by linking nursing diagnoses with nursing interventions and nursing outcomes.[1]

■ THEORY AND RESEARCH

The Holistic Caring Process (HCP)

1. Focused on establishing health and well-being, the HCP is a framework for organizing and documenting care and gives nurses the means to reflect on the entire range of nursing activities taking place within the nurse–person relationship.

2. These activities are traditionally described as the following steps: (1) assessment; (2) diagnosis, or identification of problems or needs, or pattern recognition; (3) plan of care; (4) implementation or intervention; and (5) evaluation.

3. The original concept of nursing process can be traced to the late 1950s and early 1960s when nurses in the United States sought to identify what they did as a distinct, autonomous profession within health care. In 1957, Kreuter first identified the nursing process formally as a conceptualization of an orderly approach used to conduct nursing activities.[5]

4. There have been two definitions of the nursing process: one a linear process for solving problems, and the other a circular process for describing our understanding of our encounters with clients.[6]
   a. The linear process is a step-by-step depiction of nursing work and mirrors scientific problem solving, depicting nursing as if one step is always carried out before the next.
   b. First articulated by Erikson and colleagues[7] related to the subjective experience of "being a nurse," the circular nursing process approaches nursing activities with a full understanding that every step of the process can be happening all at once and that the nurse might be addressing multiple client needs simultaneously.

5. The process is atheoretical and compatible with a variety of philosophical positions.
   a. The process has been criticized as reductionistic, steeped in positivism, emphasizing science and objectivity as the only source of knowing.
   b. Some, concerned with the use of labels and jargon, believe the nursing process serves nursing profession interests over client interests.
   c. The problem might lie, not in the process, rather in the differing philosophical perspectives used to describe it.

6. Pattern appraisal and pattern recognition are central to the nursing process. Using nursing knowledge, nurses do the following:
   a. Apply the patterns they observe to known patterns
   b. Make decisions about those patterns

   c. Act upon those decisions
   d. Then reappraise and react based on the response of the person

7. Culturally shaped, the nursing process is inseparable from the culture in which it is practiced.
   a. Engebretson and Littleton describe the nursing process from an ecological perspective as the cultural negotiation of cultural and formal knowledge, experience, and unique individual factors that both client and nurse bring to the interaction.[8]
   b. The nurse and the person enter into mutual partnership wherein they
      - Exchange expert knowledge
      - Collaborate on the analysis and interpretation of information
      - Engage in joint decision making
      - Implement mutually derived plans for action
      - Undertake an analytical appraisal of both process and expected outcomes
   c. Holistic nurses balance formal knowledge and expertise gained from nursing education and practice with philosophies of health that might not yet be fully embraced by mainstream culture (e.g., nursing defined as the "practice of presence" within the nurse–person relationship rather than the more predominant definition of nursing as "activities carried out by the nurse on behalf of the patient").

Reflective Practice

1. The HCP process is experienced within reflective practice.
2. Insights derived from the four patterns of knowing identified by Carper guide the nurse's process within the nurse–person interaction.[9]
   a. Empirical or scientific knowledge is based on objective information measurable by the senses and by scientific instrumentation.
   b. Ethical knowledge flows from the "basic underlying concept of the unity and integral wholeness of all people and of all nature."[10]
   c. Aesthetic knowledge draws on a sense of form and structure and of beauty and creativity for discerning pattern and change.

d. Personal knowledge incorporates the nurse's self-awareness and knowledge (emotional intelligence), as well as the intuitive perception of meanings based on personal experiences, and is demonstrated by the therapeutic use of self.

3. Within Johns's model of reflective practice, structured reflection providing a set of questions challenges the nurse's unexamined norms and habitual practices, allows for interpreting the nurse's subjective experience, and facilitates projection of the effects of nursing actions on the observed outcomes.[11]

4. The first author adapted Johns's questions to a reflective assignment for master's-level nursing students contemplating opportunities for implementing holistic complementary healing modalities:[12]
   a. Focus on a description of an experience that seems significant in some way. (Aesthetics)
   b. How was I feeling, and what made me feel that way? (Personal)
   c. What were the consequences of my actions on the patient, others, and myself? (Aesthetics)
   d. What knowledge did or might have informed me? (Empirics) (Cite literature)
   e. To what extent did I act for the best and in tune with my values? (Ethics)
   f. What would be the consequences of alternative actions for the patient, others, and myself? (Reflexivity)
   g. What factors might constrain me from responding in new ways? (Personal)
   h. What insights have I gained from this reflection? (Reflexivity)

Intuitive Thinking

1. The HCP involves collection and evaluation of data from both a rational, analytic, and verbal (or left brain) mode and an intuitive, nonverbal (right brain) mode.

2. Intuitive perception, sometimes described as a "gut feeling", allows one to know something immediately without consciously using reason.

3. Clinical intuition has been described as a "process by which we know something about a client that cannot be verbalized or is verbalized poorly or for which the source of the knowledge cannot be determined."[13p52]

4. Intuition, characterized by Effken as direct perception, occurs when the holistic nurse perceives in the environment higher-order variables that call for action.[14,15]

5. Expert nurses, like "smart devices," sensitive to and capable of acting immediately upon higher-order information, directly apprehend environmental information as a whole—as a complex or composite variable.

Emotional Intelligence

1. Emotional intelligence, informing the gut feeling dimension of intuition, facilitates interpretation of the nurse's perceptions[16,17]

2. McQueen describes emotional intelligence in nursing work as the assessment, expression, control, and use of emotions within the nursing intervention.[18]

3. Established on Goleman's[19] theoretical framework, Robertson[16] identifies four building blocks for cultivating emotional intelligence within the healthcare setting.
   a. Internal domains (intrapersonal)
      - Self-awareness, the ability to recognize one's emotional response pattern to specific people and situations, is demonstrated through recognizing one's own emotions and their communication (facial expression, body language, word choice, and voice tone) to create congruence between intention and message sent.
      - Self-management, the ability to modulate one's emotional response, draws from emotional awareness to manage how those emotions are expressed. This response might be expressed through *surface acting*, in which the nurse changes the outward expression to display feelings appropriate to the situation, or through *deep acting*, in which the nurse changes the deeper feelings to those appropriate to the situation.[18] The purpose is to create safety for focusing on client-centered feelings and concerns.
   b. External domains (interpersonal)
      - Social awareness demonstrates the ability to accurately perceive and

understand another's emotions even if they are expressed through a different cultural lens.

- Relationship management consciously accesses self-awareness, self-management, and social awareness to support relationship enhancement and to avoid relationship-ending confrontations.

4. Therapeutic use of self through the holistic caring process requires emotional intelligence.
5. By distinguishing empathic concern from emotional contagion, nurses adopt emotionally intelligent strategies within the holistic caring process to support healing rather than enable stagnation.

Applying Holistic Nursing Theory

1. Holistic nurses select a theoretical framework compatible with holism to guide their practice when they enact the nursing process.
2. The theory the nurse uses to guide practice is identifiable within the application of the nursing process.
3. Adaptation and expansion of the nursing process based on holistic nursing philosophy includes the person as a mutual participant in nursing care, emphasizing that the person is primary.
4. The HCP incorporates both the problem-solving components of natural science methodology and the often immeasurable caring dimension of the human science approach.[20]
5. Patterns, desired outcomes, and nursing actions are identified through a synthesis of the theory base and information gathered from the person in mutual process with the nurse.
6. Care is evaluated and documented in the language of the theory.

Taxonomies and Classifications of Nursing Practice

1. Standardization of language about nurses' activities and responsibilities affords a unified structure for the application of nursing theory and subsequent nursing research.
2. As early as the 1970s, in efforts to acknowledge nursing as a distinct, autonomous

healthcare profession nurses began developing standardized languages that would provide a way to name, label, and track those parts of nursing's work that nurses were licensed to perform.

3. The most well known of the nursing diagnoses taxonomies are these:
   a. Nursing diagnoses (NDx) delineated by the NANDA International (NANDA-I). These diagnoses name and define patterns frequently appraised by nurses as indicating a need for care.[1]
   b. Nursing Interventions Classification (NIC) is a list of activities performed by nurses for the purpose of achieving nurse–person care goals.[3]
   c. Frequently identified goals, observable and measurable throughout the course of care, are listed as the Nursing Outcomes Classification (NOC).[4]
4. Because the NDx/NIC/NOC (NNN) taxonomies are atheoretical, they can be used with a variety of nursing theories and a holistic perspective.[21]
5. Use of standardized terms also permits documentation and retrieval of nursing information in an electronic health record (EHR).
6. There is opportunity to increase our visibility and to document the positive outcomes of the assessments and interventions we carry out daily if we document our care in such a way that what we do becomes coded as part of the permanent record.
7. Currently, more than half of the nursing diagnoses and interventions listed in standard languages address the psycho-social-spiritual aspects of care; these certainly are of use to holistic nurses.
8. The HCP and nursing taxonomies give structure and language and serve to articulate and observe the outcomes of the nurse–person relationship.

■ HOLISTIC CARING PROCESS

1. Nurses who adhere to the HCP focus on the care of the whole unique person, respecting and advocating for the person's rights and choices.
2. Based on a holistic assessment and identification of the person's health patterns, decisions about care flow from collaboration

with the person, other healthcare providers, and significant others.

3. The person assumes an active role in healthcare planning and decision making by seeking the professional expertise of the nurse via various nurse–person interactions.
4. Facilitated by the nurse in the healing relationship, the person expresses health concerns and strengths—a unique health pattern—that the nurse identifies and documents in the healthcare record.
5. The person is encouraged to participate as actively as possible, taking responsibility for personal health choices and decisions for self-care.
6. The nurse must remember that the HCP is merely a tool, a framework for ordering, documenting, and discussing the nurse–person interactions; excessive reliance on structure and objectivity can reduce the person to a mere object.
7. The HCP is presented here as a six-step process including the following steps:
   a. Holistic assessment
   b. Identification of patterns/problems/needs
   c. Outcome identification
   d. Therapeutic plan of care
   e. Implementation
   f. Evaluation
8. The following sections describe each phase and then discuss documentation of nursing's work.

Holistic Assessment

The holistic registered nurse collects comprehensive data pertinent to the person's health or situation.[22]

1. Assessment is the information-gathering phase in which the nurse and the person identify health patterns and prioritize the person's health concerns.
2. A key to a holistic assessment is to appraise the overall pattern of the responses.
3. Interpersonal interaction reveals perceptions, feelings, and thoughts about health patterns/challenges/needs as identified by the person.
4. Nursing observation relies on information perceived by the five senses and intuition, while measurement provides quantifiable information obtained from instruments.

5. Within the cultural context of negotiation, the assessment phase might be seen as an "exchange of expert knowledge" wherein both the nurse and the person bring expertise to the exchange.[8]
6. During assessment of the person's bio-psycho-social-spiritual patterns, the holistic nurse looks for the overall pattern of interrelationships, uses appropriate scientific and intuitive approaches, assesses the state of the energy field, and identifies stages of change and readiness to learn.
7. All pertinent data are documented in the person's record. Assessment and documentation are continuous within the nurse–person interaction because changes in one pattern always influence the other dimensions.
8. A lack of awareness about one's own personal beliefs and patterns can subtly influence the nurse–client interaction (e.g., communication barriers relative to culture, class, age, gender, sexual orientation, education, or physical limitation) and impede holistic assessment.

Identification of Patterns/Challenges/Needs

The holistic registered nurse analyzes the assessment data to determine the diagnosis or issues expressed as actual or potential patterns/problems/needs that are related to health, wellness, disease, or illness.[22]

1. The nurse describes a person's patterns/challenges/needs based on a standardized language that is understandable to nurses, other healthcare professionals, the managed care provider, and the person receiving nursing care.
2. Nursing diagnoses (NDx) provide a universal descriptor language for common patterns identified by nurses giving care.
   a. There are currently more than 130 approved diagnoses organized under 13 domains:
   b. Health promotion, nutrition, elimination/exchange, activity/rest, perception/cognition, self-perception, role relationship, sexuality, coping/stress tolerance, life principles, safety/protection, comfort, and growth/development.

3. The diagnostic statement
   a. Nursing diagnoses, reflecting clinical judgment, describe human responses to health conditions and life processes in an individual, family, or community.
   b. Seven axes may be incorporated explicitly or implicitly in every nursing diagnostic statement:
      - The diagnostic concept
      - Subject of the diagnosis (individual, family, community)
      - Judgment (impaired, ineffective)
      - Location (anatomic)
      - Age (infant, child, adult)
      - Time (chronic, acute, intermittent)
      - Status of the diagnosis (actual, risk, wellness, health promotion)[1]
   c. Four types of NDx
      - Actual NDx exist as fact or reality in the present time.
      - Risk NDx describe a vulnerability occurring in response to exposure to factors that intensify the possibility of injury or loss.
      - Wellness NDx reflect the condition of health.
      - Health promotion NDx reflects the person's desire to increase well-being and actualize human potential.
   d. Before making a specific NDx, the nurse compares assessment data with the defining characteristics of the diagnosis, which are those behaviors or signs and symptoms (observable cues and inferences) that cluster together as manifestations of the diagnosis.
   e. After nursing diagnoses are identified and prioritized, they become the basis for the remaining steps of the nursing process.
   f. Sometimes, when none of the available NDx appears to fit the person's circumstances, the nurse must develop a diagnosis.
4. Nursing language across levels of prevention
   a. Nursing interventions associated with these diagnoses are actively selected to reduce or prevent the particular problem.
   b. Health maintenance focuses on sustaining a neutral state of health. (Health Maintenance NDx)
   c. Illness prevention or risk reduction involves behaviors aimed at actively protecting against or reducing the chances of encountering disease, illness, or accidents. (Risk NDx)
   d. Health promotion goes beyond illness prevention or health maintenance. (Health Seeking NDx)
      - Involves personal responsibility for health.
      - Individuals strive actively to improve their lifestyle to achieve high-level wellness.
5. Nursing diagnosis as a descriptive tool
   a. Nursing diagnoses are merely a descriptive tool for articulating patterns identified in the nurse–person relationship rather than a rigid, limiting diagnostic label that might constrict and stereotype care.
   b. The person's value system, not the nurse's, is the basis for holistic nursing decisions and diagnostic labeling.
   c. Impediments to a holistic nursing diagnosis result from neglecting to make the person the focus of the process and failing to have a continual focused awareness of the person as a whole. Fitting the pattern of a dynamic, changing human being into an arbitrary diagnostic statement rather than reflecting the actual pattern of the person limits the effectiveness of the HCP.

Outcome Identification

The holistic registered nurse identifies outcomes for a plan individualized to the person or the situation. The holistic nurse values the evolution and the process of healing as it unfolds. This implies that specific unfolding outcomes might not be evident immediately because of the nonlinear nature of the healing process so that both expected/anticipated and evolving outcomes are considered.[22]

1. An identified outcome is a direct statement of a goal to be achieved through the nurse–person relationship within a specific time frame; the person's significant others and other healthcare practitioners may participate in goal setting.
2. An outcome indicates the maximum level of wellness that is reasonably attainable

for the person in view of objective circumstances and the person's perceptions.

3. Reflecting the goals of the nurse–person intervention, outcome criteria outline the specific tools, tests, observations, or personal statements that determine whether the patient outcome has been achieved.

4. The Nursing Outcomes Classification (NOC) developed by the Iowa Outcomes Project at the University of Iowa provides a comprehensive taxonomy of 385 outcomes organized into 7 domains and 29 classes.

   a. Outcomes describe the expected effect or influence of the intervention on the person.

   b. Within this classification system a nursing-sensitive patient outcome is a measurable state, behavior, or perception that is responsive to nursing interventions.[4]

   c. Outcome measures can be used as indicators of individual change as well as for quantitative comparison with a greater population.

   d. The seven NOC domains are functional health, physiologic health, psychosocial health, health knowledge and behavior, perceived health, family health, and community health.

   e. If outcomes are to be achieved, the nurse must establish them with the assistance of the patient and family. The person must be motivated to establish healthy patterns of behavior.

   f. Assumptions made by the nurse concerning desired outcomes without collaboration with the person impede outcome achievement. Rigid adherence to specific outcomes by the person or the nurse can make it impossible to recognize the value of the journey with its myriad other paths and other possible outcomes.

   g. NOC classification provides common nursing language for communicating about the effectiveness of nursing actions, a language that can be recognized by providers, payers, and other healthcare professionals.

Therapeutic Care Plan

The holistic registered nurse develops a plan that identifies strategies and alternatives to attain outcomes.[22]

1. During the planning stage, nurses who use the HCP help the person identify ways to repattern her or his behaviors to achieve a healthier state.

2. The plan outlines nursing interventions, which are the specific actions that the nurse performs to help the person solve problems and accomplish outcomes.

3. The Nursing Interventions Classification (NIC) contains an alphabetic list of 542 interventions that provide a shorthand means of documenting the nursing actions included in the plan and carried out by the nurse.[3]

   a. Each intervention is listed with a label, a definition, a set of related activities that describe the behaviors of the nurse who implements the intervention, and a brief list of background readings.

   b. The NIC makes every attempt to include all direct care interventions, both independent and collaborative, that nurses perform for patients.

4. Holistic nurses incorporate complementary modalities into their practice as interventions for treating the body (biofeedback, therapeutic massage), relieving the mind (humor, imagery, meditation), comforting the soul (prayer), and supporting significant interpersonal interaction (healing presence).[23]

   a. Therapies such as acupressure, meditation, guided imagery, and therapeutic touch are listed as nursing interventions in the classification.

5. The organization of the holistic care plan reflects the priority of identified opportunities to enhance the person's health. Priorities for intervention are based on an assessment of the urgency of the threat to the person's life and safety.

6. The holistic nurse chooses interventions based on utility, relationship to the person's patterns/challenges/needs, effectiveness, feasibility, acceptability to the person, and nursing competency.

7. Holistic nursing interventions reflect acceptance of the person's values, beliefs, culture, religion, and socioeconomic background.

8. Any revision of the care plan reflects the person's current status or ongoing changes.

9. This plan is documented in the person's record.

Implementation

The holistic registered nurse implements the identified plan in partnership with the person.[22]

1. Nurses who are guided by a holistic framework approach the implementation phase of care with an awareness that
   a. People are active participants in their care.
   b. Nursing care must be performed with purposeful, focused intention.
   c. A person's humanness is an important factor in implementation.
2. During this phase, the various persons deemed appropriate—the nurse, the person, the family, or another person or agency—implement the planned strategies.[8]
3. Within the holistic framework, anything that produces a physiologic change causes a corresponding psychological, social, and spiritual alteration.
   a. Conversely, anything that produces a psychological change causes a corresponding physiologic, social, and spiritual alteration.
   b. The encounter changes the consciousness and the physiology of both the nurse and the person.
   c. Because human emotions can be translated into physiologic responses, the greatest tool or intervention for helping and healing clients is the therapeutic use of self.[24]

Evaluation

The holistic registered nurse evaluates progress toward attainment of outcomes while recognizing and honoring the continuing holistic nature of the healing process.[22]

1. Evaluation is a planned review during the nurse–person interaction to identify factors that facilitate or inhibit expected outcomes.
   a. Evaluation is a mutual process between the nurse and the person receiving care.
   b. Data about the client's bio-psycho-social-spiritual status and responses are collected and recorded throughout the HCP.
   c. The information is related to the person's patterns/challenges/needs, the outcome criteria, and the results of the nursing intervention.

d. The nurse, in collaboration with the person during the course of care, can use measures from the NOC to document the effectiveness of the nursing interventions received.
2. The goal of evaluation is to determine whether outcomes have been successful and, if so, to what extent.
   a. The nurse, person, family, and other members of the healthcare team all participate in the evaluation process.
   b. Together, they synthesize the data from the evaluation to identify successful repatterning behaviors toward wellness.
   c. During the evaluation, the person becomes more aware of previous patterns, develops insight into the interconnections of all dimensions of his or her life, and sees the benefits of repatterning behaviors.
3. The evaluation of outcomes must be continuous because of the dynamic nature of human beings and the frequent changes that occur during illness and health.
   a. It might be necessary to develop new outcomes and revise the plan of care.
   b. Factors facilitating effective outcomes or preventing solutions to problems must also be explored.
   c. Failure to recognize that all measurable outcomes might not be immediate, but are in a process of becoming, is an impediment to evaluation.
4. Evaluation of the HCP comes full circle with a self-aware appraisal of the entire nursing process by the nurse.
5. From an ecological perspective, the evaluation of the HCP extends beyond the level of the person to include the short- and long-term impact on the healthcare delivery system, the physical environment, and the greater social context.
   a. The holistic nurse must also reflect on the greater implications of the HCP for professional practice standards and for health and environmental policy.

■ DOCUMENTING THE HOLISTIC CARING PROCESS

1. The nursing care plan is a means to document and report nursing activities, to communicate nursing needs from one nurse

to another, and to evaluate nursing care outcomes.

2. The nursing care plan is a means to document that, based on nursing assessment data, a particular nursing concern (nursing diagnosis) was established and a plan (nursing orders) was prepared to address the concern.

3. The expected outcome should be identified in the care plan so that an evaluation of outcome is possible.

4. Of the several methods of documenting the nursing care plan, two are discussed here: the concept map (frequently used in teaching) and the electronic health record (EHR) commonly used in practice.

Concept Maps

1. A concept map is a diagrammatic representation of organized knowledge. In some regards, the concept map is an individual's interpretation of a real-life experience.[25]

2. Nurses might find that concept mapping is more closely aligned with the circular nursing process, whereas the traditional nursing care plan is aligned with the linear nursing process.

3. A concept map presents an "all at once" view of the client's experiences and draws out connections between events so that they are not seen as unrelated parts. Arrows on the map can be used to indicate that one concept influences another.

4. It is important for the holistic nurse to recognize that nursing documentation of care is an essential part of professional practice and to realize that virtually all institutions require documentation in a traditional format. However, the concept map may assist all of us to see our professional work differently, and certainly a concept map helps us to select priorities of care.

Electronic Health Records (EHRs)

1. The EHR is simply a clinical record in digital format.

2. Electronic records have several advantages over paper ones: The records are readable, data are easily accessed and retrieved, and more than one user may be looking at parts of the record simultaneously.

3. Additionally, electronic records can have features such as decision supports built in.

4. These EHRs frequently have care planning systems built in so that nurses can access an assessment form, collect and store data, and build a care plan based on those data.

5. EHRs also provide an ability for nurses to retrieve data from care plans to track progress and outcomes over time.

6. With the introduction of EHRs in practice, holistic registered nurses have an opportunity to advocate for inclusion of their complete, holistic plan of care in the permanent record system.

7. Holistic nurses need to understand that in an electronic system, only data entries that are codable by the computer system can be stored in a way that the data can be retrieved at a later date when one is conducting a chart review or audit or evaluating trends.

■ NOTES

1. NANDA International. (2009). *Nursing diagnoses: Definitions and classification, 2009–2011.* T. H. Herdman (Ed.). Oxford, England: Wiley-Blackwell.

2. NANDA International. (2007). *Nursing diagnoses: Definitions and classification, 2007–2008.* Philadelphia, PA: Nanda-I.

3. Bulechek, G. M., Butcher, H., & Dochterman, J. M. (2008). *Nursing Interventions Classification (NIC)* (5th ed.). St. Louis, MO: Mosby.

4. Moorhead, S., Johnson, M., Maas, M., & Swanson, E. (2008). *Nursing Outcomes Classification (NOC)* (4th ed.). St Louis, MO: Mosby.

5. Kreuter, F. R. (1957). What is good nursing care? *Nursing Outlook, 5,* 302–304.

6. Frisch, N. C., Frisch, L. E. (2011). *Psychiatric mental health nursing* (4th ed.). Clifton Park, NY: Delmar Cengage Learning.

7. Erickson, H. C., Tomlin, E. M., & Swain, M. A. P. (1983). *Modeling and role-modeling: A theory and paradigm for nursing.* Englewood Cliffs, NJ: Prentice Hall.

8. Engebretson, J., & Littleton, L. Y. (2001). Cultural negotiation: A constructivist-based model for nursing practice. *Nursing Outlook, 49,* 223–230.

9. Carper, B. A. (1978). Fundamental patterns of knowing in nursing. *Advances in Nursing Science, 1*(1), 13–23.

10. American Holistic Nurses Association. (2007). *Position statement on holistic nursing ethics.* Flagstaff, AZ: AHNA/ANA.

11. Johns, C. (1995). Framing learning through reflection within Carper's fundamental ways of knowing in nursing. *Journal of Advanced Nursing, 22,* 227.

12. Johns, C. (2007). *Engaging reflection in practice: A narrative approach* (15th ed.). Oxford, England: Blackwell Publishing.

13. Young, C. E. (1987). Intuition and nursing process. *Holistic Nursing Practice, 1*(3), 52.

14. Effken, J. A. (2001). Information basis for expert intuition. *Journal of Advanced Nursing, 34*(2), 246–254.

15. Effken, J. A. (2007). The informational basis for nursing intuition: Philosophical underpinnings. *Nursing Philosophy, 8,* 187–200.

16. Robertson, S. A. (2007). Got EQ? Increasing cultural and clinical competence through emotional intelligence. *Communication Disorders Quarterly, 29*(1), 14–19.

17. Smith, K. B., Profetto-McGrath, J., & Cummings, G. G. (2009). Emotional intelligence and nursing: An integrative literature review. *International Journal of Nursing Studies, 46*(12), 1624–1636.

18. McQueen, A. C. H. (2004). Emotional intelligence in nursing work. *Journal of Advanced Nursing, 47*(1), 101–108.

19. Goleman, D., McKee, A., & Boyatzis, R. (2002). *Primal leadership: Realizing the power of emotional intelligence.* Boston, MA: Harvard Business School.

20. Watson, J. (1985). *Nursing: Human science and human care.* Norwalk, CT: Appleton-Century-Crofts.

21. Frisch, N. C., & Kelley, J. H. (2002). Nursing diagnosis and nursing theory: Exploration of factors inhibiting and supporting simultaneous use. *Nursing Diagnosis, 13*(2), 53–61.

22. American Holistic Nurses Association & American Nurses Association. (2007). *Holistic nursing: Scope and standards of practice.* Silver Spring, MD: Nursebooks.org.

23. Frisch, N. C. (2001). Standards for holistic nursing practice: A way to think about our care that includes complementary and alternative modalities. *Online Journal for Issues in Nursing, 6*(2), Manuscript 4.

24. Krieger, D. (1981). *Foundation of holistic health nursing practice.* Philadelphia, PA: Lippincott.

25. Johnson, V., & Frisch, N. (2011). Tools of psychiatric mental health nursing: Communication, nursing process and the nurse–client relationship. In N. Frisch and L. Frisch (Eds.), *Psychiatric mental health nursing* (4th ed., pp. 99–112). Clifton Park, NY: Cengage Delmar Learning.

■ STUDY QUESTIONS
Basic Level

1. The circular view of the HCP differs from the step-by-step nursing process in which of the following ways?
   a. An emphasis on a thorough and comprehensive assessment
   b. The need to document care in the client record
   c. The evaluation of all of client needs and wants
   d. An understanding that the steps happened all at once

2. Which if the following statements is correct about standardized nursing terms, such as those found in the NANDA-I taxonomy or in the NIC and /NOC classifications?
   a. They severely limit nursing expression and documentation.
   b. They provide a shorthand means of documenting nursing care.
   c. They include only biomedical and physiologic conditions and terms.
   d. They cannot be used in electronic or digital systems.

3. Which of the following is true about using a concept map to document care?
   a. Concept maps permit depiction of relationships between and among ideas.
   b. Concept maps provide a way to code data for entry into an EHR or electronic care plan.
   c. Concept maps allow for retrieval and evaluation of outcome data over time.
   d. Concept maps require identification of a nursing theory for use in practice.

4. What is one reason nursing as a discipline developed standardized terms?
   a. To articulate those judgments, actions, and outcomes that were specific to nursing
   b. To lessen the amount of time nurses needed to document their care to provide more time for nurse–patient interaction
   c. To create a means for nursing to be included in EHRs
   d. To express the concepts and ideas of current nursing theories

5. Which of the following statements characterizes the relationship between nursing theory and nursing standardized languages?
   a. Nursing theory concepts are subsumed in the standardized languages.
   b. Standardized nursing language terms are subsumed in nursing theory.
   c. There is no relationship.
   d. Standardized terms are atheoretical and can be used with nursing theory.

Advanced Level

6. Nurse Sharon is giving postoperative care to her assigned patient, Margaret, who has had an appendectomy 4 hours ago. Margaret is awake and oriented, with stable vital signs. Margaret reports being thirsty and having abdominal discomfort. In enacting the HCP, what will be Sharon's first priority?
   a. Complete a holistic nursing assessment
   b. Develop a nurse–patient relationship through verbal interaction
   c. Attend to comfort measures
   d. Prepare a plan of care

7. Nurse Bob is a home care nurse visiting a new client, Joyce, and her family today. Joyce is an 80-year-old woman who fell and fractured her hip. She has been through extensive rehabilitation and is doing quite well. Bob takes a nursing history and learns that she is ambulating well with her walker and without assistance of family members. Joyce does report that she frequently is losing sleep at night because she has to get up to use the bathroom. Bob thinks this could be a fall risk. What is Bob's best next action?
   a. To write a NDX on the care plan of "Risk for fall, due to nighttime ambulation"
   b. To assess the physical environment of his patient's home
   c. To refer Joyce to the physical therapist for an evaluation of safety
   d. To talk with Joyce and her family about his concerns

8. Nurse Debra is charting her care plan for an oncology patient on an EHR. One of her diagnoses is "fatigue related to compromised physical condition and feelings of sadness." Debra would like to include more information in the record than the standardized terms. What is Debra's next best action?
   a. Write about the contextual nature of her diagnosis in a narrative note.
   b. Abandon the use of electronic documentation in favor of handwritten plans of care.
   c. Talk with the next nurse about her assessment.
   d. Prepare a concept map.

9. Marjorie is a nursing faculty member teaching students in a maternal-child health course. These students are also taking a course in philosophy and are exploring ideas and concepts. One of her students asks if nursing care planning is a paternalistic endeavor. As a holistic nurse, what is Marjorie's best response?
   a. Many patients are quite vulnerable, particularly at the time of childbirth, and need the caring, compassionate nurse to direct their care.
   b. The HCP must always be enacted in partnership with our patients.
   c. Patients all have differing perspectives and cultural backgrounds, but nursing principles for supporting healthy childbirth are standard.
   d. Patient safety and quality have priority in all nursing decisions.

10. Nurse Carol is a charge nurse at a nursing facility that provides assisted living and supportive care to elderly patients. One of the residents of the facility, Mrs. Smith, begins to ask Carol about healthy eating and nutrition. Carol willingly provides information. What else should she do?
    a. Interpret this resident's request as an opportunity to enhance health.
    b. Prepare a menu plan for Mrs. Smith, based on her food preferences.
    c. Teach Mrs. Smith about new ways of preparing food.
    d. Invite Mrs. Smith out to a luncheon.

Chapter 9

Self-Assessments

Barbara Montgomery Dossey, Susan Luck,
Bonney Gulino Schaub, and Lynn Keegan

■ DEFINITIONS

Healing A process of understanding and integrating the many aspects of self, leading to a deep connection with inner wisdom and an experience of balance and wholeness.

Healing awareness A person's conscious recognition of and focused attention on intuitions, subtle feelings, conditions, and circumstances relating to the needs of self or clients.

Health An individual's (nurse, client, family, group, or community) subjective sense of well-being, harmony, and unity that is supported by the experience of his or her health beliefs and values being honored; a process of opening and widening of awareness and consciousness.

Nurse healer A professional nurse who supports and facilitates a person's process of growth and experience of wholeness through an integration of body, mind, and spirit and/or who assists in the recovery from illness or in the transition to peaceful death.

Process The continual changing and evolution of one's self through life that includes reflecting on meaning and purpose in living.

Self-efficacy The belief that one has the capability of initiating and sustaining desired behaviors; having a sense of empowerment and ability to make healthful choices that lead to enduring change.

Transpersonal self The self that transcends personal, individual identity and meaning and opens to connecting with purpose, meaning, values, unitive experiences and with universal principles.

Transpersonal view The state that occurs during a person's life maturity whereby a sense of self expands.

Wellness An integrated, congruent functioning toward reaching one's highest potential.

■ HOLISTIC NURSES, HEALTHY PEOPLE, AND A HEALTHY WORLD

Holistic Nurses as Change Agents for Health and Well-Being

1. Holistic nurses are practicing at the forefront as change agents to increase the health of the nation and the world, focusing on addressing the wellness and "health span" of people.
2. Holistic nurse endeavors include using health and wellness assessments, assessing readiness to change, and implementing action plans for healthy lifestyle behaviors and approaches that lead to healthy people living in a healthy nation and on a healthy planet by 2020.
3. An urgent need exists for initiatives to help shift the focus of health care by promoting self-efficacy and empowering individuals to recognize their potential to engage in promoting their own health and well-being.
4. The Institute of Medicine, in collaboration with Robert Wood Johnson Foundation (RWJF), published the *Future of Nursing*

report in 2010, a landmark document that presents four key messages:[1]

a. Nurses should practice to the full extent of their education and training.

b. Nurses should achieve higher levels of education and training through an improved education system that promotes seamless academic progression.

c. Nurses should be full partners, with physicians and other healthcare professionals, in redesigning health care in the United States.

d. Effective workforce planning and policymaking require better data collection and information infrastructure.

Reversing Chronic Disease

1. The Centers for Disease Control and Prevention state that more than 133 million adults, or nearly half of all adults in the United States, are living with at least one chronic disease such as obesity, diabetes, and cardiovascular disease.[2] The cost of managing their care is an astounding $270 billion a year.[3] Seventy percent of today's healthcare costs are related to preventable, lifestyle-related diseases.

2. All diseases affect multiple systems of the body with heart disease and stroke as the first and third causes of mortality, respectively, accounting for one-third of all deaths in the United States.[4] Cardiovascular problems include hypertension, dyslipidemia, heart failure, congenital heart disease, peripheral vascular disease, and peripheral arterial disease. If every form of cardiovascular disease was eliminated, Americans could add another 7 years to their life expectancy.[5]

3. Risk factors that can be modified in cardiovascular disease include smoking, dyslipidemia, hypertension, physical inactivity, obesity, and diabetes. Although gender, age, and genetics are not modifiable, many lifestyle factors can be altered.

4. If the current obesity epidemic continues unchecked, 50% of the U.S. adult population will be obese, with body mass index values of 30 or higher, by 2030.[6] Based on a simulation model and data from the National Health and Nutrition Examination Survey (NHANES) series from 1988 to 2008, it has been projected that, compared with 2010, there will be "as many as 65 million more obese adults" in the United States by that year. Obesity prevalence in both men and women in their 40s and 50s would approach 60%. Using this simulation modeling based on current obesity trends in the United States and United Kingdom, investigators estimate that up to 8.5 million additional cases of diabetes, 7.3 million more cases of cardiovascular disease and stroke, and 0.5 million more cancers will occur by 2030, with major increases in healthcare costs.

Healthcare Transformation

1. In the United States, the *Healthy People 2020* initiative continues the work started in 2000 with the *Healthy People 2010* initiative for improving the nation's health. *Healthy People 2020* is the result of a multiyear process that reflects input from a diverse group of individuals and organizations.[7]

2. The leading health indicators are increased physical activity; reduced obesity, tobacco use, substance abuse, injury, and violence; increased responsible sexual behavior; improved mental health, environmental quality, immunizations, and access to health care. These health indicators were selected on the basis of their ability to motivate action, the availability of data to measure progress, and their importance as public health issues.

3. The *Healthy People 2010* vision, mission, and overarching goals provide structure and guidance for achieving the *Healthy People 2020* objectives. Although general in nature, they offer specific, important areas of emphasis where action must be taken if the United States is to achieve better health by the year 2020.

4. The *Healthy People 2020* mission strives to accomplish the following:

a. Identify nationwide health improvement priorities.

b. Increase public awareness and understanding of the determinants of health, disease, and disability and the opportunities for progress.

c. Provide measurable objectives and goals that are applicable at the national, state, and local levels.

d. Engage multiple sectors to take actions to strengthen policies and improve practices that are driven by the best available evidence and knowledge.

e. Identify critical research, evaluation, and data collection needs.

5. The *Healthy People 2020* overall goals are the following:

a. Attain high-quality, longer lives free of preventable disease, disability, injury, and premature death.

b. Achieve health equity, eliminate disparities, and improve the health of all groups.

c. Create social and physical environments that promote good health for all.

d. Promote quality of life, healthy development, and healthy behaviors across all life stages.

6. Other important endeavors toward national health are the Patient Protection and Affordable Care Act[8] and the National Prevention Strategy.[9] The following sections address the use of the Integrative Health and Wellness Assessment (IHWA) in coaching clients to be active participants in increasing health-promoting behaviors, assessing readiness to change, and establishing action plans and goals.

Holistic Nurse Coaches in Healthcare Transformation

1. Holistic nurses are participating as health and wellness coaches and integrating whole-person principles and modalities that integrate body-mind-emotion-spirit-culture-environment. (See Chapter 9 in the sixth edition of the *Holistic Nursing Handbook*.) This perspective emerges from an awareness that effective change evolves from within before it can be manifested and maintained externally.[10,11]

2. Holistic nurse coaching is a skilled, purposeful, results-oriented, and structured relationship-centered interaction with clients provided by registered nurses for the purpose of promoting achievement of client goals.[10,11]

▌INTEGRATIVE HEALTH AND WELLNESS ASSESSMENT (IHWA)

1. Holistic nurses use self-assessments and other strategies to assist individuals to learn how to prefer wellness to unhealthy habits.

2. The Integrative Health and Wellness Assessment (IHWA) Wheel has eight components:

a. Life Balance and Satisfaction

b. Relationships

c. Spirituality

d. Mental

e. Emotional

f. Physical (Nutrition, Exercise, Weight Management)

g. Environmental

h. Health Responsibility[12]

3. After the assessment for each section the holistic nurse can coach clients as well as self to identify readiness for change, priority for change, and confidence to make change and design an action to move toward desired goals and new health behaviors.

Life Balance and Satisfaction

1. Assessing our strengthens, capacities, and human potentials can attune us to our healing awareness and to recognize our feelings, attitudes, and emotions, which are not isolated but are literally translated into body changes.

2. Assessing our life balance and satisfaction acknowledges our capacity for both conscious and unconscious choices.

3. Conscious choices involve awareness and skills such as self-reflection, self-care, discipline, persistence, goal setting, priority setting, action steps, discerning best options, and acknowledging and trusting perceptions. Unconscious choices are those of which we are not aware. They stay hidden or denied unless uncovered through self-assessment, reflection, and action plans.

Relationships

1. Understanding and nurturing our relationships assists us in creating and sustaining meaningful relationships: immediate family, extended family, colleagues at work, neighbors in the community, numerous people in organizations, and now the

ever-expanding web of electronic connection with friends, colleagues, and others around the world.

2. Relationships have different levels of meaning, from the superficial to the deeply connected. We need to recognize what we personally are hoping for and what we are bringing to the variety of relationships we engage in. How do we discern and decide when we feel willing to exchange feelings of honesty, trust, intimacy, compassion, openness, and harmony?

3. Sharing life processes requires truthful and caring self-reflection, and meaningful conversations require deep, personal contemplation about what is desired and hoped for.

4. We must extend our networks to include our immediate environment and consider that what we do locally has an impact on our larger community—the nation and planet Earth.

Spiritual

1. Assessing aspects of our spiritual nature can be a vital element and driving force in how we live our lives.

2. Spirituality is considered to involve a sense of connection with an absolute, imminent, or transcendent spiritual force, however named. It includes conviction, ethical values, direction, meaning, and purpose, all valid aspects of the individual and universe.

3. This interconnectedness with self, others, nature, and God/Life Force/Absolute/ Transcendent is not necessarily synonymous with religion. Religion is the codified and ritualized beliefs and behaviors of those involved in spirituality, usually taking place within a community of like-minded individuals.

4. Spirituality involves the development of our higher self, also referred to as the transpersonal self. A transpersonal experience (i.e., transcendence) is described as a feeling of oneness, inner peace, harmony, wholeness, and connection with the universe.

Mental

1. Assessing our mental capacity helps us examine our belief systems and influences our beliefs, thoughts, behaviors, and values.

2. Our challenge is to use our cognitive capacities to perceive the world with greater clarity and to build our capacity to notice, process, and integrate both logical and intuitive thought.

3. We become more capable of focusing our attention away from fear-based, negative thought patterns and become more open and receptive to life-affirming information and patterns of thought. In this way, mental growth can occur.

Emotional

1. Assessing our emotional potential assists us in our willingness to acknowledge the presence of feelings, value them as important information to notice, and express them.

2. Emotional health implies that we have the choice and freedom to process and/or express the full spectrum of emotions including love, joy, guilt, forgiveness, fear, and anger.

3. Understanding our emotions and our response to life events has the potential to lessen chronic anxiety, depression, worry, fear, guilt, anger, denial, failure, or repression. When we are willing to confront our emotions we can experience true healing.

Physical

1. Assessing our physical potential includes three major areas:
   a. Nutrition (See Chapter 13 in the *Holistic Nursing Handbook* [6th ed.])
   b. Exercise and movement (See Chapter 14 in the *Holistic Nursing Handbook* [6th ed.])
   c. Weight management (See Chapter 22 in the *Holistic Nursing Handbook* [6th ed.])

2. Increasing nutrition, exercise, and weight awareness and choices leads to health and wellness and decreases chronic disease and stress.

Environmental

1. Assessing our environment (See the Environmental section in Figure 8-2 in the *Holistic Nursing Handbook* [6th ed.]) increases our awareness of its impact on our health and well-being.

2. The environment is the context or habitat within which all living systems participate

and interact that includes the physical body and its physical habitat, and cultural, psychological, social, and historical influences; it includes both the external physical space and a person's internal space (physical, mental, emotional, social, and spiritual experiences).

3. A healing environment includes everything that surrounds the nurse, healthcare practitioner and student, the patient/client, family, community, and significant others as well as patterns not yet understood.

4. The precautionary principle[12] can be implemented when an activity raises threats of harm to human health or the environment. Precautionary measures are taken even if some cause-and-effect relationships are not fully established scientifically. This the "better safe than sorry" principle. If there is a suspicion about a harmful environment or substance, even though all of the evidence is not in, remove the person from the situation or stop the use of suspected harmful substances. The emphasis is on *zero* contamination and pollution of our environments as acceptable, not minimal/moderate.

Health Responsibility

1. Health responsibility occurs when an individual takes an active role in making lifestyle choices to protect and improve health. The nurse can also encourage the client to complete a Personal Health Record. The client can calculate body mass index by using the body mass index calculator in *Holistic Nursing: A Handbook for Practice, 6th ed.* pages 185-186. See Figure 8-3 and Table 8-1 in the sixth edition of the *Holistic Nursing Handbook*.

2. Health responsibility includes having physical examinations and eye examinations as recommended for one's age and health status by qualified healthcare practitioners and all baseline personal physiologic parameters, personal history, family history, and any current symptoms.

3. Health responsibility also includes noting and evaluating all medications and supplements that the client takes in terms of potential interactions with other pharmaceuticals. Allergies, hospitalizations,

surgeries, and other specific medical factors are also important to note.

4. In health care, we might hear that a client/patient is *noncompliant* with medical orders. This is often a misnomer because an individual might not follow medical recommendations for many reasons. The following are common reasons for "noncompliance": too much information given at one time; lack of full understanding of the recommendations and having unanswered questions; language barriers or cognitive limitations; fear; denial; previous lack of commitment or lack of success (e.g., weight management, smoking cessation); side effects of medications; financial restraints; religious beliefs; disabilities; lack of support from significant others. In addition, usually there is an inadequate amount of time for effective patient education in clinics, doctor's offices, hospitals, and other healthcare settings when providing discharge information.

■ NOTES

1. Institute of Medicine. (2010). *The future of nursing: Leading change, advancing health* (2010). Retrieved from http://www.iom.edu/Reports/2010/The-Future-of-Nursing-Leading-Change-Advancing-Health.aspx

2. Centers for Disease Control and Prevention. Overweight and obesity: Data and statistics. http://www.cdc.gov/obesity/data/index.html

3. Snyderman, R., & Dinan, M. (2010). Improving health by taking it personally. *Journal of the American Medical Association, 303*(4), 363–364.

4. American Heart Association. (2009). *Heart disease and stroke statistics—2009 update*. Dallas, TX: Author.

5. Centers for Disease Control and Prevention. (2011). Heart disease and stroke prevention: Addressing the nation's leading killers: At a glance 2011. Retrieved from http://www.cdc.gov/chronicdisease/resources/publications/AAG/dhdsp.htm

6. Wang, Y. C., McPherson, K., Marsh, T., Gortmaker, S. L., & Brown, M. (2011). Health and economic burden of the projected obesity trends in the USA and the UK. *Lancet, 378*(9793), 815–825.

7. U.S. Department of Health and Human Services. (2010). *Healthy people 2020*. Washington, DC: Author. Retrieved from http://www.healthypeople.gov

8. Compilation of the Patient Protection and Affordable Care Act. (2010). Retrieved from http://docs.house.gov/energycommerce/ppacacon.pdf

9. U.S. Department of Health and Human Services. (2011, June 16). Obama administration releases National Prevention Strategy [News release]. Retrieved from http://www.hhs.gov/news/press/2011pres/06/20110616a.html

10. Hess, D. R., Dossey, B. M., Southard, M.E. , Luck, S., Schaub, B. G., & Bark, L. (2013). *The art and science of nurse coaching: A provider's guidelines for scope and competencies.* Silver Spring, MD: Nurses books.org.

11. Dossey, B. M., Luck, S., & Schaub, B. G. (2013). *Nurse coaching for health and wellness.* Huntington, NY: Florence Press.

12. Raffensperger, C., & Tickner, J. (1999). *Protecting public health and the environment: Implementing the precautionary principle.* Washington, DC: Island Press.

■ STUDY QUESTIONS

Basic Level

1. Which of the following happens first for holistic nurses to serve as change agents for health and well-being?
   a. Holistic nurses must begin patient/client change with evaluating both positive and negative lifestyle behaviors.
   b. Holistic nursing assessment begins with using health and wellness assessments to gauge a patient/client's readiness for change.
   c. Holistic nurses must apply for research grants to learn assessment skills.
   d. Holistic nurses present an action plan to the patient/client and discuss how to implement the plan.

2. Healing awareness has to do with which of the following?
   a. A person's conscious recognition of and focused attention on intuitions, subtle feelings, conditions, and circumstances relating to the needs of self or clients
   b. Having a sense of purpose and knowing what and what not to do
   c. A process of understanding and integrating the many aspects of self, leading to a deep connection with inner wisdom and an experience of balance and wholeness
   d. Being able to read the energy field of the patient/client with whom you care for

3. Reversing chronic disease and its ill effects includes knowing which of the following pieces of information?
   a. By the end of life all of us will have at least one chronic disease.
   b. If the current obesity epidemic continues unchecked, 80% of the U.S. adult population will be obese, with body mass index values of 30 or higher, by 2030.
   c. With awareness we can work together to eliminate chronic disease in this country.
   d. More than 133 million adults, or nearly half of all adults in the United States, are living with at least one chronic disease, such as obesity, diabetes, and cardiovascular disease.

4. Which of the following actions is associated with healthcare transformation in the United States?
   a. Each state creating a plan to improve lifestyle behaviors for its citizens
   b. How funding is allocated among the federal government and the states and how that funding is to be spent on health care
   c. Utilizing the *Healthy People 2010* vision, mission, and overarching goals to provide structure and guidance for achieving the *Healthy People 2020* objectives
   d. Doing what is right and justified to achieve a wellness lifestyle for each resident

5. Which of the following areas are included in integrative health and wellness assessments?
   a. Body, mind, and spirit
   b. Mental, spiritual, lifestyle, and work ethic
   c. Life balance and satisfaction, relationships, spiritual, mental, emotional, physical, environment, and health responsibility
   d. Physical, mental, financial, goal orientation, and health responsibility

Advanced Level

6. Which of the following issues is important to understand when working as a change agent?

a. There is an urgent need for initiatives to help shift the focus of health care by promoting self-efficacy and empowering individuals to recognize their potential to engage in promoting their own health and well-being.

b. The nurse must be aware of the entire scope of the patient/client and the funding available from the agency and government grants and services.

c. The nurse is the most important factor in creating change.

d. Healthcare providers must be aware of the limitations of funding when creating plans for patient-centered change.

7. The *Healthy People 2020* mission strives to accomplish which of the following?

a. Identify local and regional health improvement priorities

b. Provide measurable objectives and goals that are applicable at the state and local levels

c. Engage multiple sectors to take actions to strengthen policies and improve practices that are driven by the best available evidence and knowledge

d. Identify critical research, research methodology, and funding needs

8. The Integrative Health and Wellness Assessment (IHWA) includes which of the following aspects?

a. Self-assessments and other strategies to assist individuals to learn how to prefer wellness to unhealthy habits

b. A whole person assessment that has eight components

c. Teaching points for how to make the change, who to help with the change, and confidence to design an action plan to include the backup help person

d. A 12-point system to encourage the best possible health and wellness

9. What does assessing our emotional potential accomplish?

a. Assists us in our willingness to acknowledge the presence of feelings, to judge them, and to decide not to do destructive behavior again.

b. Acknowledges that we have the choice and freedom to process and/or express the full spectrum of emotions and mental attitudes

c. Allows us to become more capable of focusing our attention away from fear-based, negative thought patterns and becoming more open and receptive to different information and ways of being

d. Aids us in understanding our emotions and our response to life events with the potential to lessen varying degrees of chronic anxiety, depression, worry, fear, guilt, and other negative processes

10. For which of the following reasons is it important to practice the skill of self-assessment?

a. To begin to reverse chronic disease, reduce hospital readmissions, and correct our previously unhealthy lifestyle

b. To help us as a society all feel better and live longer, more productive lives

c. To help reverse chronic disease, play a part in the healthcare transformation, and achieve better life balance and our human potentials

d. To model health to our family and friends when we feel better ourselves

Chapter 10

Nurse Coaching

Barbara Montgomery Dossey, Susan Luck,
Bonney Gulino Schaub, and Darlene R. Hess

■ DEFINITIONS

Professional nurse coach A registered nurse who incorporates coaching skills into his or her professional nursing practice and integrates a holistic perspective. This perspective, as applied to both self and client in a coaching interaction, emerges from an awareness that effective change evolves from within before it can be manifested and maintained externally. The professional nurse coach works with the whole person utilizing principles and modalities that integrate body-mind-emotion-spirit-environment.[1]

Professional nurse coaching A skilled, purposeful, results-oriented, and structured relationship-centered interaction with clients provided by registered nurses for the purpose of promoting achievement of client goals.[1]

■ EVOLUTION OF THE FIELD OF HEALTH COACHING AND NURSE COACHING

1. Prior to 1980s: *Coach* referred to a role in the field of human performance, specifically in the field of athletics (i.e., training Olympic athletes including relaxation, imagery rehearsal, and somatic awareness practices to enhance athletic performance).

2. 1960s: Human potential movement began and coaching moved into organizational settings related to increased demand for greater productivity and enhanced employee performance, to promote employee self-development, and to measure and document the effectiveness of these initiatives in meaningful ways.

3. 1990s: Formal coaching programs, courses, and certifications emerged outside of the nursing profession.

4. 2009–2012: *The Art and Science of Nurse Coaching: The Provider's Guide to Coaching Scope and Competencies,*[1] was a 3-year development and peer-review process that clearly recognized, identified, and defined the nurse coach role, a role that has been an inherent component of nursing philosophy and practice for decades. This process resulted in endorsements from 19 nursing organizations (as of December 2012).

5. 2013: *The Art and Science of Nurse Coaching: The Provider's Guide to Coaching Scope and Competencies,*[1] published by NurseBooks.org (ANA publisher):
   a. The American Holistic Nurses Credentialing Corporation (AHNCC) used as the foundational document *The Art and Science of Nurse Coaching: The Provider's Guide to Coaching Scope and Competencies* to establish the blueprint and criteria for the AHNCC Nurse Coach Certification Examination. The first examination was offered January 2013.[2]

Note: The authors would like to acknowledge Mary Elaine Southard and Linda Bark for their collaborative work in the Professional Nurse Coaching Workgroup (PNCW) and the coauthorship of *The Art and Science of Nurse Coaching: The Provider's Guide to Coaching Scope and Competencies*[1] that is quoted in this chapter.

b. Nurses who meet the criteria and pass the AHNCC Nurse Coach Examination are recognized as a Nurse Coach–Board Certified (NC-BC). If nurses are Holistic Nurse Certified by AHNCC, they will be recognized as a Health and Wellness Nurse Coach (HWNC-BC).

■ PROFESSIONAL NURSE COACH SCOPE OF PRACTICE AND COMPETENCIES

This section is used with permission and adapted from *The Art and Science of Nurse Coaching: The Provider's Guide to Coaching Scope of Practice and Competencies.*[1]

1. *The Art and Science of Nurse Coaching: The Provider's Guide to Coaching Scope and Competencies* brings the nurse coach role in healthcare reform to the forefront.[3,4]
2. *The Art and Science of Nurse Coaching: The Provider's Guide to Coaching Scope and Competencies* demonstrates nursing's proactive stance in healthcare transformation and clarifies nursing perspectives concerning the role of the nurse coach in four key ways:
    a. Specifies the philosophy, beliefs, and values of the nurse coach and the nurse coach's scope of practice
    b. Articulates the relationship between ANA *Nursing: Scope and Standards of Practice* (2nd edition) and nurse coaching[5]
    c. Provides the basis for continued interdisciplinary conversations related to professional health and wellness coaches and lay health and wellness coaches
    d. Provides the foundation for an international certification process for professional nurse coaching
3. Professional nurse coaches are guided in their thinking and decision making by three professional resources:
    a. The second edition of the *American Nurses Association Scope and Standards of Practice*[5] outlines the expectations of the professional role of registered nurses and the scope of practice and standards of professional nurse practice and their accompanying competencies.
    b. The ANA *Code of Ethics for Nurses with Interpretive Statements*[6] lists the nine

provisions that establish the ethical framework for registered nurses across all roles, levels, and settings.
    c. The ANA *Nursing's Social Policy Statement: The Essence of Practice*[7] conceptualizes nursing practice, describes the social context of nursing, and provides the definition of nursing.
    d. The American Holistic Nurses Association and American Nurses Association *Holistic Nursing: Scope and Standards of Practice* (2nd edition)[8] provides the philosophical underpinnings of a holistic nurse coaching practice.
4. *The Art and Science of Nurse Coaching: The Provider's Guide to Coaching Scope and Competencies* is compatible with the scope and standards of practice of all nursing specialties. Nurse coaching skills can be used in all areas of nursing.

Professional Nurse Coaching Scope of Practice

1. Nurse coaches work with individuals and with groups and are found in all areas of nursing practice. They may be staff nurses, ambulatory care nurses, case managers, advanced practice nurses, nursing faculty, nurse researchers, educators, administrators, nurse entrepreneurs, or nurse coaches in full-time private practice.
2. Nurse coaching may be a primary role.
3. The depth and breadth to which registered nurses engage in the total scope of nurse coach practice depends on education, experience, role, and the population they serve.

Professional Nurse Coaching Competencies

1. *The Art and Science of Nurse Coaching: The Provider's Guide to Coaching Scope and Competencies* describes a competent level of nurse coaching practice and professional performance common to all nurse coaches.
2. Effective nurse coaching interactions involve the ability to develop a coaching partnership, to create a safe space, and to be sensitive to client issues of trust and vulnerability as a basis for further exploration.[9-13]

3. The nurse coach must be able to structure a coaching session, explore client readiness for coaching, facilitate achievement of the client's desired goals, and cocreate a means of determining and evaluating desired outcomes and goals.[1] Nurse coaching is grounded in the principles and core values of professional nursing.

Professional Nurse Coaching Core Values

1. The following five professional nurse coaching core values are adapted from and congruent with the second edition of the AHNA and ANA *Holistic Nursing: Scope and Standards of Practice*.[8]
   a. Nurse Coach Philosophy, Theories, and Ethics
   b. Nurse Coach Process
   c. Nurse Coach Communication and Coaching Environment
   d. Nurse Coach Education, Research, and Leadership
   e. Nurse Coach Self-Development (Self-Reflection, Self Assessments, Self-Evaluation, Self-Care)
2. Core Value 5 (item e in the preceding list) is worded according to a nurse coaching model. These core values and the specific nurse coaching competencies are aligned with the second edition of the ANA *Nursing: Scope and Standards of Practice*[5] and are the foundation for curriculum development and a credentialing process.[2]

The Art and Science of Nurse Coaching

1. Nurse coaches incorporate approaches to nursing practice that are holistic, integrative, and integral and that include the work of numerous nurse scholars.
2. Coaching is a systematic and skilled process grounded in scholarly evidenced-based professional nursing practice. All chapters in this core curriculum can be utilized in a nurse coaching practice.
3. At the heart of nurse coaching is support for the client's healing process as it manifests in body-mind-spirit. Nurse coaches realize that by being open and curious and asking powerful questions, the client can

be guided in this process, while at the same time having choices in determining her or his priorities for change.
4. The nurse coach lets go of trying "to fix" a client and places the nurse expert role aside to deeply listen to the client, remembering the "power of the pause" with silence and that "less is more" in the coaching conversation.
5. The quality of human caring is central to the nurse coach and client relationship. The nurse is fully present in the coaching relationship, honoring the wholeness of the patient/client in a manner that allows clients to experience a safe environment in which to express their goals, hopes, and dreams. This provides a setting where their vulnerability can be spoken and addressed.
6. Nurse coaches utilize a full spectrum of coaching to engage the client toward meeting desired goals.

Stages of Change, Motivational Interviewing, and Appreciative Inquiry

1. The Transtheoretical Model of Behavioral Change provides a way to determine what stage a client is in regarding readiness to make changes.[14] There are five stages:
   a. Precontemplation: The client is usually not ready for change and uses phrases such as "I won't" or "I can't."
   b. Contemplation: The client is thinking about change and might use the phrase "I may."
   c. Preparation: The client is preparing for action and might say "I will."
   d. Action: The client is taking action and says "I am."
   e. Maintenance: The client is maintaining and sustaining desired changes and behaviors and says "I still am."
2. Essential nurse coaching skills include being in the present moment, inquiry, reflection, motivational interviewing, and appreciative inquiry.[15-16] (See Chapter 10 in the sixth edition of *Holistic Nursing Handbook*.) These nurse coaching skills assist clients to recognize their resistance, ambivalence, and change talk.

■ NURSE COACHING PROCESS

This section is used with permission and adapted from *The Art and Science of Nurse Coaching: The Provider's Guide to Coaching Scope and Competencies.*[1] The reader is referred to this publication for specific nurse coaching competencies.

1. Note: The nursing process involves six focal areas: assessment, diagnosis, outcomes, plan, interventions, and evaluation. The nurse coach uses the "holistic nurse caring process"[17] and understands that growth and improved health, wholeness, and well-being are the result of an ongoing journey that is ever expanding and transformative.

2. In nurse coaching, there is a shift in terminology and meaning to understand and incorporate the client's subjective experience: from assessing to establishing the relationship and identifying readiness for change; from nursing diagnosis to identifying opportunities and issues; from identifying desired outcomes to helping the client establish goals; from planning to creating the structure of the coaching interaction; from intervention to empowering the client to reach goals; from evaluating to assisting the client in determining the extent to which goals have been achieved. The nurse coaching process and role of the professional nurse coach are explored in the following sections.

Establishing Relationship and Identifying Readiness for Change (Assessment)

1. In a coaching model the foundation for coaching begins during the assessment phase of the coaching interaction that establishes the relationship and identifies readiness for change.

2. The nurse coach begins with becoming fully present with self and client before initiating the coaching interaction. The session proceeds with an assessment, establishing the relationship with the client and listening to the client's subjective experience/story.

3. The nurse coach helps the client assess readiness for change. Assessment is dynamic and ongoing.

4. The nurse coach then determines whether the client's concerns are appropriate for coaching or whether the client would be better served through a referral to other services and resources.

Identifying Opportunities, Issues, and Concerns (Diagnosis)

1. The nurse coach and the client together explore assessment data to determine areas for change. There is no attempt or need to assign labels or to establish a diagnosis. Instead, the nurse coach is open to multiple and fluid interpretations of an unfolding interaction in partnership with the client.

2. This process identifies opportunities and issues related to growth, overall health, wholeness, and well-being. Opportunities for celebrating are explored. The nurse coach understands that acknowledgment promotes and reinforces previous successes and serves to enhance further achievements.

Establishing Client-Centered Goals (Outcomes)

1. The nurse coach assists the client to identify goals that will lead to the desired change. The nurse coach values the evolution and the process of change as it unfolds. The nurse coach employs an overall approach to each coaching interaction that is designed to facilitate achievement of client goals.

2. This stage involves the client in formulating goals that are specific, measurable, action-oriented, realistic, and time-lined. This leads to facilitating the client's process of self-discovery related to establishment of goals and exploration of alternative ideas and options relevant to goal setting. The nurse coach supports the client's inner wisdom, intuition, and innate ability for knowing what is best for self. The nurse coach also realizes that new goals will emerge as the client changes and evolves.

Creating the Structure of the Coaching Interaction (Plan)

1. The nurse coach develops with the client a coaching plan that identifies strategies to attain goals. The nurse coach structures the coaching interaction with a coaching agreement that identifies specific parameters of the coaching relationship, including coach

and client responsibilities. The client's potential obstacles to goal attainment and possible responses to these challenges are also explored and the plan is adjusted as desired by the client.

Empowering Clients to Reach Goals (Implementation)

1. The nurse coach supports the client's coaching plan while simultaneously remaining open to emerging goals based on new insights, learning, and achievements. The nurse coach supports the client in reaching for new and expanded goals using a variety of specific communication skills to facilitate learning and growth.

2. The nurse coach employs effective communication skills such as motivational interviewing, appreciative inquiry, deep listening, and powerful questioning as key components of the coaching interaction. In partnership with the client, the nurse coach facilitates learning and results by cocreating awareness, designing actions, setting goals, and planning and addressing progress and accountability. The nurse coach chooses interventions based on the client's statements and actions and interacts with intention and curiosity in a manner that assists the client to achieve goals. The nurse coach effectively utilizes her or his nursing knowledge and a variety of skills acquired with additional coach training.

Assisting Client to Determine the Extent to Which Goals Were Achieved (Evaluation)

1. The nurse coach partners with the client to evaluate progress toward attainment of goals. The nurse coach is aware that the evaluation of coaching (the nursing intervention) is done primarily by the client instead of by the nurse and is based on the client's perception of success and achievement of client-centered goals.

■ NOTES

1. Hess, D., Dossey, B. M., Southard, M. E., Luck, S., Schaub, B. G., & Bark, L. (2013). *The art and science of nurse coaching: A provider's guide to scope and competencies.* Silver Spring, MD: Nursesbooks.org.

2. American Holistic Nurses Credentialing Corporation. (n.d.). Certification in nurse coaching, NC-BC and HWNC-BC. Retrieved from http://www.ahncc.org/certification/nursecoachnchwnc.html

3. Weeks, J. (2010, May 12). Reference guide: Language/sections on CAM and integrative practice in HR 3590-Healthcare Overhaul. Integrator Blog. Retrieved from http://theintegratorblog.com/site/index.php?option=com_content&task=view&id=658&Itemid=189

4. U.S. Department of Health and Human Services. (2011, June 16). Obama administration releases National Prevention Strategy [News release]. Retrieved from http://www.hhs.gov/news/press/2011pres/06/20110616a.html

5. American Nurses Association. (2010). *Nursing: Scope and standards of practice* (2nd ed.). Silver Spring, MD: Nursebooks.org.

6. American Nurses Association. (2001). *Code of ethics for nurses with interpretive statements.* Silver Spring, MD: Nursesbooks.org.

7. American Nurses Association. (2010). *Nursing's social policy statement: The essence of the profession.* Silver Spring, MD: Nursesbooks.org.

8. American Holistic Nurses Association & American Nurses Association. (2013). *Holistic nursing: Scope and standards of practice* (2nd ed.). Silver Spring, MD: Nursesbooks.org.

9. Donner, G., & Wheeler, M. (2009). *Coaching in nursing: An introduction.* Indianapolis, IN: International Council of Nursing & Sigma Theta Tau.

10. Bark, L. (2011). *The wisdom of the whole: Coaching for joy, health, and success.* San Francisco, CA: Create Space.

11. Dossey, B. M., Luck, S., & Schaub, B. G. (2013). *Nurse coaching for health and wellness.* Huntington, NY: Florence Press.

12. Schaub, R., & Schaub, B. G. (2013). *Transpersonal development: Cultivating the human resources of peace, wisdom, purpose and oneness.* Huntington, NY: Florence Press.

12. Schaub, R., & Schaub, B. G. (2009). *The end of fear: A spiritual path for realists.* Carlsbad, CA: Hay House.

14. Prochaska, J., Norcross, J. C., & Di Clemente, C. C. (1995). *Changing for good. A revolutionary six-stage program for overcoming bad habits and moving your life positively forward.* New York, NY: Harper Collins.

15. Dart, M. A. (2011). *Motivational interviewing in nursing practice.* Sudbury, MA: Jones and Bartlett.

16. Southard, M. E., Bark, L., & Hess, D. (2013). Facilitating change: Motivational interviewing and appreciative inquiry. In B. M. Dossey & L. Keegan (Eds.), *Holistic nursing: A handbook for practice* (6th ed., pp. 205–219). Burlington, MA: Jones & Bartlett Learning.

17. Potter, P., & Frisch, N. C. (2013). The holistic caring process. In B. M. Dossey & L. Keegan (Eds.), *Holistic nursing: A handbook for practice* (6th ed., pp 145–160). Burlington, MA: Jones & Bartlett Learning.

■ PROFESSIONAL NURSE COACH PROGRAM WEBSITES

Bark Coaching Institute:
http://www.barkcoaching.com

International Nurse Coach Association, Integrative Nurse Coach Certificate Program (INCCP):
http://www.iNurseCoach.com

Watson Caring Science Institute and International Caring Consortium, Caritas Coaching Education Program:
http://www.watsoncaringscience.org/index.cfm/category/3/caritas-coach-education-program ccep.cfm

■ STUDY QUESTIONS

Basic Level

1. Which of the following answer choices describe professional nurse coaching accurately?
   a. Casual and informal interaction between a nurse coach and client with specific outcomes determined by the nurse coach
   b. Skilled, purposeful, results-oriented, and structured relationship-centered interaction between nurse coach and client for the purpose of promoting achievement of client goals
   c. Structured conversation between the nurse coach and client where the nurse is the expert and assists the client to stay focused on one goal at a time
   d. Casual and formal, open-ended interactions between the nurse coach and client where the nurse leads the coaching conversation for the purpose of promoting achievement of client goals

2. Nurse coaches are guided in their professional thinking and decision-making process by which three professional resources?
   a. IOM *Future of Nursing Report, Core Competencies for Interprofessional Collaborative Practice*, and U.S. Government health report
   b. National Prevention Strategy, *Healthy People 2020*, and Patient Protection and Affordable Care Act
   c. American Nurses Association *Scope and Standards of Practice*, 2nd ed.; ANA *Code of Ethics for Nurses with Interpretive Statements*; and *Nursing's Social Policy Statement: The Essence of Practice*
   d. International Coaching Federation report, International Council of Nurses report, and *International Report on Nursing*

3. In which work settings and in which professional roles do professional nurse coaches work?
   a. In ambulatory care, operating rooms, critical care, community health nursing settings, and corporate wellness programs
   b. In all work settings serving as staff nurses, ambulatory care nurses, case managers, advanced practice nurses, nursing faculty, nurse researchers, educators, administrators, nurse entrepreneurs, and in private practice
   c. In acute care and private practice as case managers
   d. In ambulatory care as staff nurses, case managers, and advanced practice nurses

4. Regarding the description and scope of professional nurse coaching practice, which of the following statements is *not* true?
   a. Nurse coaching practice is grounded in the principles and values of professional nursing.
   b. The nurse coach is limited to working with individuals or groups in outpatient work settings.
   c. The depth and breadth of nurse coaching practice depends on education, experience, and the population served.
   d. Nurse coaching can be the primary role of the nurse.

5. Effective nurse coaching and client interactions involve which of the following?
   a. Nurse coach being able to anticipate the client's ambivalence and resistance, and to give specific instructions for changing a behavior or behaviors toward a desired goal or goals
   b. Nurse coach teaching the client about specific action steps and how to sustain desired shifts in behaviors and to be linear in the exploration of ideas

c. Nurse coach's ability to develop a coaching partnership with the client, to create a safe space, and to be sensitive to client issues of trust and vulnerability as a basis for further exploration

d. Nurse coach determining the priority of the most important client goals and working in a semistructured interactive process during the coaching session

6. **Which of the following must a nurse coach be able to do?**

   a. Utilize the key coaching skills of deep listening, appreciative inquiry, and linear thinking to identify client goals

   b. Inquire how the client is in the moment and immediately use the client's spoken words to show understanding of the client's experience

   c. Use powerful questioning to show understanding of the client's experience and to evaluate the client's progress

   d. Structure a coaching session, explore client readiness for coaching, facilitate achievement of the client's desired goals, and cocreate a means of determining and evaluating desired client outcomes and goals

Advanced Level

7. **A client tells the nurse coach she wants to lose weight and feel more energetic. She has decided to begin an exercise program. Which stage of behavioral change stage is this client in?**

   a. Precontemplation

   b. Contemplation

   c. Preparation

   d. Action

8. **In which of the following ways does the nurse coach begin every coaching interaction?**

   a. Assessing the client's readiness for change

   b. Listening deeply to the client's goals and plans

   c. Establishing the client–nurse coach relationship

   d. Becoming fully present with self and client

9. **A client becomes teary during a coaching interaction and says he does not believe he will ever be able to lose the 45 pounds his nurse practitioner has recommended he lose. What would be an appropriate next step for the nurse coach?**

   a. Remain silent and continue to listen deeply to the client's concerns.

   b. Gently ask the client why he feels that way.

   c. Assure the client by telling him you believe in him.

   d. Tell the client you will coach him to success.

10. **A nurse coach is working with a client who has long-standing uncontrolled diabetes. The client volunteers that her HbA1C level at the doctor's office 2 days ago was 8.9 and she asks the nurse what she can do to lower it. What is the appropriate coaching response?**

    a. "I wouldn't worry about that. I've seen lab results much worse than yours."

    b. "That is serious. What did the doctor tell you to do?"

    c. "Do you have some ideas about how to accomplish that?"

    d. "If it's okay with you, I want to create a nutrition and exercise plan for you."

11. **The client has developed a plan to achieve his goal of improved life–work balance. The client has identified specific steps. What would be an appropriate next step for the nurse coach?**

    a. Assist the client to identify new goals to work on for the next session.

    b. Facilitate client results by addressing client accountability and progress.

    c. Partner with the client to evaluate attainment of previous goals.

    d. Use appreciative inquiry to establish a timeline for achievement of client goals.

Chapter 11

Facilitating Change: Motivational Interviewing and Appreciative Inquiry

Darlene R. Hess, Linda A. Bark, and Mary Elaine Southard

■ DEFINITIONS

Appreciative inquiry Appreciative inquiry (AI) is both a philosophy and a methodology for change. Appreciative inquiry is the study and exploration of strengths as a way to help patients and organizations function at their best. Instead of solving problems, AI is a process in which positive change is facilitated through identifying creative possibilities.

Motivational interviewing Motivational interviewing (MI) is an intervention strategy for changing behavior. The central purpose of MI is to help patients explore and eventually resolve ambivalence in reference to a current health behavior. MI emphasizes client choice and responsibility and can be used in a variety of clinical settings.

Nurse coaching Nurse coaching is skilled, purposeful, results-oriented, and structured relationship-centered interactions with clients provided by registered nurses for the purpose of promoting the health and well-being of the whole person.[1] Nurse coaching is grounded in the principles and core values of holistic nursing. Effective nurse coaching interactions involve the ability to create a coaching partnership, build a safe space, and be sensitive to client issues of trust and vulnerability as a basic foundation for further exploration.[2] Nurse coaches can structure a coaching session, explore client readiness for coaching, facilitate achievement of the client's desired goals, and cocreate a means of determining and evaluating desired outcomes and goals.[3]

Therapeutic presence Therapeutic presence is the conscious intention to be fully present for another person. Presence involves letting go of past or future concerns resulting in the creation of an opening or opportunity to reveal what is needed in the moment.[4] Presence requires awareness, authenticity, and an appreciation of being in the moment.

Transtheoretical Stages of Change Model (Transtheoretical Model) The Transtheoretical Stages of Change Model is a model of behavioral change developed by Prochaska and DiClemente in 1984.[5] The five stages of the model are precontemplation, contemplation, preparation, action, and maintenance. Interventions designed to promote behavioral change are tailored to the individual's readiness for change. Relapses and recycling through the stages frequently occur. Relapse provides valuable information to assist in further change and is not viewed as a failure.

■ INTRODUCTION

1. Nurses and other health professionals are looking for effective and cost-efficient ways to help clients make health behavior changes.
2. New approaches are needed to assist patients to achieve lasting behavior change.

This chapter concerns two holistic interventions nurses can learn and utilize in professional nursing practice to support client behavior change to enhance client health and well-being: MI and AI.

   a. MI is used when someone is ambivalent about change.

   b. AI uncovers and expands what is working in a situation rather than focusing on what is not working.

3. Nurse coaches are taking the lead in establishing models of coaching that are designed to engage clients in self-care and management of healthcare practices and outcomes.[3]

■ MOTIVATIONAL INTERVIEWING

1. MI is a research-based method of interacting with patients to elicit motivation for change.[6]

2. The fundamental premise of MI is that patients are often ambivalent to change, and ambivalence affects a patient's motivation and readiness to alter behavior.[7]

3. The Transtheoretical Model created by Prochaska and DiClemente guides MI.[6] The model purports the following:

   a. People frequently do not succeed in changing behavior on the first attempt and often experience numerous attempts before successfully changing.

   b. There are multiple stages, progression, and relapses.

   c. Underlying the progressions are the patients' prior experiences with change and how they view the pros and cons of change.

   d. Patients consider whether or not they have the skills or resources to make a change.

   e. MI is used in all aspects of behavior change.

Guiding Principles of Motivational Interviewing

MI is based on four guiding principles known by the acronym RULE:[8]

1. Resist the righting reflex: The "righting reflex" is the natural tendency of the nurse to fix a patient's problems by imposing solutions.[9] The nurse must set aside any desire to correct the course and direction of the client. The nurse must suppress what might seem like the right thing to do and instead allow the client to determine what to do.

2. Understand and explore the client's motivation: It is the client's reasons for change, and not the nurse's, that are likely to trigger change. The nurse explores the client's concerns, perceptions, and motivations. Allowing patients to tell their story and encouraging them to discuss not only their reason for change but also how they might see themselves make those changes is the core of the partnership.

3. Listen with empathy: Answers lie within the client and finding them requires listening. Empathy is typically understood as the ability to identify with the client's difficulties or feelings. The ability to express empathy enhances the ability to engage patients in making necessary health changes.

4. Empower and encourage hope and optimism: The nurse helps the client discover *how* change can happen. The nurse views the client as the expert consultant as ideas and resources for change are explored. Providing ongoing encouragement to foster the belief that the goals are achievable can help the patient carry out a plan to change behavior.

Partnering with Clients

1. By honoring client autonomy and effectively creating a collaborative partnership between patient and provider, patients become involved in identifying goals and determining how best to achieve them.

2. The nurse applying a MI strategy seeks to evoke client strengths and to activate client motivation and resources for change.

3. MI is a refined form of guiding and includes skillful informing. The process of listening and guiding patients is quite a different stance than telling patients what they "should" be doing in terms of positive healthcare practices.

4. Nurses who utilize MI understand that it is not the nurse's job to fix the patient or the patient's problems. To attempt to do so

places responsibility on the nurse and promotes either dependency on the nurse or leads to "difficult" patients who do not listen to the information or advice provided by the nurse.[10]

Communication Skills

1. To negotiate behavior change successfully, nurses must build on basic communication skills and establish a therapeutic environment.
2. Coaching clients to achieve their desired goals involves first becoming fully present.
3. Nurse coaches develop and hone specific communication techniques such as reflective listening, asking open-ended questions, and using clarifying statements. Self-awareness is a necessary component of effective partnering with clients to effect change.
4. Communication is facilitated by being self-aware of one's voice inflections, posturing, or self-talk when interacting with a patient.

See pages 208–211 in *Holistic Nursing: A Handbook for Practice* [6th ed.] for the motivational interviewing case study with an excerpt sample of a patient and nurse conversation.

■ APPRECIATIVE INQUIRY

1. AI is a way of asking questions that creates relationships based on the basic goodness in a person, situation, or organization.
2. To appreciate is to see the best in a situation or another person, while to inquire is to explore and discover.
3. Nurses can utilize AI principles and processes to assist patients to build on their inherent strengths as a way to design and create their desired future.
4. AI differs from other change processes by focusing on transformational change—change that transforms and energizes a person, situation, or organization.
5. AI is explicitly contrasted with problem solving, which the originators of AI describe as a deficit-based approach to change.[11]
6. AI enhances momentum for change and long-term sustainability and abandons the "delivery" of ideas of action planning, monitoring progress, and building implementation strategies.

7. Rather than focusing on problems that need solving, AI focuses on imagining the best or highest outcome for the organization or client.
8. With AI, "problems" are seen as opportunities to be embraced, and the inquiry is directed toward the exploration of possibilities and the creation of a new future based on what is already working—on what is good—on what is best about the situation.
9. AI has the potential to inspire patients to consider a situation previously seen as hopeless as one that can evolve to something much better.
10. AI can lead to recognition of limiting patterns of behavior so that new behaviors can be adopted.
11. AI provides a way to address the discouragement felt by patients when their successes and achievements are overlooked and the focus is instead on the dire consequences of their diagnosis or on things that have not gone well.
12. Appreciative inquiry is based on the belief that change begins the moment a question is asked. Thus, the seeds of change are implicit in the very first questions the nurse asks. The idea is that clients will move in the direction of the questions that are asked. Holistic nurse coaches who use AI pay close attention to the exact wording and the provocative potential of the questions. They know that the words they choose have an impact far beyond the words themselves.
13. Nurse coaches attend carefully to the client's story.

4-D Cycle of Appreciative Inquiry

1. The main intervention model that has come to be associated with AI is the 4-D Cycle.[12] The model consists of four components:
   a. Discovery (inquiry)
   b. Dream (imagining what could be)
   c. Design (how to)
   d. Destiny (what will be)

Figure 10-1, 4-D Cycle Model, graphically depicts this cycle and can be found in Chapter 10 of *Holistic Nursing: A Handbook for Practice*, 6th edition.

2. The 4-D process enables individuals to discover foundational strengths—their positive core. By doing this before envisioning the future (dream), articulating designs for change (design), and establishing a path forward (destiny), they create confidence and hope for the future.[13]

3. See the section "Application of Appreciative Inquiry in the Clinical Setting" in Chapter 10 of the sixth edition of *Holistic Nursing: A Handbook for Practice* to review three case studies demonstrating the use of AI in various settings.

■ NOTES

1. Hess, D. R., Dossey, B. M., Southard, M. E., Luck, S., Schaub, B. G., & Bark, L. (2013). *The art and science of nurse coaching: The provider's guide to coaching scope and competencies*. Silver Spring, MD: Nursesbooks.org.

2. Schaub, R., & Schaub, B. G. (2009). *The end of fear: A spiritual path for realists*. Carlsbad, CA: Hay House.

3. Hess, D., Bark, L., & Southard, M. E. (2010, September). *Holistic nurse coaching*. Paper presented to the National Credentialing Team for Professional Coaches in Healthcare at the Summit on Standards and Credentialing of Professional Coaches in Healthcare and Wellness, Boston, MA. Retrieved from http://www.ahncc.org/holistic nursecoaching.html

4. McKivergin, M. (2009). The nurse as an instrument of healing. In B. M. Dossey & L. Keegan (Eds.), *Holistic nursing: A handbook for practice* (5th ed., ed., pp. 721–737). Sudbury, MA: Jones and Bartlett.

5. Leddy, S. K. (2006). *Integrative health promotion: Conceptual basis for nursing practice* (2nd ed.). Sudbury, MA: Jones and Bartlett.

6. Miller, W. R., & Rollnick, S. (2002). *Motivational interviewing: Preparing people for change* (2nd ed.). New York, NY: Guilford Press.

7. Berger, B. (1999). Motivational interviewing helps patients confront change. *US Pharmacology, 24*, 88–95.

8. Rollnick, S., Miller, W. R., & Butler, C. C. (2008). *Motivational interviewing in healthcare: Helping patients change behavior*. New York, NY: Guilford Press.

9. Levensky, E. R., Forcehimes, A., O'Donohue, W. T., & Beitz, K. (2007). Motivational interviewing: An evidence-based approach to counseling helps patients follow treatment recommendations. *American Journal of Nursing, 19*(9), 37–44.

10. Dart, M. A. (2011). *Motivational interviewing in nursing practice*. Sudbury, MA: Jones and Bartlett.

11. Cooperrider, D. L., & Whitney, D. (2005). *Appreciative inquiry: A positive revolution in change*. San Francisco, CA: Berrett-Koehler.

12. Cooperrider, D. l., Whitney, D., & Stavros, J. M. (2005). *Appreciative inquiry handbook*. Brunswick, OH: Crown Custom Publishing.

13. Whitney, D. (2010). Appreciative inquiry: Creating spiritual resonance in the workplace. *Journal of Management, Spirituality, & Religion, 7*(1), 73–88.

■ STUDY QUESTIONS

Basic Level

1. **For which stage of client change was motivational interviewing designed to be used?**
   a. When the client is ready to move forward with a behavior change
   b. When the client is taking steps to change
   c. When the client is unaware of behaviors that need to change
   d. When the client is ambivalent about making a change

2. **When using motivational interviewing, how do nurses have the tendency to use a "righting reflex"?**
   a. By helping the patient create balance during a change process
   b. By solving the patients' problem for them
   c. By helping the client select the right health decision
   d. By using healing presence and deep listening

3. **Appreciative inquiry focuses on which of the following?**
   a. Problem solving and change
   b. Discovering foundational strengths
   c. Inquiring into problematic communication
   d. Organizational development

4. **Which of the following does the design phase of appreciative inquiry involve?**
   a. Setting up the structure to accomplish the vision
   b. Determining the vision of the design
   c. Seeing what is positive about the project
   d. Looking solely for resistance and barriers

5. In the destiny phase of appreciative inquiry, what is the main goal?
   a. Realize that the plan is part of the client's destiny
   b. Look for outside resources
   c. Set up the next problem to be addressed
   d. Cultivate client empowerment and continued success

Advanced Level

6. Motivational interviewing is an intervention strategy for behavior change. Which of the following principles and models guides it?
   a. The nurse coach principles
   b. The interviewing skills embedded in active listening
   c. The Transtheoretical Model by Prochaska and Di Clemente
   d. Therapeutic presence

7. Appreciative inquiry is based on which of the following concepts?
   a. The past is the most important issue to explore.
   b. Successful change begins with images of the future.
   c. Organizations and individuals should routinely explore the need for change.
   d. Ambivalence is often the main resistance to be resolved.

8. What does partnering with clients consist of?
   a. Assessing the client's hope for new outcomes
   b. Identifying and directing goals for client approval
   c. Resources for client change
   d. Pointing out discrepancies between goals and behavior

9. Which of the following is an important competency and challenge for the appreciative facilitator?
   a. Client engagement
   b. Conflicts of interest
   c. Deciding what is best for the client
   d. Owning the process

10. Which of the following choices best describes empathetic listening?
    a. A complex, multidimensional phenomenon
    b. Asking questions and waiting for the reply
    c. Determining the why of client interaction
    d. An approach to determine how to direct the client

Chapter 12

Cognitive Behavioral Therapy

Deborah Shields and Sharon S. Parker

Original Authors: Eileen M. Stuart-Shor,
Carol L. Wells-Federman, and Esther Seibold

■ DEFINITIONS

Cognition The act or process of knowing.

Cognitive Of or relating to consciousness, or being conscious; pertaining to intellectual activities (such as thinking, reasoning, imagining).

Cognitive Behavioral Therapy (CBT) A therapeutic approach that addresses the relationships among thoughts, feelings, behaviors, and physiology.

Cognitive distortions Inaccurate, irrational thoughts; mistakes in thinking.

Cognitive restructuring Examining and reframing one's interpretation of the meaning of an event.

■ THEORY AND RESEARCH

1. Historically, cognitive behavioral therapy (CBT) is rooted in the treatment of anxiety and depression; however, in the last 10 years its application has broadened greatly.
2. CBT is applied in the context of nursing practice along the wellness–illness continuum and the bio-psycho-social-spiritual domains.
3. CBT is based on the premise that stress and suffering are influenced by perception, or the way people think, and postulates that the thoughts that create stress are often illogical, negative, and distorted:
   a. These distorted negative thoughts can affect emotions, behaviors, and physiology and can influence the individual's beliefs.
   b. By changing negative illogical thoughts, specifically those that trigger and perpetuate distress, the individual can change physical and emotional states.
4. The biopsychosocial model illustrates the relationship between illogical thoughts that trigger and perpetuate stress and changes in physical and emotional states;[1] the dimension of spirituality has been added to Engel's existing model.[2]
   a. In this eclectic bio-psycho-social-spiritual model, there is a tacit understanding that stress, or the perception of threat, can lead to changes in physical, emotional, behavioral, and spiritual states.
   b. If we accept that stress causes changes in physical and emotional states and is influenced by perception, and if we accept that perception is influenced by distorted thinking patterns (negative thoughts), then we have created a link for CBT, which restructures distorted, negative thinking patterns and mind–body interactions, which influence health and illness.
   c. This link has implications for health promotion, symptom reduction, and disease management.
5. Understanding the dynamic interaction of CBT and the psychophysiology of mind–body connections is fundamental to the application of CBT in nursing.
6. CBT was first used for depression and anxiety, as a short-term treatment that focused on helping people to recognize and change automatic, distorted thoughts that trigger and perpetuate distress.[3]

7. It is now being applied successfully to reduce health-risking behaviors, physical symptoms, and the emotional sequelae of a variety of illnesses to which stress is an important causative or contributing factor.[4]
8. CBT is also useful in value clarification, the first step in establishing meaningful health goals.[4]
9. Cognitive behavioral therapy has ancient origins:
   a. A millennium ago, the Greek philosopher Epictetus described how people most often are disturbed not by the things that happen to them but by the opinions they have about those things.
   b. Theorists have advanced the modern interpretation of cognitive therapy.
   c. In the late 1960s, Beck conceptualized cognitive theory as a model to treat depression and anxiety and developed effective intervention strategies to restructure cognitive distortions.[5,6]
   d. Ellis developed the approach known as rational emotive therapy to recognize and challenge distorted thinking; he was particularly interested in uncovering those beliefs and assumptions that people hold as absolutes and that provide the lens (or filter of life experience) that causes distortions.[7,8]
10. Research on CBT continues to provide evidence of its broad application to both psychological (e.g., unipolar depression, generalized anxiety, panic disorder, social phobia, post-traumatic stress disorder, and childhood depressive and anxiety disorders) and physical health problems (e.g., chronic low back pain, diabetes, insomnia, tinnitus, sleep–wake disturbance in cancer patients, chronic pain, fibromyalgia, migraine headache, spinal cord injuries, and chronic fatigue syndrome).

■ EFFECTS OF COGNITION ON HEALTH AND ILLNESS

1. Stress (the perception of a threat to one's well-being, and the perception that one cannot cope) can cause physical, psychological, behavioral, and spiritual changes.
2. Both cognition (the way one thinks) and perception (the way one views, interprets, or experiences someone or something) are important to an understanding of cognitive restructuring:
   a. If individuals change the way they think (cognition), they can change their perception of the situation.
   b. If they change their perception of a situation so that they no longer view that situation as threatening, they might not experience stress.
   c. Thus, changing thoughts and perceptions can influence physiologic, psychological, behavioral, and spiritual processes.
3. Physiologic effects of stress:
   a. In response to a perceived threat (stress), the body gears up to meet the challenge.
   b. This perception of threat (stress) stimulates a cascade of biochemical events initiated by the central nervous system.
   c. Termed the fight-or-flight response[9] and later the stress response,[10] this heightened state of sympathetic arousal prepares the body for vigorous physical activity.
   d. Repeated exposure to daily hassles or prolonged stress activates the musculoskeletal system, increasing muscle tension.
   e. Concurrently, the autonomic nervous system, via the sympathetic branch, produces a generalized arousal that includes increased heart rate, blood pressure, and respiratory rate.
   f. There is a heightened awareness of the environment, shifting of blood from the visceral organs to the large muscle groups, altered lipid metabolism, and increased platelet aggregability.[10]
   g. The neuroendocrine system, in response to stimulation of the hypothalamic-pituitary-adrenal axis and the secretion of corticosteroids and mineralocorticoids, increases glucose levels, influences sodium retention, and increases the anti-inflammatory response in the acute phase.
   h. Figure 11-1, Stress Response, in Chapter 11 of the sixth edition of *Holistic Nursing: A Handbook for Practice*, depicts this cascade of events.[11]
   i. Over time, however, immune function decreases.[11,12]

j. There is evidence that levels of other hormones regulated by the neuroendocrine system, such as reproductive and growth hormones, endorphins, and encephalins, can be affected.[11]

k. More recently, chronic inflammation has been identified as one likely mechanism through which stress affects disease risk.[13]

   ▪ For example, C-reactive protein (CRP), an inflammatory marker, is emerging as a predictor of cardiovascular disease. McDade and colleagues investigated the contribution of behavioral and psychosocial factors to variation in CRP concentrations in a population-based sample of middle-aged and older adults.[14] They found that psychosocial stresses, as well as health behaviors such as smoking, waist circumference, and latency to sleep, were important predictors of an increased concentration of CRP.

l. Prolonged or repeated exposure to stress has been shown to cause or exacerbate disease or symptoms of diseases (e.g., angina, gastrointestinal complaints) and to influence pain perception in older adults.[12]

4. Psychological effects of stress:

   a. The psychological effects of stress are manifested by negative mood states such as anxiety, depression, hostility, and anger.

   b. These emotions (mood states) can, in turn, negatively influence a person's ability to concentrate and effectively problem solve.

   c. Research demonstrates the correlation between prolonged negative mood states and increased morbidity and mortality in several diseases (e.g., after bypass surgery, depressive symptoms were associated with an increase in infections, impaired wound healing, and poor emotional and physical recovery[15]).

   d. The link between optimism and health was made by researchers tracking the lives of a group of Harvard alumni who graduated in 1945; they found that individuals who were optimistic in college were healthier in later life. A more recent study found that a pessimistic explanatory style was significantly associated with a self-report of poorer physical and mental functioning 30 years later.[16]

   e. It is theorized that a pessimistic explanatory style or attitude, in addition to adversely affecting behavior, might weaken the immune system through a prolonged increase in sympathetic arousal.

   f. In addition, pessimists have more health-risking behaviors (i.e., smoking, alcohol misuse, sedentary lifestyle).

   g. Recognizing the influence of explanatory style on health and well-being furthers the understanding of how thoughts, feelings, behaviors, and physiology interact.

5. Social and behavioral effects of stress:

   a. In response to stress, people often revert to less healthy behaviors.[17,18]

   b. The social and behavioral pathway is best illustrated by appreciating the effect of behavior patterns on the incidence and progression of disease; how and what people eat, drink, and smoke, as well as how they take prescribed or illegal drugs, influence health.

   c. For many, stressful events can increase behaviors such as overeating or excessive intake of alcohol.

   d. As stress increases, self-control decreases; lapsing to behaviors that provide immediate gratification is more likely when stress is high.

   e. This inability to control health-risking behaviors as a result of increased stress is called the stress-disinhibition effect.[19]

   f. Behaviors such as social isolation that might be influenced by stress and negative thinking patterns have been shown to be associated with higher morbidity and mortality in the first year after myocardial infarction;[20] conversely, social support has been found to have a positive effect on health outcomes in medical settings.

   g. Positive health outcomes in labor and delivery appear to be affected by emotional support; the presence of a supportive woman during labor and delivery has been shown to reduce the need for C-section, shorten labor and delivery time, and reduce prenatal problems.[21]

6. Spiritual effects of stress:
   a. In response to stress, people can become disconnected from their life's meaning and purpose.
   b. In *Man's Search for Meaning*, Frankl draws a parallel between connection with life's meaning and survival when he describes the survivors of the World War II concentration camps.[22]
   c. A feeling of disconnection, in addition to being an effect of stress, can also be a precursor to stress.
   d. Several studies have examined the effects of spirituality, defined as connection with life's meaning and purpose, on health; increased scores on measures of spirituality correlated with increased incidence of health-promoting behaviors.[23]
   e. Other studies have explored the association between religious affiliation and health and have found a positive correlation.[24-26]

■ COGNITIVE BEHAVIORAL THERAPY

1. Cognitions, which are exquisitely sensitive to perception, can influence physiologic, psychological, social, behavioral, and spiritual processes.
2. Because of this influence, CBT is an important intervention in optimizing the positive links between mind, body, and spirit and in minimizing the negative consequences of adverse interactions.
3. CBT helps individuals reappraise or reevaluate their thinking; it is often referred to as cognitive restructuring because the intent of the intervention is to change or restructure the distortions in thinking patterns that cause stress.

Basic Principles of Cognitive Behavioral Therapy[27-29]

1. Our thoughts, not external events, create our moods.
2. The thoughts that create stress are usually unrealistic, distorted, and negative.
3. Distorted, illogical thoughts and self-defeating beliefs lead to physiologic changes and painful feelings, such as depression, anxiety, and anger.

4. By changing maladaptive, unrealistic, and distorted thoughts, individuals can change how they feel physically and emotionally.

Goals of Cognitive Behavioral Therapy

CBT trains clients to do the following:

1. Pinpoint the negative automatic thoughts and silent assumptions that trigger and perpetuate their emotional upsets.
2. Identify the distortions, irrational beliefs, or cognitive errors.
3. Substitute more realistic, self-enhancing thoughts, which will reduce the stress, symptoms, and painful feelings.
4. Replace self-defeating silent assumptions with more reasonable belief systems.
5. Develop improved social skills, as well as coping, communication, and empathic skills.

The Process of Cognitive Behavioral Therapy

1. CBT is a short-term intervention used to help modify habits of thinking that might be distorted, negative, or irrational.
2. In the context of CBT, cognitive restructuring is an approach or series of strategies that helps people assess their thoughts, challenge them, and replace them with more rational responses.
3. Importantly, cognitive restructuring does not deny affliction, suffering, misfortune, or negative feelings; there are many experiences in life where it is appropriate to feel angry, sad, depressed, or anxious.
4. The technique of cognitive restructuring is used to help people experience a broad range of feelings when they become "stuck" in powerful negative mood states.
5. The nurse provider serves as a guide in the process of CBT.
6. Unlike in biomedical interventions, the provider cannot perform this intervention to or for the client but guides the individual to do it for himself or herself.
7. There is no way to predict what will surface during the therapy or what meaning it will have to the individual; the nurse must honor the premise that each individual can best interpret his or her own experience(s), belief(s), and distortion(s).

The Steps of Cognitive Behavioral Therapy

1. Step 1: Awareness
   a. Developing awareness is the first step in a systematic approach to a restructuring of cognitive distortions.
   b. Clients are asked to bring to their conscious awareness two things:
      - First is an awareness of how habits of distorted, negative thinking and silent assumptions influence them physically, emotionally, behaviorally, and spiritually.
      - Second is awareness that a habit pattern (silent assumptions, irrational beliefs, and cognitive distortions) underlies these automatic negative thoughts.
   c. To facilitate development of awareness, a four-step approach is used to explore a stressful situation systematically. Clients are asked to:
      - Stop: Break the cycle of "awfulizing," escalating thoughts—become aware that a stress has taken place
      - Take a breath: Release physical tension, promote relaxation—become aware of physical changes that have occurred in response to stress
      - Reflect: Realize what is going on—become aware of automatic thoughts, distortions, beliefs, assumptions
      - Choose: Decide how to respond—become aware of choices in responding[30]
   d. Clients are first asked to identify their physical, emotional, behavioral, or spiritual warning signals of stress; in monitoring responses to a particular event, clients become more consciously aware of these cues.
   e. Clients are asked to record this information; although it might initially increase an individual's perception of physical pain or emotional discomfort, conscious awareness is a necessary first step in recognizing the relationship of thoughts, feelings, behavior, and biology to distorted thinking patterns. Often, clients have long ignored the cues their minds or bodies give them.
      - Becoming aware of these stress warning signs is the first step; attending to the cues is the next. Once they make this connection, clients can more easily develop skills to reduce negative mood states, unhealthy behaviors, and physical symptoms.
      - Becoming aware of stress warning signals is an important first step.
      - Although this seems very straightforward, the average person is often quite unaware of the effects of stress on the body-mind.
      - Once the client is aware of the effects of stress, he or she might be able to release tension more easily.
      - Clients build on this awareness as they proceed through cognitive restructuring.

Exhibit 11-1, Stress Warning Signals, provides a sample form for clients to use in identifying and recording their stress cues (see Chapter 11 in the sixth edition of *Holistic Nursing: A Handbook for Practice*).

Exhibit 11-2, Challenging Stress and Winning—Stop, Take a Breath, Reflect, Choose, provides a sample form for clients to use in identifying and recording their responses to particular events (see Chapter 11 in the sixth edition of *Holistic Nursing: A Handbook for Practice*).

2. Step 2: Automatic thoughts
   a. Once the client has been able to identify a stress or a stressful situation and identify the changes in the body-mind that accompany this stress, the next step is to identify the automatic thoughts.
   b. These thoughts usually occur automatically in response to a situation.
   c. Because these thoughts occur automatically and often are not in the conscious awareness of the individual, they are described as knee-jerk responses.
   d. Clients are taught a systematic approach to identifying these self-defeating automatic thoughts.
   e. Automatic thoughts have the following characteristics in common:
      - Reflex or knee-jerk responses to a perceived stressor
      - Usually negative; quick, fleeting, a kind of shorthand (e.g., *should, ought, never, always*)

- Usually not in our conscious awareness
- Frequently unrealistic, illogical, and distorted

f. Because these thoughts form so quickly, it is often difficult to notice that they have occurred.

g. Typically, people attribute the stress they experience or the feeling they have to the person or situation that is causing the stress.

h. By stopping, taking a breath, and asking the question, "What is going on here?" clients gradually become aware that their stress does not always come from an outside event or situation but might come from the way they interpret these events.

i. Automatic thoughts can be viewed as habits of thinking, inner dialogue, or perceptions, which in turn create the experience and influence the individual's physiology, emotions, and behaviors.

j. One of the most important and difficult tasks in cognitive restructuring is developing an awareness that these automatic thoughts occur.

k. Reasons that these reflex, knee-jerk responses are so pervasive:
- The body does not know the difference between things that are imagined and things that are actually experienced.
- People are always talking to themselves, and after they say something to themselves often enough, they begin to believe it.
- People rarely stop to question their thoughts or emotions.

l. For these reasons, clients need to be taught a structured way of exploring stress and uncovering these automatic thoughts; following is an exercise to uncover automatic thoughts, feelings, and physical responses:
- Stop: Break the cycle of escalating, awfulizing thoughts.
- Take a breath: Release physical tension, promote relaxation.
- Reflect: How do I feel physically? Emotionally? What are my automatic thoughts?

3. Step 3: Cognitive distortions

a. Once clients have learned to identify stressful situations; their physical, emotional, and behavioral responses to stress; and the automatic thoughts that precipitate the experience, the next step in the process is to teach clients to identify distortions in thinking.

b. Cognitive distortions are illogical ways of thinking that lead to adverse body-mind-spirit states; the problem is not that these thoughts are wrong or bad, but that people hold the beliefs so strongly.

c. Cognitive distortions are based on beliefs or underlying assumptions that are generally out of proportion to the situation; these beliefs or assumptions are usually long held, are based on life experience, and often are not in one's conscious awareness.

d. Burns identified 10 general categories of cognitive distortions that lead to negative emotional states:[31]
- All-or-nothing thinking
- Overgeneralization
- Mental filtering
- Disqualifying the positive
- Jumping to conclusions
- Magnification
- Emotional reasoning
- "Should" statements
- Labeling
- Personalization

e. Exaggerated, unrealistic, illogical, and distorted automatic thoughts are a result of deeply held silent assumptions and beliefs that are usually not in one's conscious awareness; a client is more likely to experience stress in any given situation if he or she holds these beliefs as absolutes.

f. Situations that are encountered are far more likely to precipitate stress if the world is viewed in terms of black or white (e.g., all good or all bad) than if there is room for shades of gray.

g. An important understanding for the clinician is that it is not the belief that needs to be examined, it is the degree to which the belief is held:
- All clients are entitled to their individual sets of beliefs.

- Assigning any value, right or wrong, to their beliefs is not in the nurse's purview; the nurse is simply inviting clients to examine their beliefs in the context of their stress and to assess whether the degree to which they hold these beliefs serves them well or contributes to stress.
    - Clients can very easily be alienated if they feel the nurse is making value judgments about their beliefs.
  h. The core concept is not to examine beliefs to decide whether they are right or wrong, but to decide whether they are practical or impractical.
  i. Some commonly held assumptions and beliefs are:[32]
    - If I treat others fairly, then I can expect them to treat me fairly.
    - I must always have the love and approval of family, friends, and peers to be worthwhile.
    - I must be unfailingly competent and perfect in all that I do.
    - My worth as a human being depends on my achievements (or intelligence or status or attractiveness).
  j. Everyone has a right to his or her beliefs and opinions; problems develop only when these beliefs are held as absolutes and therefore provide no room for flexibility in an imperfect world.
  k. Because these strongly held assumptions and beliefs are mostly silent or not in people's conscious awareness, it is a challenge to discover their existence and, consequently, their influence on people's thoughts, emotions, and behaviors.
  l. In addition to the systematic approach described to explore a stressful situation (stop, take a breath, reflect, and choose), Burns's Vertical Arrow Exercise is another technique that is helpful in discovering underlying assumptions and beliefs (see page 211 in Chapter 11 in the sixth edition of *Holistic Nursing: A Handbook for Practice*).
4. Step 4: Choosing effective coping
  a. The final step in the process of CBT is to help the client restructure or reframe distortions and beliefs and choose a more effective way of responding or coping.
  b. To accomplish this, one must recognize that stressful situations have two components, which Ells termed the practical problem and the emotional hook:
    - The practical problem is the situation at hand or the problem that needs to be addressed.
    - The emotional hook is the client's opinion about the problem or the individual(s) who have caused the problem. Quite often people respond to situations as if they can solve the problem by addressing the emotional hook.
  c. Effective coping requires that one attend to both the practical problem and the emotional hook; this sometimes requires two different approaches.
  d. Careful thought must be given to each stressful situation to choose the most effective coping strategy. The following list suggests a few ways to cope:[31]
    - Distraction: Worry about resolving a stress can be put off until the time is right. This is quite different from procrastination or denial because it is a necessary delay as opposed to avoidance.
    - Direct action: The problem can be dealt with directly to resolve it.
    - Relaxation: Using relaxation techniques to reduce emotional arousal is a way of coping with a stress that cannot be changed or avoided.
    - Reframing: Looking at a situation differently can help individuals cope. A glass filled halfway can be labeled either half full or half empty; this label changes the experience greatly.
    - Affirmations: Positive thoughts can be used to recondition one's thinking. Affirmations are a way of countering self-defeating silent assumptions.
    - Spirituality: A sense of connection to the universe, God, or a higher power, or connecting with what is important and meaningful in our life, can aid in coping with stress.
    - Catharsis: Emotional catharsis, either laughing or crying, can be very effective in relieving emotional distress.

- Journal writing: Using a journal to write about thoughts, feelings, and experiences is often helpful in processing emotions.
- Social support: Having supportive family, friends, and coworkers is important to effective coping and has been shown to contribute to stress hardiness.
- Assertive communication: Communication is an important skill to help in solving problems and reducing conflicts and stress.
- Empathy: Empathy is the ability to take into consideration the other person's perspective. It is an effective coping technique because it facilitates communication; it helps clients become better listeners.

Identifying Emotions

1. The way people feel emotionally is an important part of health.
2. Feelings of vigor, vitality, and general well-being are important correlates of health; conversely, feelings of anger, hostility, anxiety, or depression can contribute to ill health.
3. Many people find their emotions troubling, either because they are out of touch with them or because they feel overwhelmed by them.
4. Family and cultural influences have a great deal to do with the way emotions are experienced; many families and cultures do not encourage the expression of emotions, and individuals learn to ignore this aspect of their lives.
5. As individuals become aware of their body-mind-spirit responses to stress by identifying their emotional stress warning signals, they become aware of their feelings and emotions and the connection between these feelings and emotions and stress.
6. Feelings of depression, anger, fear, and guilt are all part of the human experience; however, individuals might need to be encouraged to acknowledge and honor these emotions.
7. Emotions are genuine, and people are entitled to the way they feel; on the other hand, emotions, particularly exaggerated

emotions, can interfere with effective problem solving.
8. Individuals need to be guided through the process of recognizing their emotions and the thoughts that underlie these feelings.
9. It is important to distinguish healthy fear from neurotic anxiety.
10. Thoughts underlying healthy fear are realistic, keep one alert, and warn one of dangers.
11. Neurotic anxiety is related to thoughts that are distorted and unrealistic and often contain "what ifs."
12. The nurse must guide the client in discovering the thoughts that are behind the emotion; in this way, the nurse can facilitate a process of challenging the thoughts and dealing with the emotions.
13. When feelings are ignored, denied, or suppressed, they often become intertwined with stress and clients sometimes have difficulty identifying either the emotion or the automatic thoughts related to the emotion.
14. Cognitive restructuring allows individuals to become aware of the emotions, the automatic thoughts related to a particular emotion, and the connection with stress; reflecting on these underlying themes often helps individuals to explain why they feel as they do and, in turn, to choose a more effective coping mechanism.
15. Another danger in denying feelings is that individuals can become trapped in one of these emotional states so that the mind becomes a filter, letting into conscious awareness only material that confirms or reinforces their mood; through cognitive restructuring, they can learn to reduce the frequency, length, and intensity of these feelings.
16. The nurse helps the client become aware of the relationship of these emotional themes to stress triggers and cognitive distortions through stress awareness exercises.
17. Because clients have often spent so many years ignoring their emotional cues, they sometimes have difficulty recognizing either the thoughts or the emotions that are related to stressful situations; keeping a diary or journal reflecting thoughts and feelings about stressful events has been found to be a valuable tool clients can use to identify automatic thoughts and underlying emotions.

18. In addition to understanding stressors and common themes that trigger stress, acknowledging and honoring emotions are important to a healthy sense of self.
19. Healthy self-esteem, in turn, is an important ingredient in stress hardiness or the ability to greet stressful events as challenges to be met rather than as threats to be feared.

Developing Communication Skills

1. People who have problems with communication usually experience: [33]
   a. Disparity between what they say (statement) and what they want (intent)
   b. Confusion about or resistance to stating clearly how they feel, what they want, or what they need (assertiveness); there is either a tendency to deny their own feelings (passiveness) or to be indifferent toward the feelings of others (aggressiveness)
   c. Inability to listen

Principles of Effective Communication

1. It is important to match the statement with the intention. It is important to be clear. Matching statements with intentions is an art and a skill; it requires that individuals recognize their automatic thoughts, emotions, and cognitive distortions and take responsibility for their part of the conversation.
2. Effective communication requires one to be assertive. An assertive statement expresses one's feelings and opinions and reaffirms one's identity and rights; it is not judgmental.
   a. The general format of an assertive statement is "I feel [label the emotion] when you [label the behavior] because [provide an explanation]." The formula requires that all three elements be included.
   b. Cognitive restructuring facilitates assertive communication because it requires clients to identify their thoughts and feelings.
3. Effective communication takes practice as well as patience with oneself and with others.

Developing Empathy Skills

1. Empathy can be facilitated through active listening. This technique requires conscious, nonjudgmental awareness; it helps to clarify the issues involved and can deescalate many emotional exchanges.
2. Rogers suggested using the phrase "You sound [emotion] about [situation]" as a way to facilitate communication and gain awareness of another person's perspective. [34]
3. Instead of becoming hooked by a defensive emotional reaction, clients can learn to operate from empathy using the four-step approach: Stop, take a breath, reflect, choose.

Active Listening

1. When a client uses the skill of active listening the other person often feels heard, which can help to defuse further emotional arousal and defensive behavior; in addition, he or she now has an opportunity to clarify any misunderstanding.
2. Active listening allows the client to buy time to obtain a better perspective on what the other person is thinking and feeling; clients can then choose how they want to respond. This can be a time to use assertive communication or problem solving or a time to step away from the interaction until emotions and defenses have settled.
3. Active listening allows reflective, empathic, objective, and nonjudgmental communication.
4. Coaching clients to use cognitive restructuring skills that include active listening techniques facilitates effective communication, in turn reducing conflict and stress.
5. Acceptance is facing the fact that some situations or people cannot be changed or avoided and letting go of resentment. Forgiveness is often a part of acceptance.
6. Coping successfully means gaining the wisdom to achieve the delicate balance between acceptance and action, between letting go and taking control. It is the art of choosing the right strategy at the right time.
7. When clients feel that they can cope effectively, the harmful effects of stress are buffered; the situation is perceived not as a threat but as a challenge. This subtle difference has profound physiologic, psychological, behavioral, and spiritual effects and allows people facing great adversity (such as illness) to see the opportunity the situation presents.

8. Clients need to recognize that coping is the art of finding a balance between acceptance and action, between letting go and taking control.
9. Cognitive restructuring helps clients distinguish these differences by providing a format for observing or objectifying their experiences; in so doing, they gain a sense of control that minimizes or buffers the harmful effects of stress.

■ COGNITIVE BEHAVIORAL THERAPY IN CHILDREN AND ADOLESCENTS

1. CBT is an effective treatment modality for children and adolescents, but it is modified to take into consideration the unique developmental needs of this population. The same basic principles discussed previously are applied, but factors such as cognitive, social, and emotional maturity are taken into consideration.
2. Adults can reflect on their thought processes, identify their responses to stressful situations, and develop alternative strategies; children often do not have the capacity for this mental activity.
3. Families and school personnel should also be included in the treatment plan, to promote continuity and support across the environments where children spend most of their time.[35]
4. Children and youth are less likely to identify a need for treatment; a critical factor in implementing CBT is engaging them in treatment interventions that are fun and build on their specific interests and strengths.

Techniques for Working with the Younger Child[35]

1. To help children identify the somatic manifestations of anxiety, have them trace their body shape on a large piece of paper and then color the areas where they might feel different when they are anxious.
2. Read children's books that discuss different emotions.
3. Create a reward list (tangible or social) based on the child's interests and developmental level.

4. Actively include family members in the treatment plan so that they can gradually integrate strategies into the family's routine.

Techniques for Working with Adolescents

1. Make a collage from teen magazines with images that display different emotional states.
2. Invite the youth to participate by using examples from the teen's life (e.g., interest in a sport or other activity).
3. Provide age-appropriate rewards.

■ APPLICATION OF THE GENERAL PRINCIPLES OF CBT

1. CBT is most useful for individuals, not for relationship problems or interpersonal conflict.[36]
2. The nurse must be imaginative and tenacious; CBT requires constant shifting between technique and process.
3. The therapy combines problem resolution using cognitive and behavioral techniques with empathic focus on the client's feelings.
4. The process requires the skills of presence, intention, and communication.
5. Several attempts and several different ways of looking at a situation can be required before a client recognizes the automatic thoughts and underlying beliefs involved.
6. CBT can be used in both inpatient and outpatient settings, but the goals and process are different in these settings:
   a. Outpatient goals are generally to restructure cognitive distortions to enhance a variety of self-management skills and healthy lifestyle behaviors, which in turn help to promote health, reduce symptoms, or manage illness. Outpatient CBT can be provided either individually or in a group.
   b. Inpatient goals are typically confined to assisting the patient to cope more effectively with those stresses that arise during hospitalization for an acute illness; in this context, the nurse must remember that he or she is viewing the patient from a cross-sectional perspective (through one episode in the continuum of the patient's life).

- Patients brought to this hospital experience a reliance on long-standing coping styles—some adaptive, some maladaptive, and many influenced by cognitive distortions; in view of the short hospital stay and critical needs during this time, long-standing maladaptive coping patterns are best left to be addressed after discharge from the hospital.

- In the hospital, CBT can be integrated into communications that occur each day. Each interaction can be an occasion to assist patients in identifying the relationship of thoughts, feelings, and behaviors to biology as it applies to their current symptoms and illness.

- The nurse can utilize the structure of CBT to assist the patient in identifying distorted thinking patterns and realistically appraising the situation as well as in seeing opportunity in adversity. Thus, the patient can often choose a more realistic and less stressful way to view the situation. This, in turn, can decrease physical and emotional symptoms.

- Hospitalization can be a time of opportunity despite its difficulties; because hospitalization usually occurs when individuals are in need or crisis, they often feel vulnerable and might be more open to exploring different ways of thinking. They might be more open to discussing the role that negative thoughts, pessimism, and stress play in their illness or the role that enhanced self-management skills would play in promoting wellness.

7. The holistic nurse integrates CBT to support clients at all stages of health. (See Chapter 11 in the sixth edition of *Holistic Nursing: A Handbook for Practice* for a description of the holistic caring process.)

■ NOTES

1. Engel, G. (1980). The clinical application of the biopsychosocial model. *American Journal of Psychiatry, 137,* 535–544.

2. Stuart, E. M. (1989). Spirituality in health and healing: A clinical program. *Holistic Nursing Practice, 3,* 35–36.

3. Beck, A. T. (1961). A systematic investigation of depression. *Comprehensive Psychiatry, 2,* 163–170.

4. Benson, H., & Stuart, E. M. (1993). *The wellness book: A comprehensive guide to maintaining health and treating stress-related illness.* New York, NY: Fireside, Simon & Schuster.

5. Beck, A. T. (1979). *Cognitive therapy.* New York, NY: New American Library.

6. Beck, A. (2000). *Prisoners of hate: The cognitive basis of anger, hostility and violence.* New York, NY: Harper Collins.

7. Ellis, A. (1962). *Reason and emotion in psychotherapy.* New York, NY: Lyle Stuart.

8. Ellis, A. (2000). A critique of the theoretical contributions of nondirective therapy. *Journal of Clinical Psychology, 56,* 897–905. (Original work published in 1948 *Journal of Clinical Psychology, 4,* 248–255)

9. Cannon, W. B. (1914). The emergency function of the adrenal medulla in pain and the major emotions. *American Journal of Physiology, 33,* 356–372.

10. Selye, H. (1982). Handbook of stress: Theoretical and clinical aspects. In L. Goldberger & S. Breznitz (Eds.), *History and present status of stress concept* (pp. 7–20). New York, NY: Free Press.

11. Bartol, G. M., & Courts, N. F. (2005). The psychophysiology of bodymind healing. In B. Dossey, C. Guzetta, & L. Keegan (Eds.), *Holistic nursing: A handbook for practice* (pp. 111–133). Sudbury, MA: Jones and Bartlett.

12. Graham, J. E., Robles, T. F., Kiecolt-Glaser, J. K., Malarkey, W. B., Bissell, M.G., & Glaser, R. (2006). Hostility and pain are related to inflammation in older adults. *Brain, Behavior, and Immunity, 20,* 389–400.

13. Ranjit, N., Diez-Roux, A. V., Shea, S., Cushman, M., Seeman, T., Jackson, S. A., & Ni, H. (2007). Psychosocial factors and inflammation in the multi-ethnic study of atherosclerosis. *Archives of Internal Medicine, 167,* 174–181.

14. McDade, T. W., Hawkley, L. C., & Cacioppo, J. T. (2006). Psychosocial and behavioral predictors of inflammation in middle-aged and older adults: The Chicago Health, Aging, and Social Relations Study. *Psychosomatic Medicine, 68,* 376–381.

15. Doering, L. V., Moser, D. K., Lemankiewicz, W., Luper, C., & Khan, S. (2005). Depression, healing, and recovery from coronary artery bypass surgery. *American Journal of Critical Care, 14,* 316–324.

16. Maruta, T., Colligan, R. C., Malinchoc, M., & Offord, K. P. (2002). Optimism-pessimism assessed in the 1960s and self-reported health status 30 years later. *Mayo Clinic Proceedings, 77,* 748–753.

17. Steptoe, A., Wright, C., Kunz-Ebrecht, S. R., & Iliffe, S. (2006). Dispositional optimism and health behaviour in community-dwelling older

people: Associations with healthy ageing. *British Journal of Health Psychology, 11,* 71–84.

18. Steptoe, A., Wardle, J., Pollard, T. M., Canaan, L., & Davies, J. G. (1996). Stress, social support and health-related behavior: A study of smoking, alcohol consumption and physical exercise. *Journal of Psychosomatic Research, 41,* 171–180.

19. Marlatt, G. (1985). Relapse prevention: Theoretical rationale and overview of the mode. In G. Marlatt & J. Gordon (Eds.), *Relapse prevention* (pp. 280–350). New York, NY: Guilford.

20. Lesperance, F., & Frasure-Smith, N. (2007). Depression and heart disease. *Cleveland Clinic Journal of Medicine, 74*(Suppl. 1), S63–S66.

21. Hodnett, E. D., Gates, S., Hofmeyr, G. J., & Sakala, C. (2003). Continuous support for women during childbirth. *Cochrane Database of Systematic Reviews, 2,* CD003766.

22. Frankl, V. (1963). *Man's search for meaning.* Boston, MA: Beacon Press.

23. Harvey, I. S., & Silverman, M. (2007). The role of spirituality in the self-management of chronic illness among older Africans and whites. *Journal of Cross-Cultural Gerontology, 22,* 205–220.

24. Masters, K. S., & Spielmans, G. I. (2007). Prayer and health: Review, meta-analysis, and research agenda. *Journal of Behavioral Medicine, 30*(4), 329–338.

25. Curlin, F. A., Sellergren, S. A., Lantos, J. D., & Chin, M. H. (2007). Physicians' observations and interpretations of the influence of religion and spirituality on health. *Archives of Internal Medicine, 167,* 649–654.

26. Yuen, E. J. (2007). Spirituality, religion, and health. *American Journal of Medical Quality, 22,* 77–79.

27. Burns, D. D. (1999). *The new mood therapy.* New York, NY: William Morrow Paperbacks.

28. Childress, A. R., & Burns, D. D. (1981). The basics of cognitive therapy. *Psychosomatics, 22,* 1017–1027.

29. Webster, A. (1993). How thoughts affect health. In H. Benson & E. Stuart (Eds.), *The wellness book.* New York, NY: Fireside, Simon & Schuster.

30. Stuart, E., Webster, A., & Wells-Federman, C. (1993). Coping and problem solving. In H. Benson & E. Stuart (Eds.), *The wellness book.* New York, NY: Fireside, Simon & Schuster.

31. Burns, D. (1989). *The feeling good handbook: Using the new mood therapy in everyday life.* New York, NY: William Morrow.

32. Ellis, A. (1999). *How to make yourself happy and remarkably less disturbable.* Lafayette, CO: Impact Publishers.

33. Caudill, M. A. (2008). *Managing pain before it manages you* (3rd ed.). New York, NY: Guilford Press.

34. Rogers, C. (1951). *Client-centered therapy.* Boston, MA: Houghton Mifflin.

35. Kingery, J. N., Roblek, T. L., Suveg, C., Grover, R. L., Sherrill, J. T., & Bergman, R. L. (2006). They're not just "little adults": Developmental considerations for implementing cognitive-behavioral therapy with anxious youth. *Journal of Cognitive Psychotherapy: An International Quarterly, 20,* 263–273.

36. Burns, D. D. (1993). *Ten days to self-esteem.* New York, NY: William Morrow.

■ STUDY QUESTIONS

Basic Level

1. Which of the following choices would be appropriate for a nurse to say to a person during an anxiety attack?
   a. "Why are you acting so anxious?"
   b. "Calm down. There's nothing to get upset about."
   c. "I will stay with you."
   d. "If you don't watch out, you will lose control again."

2. What is the primary focus of cognitive behavioral therapy?
   a. Providing psychoeducation related to etiology and treatment of the illness
   b. Identifying the interplay of maladaptive behavioral, emotional, and cognitive responses
   c. Modifying maladaptive behaviors through operant conditioning
   d. Identifying the interplay of maladaptive behaviors and unresolved instinctual urges

3. Which of the following answer choices best describes the causes of stress?
   a. Real or perceived threat to one's well being
   b. Unconscious thoughts of harm
   c. Unreliable family and friends
   d. Uncontrollable events

4. CBT is considered effective treatment for which of the following?
   a. Anxiety and depressive disorders
   b. Schizophrenia
   c. Suicidal ideation
   d. Bipolar disorder

5. Physiologic effects of stress include which of the following?
   a. Increase in immune response
   b. Decreased awareness of the environment
   c. Decrease in muscle tension
   d. Increase in heart rate, blood pressure, and respiratory rate

Advanced Level

6. What is the first step in a systematic approach to guide clients to a restructuring of their cognitive distortion should be pulled up cognitive distortions?
   a. Developing awareness
   b. Choosing effective coping
   c. Identifying automatic thoughts
   d. Identifying cognitive distortions

7. When a person reframes his or her way of thinking, which of the following is an appropriate question to ask?
   a. Why me?
   b. Is this thought helpful?
   c. If I treat others fairly, shouldn't they do the same to me?
   d. Why does this always happen to me?

8. What must a person attend to for effective coping?
   a. Both the practical problem and the emotional hook
   b. Only the emotions surrounding the problem
   c. Solving the problem immediately
   d. Avoidance of relaxation techniques until the problem is dealt with

9. To break the cycle of escalating negative thoughts, what is a client asked to do?
   a. Take a breath, stop, reflect, and journal.
   b. Choose how to respond and then reflect on how that choice worked.
   c. Stop, breathe, reflect, and choose a coping method.
   d. Cope as usual and reflect on effectiveness.

10. When developing an affirmation, a client is guided to do which of the following?
   a. Explore the literature.
   b. Formulate a goal.
   c. Join a support group.
   d. Focus on the stress and determine how it was handled in the past.

11. Cognitive behavioral therapy would be most useful for which of the following people?
   a. A married couple experiencing relationship problems
   b. A middle-aged man having problems with his boss
   c. A 25-year-old woman experiencing negative thoughts about her abilities
   d. A single mother experiencing difficulty with her adolescent son

12. The AHN-BC has been called to the surgical ICU to evaluate Mrs. Hall, a 63-year-old woman who just learned she is living with colon cancer. What can CBT provide for Mrs. Hall?
   a. A diversion for her stress
   b. An opportunity to cognitively restructure her distorted thinking
   c. Emotional freedom
   d. An opportunity to discuss her fears

Chapter 13

Self-Reflection

Jennifer L. Reich and
Jackie D. Levin

■ DEFINITIONS

Consciousness Information in the form of pattern and meaning.

Deliberative mutual patterning Coparticipative process of nurse with client patterning and/or repatterning the unified human-environmental fields to promote health and inner coherence as the client defines it.

Habitual patterning Automatic noncritical responses to thoughts, feelings, situations, and ideas.

Inner coherence Internal harmony, synchronization, and order in a system.

Intention Focusing attention from a place of conscious awareness.

Mind-body-spirit complex Integrated unified aspects of being human.

Pattern appraisal/appreciation Continuous process of recognizing the manifestation of the human and environmental fields as they are expressed.

Reflective practice Continuous mutual process of inner awareness/self-reflection of internal and external pattern manifestation as it is occurring.

Self A principle that underlies and organizes subjective experience.

Self-centering Practice of coming into balance, aware of the forces that are pulling us one way and then the other.

Self-reflection Inner awareness of our thoughts, feelings, judgments, beliefs, and perceptions.

Unknowing A state of being that is open to not-knowing.

■ THEORY AND RESEARCH

Nursing Theory Related to Self-Reflection

1. Self-reflection is both a self-care and a therapeutic clinical practice that integrates the critical thinking mind with the intelligent compassion of the heart.[1-3]
2. Self-reflection is a skill that requires focus and practice to develop inner awareness of one's thoughts, feelings, sensations, judgments, and perceptions.
3. As a practice, self-reflection requires the holistic nurse to face his or her inner self with honesty, compassion, curiosity, and humor; for without this practice, we can become captive to our own and others' habitual perceptions and automatic responses.
4. Self-reflection is highlighted in the *Holistic Nursing: Scope and Standards of Practice* under Practice Standards and Self-Care Standards,[4] acknowledging its acceptance as not only for personal awareness, but for clinical awareness as well.
5. Self-reflection is an act of service. The time spent observing one's thoughts and beliefs prepares the nurse for the safe and deep relationship to self and others.

Research

1. Nursing theory, integral to self-reflection, is incorporated in theories at all levels on the ladder of abstraction.
   a. Elizabeth Barrett's Power Theory formulates that "power is the capacity to participate knowingly in change."[5p48]
   b. Self-reflection also consists of appraising "four inseparable dimensions—awareness, choices, freedom to act intentionally, and involvement in creating change."[5p49]
2. Barbara Dossey developed her Theory of Integral Nursing (TIN) as praxis, theory in action.[6] (See Chapter 1 in the sixth edition of the *Holistic Nursing: A Handbook for Practice*.)
   a. One component of TIN is represented in a model with four quadrants. Each of the quadrants, the "I" individual interior (personal/intentional), the "It" individual exterior (objective, behavioral), the "We" (collective interior), and the "Its" (collective exterior), formulate how we view and describe our reality. Dossey explains that the development of the "I," or self-awareness, is critical to becoming a healthy nurse.
3. Margaret Newman's Theory of Health as Expanding Consciousness (HEC) defines "consciousness as the *information* of the system: The capacity of the [human] system to interact with the environment [system]."[7p33]
   a. Health is not defined by the presence or the absence of disease, but rather by the transformation through chaos to a higher order of complexity and understanding.
   b. Chaos brings uncertainty, which is a component of unknowing pattern appreciation essential to the practice self-reflection in action.
4. Jean Watson expresses that a caring science perspective is rooted in a relational ontology of being-in-relation, with unity and connectedness composing the worldview.
   a. Caring science embraces multiple approaches to inquiry and is open to exploring other ways of knowing such as aesthetic, poetic, personal, intuitive, and spiritual among others.[8]
   b. Self-reflection as a process can assist the holistic nurse to access these realms.
5. Martha Roger's Science of Unitary Human Beings (SUHB) describes several important concepts essential to self-reflection.
   a. The concepts of wholeness and openness regard the person as an "irreducible, indivisible, multidimensional (now called pandimensionality) energy field identified by pattern and manifesting characteristics that are specific to the whole and which cannot be predicted from the knowledge of its parts."[9p7]

Examples of reflective practice in action can be found in Chapter 12 in the sixth edition of the *Holistic Nursing: A Handbook for Practice*.

Self-Reflection Strategies

1. Dreams: Dreams often represent parts of ourselves that are still hidden from our conscious awareness. The messages are presented through metaphor and symbols. With reflective practice, the nurse can begin to decode the messages for growth and self-understanding. Using dreamwork as a self-reflective practice:
   a. Keep a journal or notebook by your bed.
   b. Upon waking, remain in the same position to remember your dream.
   c. Write down the dream or parts of the dream.
   d. Circle words, phrases, numbers, animals, characters, and the overall feelings that have significance to/for you.
   e. Reflect on how these images have meaning to your current life.
2. Exercise and physical activity
   a. Exercise can be a pathway to self-reflection.
   b. Physical activity has both physiologic benefits and mental health benefits.
   c. Some exercise practices combine breath work, meditation, and physical movement to deepen awareness of the present moment.
3. Reflective writing
   a. Reflective writing can take many forms.
      - For example: Poetry and story writing, journaling
   b. Journaling can be a tool for recording creative ideas and insights.
      - Can help nursing students understand relationships between theory and practice.[10]

4. Storytelling
   a. Stories are a human experience that help us receive information as well as create meaning and structure around it.[11]
   b. Listeners of story can transcend normal waking consciousness and change their experience of reality.
      - Storytelling trance[12]

See pages 257–258 in *Holistic Nursing: Handbook for Practice* (6th edition) for a Case example: Diane's Story.

5. Listening, metaphors, and images
   a. Listening occurs on multiple levels simultaneously.
   b. Three basic levels of listening are:
      - Listening to the person's words from your point of view or beliefs
      - Listening deeply to words without judgment
      - Listening to the greater environmental field of language and messages beyond the words
   c. When listening on all depths simultaneously, one is tuning into body language, tone, pace, and the metaphoric and symbolic language as well as to synchronistic events occurring in the environment.
   d. A metaphor is the use of one image, word, or phrase to represent something else. This level of listening requires the holistic nurse to entrain herself to the unity of experience in the mutual process of pattern appreciation and pattern recognition.
6. The medicine walk
   a. The medicine walk is an indigenous practice of going into nature with a question or intention for insight into a problem or personal dynamic. The medicine walk involves three phases:
      - *Preparation* readies the individual for the coming journey within the context of a supportive community.
      - *Solo time* involves going out on the medicine walk. The individual takes a walk by himself or herself with a particular focus, intention, or question.
      - *Returning to community* is done through sharing the story of the walk. The story, witnessed by trusted others or through journaling, can be told in first or third person.

See instructions and a case example of the Mini Medicine Walk (on pages 256 in Chapter 12 of the sixth edition of *Holistic Nursing: Handbook for Practice*).

7. Mindfulness meditation
   a. Mindfulness is moment-to-moment awareness, and mindfulness meditation is the practice of being awake and aware of one's breaths, thoughts, feelings, and sensations as they occur.
      - Formal practice
         - Locating a quiet place where one can spend 20 minutes undisturbed and focus on breathing.
         - When the mind wanders from the breath, the individual notices where it has gone to, like "memory, future, thought, sensation, idea," and brings it back to the breath.
      - Informal practice
         - Using everyday activities to practice mindfulness such as when washing the dishes, simply attending to the sensations of soap on the hands, sponge working against the surface of the pot, and the temperature of the water.
         - The individual softly smiles and allows the moment to be experienced with a sense of joy and restfulness.

■ NOTES

1. Asselin, M. E. (2011). Reflective narrative: A tool for learning through practice. *Journal for Nurses in Staff Development, 27*(1), 2–6.
2. Forniers, S. G., & Peden-McAlpine, C. (2007). Evaluation of a reflective learning intervention to improve critical thinking in novice nurses. *Journal of Advanced Nursing, 57*(4), 410–421.
3. Siegel, D. (2010). *Mindsight: The new science of personal transformation.* New York, NY: Bantam Books.
4. American Holistic Nurses Association & American Nurses Association. (2007). *Holistic nursing: Scope and standards of practice.* Silver Spring, MD: Nursebooks.org.
5. Barrett, E. (2010). Power as knowing participation in change: What's new and what's next. *Nursing Science Quarterly, 23*(1), 47–54.
6. Dossey, B. M. (2009). Integral and holistic nursing. In B. M. Dossey & L. Keegan (Eds.), *Holistic nursing: A handbook for practice* (5th ed., pp. 3–46). Sudbury, MA: Jones and Bartlett.

7. Newman, M. A. (1994). *Health as expanding consciousness*. New York, NY: National League for Nursing Press.

8. Watson, J. (n.d.). Caring science: Ten caritas processes. Watson Caring Science Institute. Retrieved from http://www.watsoncaringscience.org/index.cfm/category/61/10-caritas-processes.cfm

9. Rogers, M. (1992). Nursing science and the space age. *Nursing Science Quarterly, 5*(1), 34.

10. Van Horn, R., & Freed, S. (2008). Journaling and dialogue pairs to promote reflection in clinical nursing education. *Nursing Education Research, 29*(4), 220–225.

11. Smith, M. C. (1992). Metaphor in nursing theory. *Nursing Science Quarterly, 5*(2), 48–49.

12. Sturm, B. (1999). The enchanted imagination: Storytelling's power to entrance listeners. *School Library Media Research, 2*. Retrieved from http://www.ala.org/ala/mgrps/divs/aasl/aaslpubsandjournals/slmrb/slmrcontents/volume21999/vol2sturm.cfm

■ STUDY QUESTIONS

Basic Level

1. Self-reflection is inherent in all of the following nursing theories except which one?
   a. Story Theory
   b. Science of Unitary Human Beings
   c. Theory of Integral Nursing
   d. Theory of Dynamic Transformation

2. Which of the following answer choices best represents how Margaret Newman's theory defines health?
   a. The capacity to participate knowingly in change
   b. Transformation through chaos to a higher order of complexity and understanding
   c. Being-in-relation, with unity and connectedness composing the worldview
   d. The person as an irreducible, indivisible, and multidimensional energy field

3. Which of the following exercises is usually not part of a self-reflection practice?
   a. Mindfulness meditation
   b. Medicine walk
   c. Physical exercise and movement
   d. Carefree jogging

4. Which of the following terms is defined as "focusing attention from a place of conscious awareness"?
   a. Reflective practice
   b. Self-centering
   c. Intention
   d. Patterning

5. Which of the following choices best describes habitual patterning?
   a. A coparticipative process
   b. Automatic noncritical responses
   c. Pausing to reflect on thoughts and feelings
   d. Unknowing

Advanced Level

6. In which of the following answers is the holistic nurse using Barrett's Power as Knowing Participation in Change Theory to respond to a patient's request for help with stress?
   a. The holistic nurse gives the patient a prescription for meditation.
   b. The holistic nurse first listens to the patient describe her experience of stress.
   c. The holistic nurse recognizes that the patient and nurse are in the We quadrant of the theory.
   d. The holistic nurse refers the patient to a dream therapist.

7. The holistic nurse comprehends which of the following to be an aspect of *inner coherence*?
   a. Information in the form of pattern and meaning
   b. Internal harmony, synchronization, and order in a system
   c. A state of being that is open to not-knowing
   d. A principle that underlies and organizes subjective experience

8. A holistic nurse is assessing a 35-year-old first-time mother who is worried about breastfeeding. Which of the following answer choices demonstrates that the nurse is using holistic pattern knowing and appreciation?
   a. The nurse is aware that older first-time mothers commonly have difficulty breastfeeding, so she teaches the mother a breastfeeding technique.
   b. The nurse tells the mother a story about when she had difficulty breastfeeding her own daughter.
   c. The nurse leaves the room to get the breastfeeding expert on the unit.
   d. The nurse is aware that the mother's worry is the manifested aspects of the person and there are underlying unseen patterns contributing to this emotion.

9. All of the following are part of a self-reflective practice except which one?
   a. Writing down a dream and looking for symbolic meanings
   b. Choosing a question to focus on while walking in the park
   c. Informing another nurse that her technique for leading the support group could use more quiet time
   d. Being present to another's story and listening to the meanings beneath the words

10. How does the reflective practitioner become the therapeutic milieu?
    a. By modeling spaciousness and coherence
    b. By fostering a sense of dependence
    c. By writing a story about his own fears
    d. By sharing personal belief systems

Chapter 14

Nutrition

Karen Avino and Susan Luck

Original Author: Susan Luck

■ DEFINITIONS

Antioxidants Substances that limit free radical formation and damage by stabilizing or deactivating free radicals before they attack cells.

Diabesity A popular term for the common clinical association of type 2 diabetes mellitus and obesity.

Epigenetics The study of changes produced in gene expression caused by mechanisms other than changes in the underlying DNA sequence.

Free radicals Electrically charged molecules with an unpaired electron capable of attacking healthy cells in the body, causing them to lose their structure and function.

Glycemic index An index that classifies carbohydrate foods according to their glycemic response (effect on blood glucose levels), which varies with fiber content, starch structure, food processing, and presence of proteins and fats.

HDL High-density lipoprotein form of cholesterol associated with reduced risk of atherosclerosis.

Homocysteine An amino acid found in the blood and intermediate product of methionine metabolism.

Leptin A peptide hormone neurotransmitter produced by fat cells and involved in the regulation of appetite.

LDL Low-density lipoprotein form of cholesterol strongly associated with increased risk of atherosclerosis.

Metabolic syndrome A collection of heart disease risk factors that increase the chance of developing heart disease, stroke, and diabetes. The condition is also known by other names including Syndrome X and cardiometabolic and insulin resistance syndrome.

Mineral An inorganic trace element or compound that works in synergy with other compounds and is essential for human life.

Nutrigenomics The study of the effects of foods and food constituents on gene expression. It is about how our DNA is transcribed into mRNA and then to proteins and provides a basis for understanding the biological activity of food components.

Nutraceuticals Food, or parts of food, that provide medical or health benefits, including the prevention and treatment of disease.

Obesogens Identifiable industrial pollutants contributing to the obesity epidemic by increasing fat cells in the body and altering metabolism and feelings of hunger and fullness.

Optimal nutrition Adequate intake of nutrients for health promotion and disease prevention.

Organic food Food from plants and animals that have been grown without the use of synthetic fertilizers or pesticides and without antibiotics, growth hormones, and feed additives.

Phytochemicals Biologically active compounds found in foods and plants.

Phytoestrogens Compounds found in plants that have some estrogenic or antiestrogenic activity.

Probiotic Formulation containing beneficial living microorganisms that maintain health as part of the internal ecology of the digestive tract.

Vitamin An organic substance necessary for normal growth, metabolism, and development of the body; acts as a catalyst and coenzyme, assisting in many chemical reactions while nourishing the body.

Xenoestrogens Synthetic, environmental, hormone-mimicking compounds found in many pesticides, drugs, plastics, and personal care products.

■ THEORY AND RESEARCH

1. Dietary habits play a role in almost all health problems, including inflammation and pain, digestive and gastrointestinal disturbances, allergies and food sensitivities, fatigue, mood disorders, and immune dysfunction.
2. Many foods produced today are processed and denatured, depleted of nutrients, and often contain toxic chemicals including additives, preservatives, pesticides, hormones, and antibiotics. The changes to our food supply contribute to a rising number of chronic health issues including learning disabilities, obesity, diabetes, atherosclerosis, heart disease, hypertension, immune and autoimmune diseases, and various cancers.[1] A nurse's role is to coach and educate individuals and communities in nutrition and lifestyle changes that affect long-term health goals and health policy.
3. Current research supports healthful dietary patterns, such as the Mediterranean diet, which includes whole grains, legumes, nuts, vegetables, fruits, olive oil, and fish and is associated with a decrease in chronic disease and death from all causes. The harmful

effects of trans and certain saturated fats, refined carbohydrates, high-fructose corn syrup, and many food additives are well documented in the medical literature.

Current Health Crisis

1. In 2009, the American Heart Association, the Centers for Disease Control and Prevention, and the National Institutes of Health reported the economic costs of cardiovascular disease and stroke in the United States was estimated at $475.3 billion and nutrition's relationship to chronic disease includes metabolic syndrome, obesity, and diabetes.[2]
2. Obesity and metabolic syndrome affect cardiovascular pathologies and are characterized by visceral obesity, insulin resistance, hypertension, chronic inflammation, and thrombotic disorders contributing to endothelial dysfunction and to accelerated atherosclerosis.
3. Studies suggest that weight loss is the key to reduce diabetes risk and that sugar intake significantly contributes to ill health and increases triglycerides and cholesterol levels.
4. Hypertriglyceridemia is a common lipid abnormality in persons with visceral obesity, metabolic syndrome, and type 2 diabetes.
5. Obesity is a contributing cause of heart disease, stroke, diabetes, and some types of cancer, the leading causes of death in the United States. Obesity health risks include sleep apnea, asthma and breathing problems, limited mobility, inflammation, early deterioration of joints leading to arthritis, osteoporosis and hip fractures, and pregnancy problems.
6. Children of obese parents are at a higher risk for obesity.[3]

Emerging Research in the Study of Obesity

1. Environmental toxins, or *obesogens*, are stored in fat tissue and can influence and interfere with healthy fat cell signaling and metabolism. Overeating can interfere with cell signaling messengers that control feelings of satiety after eating. For healthy fat metabolism, leptin maintains normal body weight, energy expenditure, and glucose homeostasis by reducing appetite and

stimulating fat burning. There is a relationship between leptin and perceived hunger, and in obesity leptin resistance develops, making losing weight increasingly difficult.

2. Fat regulates how the body burns fuel for energy used by muscle. Adiponectin is produced to curb appetite and burn fat; obese individuals have an adiponectin deficiency. Adipokines encourage the inflammatory response, which further affects fat metabolism and homeostasis.[4] Weight loss is associated with reduced inflammation systemically.[4] The obesogen hypothesis proposes that perturbations in metabolic signaling that result from exposure to environmental chemicals known as endocrine disruptors, and stored in the body's adipose tissue, exacerbate the effects of imbalances, resulting in obesity.[5]

3. Effective health promotion programs include awareness practices, exercise, behavioral motivation for change, and nutrition education. An individual's metabolism, environment, genetics, emotional health, social networks, life stressors, and culture must be considered in evaluating nutritional needs and nutritional goals.

4. Without proper nutrient synergy and healthy cellular communication, the end result is diminished function that often results in decreased energy output, inflammation, and lowered immune response. Essential macronutrients and micronutrients include carbohydrates, proteins, fats, vitamins, and minerals, and essential fatty acids.

Food as Energy

1. In a nutrient-deficient diet, on a molecular level, enzymes become depleted, and then eventually change the cells. Overt signs and symptoms appear, but routine laboratory tests do not uncover nutritional deficiencies. Undiagnosed nutrient deficiencies over many years leave the body more vulnerable to illnesses to which the individual might be genetically predisposed and to immune system compromise.

2. The Nurses' Health Study found that a low-carbohydrate diet high in vegetables and with a larger proportion of proteins and oils coming mostly from plant sources decreases mortality. In contrast, a low-carbohydrate diet with largely animal sources of protein and fat increases mortality.[6]

An Integrative Functional Health Model

The Integrative Functional Health Model (IFHM) is a unique nursing model that expands on the functional medicine model, and views health and balance as a dynamic interaction and interconnectedness between the individual and his or her environment.

Foundations of a Nurse-Based Functional Health Model

1. Interconnectedness: Includes the mind, body, and spiritual dimensions of physiologic factors.

2. Energy field principles and dynamics: An understanding of how thoughts, stress, toxic environments, and a nutrient-deficient diet can disrupt human energy fields, impair optimal functioning, and contribute to disease.

3. Patient-centeredness: Honors and emphasizes the individual's unique history, beliefs, and story rather than a medical diagnosis and disease orientation.

4. Biochemical individuality: Recognizes the importance of variations in metabolic function that derive from unique genetic and environmental vulnerabilities and strengths among individuals.

5. Health on a wellness continuum: Views health as a dynamic balance on multiple levels and seeks to identify, restore, and support our innate reserve as the means to enhance well-being and healing throughout the life cycle.

6. Optimization of our internal and external healing environments: Holds the worldview that human health is the microcosm of the macrocosm in the web of life.

Overview of Clinical Nutrition

Changes to the U.S. food supply contribute to health problems including atherosclerosis, heart disease, hypertension, diabetes, and various cancers. Basic essential nutrient requirements are unavailable for healthy cell signaling and to meet the demands and needs of people throughout the various stages of life, beginning with prenatal development and continuing into old age.

The Standard American Diet

1. Nutrient deficiencies most often result from a high intake of processed and refined foods.
2. The American Heart Association (2009) report estimated that an adult consumes 22 teaspoons of sugar per day; and teens eat 34 teaspoons of sugar and high-fructose corn syrup each day. [7] Fructose is metabolized primarily in the liver, which favors the formation of fats and results in elevated triglycerides, with increased risk of metabolic syndrome.
3. The standard American diet (SAD) consists of refined products such as white bread and white rice, deficient in 28 essential nutrients including essential vitamins (in particular the B vitamins), minerals, protein, and fiber, all contained in the whole grain prior to processing.

Clinical Nutrition Research

1. The American Heart Association recommends pharmaceutical-grade omega-3 essential fatty acids (EFAs) to prevent heart disease and stroke and lower triglycerides. It is recommended in the treatment of arthritis, diabetes, obesity, cancer, immune and autoimmune disorders, cognitive function, and a variety of women's health problems.[8]
2. Mortality rates for certain cancers and cardiovascular disease are higher among those who consume the standard American diet than among those who consume Asian, Scandinavian, or Mediterranean diets.[9] Figure 13-1, Mediterranean Diet Pyramid, is found on page 269 in Chapter 13 in *Holistic Nursing: A Handbook for Practice* (6th edition).
3. Research demonstrates the cardioprotective effects of several dietary nutrients, including fiber (both soluble and insoluble), antioxidants (vitamins C and E, beta-carotene, selenium, coenzyme Q10), folic acid, and omega-3 essential fatty acids.
4. Homocysteine levels diagnostics assess increased risk for cardiovascular disease and stroke.
   a. Elevated homocysteine levels result from subclinical deficiencies of the B

vitamins, including folic acid, vitamin B_6 and vitamin B_{12}.
   b. Deficiencies in these nutrients, especially vitamin B_6 (pyridoxine), are also associated with diabetes, heart disease, depression, anxiety, and premenstrual syndrome.[10]
5. Heart disease is responsible for 45% of all deaths among women, and nearly 40% of all females are expected to develop cancer at some point in their lifetime. Women can lower their risk by 43% over a 10-year period[11] by improving their blood lipid and fatty acid profiles by consuming a combination of essential fatty acids including eicosapentaenoic acid (EPA), docosahexaenoic acid (DHA), and gamma-linolenic acid (GLA) derived from fish oils and certain vegetable oils.

Exhibit 13-1, Hypoglycemic Diet Plan, reviews guidelines and a sample meal plan; this diet plan assists in weight loss, blood glucose regulation, energy maintenance, nutrient needs, and satiation (found on page 268 in Chapter 13 of *Holistic Nursing: A Handbook for Practice* [6th edition]).

Review of Nutrient Sources

1. Carbohydrates: Carbohydrates are the main source of energy for all body functions, aiding in digestion, assimilation, and metabolism of proteins and fats.
   a. Simple carbohydrates include refined white flour products, white rice, white table sugar (dextrose), honey, fruit sugars (fructose), and milk sugars (lactose).
   b. Complex carbohydrates are found in whole grains, legumes, and vegetables and also contain protein, vitamins, minerals, and fiber. Complex carbohydrates supply the body with essential nutrients and amino acids and provide longer-lasting energy than do simple carbohydrates.[12]
2. Fiber: Dietary fiber is plant material that is left undigested. It contains polysaccharides.
   a. Fiber can be subdivided into soluble fiber and insoluble fiber. Food sources of dietary fiber are classified according to whether they contain predominantly soluble or insoluble fiber. Plant foods usually contain a combination of both types of fiber.

- Insoluble fiber includes pectin and cellulose, hemicellulose, and lignins[13] and is present in fruits, leafy vegetables, whole grains and brans, and beans.
- Soluble fiber is a gelatin-like substance, such as the mucilage found in oatmeal and legumes.

b. The Western diet, low in fiber content, has increased digestive problems; dietary fiber is not digested but increases fecal bulk and weight passing waste products, toxins, and metabolic by-products to be eliminated.

c. Fiber also is important in modulating insulin response and thereby stabilizing blood glucose levels.

d. Complex-carbohydrate foods offer fiber and are also good sources of protein, vitamins, and minerals.

e. A low-fat, high-fiber diet for prevention of heart disease, diabetes, obesity, digestive disorders, and cancer is recommended. Fiber-rich diets help lower blood cholesterol levels, stabilize blood glucose levels, and are heart healthy.

f. At least half of all grains consumed daily should be whole and unrefined. Fiber intake is recommended to be 25 grams per day for women and 28 grams per day for men. One study states that achieving these goals can reduce a person's risk of dying from heart disease, infections, and respiratory diseases. [14]

3. Protein: Protein is the second most plentiful substance in the body (after water) and constitutes approximately one-fifth of the body's weight. It builds the rigid structures such as bone, solid organs, and blood vessels. Protein is essential for the growth and maintenance of all body tissues, including muscle, skin, hair, nails, and eyes. Hormones, chemicals such as antibodies, and enzymes are composed of protein.

a. Protein molecules, essentially composed of amino acids, form long chains and branched structures of amino acids that contain nitrogen, carbon, hydrogen, and sometimes sulfur. Twenty-two amino acids are required to build protein; half of these are produced in the body when adequate nutrients are available, and eight are considered essential.

b. Excessive protein consumption taxes the kidneys and digestive system; consumption of a large quantity of animal protein is associated with increased risk of cardiovascular disease and breast, colon, and prostate cancers.

c. Plant foods such as whole grains, legumes, seeds, and nuts provide excellent protein, but this protein is incomplete, and these foods must be combined with others to provide all of the essential amino acids. Foods can be combined to make complete proteins, such as by pairing beans with brown rice.

d. All animal proteins including red meat, poultry, seafood, eggs, and dairy are complete proteins that can also be obtained through plant foods including soy, lentils, amaranth, buckwheat, and quinoa.

e. The recommended daily protein allowance for health maintenance in the United States is 0.8 grams per kilogram of body weight. Men and women who body build require up to 1.2 grams per kilogram of body weight per day.[15]

4. Lipids: Lipids are a group of fats that account for more than 10% of body weight in most adults and serve as a source of energy.

a. Current recommendations call for 20% of total calories from fat and less than 10% from saturated fats. The RDA for dietary fat to ensure the intake of essential fatty acids is 25 grams.

b. Fats are calorie rich and contain approximately 9 calories per gram.

c. Essential fatty acids (EFA) are found in both monosaturated and polyunsaturated fats.

- Monosaturated fats include olive, peanut, avocado, and canola oils.
- Polyunsaturated fats (PUFAs) are found in safflower, sunflower, corn, sesame, and soy oils.

d. EFAs form a structural part of all cell membranes that hold proteins and signals bioelectrical currents that transmit messages. EFAs shorten the time required for the recovery of fatigued muscles after exercise by facilitating the conversion of lactic acid to water and carbon dioxide.[16] EFAs act as precursors to hormone-like substances called prostaglandins, which mediate inflammatory processes and immune responses.

e. Fats can be divided into two main classes: omega-3 fatty acids and omega-6 fatty acids.

- Omega-3 essential fatty acids regulate immune and inflammatory responses and contain high concentrations of linoleic acid. They are necessary for normal growth and development throughout the life cycle. Omega-3 essential fatty acids are found in high concentrations in fish, fish oils, flax seeds, and walnuts.

f. Research shows that EFAs can lower blood pressure, lower cholesterol and triglyceride levels, and reduce the risk of heart disease and stroke.

g. High concentrations of DHA are found in the brain, and a deficiency of this omega-3 essential fatty acid component can lead to impaired learning and decreased cognitive function. Other EFA deficiency symptoms include poor immune response, dry skin and hair, behavioral changes, menstrual irregularities, and arthritic and inflammatory conditions.

h. Table 13-1, Dietary Goals and Recommendations, in Chapter 13 of *Holistic Nursing: A Handbook for Practice* (6th edition) serves as a guide for general dietary goals and recommendations.[16]

5. Vitamins: Vitamins regulate metabolism and assist in biochemical processes that release energy from digested food. Vitamins are coenzymes that activate the chemical reactions continually occurring in the body.

a. Vitamins are divided into two major groups: water soluble and fat soluble.

- Water-soluble vitamins such as vitamin C and the B complex must be taken into the body daily and are excreted within 1 to 4 days; excessive quantities of water-soluble vitamins are excreted rather than stored; therefore, seldom are they associated with toxicity problems.

- Fat-soluble vitamins are absorbed into the blood along with dietary fats; they are insoluble in water and are transported via the lymphatic vessels and stored in the body's adipose tissue and in the liver.

b. Table 13-2, Fat-Soluble and Water-Soluble Vitamins, in Chapter 13 of *Holistic Nursing: A Handbook for Practice* (6th edition) provides more information about vitamins and their food sources.

6. Minerals: Minerals are essential components of all cells and function as coenzymes and for proper composition of body fluids, formation of blood and bone, and maintenance of healthy nerve function.

a. Some minerals compete with others minerals for absorption, while others enhance the absorption of other minerals; for example, too much calcium can decrease the absorption of magnesium. Therefore, these minerals should be consumed in the proper ratio to maintain balance.

b. Minerals are classified as either major minerals or trace minerals.

- Major minerals include calcium, magnesium, phosphorus, potassium, sodium, and chloride.

- Trace minerals include arsenic, boron, chromium, cobalt, copper, fluoride, iodine, iron, manganese, molybdenum, nickel, selenium, silicon, tin, vanadium, and zinc.[17,18]

c. Long-term therapeutic doses of one or more trace minerals at the expense of other minerals might result in secondary deficiencies that could impair immunological or antioxidant processes.

d. Cell-mediated immunity, antibody response, and other immune responses can be impaired by marginal deficiencies in trace minerals. For example, borderline zinc deficiency is associated with depletion of lymphocytes and lymphoid tissue atrophy. Excessive long-term consumption of competing minerals, such as iron, might suppress immune response by producing a secondary deficiency of zinc.

e. Nutrient intake through food consumption depends on many factors, including the quality of the soil in which the foods were grown, use of fertilizers, and genetic engineering of foods.

f. Consumption of a wide variety of fresh fruits and vegetables and unprocessed whole foods, locally grown and organic whenever possible, is recommended.

g. Table 13-3, Major Minerals and Trace Elements, in Chapter 13 of *Holistic Nursing: A Handbook for Practice* (6th edition) provides further information on minerals and their food sources.

7. Antioxidants: Some vitamins and minerals function as antioxidants such as vitamins C and E, beta-carotene (a precursor of vitamin A), coenzyme Q10, alpha lipoic acid, vitamin D, and the trace mineral selenium. Antioxidants protect the body from the formation of free radicals that can damage healthy cells and suppress the immune system to defend against organisms, toxins, and metabolic by-products, all of which can lead to degenerative or infectious disease.

a. Glutathione, manufactured by the body, is a powerful antioxidant composed of the amino acids cysteine, glycine, and glutamic acid. Liver stores of glutathione can be depleted by disease processes, malnutrition, and poor-quality nutrient intake. Dietary amino acids are essential to glutathione synthesis. Lifestyle factors that affect efficient utilization of glutathione include stress, alcohol, cigarette smoking, excessive pharmaceutical use, drug abuse, and aging.[18]

8. Phytonutrients: Plant-based chemicals and nutrients, phytochemicals contain protective, disease-preventing compounds and form part of plants' immune system. They offer built-in protection from disease, injuries, insects, drought, excessive heat, ultraviolet rays, and poisons or pollutants in the air or soil.

a. Plant nutrients and their bioactive components have been studied for the treatment of cancer, diabetes, cardiovascular disease, and hypertension because they have been shown to exhibit potent antioxidant properties and to modulate many processes including cellular protection, healthy cell signaling, cancer cell replication and apoptosis (cancer cell death). They can decrease cholesterol levels.[19]

b. To ensure adequate amounts of nutrients and phytochemicals are obtained from fruits and vegetables, it is recommended that people eat a minimum of five to seven portions daily of a variety of foods from the following color groups: red, orange, yellow-green, and blue-purple.

Digestion, Absorption, Assimilation

1. Assessing nutrition includes how humans digest, absorb, assimilate, and eliminate foods.

a. The gastrointestinal tract is lined with mucosal tissue that secretes enzymes and protective antibodies. Absorbing food is the process of bringing the nutrients from the gastrointestinal tract to the rest of the body's tissues. The proper absorption and utilization of nutrients depend on a complex orchestration of processes in the digestive tract, and therefore it is essential to maintain the health and balance of this system.[20]

b. The gastrointestinal tract also contains billions of friendly microflora that assist in metabolic processes while maintaining the integrity of the mucosal lining. The microflora include strains of *Lactobacillus* and acidophilus and assist in synthesizing B vitamins, digesting proteins, balancing intestinal pH, reducing serum cholesterol, strengthening the immune system in the gut, preventing parasites and overgrowth of yeast, and maintaining bowel regularity. The most common reason for the destruction of microflora in the gastrointestinal tract is from the use of antibiotics. Beneficial bacteria must be replaced by probiotic supplementation following antibiotic therapy.[21]

c. For those with food sensitivities, removing "triggers" from the diet for a minimum of 21 days can be an important dietary intervention. Wheat, gluten, lactose, and casein products are the most common foods to eliminate, and this elimination often can relieve many common gastrointestinal problems including constipation, bloating after consuming, and irritable bowel syndrome.[22]

◼ EATING TO PROMOTE HEALTH

1. Increasing awareness of how diet can affect health and well-being is an essential component in nutrition coaching and education.

2. Nurses can use the following questions as a guideline. Ask clients to sit down in a quiet place and plan a day's menu by asking themselves these questions:
   a. What does my body need to enhance wellness?
   b. What are my past eating patterns? Which do I want to keep? Which do I want to change?
   c. What are my activity levels, and how should I include foods that meet my needs?
   d. How do I need to plan for psychological factors?
   e. What factors, unique to me, influence my food planning?

Stress and Nutrient Needs

1. Stress causes consequences in our lives and affects our health. It can necessitate increased nutrient intake to support normalization of stress-induced biochemical changes, increased nutrient needs, and natural resistance to stress responses.
   a. Research increasingly supports the critical role in disease played by stress-induced hormones, including elevated cortisol levels, which induce inflammation, sleep disturbances, and obesity.
   b. Removing inflammatory triggers calms the inflammatory chemicals and cytokines produced by stress.
   c. Chronic inflammation plays a role in diabetes, osteoporosis, hypertension, cardiovascular disease, infectious disease, gastric ulcer, cancer, immune system disturbances, and gastrointestinal, skin, endocrine, and neurologic disorders.
2. Chronic stress has been shown to affect behavior and has been linked to anxiety states and depression. The vulnerability of a particular bodily system to stress is determined by genetic makeup and constitution and might be influenced by nutritional and environmental factors.
3. A healthy diet rich in whole foods that contain antioxidants, B vitamins, essential fatty acids, and trace minerals can mediate the stress response and support overall health and well-being throughout life.

Eco Nutrition

1. In the United States, breast cancer is the second most common cause of cancer-related deaths in women.
   a. Research indicates that poor nutrient intake, chronic stress, inflammatory processes, and obesity are all risk factors.
   b. Evidence shows that another risk factor for breast cancer is chemical exposure to xenotoxins[23] found in certain pesticides, drugs, and plastics, and occupational exposures.[24] Xenoestrogens accumulate in the fatty tissues of the body and can interact with estrogen receptor sites in the breast, enhancing breast cell proliferation.
   c. Women with breast cancer often have higher concentrations of pesticides in their blood and fatty tissues than do healthy women.[25]
2. In women, fat intake and obesity are primary risk factors associated with cardiovascular disease, diabetes, and cancer.
3. Studies associate a high-fat, low-fiber diet with an increased risk of developing cancer of the colon, prostate, and breast.
4. Weight loss plans that support a low-fat, high-fiber whole foods diet, stress reduction, and exercise are part of a comprehensive preventative health approach.
5. Studies suggest a relationship between the incidence of cancer and quantity of fresh fruits and vegetables consumed.
   a. The fiber, antioxidants, and other plant-derived substances, or phytonutrients, in fresh foods are believed to contain cancer-protective properties.
   b. Fruits and vegetables, rich in fiber, are thought to influence hormone levels by facilitating the fecal excretion of estrogen metabolites, which at high levels can pose a risk for many women.[26]
   c. Other anticancer vegetables are cruciferous (watercress, broccoli, cauliflower, Brussels sprouts), which contain isothiocynates, such as sulforophane, and are rich in indoles, which help in liver detoxification, aid in the removal of carcinogens and environmental toxins, and play a role in cancer prevention.[27,28]
6. Cancer prevention tips and a whole food nutrition plan can be found in Chapter

13 of the sixth edition of *Holistic Nursing: A Handbook for Practice.*

Osteoporosis

1. Osteoporosis often is the result of lack of exercise and deficiencies of several key nutrients, of which calcium is but one. Other essential nutrients, including vitamin D_3, vitamin K, magnesium, boron, and other trace minerals, must be available in the proper balance to facilitate calcium reabsorption and uptake into the bone.
   a. Beyond maintaining healthy bones (and preventing rickets), vitamin D is a pro-hormone that has hundreds of receptor sites on every cell.
   b. Common dietary risk factors for osteoporosis and guidelines for healthy bones can be found in Chapter 13 of the sixth edition of *Holistic Nursing: A Handbook for Practice.*
2. Supplement recommendations for healthy bones:
   a. The recommended ratio of calcium to magnesium is 2:1 (800–1200 mg calcium to 400–600 mg magnesium per day). The daily amount of vitamin D_3 depends on exposure to sunlight, genetics, skin pigmentation, geographical location, and individual physiologic requirements.
   b. Testing 25-hydroxyvitamin D levels is recommended.
   c. It is recommended that vitamin D levels be maintained above 40.[29]
   d. Other nutrients that help maintain bone mass include vitamin K, boron, vitamin B_6, manganese, folic acid, vitamin C, and zinc.[29]

Nutrition and Healthy Aging

1. The National Health and Nutrition Examination Survey revealed that the nation's older citizens remain at high risk of macronutrient and micronutrient deficiencies such as B_{12}, resulting in accelerated aging. Inadequate nutrition and protein deficiencies, for example, can lead to increased muscle loss, cognitive decline, fatigue, and immune system impairment.

2. Medical foods such as whey protein powder, high in glutamine and other amino acids, have been shown to improve protein stores and rebuild muscle mass.[30]
3. Antioxidants that counteract the detrimental effects of oxidative stress can help prevent Alzheimer's disease.[31]
   a. Research indicates that vitamin D might be involved in neuroprotection, control of pro-inflammatory cytokine-induced cognitive dysfunction, and synthesis of calcium-binding proteins.[32]
   b. The role of vitamin D receptors in the pathophysiology of cognitive decline, incidence of Alzheimer's disease, and vascular dementia and/or cognitive decline with respect to previous plasma 25-hydroxyvitamin D concentration has been observed in several studies.[33]
4. In the evaluation of older adults, psycho-social factors must be considered when addressing nutrition needs and goals, including economics, ability to shop and prepare meals, and social support networks. Other issues to be considered include chewing difficulties, impaired cognitive function and forgetting to eat, social isolation and apathy in food preparation, and inability to shop or carry packages.
   a. Impaired memory in elderly people often is related to the effect of B vitamins, vitamin D, antioxidant, and essential fatty acid deficiencies.
   b. Undetected hypochlorhydria, a deficiency of hydrochloric acid in the stomach, leads to bacterial overgrowth in the small bowel and results in impaired digestion and absorption of essential nutrients, including vitamins B_6 and B_{12}.[34]
5. One of the hallmarks of biologic aging is altered glucose metabolism, which affects many age-related diseases, including heart disease, inflammatory disorders, dementia, and diabetes.
6. Weight management guidelines can be found in Chapter 13 of *Holistic Nursing: A Handbook for Practice* (6th edition).

Eating with Awareness

1. Taking time for the eating experience can help to reduce cravings, control portion

sizes, enhance the eating experience, improve digestion and overall health, and engender a sense of well-being. Nurse coaches can recommend the following guidelines to their clients: Eat in a setting where you feel relaxed, chew thoroughly, eat mindfully, and choose foods to support your health and well-being.

2. Healthy nutrition choices can be found in Chapter 13 of *Holistic Nursing: A Handbook for Practice* (6th edition).

Nutrition Guidelines for Maintaining Healthy Cholesterol Levels

1. Oatmeal, oat bran, and high-fiber foods: Contain soluble fiber, which reduces low-density lipoprotein (LDL). Soluble fiber is also found in such foods as kidney beans, apples, pears, barley, and prunes. Five to 10 grams or more of soluble fiber a day decreases LDL cholesterol.

2. Fish and omega-3 fatty acids: Eat fatty fish with its high levels of omega-3 fatty acids. Omega-3 fatty acids reduce the risk of sudden death.
   a. The highest levels of omega-3 fatty acids are in the following fish: mackerel, lake trout, herring, sardines, wild salmon, halibut.
   b. Most farm-raised fish are high in chemicals including hormones and antibiotics.
   c. Other plant sources of omega-3 EFAs are walnuts and ground flaxseeds.

3. Walnuts, almonds, and other nuts: Nuts can reduce blood cholesterol. Rich in polyunsaturated fatty acids, walnuts also help keep blood vessels healthy. Replace foods high in saturated fat with a handful (1.5 ounces, or 42.5 grams) a day of nuts such as almonds, hazelnuts, peanuts, pecans, some pine nuts, pistachio nuts, and walnuts to reduce the risk of heart disease.

4. Olive oil: Olive oil contains a potent mix of antioxidants (hydroxytyrosol) that can lower "bad" (LDL) cholesterol but leave "good" (HDL) cholesterol untouched, reducing the risk of coronary heart disease. Olive oil is rich in monounsaturated fats, most notably oleic acid that helps in the production of antioxidants. The FDA recommends using 2 tablespoons (23 grams)

of olive oil a day in place of other fats to receive heart-healthy benefits.

Other Important Health-Promoting Tips

1. Drink four to six glasses of liquid daily including spring or filtered water or herbal teas.
2. Cook and prepare food in cast-iron or stainless steel cookware (avoid aluminum).
3. Chew foods slowly and thoroughly.
4. Eat smaller, simpler meals.
5. Include fiber with each meal.
6. Exercise daily.
7. Reduce stress through yoga, meditation, deep breathing, relaxation practice, and visualization.
8. Avoid alcohol, caffeine, smoking, recreational drugs, and over-the-counter drugs.
9. Get sufficient rest and sleep.
10. A description of the holistic caring process is found in Chapter 13 of *Holistic Nursing: A Handbook for Practice* (6th edition).

■ NOTES

1. Miller, M., Stone, N. J., Ballantyne, C., Bittner, V., Criqui, M. H., Ginsberg, H. N.,...Council on the Kidney in Cardiovascular Disease. (2011). Triglycerides and cardiovascular disease: A scientific statement from the American Heart Association. *Circulation, 123*(20), 2292–2333.
2. R. Solá, M. Fitó, R. Estruch, et al., "Effect of a Traditional Mediterranean Diet on Apolipoproteins B, A-I, and Their Ratio: A Randomized, Controlled Trial," *Atherosclerosis* 218, no. 1 (September 2011): 174–180.
3. C. Ogden and M. Carroll, "Prevalence of Obesity Among Children and Adolescents: United States, Trends 1963–1965 Through 2007–2008," *Health E-Stat.* Retrieved from http://www.cdc.gov/nchs/data/hestat/obesity_child_07_08/obesity_child_07_08.pdf
4. Basoglu, O. K., Sarac, F., Sarac, S., & Uluer, H. (2011). Metabolic syndrome, insulin resistance, fibrinogen, homocysteine, leptin, and c-reactive protein in obese patients with obstructive sleep apnea syndrome. *Annals of Thoracic Medicine, 6*(3), 120–125.
5. Grün, F., & Blumberg, B. (2009). Minireview: The case for obesogens. *Molecular Endocrinology, 23*(8), 1127–1134.
6. Jones, J. L., Comperatore, M., Barona, J., Calle, M. C., Andersen, C., McIntosh, M.,...Fernandez, M. L. (2012). A Mediterranean-style, low-glycemic-load diet decreases atherogenic lipoproteins and reduces lipoprotein (a) and oxidized

low-density lipoprotein in women with metabolic syndrome. *Metabolism, 61*(3), 366–372.

7. National Research Council, *Recommended Daily Allowance*, 10th ed. (Washington, DC: National Academy Press, 1989).

8. Salas-Salvado, J., Bullo, M., Babio, N., Martínez-González, M. Á., Ibarrola-Jurado, N., Basora, J.,...PREDIMED Study Investigators. (2011). Reduction in the incidence of type 2 diabetes with the Mediterranean diet. *Diabetes Care, 34,* 14–19.

9. Jones, J. L., Fernandez, M. L., McIntosh, M. S., Najm, W., Calle, M. C., Kalynych, C.,...Lerman, R. H. (2011). Mediterranean-style low-glycemic-load diet improves variables of metabolic syndrome in women, and addition of a phytochemical-rich medical food enhances benefits on lipoprotein metabolism. *Journal of Clinical Lipidology, 5*(3), 188–196.

10. Clarke, R., Smulders, Y., Fowler, B., & Stehouwer, C. D. (2005). Homocysteine, B vitamins, and the risk of cardiovascular disease. *Seminars in Vascular Medicine, 5*(2), 75–76.

11. Galli, C., & Risé, P. (2009). Fish consumption, omega 3 fatty acids and cardiovascular disease: Science and the clinical trials. *Nutrition and Health, 20*(1), 11–20.

12. Boyle, P. J., & Zrebiec, J. (2007). Management of diabetes-related hypoglycemia. *Southern Medical Journal, 100*(2), 183–194.

13. Mente, A., de Koning, L., Shannon, H. S., & Anand, S. S. (2009). A systematic review of the evidence supporting a causal link between dietary factors and coronary heart disease. *Archives of Internal Medicine, 169*(7), 659–669.

14. Park, Y., Subar, A. F., Hollenbeck, A., & Schatzkin, A. (2011). Dietary fiber intake and mortality in the NIH-AARP Diet and Health Study. *Archives of Internal Medicine, 171*(12), 1061–1068.

15. Deminice, R., Portari, G. V., Marchini, J. S., Vannucchi, H., & Jordao, A. A. (2009). Effects of a low-protein diet on plasma amino acid and homocysteine levels and oxidative status in rats. *Annals of Nutrition and Metabolism, 54*(3), 202–207.

16. Barberger-Gateau, P., Samieri, C., Féart, C., & Plourde, M. 2011). Dietary omega 3 polyunsaturated fatty acids and Alzheimer's disease: Interaction with apolipoprotein E genotype. *Current Alzheimer Research, 8*(5), 479–491.

17. J. Thompson, "Vitamins, Minerals and Supplements: Overview of Vitamin C (5)," *Community Practice* 80, (1) (2007): 35–36.

18. P. Chen, J. Stone, G. Sullivan, J. A. Drisko, and Q. Chen, "Anti-Cancer Effect of Pharmacologic Ascorbate and Its Interaction with Supplementary Parenteral Glutathione in Preclinical Cancer Models," *Free Radical Biology and Medicine* 51, (3) (2011): 681–687.

19. C. Martin, E. Butelli, K. Petroni, and C. Toneli, "How Can Research on Plants Contribute to Promoting Human Health?" *Plat Cell* 23, no. 5 (2011): 1685–1699.

20. Wallace, T. C., Guarner, F., Madsen, K., Cabana, M. D., Gibson, G., Hentges, E., & Sanders, M. E. (2011). Human gut microbiota and its relationship to health and disease. *Nutrition Review, 69*(7), 392–403. doi:10.1111/j.1753-4887.2011.00402

21. B. N. Ames, "Optimal Micronutrients Delay Mitochondrial Decay and Age-Associated Diseases," *Mechanisms of Ageing and Development* 131, 7–8 (2010): 473–479

22. Guandalini, S., & Newland, C. (2011). Differentiating food allergies from food intolerances. *Current Gastroenterology Reports, 13*(5), 426–434.

23. Nahleh, Z. (2011). Breast cancer, obesity and hormonal imbalance: A worrisome trend. *Expert Review of Anticancer Therapy, 11*(6), 817–819.

24. Labrèche, F., Goldberg, M. S., Valois, M. S., & Nadon, L. (2010). Postmenopausal breast cancer and occupational exposures. *Occupational and Environmental Medicine, 67*(4), 263–269.

25. Teitelbaum, S. L., Gammon, M. D., Britton, J. A., Neugut, A. I., Levin, B., & Stellman, S. D. (2007). Reported residential pesticide use and breast cancer risk on Long Island, New York. *American Journal of Epidemiology, 165*(6), 643.

26. Sonestedt, E., Gullberg, B., & Wirfalt, E. (2007). Both food habit change in the past and obesity status may influence the association between dietary factors and postmenopausal breast cancer. *Public Health and Nutrition, 5,* 1–11.

27. Hanf, V., & Gonder, U. (2005). Nutrition and primary prevention of breast cancer: Foods, nutrients and breast cancer risk. *European Journal of Obstetrics, Gynecology and Reproductive Biology, 123*(2), 139–149.

28. American Institute for Cancer Research. (n.d.). Homepage. Retrieved from http://www.aicr.org/

29. Barnard, K., & Colón-Emeric, C. (2010). Extraskeletal effects of vitamin D in older adults: Cardiovascular disease, mortality, mood, and cognition. *American Journal of Geriatric Pharmacotherapy, 8*(1), 4–33.

30. Katsanos, C. S., Chinkes, D. L., Paddon-Jones, D., Zhang, X., Aarsland, A., & Wolfe, R. R. (2008). Whey protein ingestion in elderly results in greater muscle protein accrual than ingestion of its constituent essential amino acid content. *Nutrition Research, 28*(10), 651–658.

31. Wellan, M. S. (2007). Prevention, prevention, prevention: Nutrition for successful aging. *Journal of the American Dietetic Association, 107*(5), 741–743.

32. Liu, Q., , Xie. F., Rolston, R., Moreira, P. I., Nunomura, A., Zhu, X.,....... Perry, G. (2007). Prevention and treatment of Alzheimer's disease and

aging: Antioxidants. *Mini Reviews in Medicinal Chemistry, 7*(2), 171–180.

33. Donini, L. M., . De Felice, M. R. & Cannella, C. (2007). Nutritional status determinants and cognition in the elderly. *Archives of Gerontology and Geriatrics, 44*(Suppl. 1), 143–153.

34. Morris, M. S., Selhub, J., Morris, M. S., Jacques, P. F. & Rosenberg, I. H. (2007). Folate and vitamin B-12 status in relation to anemia, macrocytosis, and cognitive impairment in older Americans. *American Journal of Clinical Nutrition, 85*(1), 193–200.

■ STUDY QUESTIONS

Basic Level

1. In which of the following conditions does chronic inflammation play a role?
   a. Diabetes
   b. Cardiovascular disease
   c. Endocrine and neurologic disorders
   d. All of the above

2. Which of the following is an unhealthy fat in the diet?
   a. Avocado
   b. Walnuts
   c. Olive oil
   d. Cottonseed oil

3. Soluble fiber is found in which of the following foods?
   a. Lettuce
   b. Apples
   c. Whole grains
   d. Legumes

4. Effective weight loss plans include the following except which one?
   a. Low-fat, high-fiber whole foods diet
   b. Stress reduction
   c. Exercise
   d. Less than 6 hours of sleep per night

5. High-fructose corn syrup ultimately increases risk for which of the following conditions?
   a. Metabolic syndrome
   b. Cancer
   c. High blood pressure
   d. Cognitive decline

6. Research demonstrates that the use of omega-3 essential fatty acids supplementation supports all of the following except which one?
   a. Prevention of heart disease
   b. Lowering of triglycerides
   c. Enhancing cognitive function
   d. Improving digestive function

Advanced Questions

7. An older adult is consulting with you for a wellness visit. In terms of nutrition, you are aware that older adults are often deficient in which of the following nutrients?
   a. vitamin B_{12}
   b. Vitamin D
   c. Omega-3 essential fatty acids
   d. All of the above

8. You are providing health coaching to a 30-year-old female client who recently increased her physical activity and is exhibiting signs of hypoglycemia. Recommendations for a hypoglycemic diet include the following except which one?
   a. Eliminate all refined carbohydrates.
   b. Consume several smaller meals throughout the day.
   c. Have an unlimited intake of fruits.
   d. Increase fiber.

9. A 49-year-old client reports she is in good health, is perimenopausal, is a marathon runner, and that she has a family history of osteoporosis. Which lifestyle behavioral changes would you want to be certain to share with the client? ?
   a. Reducing high intake of animal protein
   b. Limiting intake of carbonated beverages
   c. Decreasing exercise
   d. Reducing intake of antacids (low HCl that can occur with aging)

10. Obtaining clients' vitamin D levels is important because research findings show that vitamin D deficiency is associated with an increased risk for which of the following conditions?
    a. Multiple sclerosis
    b. Cognitive impairment
    c. Breast cancer
    d. All of the above

Chapter 15

Exercise and Movement

Francie Halderman and
Christina Bergh Jackson

■ DEFINITIONS

Aerobic exercise Sustained muscle activity within the target heart rate range that challenges the cardiovascular system to meet the muscles' needs for oxygen.

Endurance The period of time the body can sustain exercise or movement.

Fitness Fitness comprises flexibility, endurance, strength, and balance. It includes the ability to carry out daily tasks with vigor and alertness, without undue fatigue, and with ample reserve to enjoy leisure pursuits.

Flexibility The ability to use a joint throughout its full range of motion and to maintain some degree of elasticity of major muscle groups.

Maximal heart rate The rate of the heart when the body is engaged in intense physical activity.

Mindful movement Movement with intention to notice present moment sensations, thoughts, feelings, and emotions with a nonjudgmental and compassionate attitude. A focus on full, rhythmic breathing is incorporated to enhance mindful awareness.

Moderate-intensity activity Activity that induces an intermediate change in breathing and heart rate from a person's baseline.

Posture Pose or placement of parts of the body in spatial relationships.

Resting heart rate The heart's rate when the body is at rest.

Strength training The use of weights or opposing forces during activity to strengthen muscle groups; usually accomplished with intentional repetitive movements.

Target heart rate The safe rate for the heart during exercise that produces health benefits.

Vigorous-intensity activity Activity that induces large changes in breathing and heart rate.

■ THEORY AND RESEARCH

Exercise and Movement

1. Exercise and movement positively affect both physical and mental health and are effective interventions to promote wellness and prevent illness.[1-3]
2. Exercise and movement are the physical expression of the whole person.
3. A person's energy expenditure reflects patterns that are intertwined with his or her body-mind-spirit.
4. Exercise plays an integral role not only in disease prevention but also in health promotion and well-being.
   a. Physical activity can release endorphins resulting in a sense of well-being and can elevate mood and promote a positive outlook.
   b. Exercise lowers the risk of chronic disease by exerting anti-inflammatory influences that prevent diabetes, cardiovascular disease, arthritis, osteoporosis, chronic obstructive pulmonary disease, several types of cancer, and premature mortality.
   c. Even moderate exercise improves immunity and protects against upper-respiratory illness, the most prevalent infectious disease worldwide.

Old and New Fitness Paradigms

1. A new paradigm of fitness is emerging that emphasizes enjoyment, engagement, and adherence.
2. Qualities of the old fitness paradigm:
   a. Focused on "compliance," or getting someone to conform or comply with a regimen.
   b. A person exercised out of a sense of obligation.
   c. Sometimes perceived as rigorous or with dread.
   d. Competitive with comparison to others.
   e. Body focused and achievement oriented.
   f. Regimented routines.
   g. Compartmentalized schedule: "all or nothing" view.
3. Qualities of the new fitness paradigm:
   a. Focuses on engagement and adherence model.
   b. Promotes movement that is enjoyable and fun for the individual (enhancing sustainability).
   c. Encourages mindfulness of one's internal state as well as the external environment.
   d. Goal is to promote self-awareness, self-acceptance, and achieve one's personal best.
   e. Uses awareness of breath to energize and calm the body and mind throughout movement.
   f. Incorporates many types of activities such as aerobic, nonaerobic, group, and individual practices.
   g. Awareness of cumulative effects of activities throughout the week: "some better than none."

Fitness

1. The primary purpose of exercise is to produce fitness. The following are the four basic components of fitness:
2. Flexibility is the ability to use a joint throughout its full range of motion and to maintain some degree of elasticity of major muscle groups. Benefits include:
   a. Increased resistance to muscle and joint injury.
   b. Prevention of mild muscle soreness if flexibility exercises are done before and after vigorous activity.

3. Muscle strength is the contracting power of a muscle. Benefits include:
   a. Daily activities become less strenuous as muscles become stronger.
   b. Strong abdominal and lower back muscles help prevent lower back problems.
   c. Appearance improves as muscles become firmer.
4. Cardiorespiratory endurance is the ability of the circulatory and respiratory systems to maintain blood and oxygen delivery to the exercising muscles. Benefits include:
   a. Increased resistance to cardiovascular diseases.
   b. Improved ability to maintain activity levels (endurance).
   c. High-energy return from daily activities.
5. Postural stability is the body's ability to balance and stay balanced during dynamic action. This is important because:
   a. Balance declines naturally with age.
   b. Exercise and movement practices can assist with fall prevention.
   c. Yoga, standing Pilates, and tai chi assist with fall prevention integration of neuromuscular and sensory responses.

Holism of the New Fitness Paradigm

1. Flexibility, strength, endurance, and balance refer not only to the physical body but to the whole person and body-mind-spirit. These four qualities help integrate all aspects of one's life in a unified whole.
2. Movement practices from Eastern traditions have embraced this understanding for several thousand years, and in this sense the paradigm is not new.
3. However, adaptations of these traditions have developed as the practices came to the West. Practices such as yoga have become "westernized" in that styles now range from meditative and restorative to athletic and achievement-oriented practice.
4. In general, practices with pacing of movements and postures that are slow, flowing, meditative, and mindful might be more conducive to relaxation and positive parasympathetic response while promoting endurance, balance, strength, and flexibility.[4]
5. Mindful movement helps integrate awareness of breath, sensations, thoughts, and feelings.

Movement Modalities

1. Modalities from Eastern traditions such as yoga, tai chi, and qi gong have become increasingly available and help cultivate mindfulness in movement.
    a. These practices employ rhythmic patterns and sequences of movement and/or holding postures or poses along with mindful breathing.
    b. They help enhance present moment awareness of what is happening in one's interior environment of sensations, thoughts, emotions, feelings, and energy flow, as well as awareness of the exterior environment.
    c. Movement modalities help cultivate a greater sense of connection with oneself and interconnectedness with others.
    d. These practices can support connection to one's spirituality (for example, the word *yoga* means union and "yoked back," or reunited with one's source instead of a separate sense of self).
2. Movement practices can promote health, wellness, and support disease prevention.
3. Research supports the following:
    a. Yoga improves glucose regulation, balance, flexibility, and stress reduction. It can reduce mild to moderate depression, certain kinds of musculoskeletal pain, and fatigue.
    b. Mindful movement can regulate the body's hormonal response to stress and promote feelings of acceptance and well-being.
    c. In combination with aerobic exercise and strength training, movement practices can provide enjoyment that leads to sustained behavior change over time.

Recommendations for Physical Activity

1. In 2008, the U.S. Department of Health and Human Services (DHHS) released the *Physical Activity Guidelines for Americans* (PAG) that serve as the first-ever national guidelines for exercise and movement.[5]
2. Table 14-2, Fitness Paradigms, illustrates weekly recommendations for aerobic activity and muscle-strengthening activity by age group. (See Chapter 14 in *Holistic Nursing: A Handbook for Practice* [6th edition].)

3. In addition to the DHHS PAG guidelines, research supports a new trend in cardiovascular fitness called peak interval training (PIT).[6] PIT involves alternating cycles of short bursts of vigorous activity (1–3 minutes) with several minutes of moderate or mild activity, and repeating for 20 minutes.

Adherence

1. Fewer than 20% of adult Americans meet the U.S. physical activity guidelines for both aerobic and muscle-strengthening activities.[7] The holistic nurse should know the following:
    a. General considerations
        ▪ The benefits of exercise are cumulative, and just 10 minutes of sustained vigorous activity can be beneficial and count toward the weekly guideline totals.
        ▪ Motivational interviewing techniques can be used to assess the person's phase of readiness and level of intrinsic motivation (see Chapter 10 in *Holistic Nursing: A Handbook for Practice* [6th edition]).
        ▪ Supporting a client to identify barriers and creatively address them will increase likelihood of engagement and adherence over time.
    b. The following factors are known to enhance adult adherence to exercise and movement over time:
        ▪ Selecting a variety of activities that, in combination, meet the total weekly activity guidelines.
        ▪ Client ability to self-select the level, intensity, and type of exercise.[8.]
        ▪ Self-selection of activities that are enjoyable and fun.[8]
2. Table 14-3, Adherence Factors, reviews additional factors that both positively and negatively affect exercise adherence in adults. (See Chapter 14 in *Holistic Nursing: A Handbook for Practice* [6th edition].)

Cultural and Socioeconomic Factors

1. A person's cultural background includes his or her beliefs, practices, values, and preferences. The meaning and purpose of exercise can be culturally and economically

influenced and affect engagement and adherence.[9]

2. The holistic nurse:

   a. Discusses relevant cultural and economic factors with clients to identify how they might affect choice of activities or how they might present barriers.

   b. Where economic disparities exist, finds creative ways to meet client needs

      ▪ Community centers and churches sometimes offer free programs. This is beneficial for those who are motivated to exercise in groups.

      ▪ Public television and basic cable channels frequently offer yoga and cardiovascular workout shows for those motivated to exercise individually or who might otherwise need to workout at home.

      ▪ Libraries frequently offer free DVD rentals including those for health and fitness.

      ▪ Clients can access online exercise and movement classes as well as support groups and blogs that foster community and virtual support.

   c. Advocates for justice to reduce disparities in access to healthy environments.

   d. Supports the *Healthy People 2020* goals for exercise and well-being for all populations.[7]

▪ SPECIAL CONDITIONS AND POPULATIONS

Aging Populations

1. Fewer than one-third of older Americans meet the guidelines for physical activity despite the benefits that exercise and movement provides for physical, mental, and cognitive function.[10,11]

2. Older Americans who exercise have less risk for diabetes, falls and fractures, osteoporosis, cardiovascular disease, and some forms of cancer.[8]

3. Consistent evidence shows that health providers *fail to recommend* exercise and movement to older patients on a routine basis.[12]

4. Older populations have better exercise adherence when exercise is recommended and emphasized by medical professionals.[12]

5. Telephonic support for the frail elderly has been an effective follow-up method to improve adherence.[13]

6. Every healthcare encounter with older patients should include some discussion on starting, maintaining, and/or evaluating a fitness plan whenever possible.

Cardiovascular Disease

1. Currently one in three Americans have some form of cardiovascular disease.[14]

2. Heart disease and stroke are, respectively, the first and third leading causes of death in the United States.[14]

3. Regular exercise lowers the risk of heart disease and stroke and with medical supervision offers benefits after a cardiovascular event.[15]

4. Recommendations for evaluation for exercise should begin immediately after the cardiac event (in combination with diet and smoking cessation if applicable).[15]

5. Early behavioral interventions including exercise prescriptions and counseling should be given as high a priority as medications and invasive procedures.

Depression and Anxiety

1. Yoga has been found to be effective in reducing depression and anxiety in populations with and without existing disease.[4]

   a. Yoga promotes stress reduction by lessening stimulation of the sympathetic nervous system (SNS).

2. Lower-intensity exercise reduces cortisol levels while sustained high-intensity exercise increases cortisol release as if the body were responding to ongoing stress.[4]

3. Moderate exercise alone has been shown to be as effective as antidepressant medication for major depressive disorder (MDD).[16]

4. Clinicians should integrate exercise as an intervention on a routine basis to promote overall physical and mental well-being.

Diabetes

1. People with type 2 diabetes have more health risks than the general population.

2. Exercise improves glycemic control, yet many in the diabetic population remain sedentary despite well-established benefits of exercise for morbidity and mortality.[17]

3. Patients with diabetes have moved from the preaction stage (without exercise) to the maintenance phase by linking exercise with enjoyment and achieving their life goals.[18]

4. As patients with diabetes exercised over time, their motivation changed from extrinsic to intrinsic, leading to sustained behavioral change and overall improvement with self-management of diabetes.[18]

5. Holistic nurses can engage clients with type 2 diabetes to do the following:
   a. Identify their life goals and pleasurable activities.
   b. Relate the benefits of exercise with greater ability to manage overall health and achieve their goals.

6. Holistic nurses can inform clients that initial adherence can generate even stronger motivation over time.

Eating Disorders

1. Both anorexia nervosa and bulimia nervosa commonly involve a type of dysfunctional and excessive exercise behavior called exercise dependence.[19]

2. Vigorous and compulsive exercise is used as a compensatory mechanism to control weight or shape.

3. Missing a workout can cause extreme guilt and anxiety, and excessive exercise can interfere with important life activities.

4. People with bulimia nervosa can have body weights in the normal or overweight range whereas signs of malnutrition might be present in those with anorexia nervosa.

5. Of all mental disorders, anorexia nervosa has the highest mortality rate.[20]

6. Excessive exercise should *not* be reinforced for people with known eating disorders, and follow-up with a mental health specialist is important because of the serious nature of these conditions.

7. Further inquiry into eating habits, body image, and other physical or emotional symptoms might be warranted for someone who demonstrates exercise dependence.

Musculoskeletal Pain

1. Movement modalities can be particularly helpful for several types of musculoskeletal pain because the slow, rhythmic movement and postures promote balance, strength, and endurance while preserving joint flexibility.

2. Clients with osteoarthritis and rheumatoid arthritis can benefit from modified aerobic and strengthening exercises.[21]

3. During episodes of joint inflammation, the intensity of activity can be decreased to avoid joint damage and decrease pain.

4. Research supports use of yoga and tai chi to reduce pain ranging from arthritis to low back pain, and these modalities can improve depression and self-efficacy.[22,23]

Osteoporosis

1. Osteoporosis can lead to fractures of the vertebrae and hips, which can cause loss of function, disability, and death.[24]

2. Exercise is widely acknowledged as an essential preventive strategy to avoid osteoporosis.

3. Exercise can significantly increase bone strength in children but not adults; therefore, exercise in childhood is essential for prevention later in life.[25]

4. Exercise in older adults can prevent rapid loss of bone and reduce the risk of falls and fractures by improving muscle strength, flexibility, and mobility.[24]

5. Movement modalities are useful interventions in conjunction with exercise for those who have osteoporosis.

Trauma

1. Avoidance of exercise and movement can be the result of past physical or emotional trauma.

2. As the seminal book *Waking the Tiger: Healing Trauma* describes, the body's immediate response to trauma might include the fight, flight, or freeze response.[26]
   a. When unable to fight or run away, a person might freeze or become immobilized as a survival mechanism.
   b. If there is no way to release the bound tension in the nervous system after the

event is over, the immobility can become chronic.

c. Significant immobility and lack of exercise can be presenting symptoms of the fear response from trauma.[26]

d. Movement and exercise can play an integral role in unwinding the tension held in the nervous system in conjunction with support from a trauma-informed mental health professional.

■ THERAPEUTIC CARE PLAN AND INTERVENTIONS

Holistic Assessment

1. In preparing to use exercise and movement interventions, the nurse assesses the following parameters:

   a. The client's motivation, phase of readiness, and ability to make the necessary lifestyle changes in the areas of exercise and movement (see Chapter 10 in *Holistic Nursing: A Handbook for Practice* [6th edition]).

   b. The client's history of exercise and movement, any positive associations and past enjoyment of activities, and any modalities about which the client might be curious.

   c. Perception of barriers to perform exercise and movement.

   d. Cultural, socioeconomic, and environmental factors.

   e. Support systems that can enhance adherence.

Identification of Patterns/ Challenges/Needs

1. The following are patterns/challenges/ needs (see Chapter 7 in the sixth edition of *Holistic Nursing: A Handbook for Practice*) compatible with exercise and movement interventions:

   a. Altered nutrition

   b. Altered circulation

   c. Altered oxygenation

   d. Altered coping

   e. Altered physical mobility

   f. Sleep pattern disturbance

   g. Altered activities of daily living

   h. Disturbance in body image

   i. Disturbance in self-esteem

   j. Potential hopelessness

   k. Potential powerlessness

   l. Pain

   m. Anxiety

Outcome Identification

1. Figure 14-1, Nursing Interventions: Exercise and Movement, guides the nurse in client outcomes, nursing prescriptions, and evaluation for the use of exercise and movement as nursing interventions. (See Chapter 14 in *Holistic Nursing: A Handbook for Practice* [6th edition]).

2. Figure 14-2, Evaluation of the Client's Subjective Experience with Exercise and Movement Interventions, can be found in Chapter 14 of *Holistic Nursing: A Handbook for Practice* (6th edition).

3. Before the session:

   a. Create a safe environment in which the client feels comfortable discussing the needs of his or her physical body from a physical movement perspective.

   b. Clear your mind of other client or personal encounters to be fully present when meeting with the client.

   c. Bring intention for wholeness and highest good of the person to the session and respect for his or her healing process and choice.

4. At the beginning of the session:

   a. Take and record any necessary physical assessment data (e.g., height, weight, skinfold thickness measurements, hip–waist ratio, blood pressure, data on range of motion and mobility limitations).

   b. Guide the client as he or she discloses past habit patterns that affect exercise behavior.

   c. Assess the client's phase of readiness and level of motivation.

5. During the session:

   a. Ascertain the client's current weekly exercise pattern and practice.

   b. Be alert to psychological clues that might relate to exercise behavior or extremes (i.e., completely sedentary or excessive exercise dependence).

   c. Help the client identify any barriers that prevent starting or maintaining a program. Guide his or her exploration of creative solutions and available resources.

d. Assist the client to explore multiple types of activities that are enjoyable and cumulative throughout the week.

e. Discuss rhythmic breathing and awareness of full breathing during movement to increase attention to mindful movement practice.

f. Support the client to develop an individualized exercise and movement program.

g. Ensure that the teaching is at the client's cognitive and emotional levels.

6. At the end of the session:

a. Have the client identify the options presented that best fit his or her lifestyle.

b. Work with the client to establish written attainable goals and target dates.

c. Give the client specific affirmations to use to support these goals.

d. Give the client handout material or refer to pertinent resources to reinforce the teaching.

e. Use the client outcomes that were established before the session (see Figure 14-1) and the client's subjective experiences (see Figure 14-2) to evaluate the session.

f. Schedule a follow-up session.

■ HOLISTIC CARING PROCESS

Benefits that Contribute to Well-Being

1. Many rewards of exercise and physical activity are realized immediately and others are realized over time. Mental and spiritual improvements include beneficial changes in the following areas:

a. Mental attitude and outlook on life

b. Ability to cope with stress

c. Ability to avoid or control mild depression

d. Sleep patterns

e. Strength and endurance

f. Eating habits

g. Appearance and vitality

h. Posture

i. Physical stamina as you age

Getting Started

1. The holistic nurse practices the following and guides others to:

a. Learn about the different types of exercise and movement programs available in the area.

b. Consult a physician or exercise authority. If clients are older than 35 years, have never seriously exercised, have a disability or chronic illness, or are pregnant, they should obtain guidance to avoid injuries or complications.

c. Warm up and cool down. Stretching exercises are essential before and after each activity or period of exercise.

d. Wear shoes with proper support for the activity and choose proper ground surfaces for activities.

e. Establish an exercise routine.

f. Evaluate the program periodically. Clients should determine if they are making progress. If they want to go further, they can set new goals.

g. Create competition for themselves only if it benefits them. If clients allow too much competition, exercise can become more of a burden than a joy.

Safety

1. To reduce risks associated with exercise, clients must know not only how often and how long to exercise but also how vigorously to exercise.

2. Although the target pulse range allows for a heart rate within 60–80% of maximal capacity, the American Heart Association guidelines state that regular exercise of a moderate level, or from 50–75% of maximal capacity, appears to be sufficient.

3. Maintaining the target pulse rate during physical exercise for 15–30 minutes three to five times per week reduces the risk of overexertion, enhances enjoyment, and results in cardiovascular fitness.

4. Each person can informally assess whether activity is vigorous or moderate based on his or her body's response.

a. If one can talk but not sing while exercising, that person has reached *moderate intensity*.

b. If one can say only a few words and then needs to catch his or her breath while exercising, that person has reached *vigorous intensity*.

5. Clients must always warm up for at least 5 to 10 minutes and cool down after exercising.

6. They should stop if any one of the following occur:
   a. Something hurts.
   b. Significant fatigue occurs.
   c. They feel dizzy or nauseated.
7. To ease the heart rate into the training range, clients should begin with 10 minutes of low-intensity, warm-up exercise. To cool down, they should do 10 minutes of the same slow activity.

■ NOTES

1. Dishman, R. K., & O'Connor, P. J. (2009). Lessons in exercise neurobiology: The case of endorphins. *Mental Health and Physical Activity, 2*(1), 4–9.2.

2. Stathopoulou, G., Powers, M. B., Berry, A. C., Smits, J. A. J., Otto, M. W. (2006). Exercise interventions for mental health: A quantitative and qualitative review. *Clinical Psychology: Science and Practice, 13*(2), 179–193.

3. Nieman, D. (2007). Moderate exercise improves immunity and decreases illness rates. *American Journal of Lifestyle Medicine,* 1–8. Retrieved from http://ajl.sagepub.com/content/early/2011/04/26/1559827610392876

4. Ross, A., & Thomas, S. (2010). The health benefits of yoga and exercise: A review of comparison studies. *Journal of Alternative and Complementary Medicine, 16*(1), 3–12.

5. U.S. Department of Health and Human Services, Office of Disease Prevention and Health Promotion. (2008). *2008 Physical Activity Guidelines for Americans.* ODPHP Publication No. U0036. Retrieved from http://www.health.gov/paguidelines/pdf/paguide.pdf

6. Wisloff, U., Stoylen, A., Loennechen, J. P., Bruyold, M., Rognmo, O., Per Mangus, J.,...Skjaerpe, T. (2007). Superior cardiovascular effect of aerobic interval training versus moderate continuous training in heart failure patients. *Circulation, 115,* 3086–3094.

7. U.S. Department of Health and Human Services. (2010). *Healthy People 2020: Physical Activity: Overview.* HealthyPeople.gov. Retrieved from http://healthypeople.gov/2020/topicsobjectives2020/overview.aspx?topicid=33

8. Larson, J. S., & Winn, M. (2010). Health policy and exercise: A brief BRFSS study and recommendations. *Health Promotion Practice, 11*(2), 268–274.

9. Saint Onge, J. M., & Krueger, P. M. (2011). Education and racial-ethnic differences in types of exercise in the United States. *Journal of Health and Social Behavior, 52*(2), 197–211. Retrieved from http://hsb.sagepub.com/content/52/2/197.abstract

10. Resnick, B., Ory, M. G., Hora, K., Rogers, M. E., Page, P., Chodzko-Zajko, W.,...Bazzarre, T. L. (2008). The Exercise Assessment and Screening for You (EASY) tool: Application in the oldest population. *American Journal of Lifestyle Medicine, 2*(5), 432–440.

11. Zoeller, R. F., Jr. (2010). Exercise and cognitive function: Can working out train the brain too? *American Journal of Lifestyle Medicine, 4*(5), 397–409.

12. Dauenhauer, J. A., Podgorski, C. A., & Karuza, J. (2006). Prescribing exercise for older adults: A needs assessment comparing primary care physicians, nurse practitioners, and physician assistants. *Gerontology and Geriatrics Education, 26,* 81–99.

13. Peterson, M. J., Sloane, R., Cohen, H. J., Crowley, G. M., Pieper, C. F., & Morey. M. C. (2007). Effect of telephone exercise counseling on frailty in older veterans: Project LIFE. *American Journal of Men's Health, 1*(4), 326–334.

14. U.S. Department of Health and Human Services. (2010). Healthy People 2020: Heart Disease and Stroke. HealthyPeople.gov. Retrieved from http://healthypeople.gov/2020/topicsobjectives2020/overview.aspx?topicid=21

15. Chow, C. K., Jolly, S., Rao-Melacini, P., Fox, K. A., Anand, S. S., & Yusuf, S. (2010). Association of diet, exercise, and smoking modification of early cardiovascular events after acute coronary syndromes. *Circulation, 121,* 750–758.

16. Blumenthal, J. A., Babyak, M. A., Doraiswamy, P. M., Watkins, L., Hoffman, B. M., Barbour, K. A.,...Sherwood, A. (2007). Exercise and pharmacotherapy in the treatment of major depressive disorder. *Psychosomatic Medicine, 69,* 587–596.

17. American Association of Diabetes Educators. (2008). Position statement: Diabetes and exercise. *Diabetes Educator, 34*(1), 37–40.

18. Fortier, M. S., Sweet, S. N., Tulloch, H., Blanchard, C. M., Sigal, R. J., Kenny, G. P., & Reid, R. D. (2011). Self-determination and exercise stages of change: Results from the Diabetes Aerobic and Resistance Exercise Trial. *Journal of Health Psychology,* 1–13. doi:10.1177/1359105311408948

19. Cook, B. J., & Hausenblas, H. A. (2008). The role of exercise dependence for the relationship between exercise behavior and eating pathology: Mediator or moderator? *Journal of Health Psychology, 13*(4), 495–502.

20. Miller, C. A., & Golden, H. H. (2010). An introduction to eating disorders: Clinical presentation, epidemiology, and prognosis. *Nutrition in Clinical Practice, 25*(2), 110–115.

21. Herbert, W. G., Humphrey, R., & Myers, J. N. (Eds.). (2010). *ACSM's resources for clinical exercise physiology: Musculoskeletal, neuromuscular, neoplastic, immunologic, and hematologic conditions* (2nd ed.). Baltimore, MD: Lippincott Williams & Wilkins.

22. Wang, C., Schmid, C. H., Hibberd, P. L., Kalish, R., Roubenoff, R., Rones, R., & McAlindon, T. (2009). Tai chi is effective in treating knee osteoarthritis: A randomized controlled trial. *Arthritis Care & Research, 61*(11), 1545–1553.

23. Tekur, P., Singphow, C., Nagendra, H. R., & Raghuram, N. (2008). Effect of a short-term intensive yoga program on pain, functional disability and spinal flexibility in chronic low back pain: A randomized control study. *Journal of Alternative and Complementary Medicine, 14*(6), 637–644.

24. Tuzun, S., Aktas, I., Akarirmak, U., Sipahi, S., & Tuzun, F. (2010). Yoga might be an alternative training for the quality of life and balance in postmenopausal osteoporosis. *European Journal of Physical and Rehabilitation Medicine, 46*(1), 69–72.

25. Nikander, R., et al. (2010). Targeted exercise against osteoporosis: A systemic review and meta-analysis for optimizing bone strength throughout life. *BMC Medicine, 8*(47). Retrieved from http://www.biomedcentral.com/1741-7015/8/47

26. Levine, P. A. (1997). *Waking the tiger.* Berkeley, CA: North Atlantic Books.

▪ STUDY QUESTIONS

Basic Level

1. You know that people often perceive barriers that interfere with regular physical activity, so you teach your clients which one of the following details to reduce barriers?
   a. If they buy a home gym system, they will be more likely to participate regularly.
   b. If they weigh themselves daily, they will be motivated to exercise regularly.
   c. If they keep a written record of their physical activity, they will be more motivated.
   d. Even if they exercise only 10 minutes at a time, the positive effects are cumulative.

2. Which of the following answer choices best describes mindful movement?
   a. The use of rhythmic, interval breathing throughout the movement
   b. Rigorous and deep concentration throughout the activity
   c. Awareness of one's breath, sensations, thoughts, and feelings throughout the movement
   d. Knowing that one is body-mind-spirit while running, stretching, or lifting weights

3. You incorporate the four basic components of fitness into your planning with clients. This means you include which of the following components?
   a. Flexibility, muscle strength, cardiorespiratory endurance, and postural stability (balance).
   b. Body mass index, cardiorespiratory endurance, fixed point balance, and anaerobic conditioning.
   c. Endurance, motivation, readiness, and adherence.
   d. Skinfold fat analysis, balance, aerobic capacity, and nutritional intake.

4. In evaluating research evidence relating to various types of exercise, what do you learn about yoga?
   a. Yoga is ideal for promoting bone growth in those with osteoporosis.
   b. Yoga has been shown to help reduce anxiety, depression, and certain types of joint and musculoskeletal pain.
   c. Yoga delivers excellent aerobic fitness.
   d. Yoga is not effective for those with depression.

5. In practicing self-care for stress reduction, you jump back into the vigorous running and power yoga schedule you maintained several years ago when you were in high school. Within weeks you develop a recurrence of plantar fasciitis and feel more stressed than ever. Which of the following courses of action shows that you will start to base your self-care on the more recent evidence on the benefits of exercise?
   a. Pushing through the pain, knowing it can take a while to become reconditioned.
   b. Scheduling an appointment with a specialist for a full battery of lab work and stress tests.
   c. Starting to save money so that you can join a swim club instead of running.
   d. Stopping the running and power yoga for now, and engaging in a gentle yoga practice along with stationary biking to build endurance.

Advanced Level

6. As clinical director of a senior center, you are alarmed at the lack of physical fitness among your clients. In reviewing the literature, you realize which of the following facts?
   a. Geriatric clients do not experience enough health risk reduction benefits to warrant a regular exercise program.
   b. The focus for older adults should be on community-building activities rather than fitness-oriented activities.
   c. Healthcare providers often fail to recommend exercise and movement to older clients.
   d. It is unrealistic to expect frail older adults to adhere to exercise and movement programs.

7. In your work with clients, you know that the best time to discuss exercise and movement benefits and options is when?
   a. Only when they present with a specific problem that could be helped by exercise.
   b. With every possible healthcare encounter.
   c. When clients are fully recovered from illness.
   d. When clients indicate a high level of motivation and readiness.

8. You are working with a client who exhibits low levels of motivation and readiness to engage in exercise. Which of the following is your best next step?
   a. Wait for a better time to discuss exercise.
   b. Avoid engaging the client because this will make him more resistant to exercising.
   c. Use the research evidence to make the client aware of the risks of inactivity and share information on exercise and movement practices that work for most people in the population.
   d. Explore with the client the types and levels of activities that are most appealing to him and whether there are any personal barriers to perform them.

9. In applying the new fitness paradigm to your clients, you decide to do which of the following?
   a. Stress the importance of regular compliance to ensure consistency.
   b. Suggest that clients compete with an "exercise buddy" to enhance motivation.
   c. Encourage clients to use a variety of movement activities to enhance enjoyment and achieve cumulative exercise amounts per week.
   d. Enhance client mindfulness by asking them to journal after each exercise activity and track progress.

10. You are working with a client who is moderately depressed and taking antidepressant medication. Based on research evidence and holistic philosophy, which of the following plans makes the most sense?
    a. Continuing the medication for now and increasing levels of regular exercise and activity while exploring additional healing options with the client.
    b. Prescribing seated meditation, St. John's wort, and aerobic exercise.
    c. Providing nutritional counseling, recommending joining a gym, adding St. John's wort, and suggesting lowering the dose of antidepressant.
    d. Recommending the client stop seeing the psychiatrist and discontinue the medication immediately because they are not helping, and prescribing a regular exercise regimen and adding social supports.

Chapter 16

Humor, Laughter, and Play

Deborah Shields

Original Author: Patty Wooten

■ DEFINITIONS

Humor A quality of perception and attitude toward life that enables an individual to experience joy even when facing adversity; a perception of the absurdity or incongruity of a situation.

Laughter A physical behavior that occurs in response to something that is perceived as humorous, amusing, or surprising. This behavior engages most of the muscle groups and organ systems in the body. Laughter is often preceded by physical, emotional, or cognitive tension.

Play A spontaneous or recreational activity that is performed for sheer enjoyment rather than to reach a goal or produce a product. Playfulness is a mood or attitude that infuses the individual with a sense of joy and positive emotions.

■ THEORY AND RESEARCH

1. Complex phenomenon; essential part of human nature
2. Found in some measure, throughout history, in every culture or society
3. A sense of humor is:
   a. A perspective on life—a way of perceiving the world
   b. A behavior that expresses that perspective
   c. Helpful in tolerating and coping with life challenges
4. *Humor*: A word of many meanings
   a. Derived from the Latin word *umor*, meaning liquid or fluid

   b. Middle Ages: *Humor* referred to an energy that was thought to interact with a body fluid and an emotional state. This energy was believed to influence health and disposition and was an early recognition of the energy links between the mind and the body. *Sanguine humor* was cheerful and associated with blood; *choleric humor* was angry and associated with bile; *phlegmatic humor* was apathetic and allied with mucus; *melancholic humor* was depressed and related to black bile.
5. Vera Robinson, nurse educator: Compiled one of the earliest and most extensive reviews of humor and its use by health professionals as part of her doctoral thesis.[1] First published in 1977; updated and released again in 1991—a summary of findings on humor from different perspectives:
   a. Humanities and the literature of the world, from the time of the ancient Greeks to the present, have been concerned with the nature of comedy and laughter.
      ■ Comedy: Reveals people's imperfections, gives them courage to face life, and leaves them more tolerant; expresses "the absurdity of it"[2]
      ■ Tragedy: Is idealistic and expresses "the pity of it"[2]
   b. Philosophical perspective: Early philosophers were concerned with the nature of humor in relation to the issues of good and evil and the nature of humans.
      ■ Plato and Aristotle felt that laughter arose from enjoyment of the misfortunes of others and that comedy was an imitation of people at their worst.

- Other philosophers viewed laughter as a valuable asset in correcting the minor follies of society.
  c. Psychological perspective: Sigmund Freud set forth the psychoanalytic view of humor:
    - Civilization has led to repression of many basic impulses, and joking is a socially acceptable way of satisfying these repressed needs; humor is determined by the present stimulus situation.
    - There are four major types of jokes: the sexual joke, the aggressive and hostile joke, the blasphemous joke, and the skeptical joke.
    - Joking activity serves to preserve psychic energy.
    - Differentiated source of pleasure between wit (an economy of inhibition); the comic effect (an economy of thought); and humor (an economy of feelings).[3]
  d. Other psychologists assert that humor is not simply determined by the present stimulus situation but also depends on recollections of the past and anticipation of the future. Harvey Mindess proposed the liberation theory of humor. Humor and laughter are agents of psychological liberation, freeing us from the constraints and restrictive forces of daily living and, in doing so, make us joyful.[4]
  e. Anthropological perspective describes the use of humor within various cultures or ethnic groups. Humor is universal, but the culture, society, or ethnic group in which it occurs influences the style and content of humor and the situations in which humor is used and is considered appropriate.
  f. Sociological perspective explores exactly how humor is used within society:
    - Humor is a social relationship and occurs in a social environment.
    - Promotes group cohesion, initiates relationships, relieves tension during social conflict, and can be a means of expressing approval or disapproval of social action.[5-7]
    - Joking relationships within organizations serve to minimize stress and release antagonism.

Three Major Theories of Humor

1. Superiority Theory: Asserts that people laugh at the inferiority, stupidity, or misfortunes of others so that they can feel superior to them. This type of laughter can be cruel and scornful or can reflect warmth and empathy. In the Superiority Theory, humor can be viewed as a continuum from laughing at no one (nonsense jokes), to laughing at a specific person or group (jokes about morons or ethnic groups), to laughing with others in general at people's foibles (Charlie Chaplin's humor), to laughing at oneself, the most therapeutic of all.
2. Incongruity Theory: Asserts that humor holds that a sudden shock or unexpectedness, an incongruity, ambivalence, or conflict of ideas or emotions, is necessary to produce the absurdity provoking a burst of laughter.
3. Relief or Release Theory: Proposes that humor and laughter provide a release of tension and can be cognitive, emotional, and/or a release of nervous energy and physical tension.
   a. Reflections
      - Theories and perspectives on humor overlap: Some describe the nature of humor, while others describe the function of humor.
      - Diversity demonstrates the complexity of humor, laughter, and play and the ways these phenomena serve people.
      - More information about the influence of humor in people's lives can be obtained from the *International Society for Humor Studies*.

■ THERAPEUTIC HUMOR

1. Modern dictionaries define *humor* as the quality of being laughable or comical, or as a state of mind, mood, and spirit.
2. Our sense of humor gives us the ability to find delight and experience joy even when facing adversity.
3. Humor is a flowing energy, involving and connecting the body, mind, and spirit.
4. Humor can take many forms: jokes, cartoons, amusing stories, outrageous sight gags, funny songs, whimsical signs, bloopers,

"daffynitions," and physical slapstick antics. These humorous techniques stimulate the auditory, visual, or kinesthetic senses.

5. The term *to heal* comes from the Anglo-Saxon word *haelen*, which means to bring together and make whole. Bringing together the body, mind, and spirit can be healing. Humor, laughter, and the resulting emotion, mirth, unite the body, mind, and spirit.
   a. Humor is a cognitive activity engaging the mind.
   b. Laughter is a physical activity involving the body.
   c. Mirth is an emotional state that lifts the spirit.[8]
      - Sharing humor and laughter with clients and colleagues can have profound healing potential.
      - Finding a humorous perspective on one's problems, or experiencing the relaxing effects of laughter, can be an effective stress management technique that helps one stay healthy.
      - Therapeutic humor can be divided into three basic categories: hoping humor, coping humor, and gallows humor.

Hoping Humor: The Courage to Face Challenges

1. The ability to hope for something better enables human beings to cope with difficult situations.[9]
2. Hoping humor laughs in spite of the overwhelming circumstances and reflects an acceptance of life with all its dichotomies, contradictions, and incongruities.
3. This type of humor is usually warm and gentle and accepts the reality of the situation.
4. Hoping humor can also be used to sustain the spirit during the shock and trauma of natural disasters.
5. People create humor to literally laugh in the face of their loss; both disaster victims and those who offer professional assistance use humor to provide hope and courage as they deal with the overwhelming task of recovery.
6. Nurses and other professional caregivers use hoping humor to acknowledge their own reality and to laugh in spite of the pressure and demands.

Coping Humor: A Release for Tension

1. Illness and trauma cause stress and suffering; they present many challenges and can disrupt our ability to function smoothly.
2. Coping describes what people do to minimize this disruption and attempt to regain some control.
3. To cope effectively, people must change how they think and how they behave.
4. Coping humor can be used as a tool to change perspective, release physical and emotional tension, and regain a sense of control.
5. Clients can use coping humor to laugh about uncomfortable and embarrassing moments. Although they might not always be able to control their external reality, they can use humor to control how they perceive their situation and use their ability to laugh about it to provide some sense of empowerment.[10-12]
6. Coping humor often expresses anxiety or frustration about things that are out of one's control.
7. Caregivers also create humor to help release feelings of hostility or frustration created by patients or other professionals.
8. Coping humor is a socially acceptable form of expressing hostility, but it should be used with caution; it can be viewed as disrespectful and hurtful if overheard by someone who either identifies with the person being laughed at or feels that this type of humor is offensive and inappropriate for health professionals.[13-14]

Gallows Humor: Protection from Pain

1. Gallows humor is often used by professionals who work in situations that are horrifying or tragic. Every day these people cope with the reality and horror of illness, suffering, and death and, because of their caring and compassion, are more likely to feel the impact of the suffering they witness.
2. Caregivers often use humor as a means of maintaining some distance from the suffering to protect themselves from empathic pain.[15-16]
3. Gallows humor provides protection from the emotional impact of witnessing tragedy, death, and disfigurement.

4. Gallows humor acknowledges the disgusting or intolerable aspects of a situation and then attempts to transform them into something lighthearted and amusing. People's ability to laugh in this type of situation provides them with a momentary release from the intensity of what might otherwise be overwhelming. They are able to maintain their balance and professional composure so that they can continue to offer their therapeutic skills.

5. Gallows humor, so therapeutic for staff, might not be appreciated by clients or their families.

■ SHARING HUMOR

1. Always a risky venture because people vary greatly in what they find funny and which topics they consider too serious to laugh about; opinions vary about how or even if humor improves quality of life.

2. Exhibit 15-1, Concerns and Cautions About Using Humor in Healthcare Settings, reviews additional factors to consider when using humor. (See Chapter 15 in *Holistic Nursing: A Handbook for Practice* [6th edition].)

■ LAUGHTER

Cathartic Laughter

1. For some people, laughter is a whole-being experience.

2. It is said that laughter is a smile that engages the entire body.

3. Laughter, an experience that begins as the corners of the mouth turn up slightly. Then, the muscles around the eyes engage and a twinkling can be seen in the eyes. Next, the person begins to make noises, ranging from controlled snickers, escaped chortles, and spontaneous giggles to ridiculous cackles, noisy hoots, and uproarious guffaws. The chest and abdominal muscles become activated. As the noises get louder, the person begins to bend the body back and forth, sometimes slapping the knees, stomping the feet on the floor, or elbowing another person nearby. As laughter reaches its peak, tears flow freely. All of this continues until the person feels so weak and exhausted that he or she must sit down or fall down.

4. Not everyone experiences such intense laughter every time they are amused. Concerns include how others might judge this behavior, the need to maintain a dignified image, feeling that others might be offended by laughter, and cultural taboos on such behavior.

Sounds of Laughter

1. Laughter has different tones and rhythms, almost as if the laughter were coming from different parts of the body; as we listen, these sounds can give us a clue as to why the person is laughing.

2. Common laughter sounds:

   a. *Tee hee* laugh is often a high-pitched titter that seems to come from the top of the head.
      - Arises when a person is very nervous and tries to disguise his or her anxiety with laughter.
      - This laughter acts as a safety valve and allows the person to release a little steam before he or she explodes from built-up pressure.

   b. *Heh heh* laugh is a shallow, almost hollow sound that comes from the throat area.
      - Occurs when a person feels socially obligated to laugh at a joke that is not really considered funny

   c. *Ha ha* laugh emanates from the heart space with a warm resonance and palpable sincerity.
      - Occurs when someone is truly amused or delighted by the humorous stimuli.
      - The kind of laugh that occurs during deep insight or peaceful, joy-filled moments, such as during meditation.

   d. *Ho ho* laugh is the deep belly laugh, the kind in which a person really begins to let go of control and surrender to the experience of deep joy and amusement.
      - The whole body is engaged in movement, which usually continues until exhaustion.
      - The laughter can be deep and so prolonged that the person is left gasping for air and exhausted.

- After the laughter, as the person becomes quiet, a warm glow fills his or her body; there is a lighter, almost buoyant feeling and the mind is less filled with worry, fear, and anger.
- During this after-laughter time, the body feels energized yet relaxed and the person is no longer aware of any pain that was previously felt.
- If this laughter was shared with others, the person feels a sense of connection and trust.
- During these moments one's problems do not feel oppressive; one feels safe and at peace with the world.
- As this occurs the body is making subtle, or sometimes profound, changes at a molecular level that have a powerful impact on the immune system and can enhance the ability to heal.

The Healing Energy of Laughter

1. Laughter is the best medicine seems a widely accepted truth that is now being explained by scientific research.
2. Norman Cousins enlightened the medical community about the healing potential of laughter in his book *Anatomy of an Illness*.[17]
   a. In 1968, Cousins was diagnosed with ankylosing spondylitis; his case was so extreme that he soon experienced great difficulty and pain in moving his joints and was told that his prospect for recovery was very bleak. Because of discomfort and fatigue, he was unable to travel or play tennis, activities that brought him great joy and satisfaction.
   b. Cousins refused to accept his grim prognosis and decided to take charge of his own treatment, working in partnership with his physician. He reasoned that, if negative emotions had played any part in predisposing him to illness, then perhaps positive emotions could aid in his recovery and sought activities that increased his positive emotions, such as faith, hope, festivity, determination, confidence, joy, and a strong will to live.
   c. Cousins used laughter to create positive emotions; he watched films of the Marx Brothers and *Candid Camera*, had nurses read to him from humorous books, and played practical jokes and told jokes.
   d. Cousins began feeling better and objective testing (i.e., sedimentation rates) improved; after several months of this "humor therapy," his illness resolved and never returned.
   e. Despite differing views related to his recovery (i.e., it would have happened anyway; the results were not scientifically significant and represent the observations of a single case), Cousins dedicated the remainder of his life to trying to understand just how his healing occurred.
   f. As an adjunct professor at UCLA (LA), he established a "humor task force" to coordinate and support clinical research into laughter. Today there is scientific research providing evidence for the specific physiologic changes that his individual story suggests.

Physiologic Response to Laughter

1. Berk and Tan were part of Cousins's humor task force. Their research shows that mirthful laughter can have the following effects:
   a. Increase the number and activity of natural killer cells, which attack viral-infected cells and some types of cancer cells.
   b. Increase the number of activated T cells; these cells are "turned on and ready to go."
   c. Increase the level of the antibody IgA, which fights upper respiratory tract infections.
   d. Increase the levels of gamma interferon, a lymphokine that activates many immune components.
   e. Increase levels of complement 3, which helps antibodies to pierce infected cells.
   f. Decrease levels of stress hormones (cortisol, dopamine, epinephrine) that weaken the immune response.[18-20]
   g. This research helps us to better understand the mind–body connection. The emotions and moods we experience directly affect our immune system. If we have a well-developed sense of humor, we are more likely to appreciate the amusing incongruities of life and experience more moments of joy and delight.

These positive emotions can create neurochemical changes that buffer the immunosuppressive effects of stress.[19-26]

2. William Fry began his research into the physical effects of laughter in the 1950s.[27]
   a. Laughter causes the heart rate to elevate, sometimes reaching rates of above 120 beats per minute; respiratory rate and depth and minute volume also increase while the residual volume decreases.
   b. Coughing often occurs during laughter, dislodging mucus plugs.
   c. Peripheral vascular flow is increased as a result of vasodilatation.
   d. Systolic blood pressure is elevated during vigorous laughter but falls below resting levels after the laughter.

3. Extensive research shows that some emotions can create a toxic environment within the body (rage, depression, anxiety) where illnesses such as coronary artery disease, hypertension, and slower wound healing result.[28, 29] These toxic emotional states have been shown to increase the production of proinflammatory cytokines that can lead to arthritis, osteoporosis, cardiovascular disease, and type 2 diabetes. Most studies surrounding the therapeutic effects of humor and laughter focus on the ability of laughter, humor, and play to modulate our emotional experiences.[30-32]

4. Psychoneuroimmunology explores the connections and communication patterns linking the nervous, endocrine, and immune systems.
   a. Research in psychoneuroimmunology shows that the body's own healing system responds favorably to positive attitudes, thoughts, moods, and especially to emotions (e.g., love, hope, optimism, caring, intimacy, joy, laughter, and humor) and responds negatively to negative ones (hate, hopelessness, pessimism, indifference, anxiety, depression, loneliness, etc.).[33]

5. Candace Pert notes that emotions, which are registered and stored in the body in the form of chemical messages, are the most influential connection between the mind and the body. The emotions one experiences in connection with one's thoughts and daily attitudes—and, more specifically, the neurochemical changes that accompany these emotions—have the power to influence health.[34,35]

6. Kubzansky and Thurston, in a 15-year prospective study, show that individuals with higher levels of positive emotion reduced their risk of coronary artery disease.[36]

7. Jacqueline Dowling studied children with cancer.[37] Children with high scores for sense of humor had better psychosocial adjustment to cancer stressors (fatigue, pain, nausea) than those with lower scores; as cancer stressors increased, those children with high humor scores had fewer incidents of infection.

8. A new question is now being asked in the field of psychoneuroimmunology research: Can one's emotional state influence the expression of genes? Preliminary research in the field of epigenetics indicates this is possible.
   a. Several studies from Japan focus on the effect of humor and laughter on diabetes.
   b. Hayashi discovered that the expression of the prorenin receptor gene was less expressed in diabetic patients than in nondiabetic subjects. The decreased expression of this gene among diabetics contributes to increased levels of prorenin concentrations that lead to the release of angiotensin, which triggers vasoconstriction and microvascular problems.
   c. Researchers also found that this prorenin receptor gene was up-regulated significantly after watching a comedy show, thus contributing to a lower level of prorenin and angiotensin and perhaps the vasoconstriction they cause.[38]
   d. This same research team analyzed 41,000 genes and found that 39 of them were up-regulated for at least 90 minutes after watching a comedy video. Four hours after the comedy, 27 genes were still up-regulated and 14 of these genes were related to natural killer cell activity.[39,40]
   e. These studies support the findings of Berk and Tan in 1989 when they measured increased numbers and activity of natural killer cells.[41]

9. Hob Osterlund at Queen's Medical Center in Honolulu together with the University of Hawaii designed a study to compare changes in symptoms related to cancer

and chemotherapy, immune function, and emotional stress levels in two groups of patients who view a humorous or nonhumorous DVD.
   a. A reference to the article is found on Osterlund's website: www.ChuckleChannel.com.
   b. Chuckle Channel is a video resource company that provides hospitals with site-licensed wholesome comedy clips for patient viewing when broadcast through an in-house video programming system.
10. Summary Thought: Humor and laughter are effective methods to modulate our emotional experience probably because of humor's ability to trigger the experience of joy (a strong positive emotion) even in the midst of negative emotion. Studies are showing that almost any program that reduces chronic negative emotion and/or increases daily positive emotion can be expected to support better health.

■ PLAYFULNESS

The Power of Playfulness

1. Play is defined as activities that are amusing, fun, or otherwise enjoyable in their own right—there is joy in the moment.
2. The key to improving our sense of humor is the rediscovery of the playfulness we had as children.
3. Playfulness enhances spontaneity and enjoyment.
4. Playing is as old as humankind.
5. Children use their imagination to invent a reality that meets their needs; as we grow older our ability to open ourselves to moments of playfulness becomes constrained.
   a. Adults are focused on the business at hand.
   b. Playfulness might not fit the image of a proper adult.
6. Scientists believe that the intense sensory and physical stimulation that comes from playing is critical to the growth of cerebral synapses and thus to proper motor development.
7. Early childhood play is one way that humans practice socialization skills and mimic cultural rituals; people create connections with others and build trust.

8. Creative people are playful, experimental, and willing to take risks.
9. In serious situations such as illness or injury, which can require a change in lifestyle or other adaptation, creative problem solving can be a great help. Creative solutions are more likely to come when people are in a relaxed, even playful mood.

■ HUMOR AND STRESS MANAGEMENT

1. One of the main reasons humor exists might be that it helps people adapt to the stresses in their lives.
2. Human beings' superior intellectual capacities lead to high stress.
3. Stress is our perception of the event (Selye); it is people's interpretation of events that causes stress.
4. A sense of humor helps people to view difficult circumstances in a less stressful way.
5. People respond differently to the same environmental stimuli; some seem to cope with stress better than others do.
6. Three "hardiness factors" that can increase a person's resilience to stress and prevent burnout (Kobassa):
   a. Commitment to oneself and one's work
   b. Internal locus of control—belief that one is in control of the choices in one's life
   c. View change as challenging rather than as threatening
7. Humor can be an empowerment tool; it gives people a different perspective on their problems, and with an attitude of detachment, they feel a sense of self-protection and control in their environment.
8. Powerlessness is a current theme in burnout. It is reasonable to assume that, if the locus of control is strongly internal, a person will feel a greater sense of power and thus be more likely to avoid burnout.[42]

■ HUMOR AND LOCUS OF CONTROL

1. Wooten conducted research that documented changes in locus of control and appreciation of humor related to a humor training course.
2. Assessed the locus of control in 231 nurses divided into an experimental and a control group.

3. The experimental group completed a 6-hour humor training course, in which they were given permission and techniques for appropriate use of humor with patients and coworkers. The control group had no such humor training.

4. Both groups were pretested and the same survey tools were readministered 6 weeks later to determine changes in locus of control and appreciation of humor.

5. Data analysis indicated that there was a significant decrease in the score for external locus of control in the experimental group ($P < .0063$, two-tailed) and no significant change for the control group.

6. No significant differences were found in the initial locus of control scores for the experimental and the control groups.

7. This study indicates that, if people are encouraged and guided in using humor, they can gain a sense of control in their lives.

8. Further research is needed to determine how long these effects persist.[43]

Ho Ho Holistic Health

1. Humor, laughter, and play contribute to our health and well-being in many ways.
2. Humor, as a cognitive process, is primarily a mental activity.
3. The behavior of laughter affects the whole body, from cells to entire organ systems.
4. Play and a playful spirit fill us with joy, connect us with others, and keep us focused on the present moment.
5. The interaction of body, mind, and spirit with humor, laughter, and play forms the "Aha, Ha Ha, Ahhhh" continuum:
   a. The mind says, Aha! I get the joke.
   b. The body says, Ha Ha!
   c. The spirit says, Ahhhh, everything feels much better now.

■ HOLISTIC CARING PROCESS

Holistic Assessment

1. In preparing to use humor, laughter, and play interventions, the nurse assesses the following parameters:
   a. The client's ability and willingness to smile and laugh
   b. The client's attitude toward using laughter and play in the current situation

c. The client's history of using humor, laughter, and play in other circumstances
d. The client's visual, auditory, cognitive, and physical limitations
e. The client's preferred style of humor (e.g., jokes, cartoons, stories, comedy movies, animated cartoons, stand-up comedy, funny songs)
f. The client's favorite comedy artists—performers, writers, cartoonists, and so on
g. The client's feelings about previous experiences with humor and play
h. The client's preferred playful activities

2. Identification of patterns/challenges/needs: The patterns/challenges/needs compatible with interventions for humor, laughter, and play are as follows:
   a. Altered parenting, actual or potential
   b. Social isolation
   c. Ineffective individual and family coping
   d. Activity intolerance, actual or potential
   e. Deficit in diversion activity
   f. Impaired physical mobility
   g. Powerlessness
   h. Disturbance in self-concept: altered self-esteem, role performance, personal identity
   i. Altered sensation or perception: visual, auditory, kinesthetic, gustatory, tactile, olfactory
   j. Altered thought processes
   k. Anxiety
   l. Pain
   m. Fear
   n. Potential for violence: self-directed or directed at others

3. Exhibit 15-2, Nursing Interventions: Play and Laughter, guides the nurse in outcomes, nursing prescriptions, and evaluation for the use of humor, laughter, and play as a nursing intervention. (See Chapter 15 in *Holistic Nursing: A Handbook for Practice* [6th edition].)

Therapeutic Care Plan and Interventions

1. Before the session:
   a. Assess your own ease and comfort with using humor and play as a therapeutic intervention.
   b. Practice smiling in front of a mirror: First scowl, and then smile. Feel the difference.

c. Evaluate your ability to respond to humor or engage in playful activity for your own personal pleasure.

d. Increase awareness of your own preferred humor style, artist, writer, performer.

e. Allow yourself to laugh with abandon at things you find funny.

f. Become familiar with the content and variety of humorous items and playful activities that are available for you to use.

g. Ensure that all supplies and equipment are in working condition.

h. Improve your ability to tell a good joke. Remember these tips: Keep it short—less than 2 minutes. Be sure you can remember the whole joke before you start. Let your body, face, and voice become animated as you tell the joke. Pause occasionally as you deliver the material; create a brief and concise setup for the punch line; pause before delivering the punch line; speak the punch line clearly and with punch!

i. Review the client's chart or consult with others to assess changes in the client's situation since you last met.

j. Sense your own needs and stress level. Give yourself permission to be silly and playful.

2. At the beginning of the session:

a. Assess the client's status according to the assessment parameters.

b. Record vital signs and ask the client to assess pain, anxiety, tension, or other target symptoms on a numerical scale (1 = comfortable, 10 = extremely uncomfortable).

c. Describe to the client the benefits that humor, laughter, and play have on the body (physiologic), mind (psychological), and spirit (emotional and energy level).

d. Provide the client with appropriate materials to match his or her preference and some instructions for use.

3. During the session:

a. Use all interventions with sensitivity to the client's needs, responses, and difficulties.

b. Provide support for the client through your physical presence, encouragement, or time alone if the client wants to read or watch a videotape.

c. Remember that humor is contagious and social. Interventions can be most effective if used within a group (e.g., family and friends) rather than individually.

d. Remember that humor and play are spontaneous and therefore are most successful when not precisely planned.

4. At the end of the session:

a. Record vital signs and ask the client to reevaluate the pain, tension, or target symptom on a scale of 1 to 10.

b. Discuss the intervention with the client and obtain feedback for future sessions.

c. Answer any questions the client might have.

d. Encourage the client to continue using the intervention at home and to explore other possible variations.

e. Use Client Outcomes (Exhibit 15-2) and the Evaluation of the Client's Subjective Experience with Humor, Laughter, and Play (Exhibit 15-3), in *Holistic Nursing: A Handbook for Practice* (6th edition) to evaluate the session.

f. Schedule a follow-up session.

Specific Interventions: Humor, Laughter, and Play

1. Humor interventions can be packaged in many different ways—as humor rooms, comedy carts, humor baskets, laughter libraries, or caring clown programs.

2. The individual caregiver can adapt these programs to meet the specific needs of clients.

3. Suggestions for starting a humor program:

a. Create a scrapbook of cartoons; consider the audience that will read this scrapbook.

b. Develop a file of funny jokes, stories, cards, bumper stickers, poems, and songs.

c. Collect or borrow funny books, DVDs, videos, and audiocassettes of comedy routines.

d. Keep a file of local clowns, magicians, storytellers, and puppeteers; invite them to entertain at your facility, at the patient's home, or at a group function.

e. Collect toys, interactive games, noise-makers, and costume items and keep them available for play.

f. Create a humor journal or log to record funny encounters or humorous discoveries.

g. Establish a bulletin board in your facility or on your refrigerator at home. Post cartoons, bumper stickers, and funny signs. If the display is public, you must consider the sensitivities of the audience and be careful to exclude potentially offensive (e.g., ageist, sexist, ethnic) material.

h. Subscribe to a humorous newsletter or journal to collect new ideas and inspiration.

i. Educate yourself about therapeutic humor:
   - Communication studies have shown that people take in 7% of other people's words, 38% of their vocal characteristics, and 55% of their nonverbal signals.[44]
   - Applying these concepts in the creation and communication of humor can make your efforts even more effective.
   - Because the client will notice less than 10% of your words, choose them carefully.

j. Develop a collection of zingy one-liners, clever riddles, funny stories, and brilliant jokes for every occasion.

k. Vocal characteristics are five times more important than words alone; try to change the pace and tone of your voice, or speak with an accent, and your words will have more impact.

l. The most powerful communication tool we have is the ability to communicate nonverbally; facial expressions, physical gestures, costuming, props, and the way we walk or stand or reach for something are nonverbal communication techniques that provide the greatest impact on our audience.

m. Suggestions for humor program packages:
   - Laughter libraries offer a selection of funny and informative books about humor and health; audiocassettes, DVDs, and videos are usually a part of this collection.
   - A humor room is a place where clients, their families, and staff can gather to laugh, play, and relax together.
   - A comedy cart is a mobile unit with many of the same supplies available in a humor room.
   - A humor basket is probably the easiest therapeutic humor program to create and is an appropriate place to start if time and resources are limited.
   - Bedside clowning attempts to distract patients from their problems to help them forget their pain.[43]
   - Scan the local TV program schedule and create a list of humorous entertainment options; post this list in a common area.
   - When using closed-circuit video, be sure to obtain permission for use if the material is copyrighted. In some situations, a license must be purchased to show these films to large audiences.

4. Exhibit 15-4, Supplies for Humor Programs, guides the nurse in gathering supplies for use in a humor therapy program. (See Chapter 15 in *Holistic Nursing: A Handbook for Practice* [6th edition].)

Evaluation

1. With the client, the nurse determines whether the client outcomes for humor, laughter, and play were successfully achieved (Exhibit 15-2).

2. To evaluate the session further, the nurse might again explore the subjective effects of the experience with the client using the evaluation questions in Exhibit 15-3.

▣ NOTES

1. Robinson, V. (1952). *Humor and the health professions*. Thorofare, NJ: Slack.

2. Kronenberger, L. (1952). *The thread of laughter*. New York, NY: Knopf.

3. Freud, S. (1961). Jokes and their relation to the unconscious. In *The complete psychological works of Sigmund Freud* (Vol. 8). London, England: Hogarth Press. (Original work published 1905)

4. Mindess, H. (1971). *Laughter and liberation*. Los Angeles, CA: Mansh.

5. Dean, R., Kinsman, A., & Gregory, D. (2005). More than trivial: Strategies for using humor in palliative care. *Cancer Nursing, 28*(4), 292–300.

6. Borod, M. (2006). SMILES: Toward a better laughter life: A model for introducing humor in

the palliative care setting. *Journal of Cancer Education, 2*(1), 30–34.

7. Walter, M., Hanni, B., Haug, M., Amrhein, I., Krebs-Roubicek, E., Muller-Spahn, F.,...Savaskan, E. (2007). Humour therapy in patients with late-life depression or Alzheimer's disease: A pilot study. *International Journal of Geriatric Psychiatry, 22*(1), 77–83.

8. Wooten, P. (2000). *Compassionate laughter* (2nd ed.). Santa Cruz, CA: Jest.

9. Olsson, H., Backe, H., Sorensen, S., & Kock, M. (2002). The essence of humour and its effects and functions: A qualitative study. *Journal of Nursing Management, 10*(1), 21–26.

10. Johnson, P. (2002). The use of humor and its influences on spirituality and coping in breast cancer survivors. *Oncology Nursing Forum, 29*(4), 691–695.

11. Christie, W., & Moore, C. (2005). The impact of humor on patients with cancer. *Clinical Journal of Oncology Nursing, 9*(2), 211–218.

12. Joshua, A., Cotroneo, A., & Clarke, S. (2005). Humor and oncology. *Journal of Clinical Oncology, 23*(3), 645–648.

13. Scholl, J. C., & Ragan, S. L. (2003). The use of humor in promoting positive provider–patient interactions in a hospital rehabilitation unit. *Health Communication, 15*(3), 321–330.

14. Scholl, J. (2007). The use of humor to promote patient-centered care. *Journal of Applied Communication Research, 35*(2), 156.

15. Klein, A. (1998). *Courage to laugh*. Los Angeles, CA: Tarcher.

16. Garrick, J. (2006). The humor of trauma survivors: Its application in a therapeutic milieu. *Journal of Aggression, Maltreatment, and Trauma, 12*(1), 169–182.

17. Cousins, N. (1979). *Anatomy of an illness*. New York, NY: W. W. Norton.

18. Berk, L. S., Felten, D., Tan, S., Bittman, B., & Westengard, J. (2001). Modulation of neuroimmune parameters during the eustress of humor-associated mirthful laughter. *Alternative Therapies Health Medicine, 7*(2), 62–72, 74–76.

19. Bennett, M., Zeller, J. M., Rosenberg, L., & McCann, J. (2003). The effect of mirthful laughter on stress and natural killer cell activity. *Alternative Therapy Health Medicine, 9*(2), 38–45.

20. Takahashi, K., Iwase, M., Yamashita, K., Tatsumoto, Y., Ue, H., Kuratsune, H.,...Takeda, M. (2001). The elevation of natural killer cell activity induced by laughter in a crossover designed study. *International Journal of Molecular Medicine, 8*(6), 645–650.

21. Martin, R. (2001). Humor, laughter, and physical health: Methodological issues and research findings. *Psychological Bulletin, 127,* 504–519.

22. Lefcourt, H., & Martin, R. (1986). *Humor and life stress.* New York, NY: Springer-Verlag.

23. Wooten, P. (1996). Humor: An antidote for stress. *Holistic Nursing Practice, 10*(2), 49–55.

24. Bennett, M., & Lengacher, C. (2006, March). Humor and laughter may influence health: I. History and background. *Evidence-Based Complementary and Alternative Medicine,* 61–63.

25. Bennett, M., & Lengacher, C. (2006, June). Humor and laughter may influence health: II. Complementary therapies and humor in a clinical population. *Evidence-Based Complementary and Alternative Medicine,* 187–190.

26. Bennett, M., & Lengacher, C. (2007, May). Humor and laughter may influence health: III. Laughter and health outcomes. *Evidence-Based Complementary and Alternative Medicine.*

27. Fry, W. (1992). The physiological effects of humor, mirth, and laughter. *Journal of the American Medical Association, 267,* 1857–1858.

28. Biing-Jiun, S. et. al. (2008).

29. Glaser, R., Kiecolt-Glaser, J. K. (2002). Depression and immune function: Central pathways to morbidity and mortality. *Journal of psychosomatic research, 53*(4), 873–876.

30. Glaser, R., Kiecolt-Glaser, J. K., Preacher, K. J., MacCallum, R. C., Atkinson, C., & Malarkey, W. B. (2003, January). Chronic stress and age-related increases in the proinflammatory cytokine IL-6. *Proceedings of the National Academy of Sciences of the United States of America, 100*(15), 9090–9095.

31. Graham, J., Christian, L., & Kiecolt-Glaser, J. (2006). Stress, Age, and Immune Function: Toward a Lifespan Approach. *Journal of Behavioral Medicine, 29*(4), 389–400.

32. Kendall-Tackett, K. A. (2009). Psychological trauma and physical health: A psychoneuroimmunology approach to etiology of negative health effects and possible interventions. *Psychological Trauma, 1,* 35–48.

33. McGhee (2010). *Humor: The Lighter Path to Resilience and Health.* Bloomington, Indiana: AuthorHouse.

34. Pert, C. (1997). *Molecules of emotion.* New York, NY: Scribner's.

35. Glaser, R., Kiecolt-Glaser, J. K. (2005). Stress-induced immune dysfunction: Implications for health. *Nature reviews. Immunology, 5*(3), 243–251.

36. Kubzansky, L., & Thurston, R. (2007). Emotional vitality and incident coronary heart disease. *Archives of General Psychiatry, 64,* (12), 1393–1401.

37. Dowling, J. S. (2002). Humor: A coping strategy for pediatric patients. *Pediatric Nursing, 28*(2), 123–131.

38. Hayashi, T., Urayama, O., Hori, M., Sakamoto, S., Nasir, U. M., Iwanaga, S.,...Murakami, K. (2007).

Laughter modulates prorenin receptor gene expression in patients with type 2 diabetes. *Journal of Psychosomatic Research, 62,* 703–706.

39. Hayashi, T., Tsujii, S., Iburi, T., Tamanaha, T, Yamagami, K., Ishibashi, R.,...Murakami, K. (2007). Laughter up-regulates the genes related to NK cell activity in diabetes. *Biomedical Research, 28*(6), 281–285.

40. Matsuzaki, T., Nakajima, A., Ishigami, S., Tanno, M., & Yoshino, S. (2006). Mirthful laughter differentially affects serum pro and anti-inflammatory cytokine levels depending on the level of disease activity in patients with rheumatoid arthritis. *Rheumatology, 45,* 182–186.

41. Berk, L. (1989). Neuroendocrine and stress hormone changes during mirthful laughter. *American Journal of Medical Sciences, 298,* 390–396.

42. Maslach, C. (2001). Job burnout: New directions in research and intervention. *Current Directions in Psychological Science, 12,* 189–192.

43. Wooten, P. (1992). Does a humor workshop affect nurse burnout? *Journal of Nursing Jocularity, 2*(2), 42–43.

44. Beckman, H., Regier, N., & Young, J. (2007). Effect of workplace laughter groups on personal efficacy beliefs. *Journal of Primary Prevention, 28,* 167–182.

▨ STUDY QUESTIONS

Basic Level

1. Which of the following answer choices best defines *humor*?
   a. A willingness to laugh
   b. An ability to recognize and appreciate the absurdity of a situation
   c. An ability to tell jokes and make people laugh
   d. A time of playfulness

2. Which of the following answer choices best characterizes therapeutic humor programs?
   a. Inappropriate for seriously ill or terminal patients
   b. Most effective when created by one or two enthusiastic staff members
   c. Usually limited to the pediatric department
   d. Helpful to patients, family, and staff

3. What is the difference between hoping humor and coping humor?
   a. There is no difference between hoping and coping humor.
   b. Hoping humor is used any time and coping humor is used during stress.
   c. Hoping humor reflects an acceptance of life while coping humor releases tension.
   d. Hoping humor makes others feel good and coping humor makes you feel good.

4. In preparing to use humor, laughter, and play interventions, what does the holistic nurse assess?
   a. Client's financial status
   b. Supplies available on the laughter cart
   c. Availability of the local clown group
   d. Client's cognitive limitations

5. The holistic nurse observes a person telling a client a joke. Which laughter sound indicates to the nurse that the client is uncomfortable?
   a. Ho ho
   b. Heh heh
   c. Tee hee
   d. Ha ha

6. The client tells the holistic nurse a joke that he finds uncomfortable. What is the nurse's best response?
   a. Laugh
   b. Say nothing
   c. Be honest with the client
   d. Tell a joke of his own

7. Which of the following is a guideline for appropriate use of humor with clients?
   a. Humorous interventions should occur after the client's physical or emotional needs are met.
   b. If the client does not respond with observable laughter, the intervention should be discontinued.
   c. Initiate humorous intervention within the first 20 minutes of meeting a client to establish the connection of shared laughter.
   d. If a client seems offended by your humor, keep trying a different joke or prop until you get a laugh.

Advanced Level

8. The AHN-BC has just started as the educator in the ED. She enters the break room and sees the following cartoon: A patient is carried into an emergency room by army of body lice, who chant, "Save our host. Save our host." Which of the following responses best illustrates her understanding of this type of humor?
   a. Hoping humor decreases stress.
   b. Gallows humor offers distance from suffering.
   c. Therapeutic humor prevents burnout.
   d. Coping humor is appropriate in emergencies.

9. How does an AHN-BC evaluate a client's subjective response to a humor intervention?
   a. Compares pre- and postintervention blood pressure
   b. Schedules additional interventions
   c. Observes the client's body language
   d. Explores any shifts that the client notices

10. What does the AHN-BC who works with people living with immunosuppressive challenges understand laughter interventions might do?
    a. Increase the number and activity of natural killer cells
    b. Down-regulate angiotensin
    c. Stabilize the emotions
    d. Decrease IgA

11. Utilizing her knowledge of holistic communication in planning a humor program, the AHN-BC determines that which of the following interventions will be most appropriate for the pediatric clinic?
    a. Employ a play therapist
    b. Have comic cartoons playing in the waiting room
    c. Post a drawing board with colorful crayons available
    d. Help the staff to develop funny one-liners

12. The AHN-BC understands that humor interventions enhance resilience by which mechanism?
    a. Stimulating laughter to external stimuli
    b. Strengthening the internal locus of control
    c. Negating bad news
    d. Improving strength

13. Mr. H states that he has found the humor cart lacking in certain materials. The AHN-BC understands that his statement contributes to the humor program evaluation in which way?
    a. Suggesting what materials are needed
    b. Offering his descriptions of the experience
    c. Indicating that the program needs revision
    d. Reflecting his general discomfort with humor

Chapter 17

Relaxation

Dorothy M. Larkin and
Jeanne Anselmo

■ DEFINITIONS

Autogenic training Developed by Johannes Schultz and Wolfgang Luthe, this practice teaches relaxation through the repetition of phrases that influence muscle relaxation by bringing an awareness of sensations and feelings of warmth, heaviness, and relaxation to the body.

Biofeedback The use of technology or monitors that augment and feed back usually imperceptible signals from the person's psychophysiologic processes for the purpose of cultivating the ability to influence or change stress-related patterns or symptoms. This self-regulation process, which is usually paired with a relaxation practice, offers the person an opportunity to be an active participant in his or her own healing and health maintenance.

Hypnosis A process for focused awareness and expanded consciousness with diminishing perception of peripheral sensations, thoughts, and feelings.

Mantra A word, short phrase, or prayer that is repeated either silently or aloud as a focus of concentration during the practice of meditation.

Meditation Originally based in spiritual traditions, the practice of awareness, focus, and concentration while maintaining a passive yet awake attitude; evolves with discipline and practice and is known to provide health benefits as well as being a road to personal and spiritual transformation.

Pain (medical definition) Localized sensation of hurt, or an unpleasant sensory and emotional experience associated with actual or potential tissue damage, or described in terms of such damage.

Pain (nursing definition) A subjective experience including both verbal and nonverbal behavior.

Power Barrett's theory of power as knowing participation in change is being aware of what one is choosing to do, feeling free to do it, and doing intentionally.

Progressive muscle relaxation The process of alternately tensing and relaxing muscle groups to become aware of subtle degrees of tension and relaxation; originally developed by Edmund Jacobson.

Relaxation (psychophysiologic definition) A psychophysiologic experience characterized by parasympathetic dominance involving multiple visceral and somatic systems; the absence of physical, mental, and emotional tension; the opposite of Canon's fight-or-flight response and Selye's general adaptation syndrome.

Relaxation response An alert, hypokinetic process of decreased sympathetic nervous system arousal that can be achieved in a number of ways, including through breathing exercises, relaxation and imagery exercises, biofeedback, and prayer. A degree of discipline is required to evoke this response, which increases mental and physical well-being.

Self-hypnosis An approach for voluntarily fostering a consciousness process for the purpose of influencing one's thoughts, perceptions, behaviors, or sensations.

Stress (psychophysiologic definition) The felt experience of overactivity of the sympathetic nervous system.

■ THEORY AND RESEARCH

1. Relaxation is an ancient art with many modern interpretations.
2. Relaxation has been defined in medical and scientific terms as a psychophysiologic state characterized by parasympathetic dominance involving multiple visceral and somatic systems. It is also defined as the absence of physical, mental, and emotional tension, and the opposite of Canon's fight-or-flight response.
3. Relaxation can also be described as an experience of calm, comfort, deep rest, natural nurturing, inner connectedness, renewal, and openness that every living creature instinctively and intuitively knows how to access.
4. Stress-related illnesses account for 75–80% of illness in modern life
5. Exhibit 16-1, Clinical Benefits of Relaxation, outlines the usefulness of relaxation interventions for people in all stages of health and illness.[1] (See Chapter 16 in *Holistic Nursing: A Handbook for Practice* [6th edition]. All references to *Holistic Nursing* are for the sixth edition.)
6. Relaxation is not new to nursing. Florence Nightingale counseled her nurses to support patients' rest and well-being by reducing unnecessary noise, not awakening patients out of their first sleep, and protecting patients from unnecessary disturbances such as conversations of doctors or friends within earshot and the disturbing rustling of crinolines. She advised that "all hurry or bustle is peculiarly painful to the sick."[2]
7. Today, nurses offer relaxation practices in self-care circles for themselves and their colleagues, as well as for clients in hospitals, community and adult education programs, outpatient clinics, and homeless shelters, to promote a variety of personal benefits.
8. Exhibit 16-2, Whole Self Benefits of Relaxation, can be found in Chapter 16 of *Holistic Nursing: A Handbook for Practice* (6th edition).

Cross-Cultural Context

1. Relaxation practices are found throughout time in all cultures around the world.
2. These practices can be mediated through the use of herbs, acupuncture, movement, or prayer. Evidence of the power, impact, and importance of relaxation and the use of breath can be seen in shamanic healing, yoga, and meditation.
3. Modern research supports the efficacy of relaxation in the areas of psychoneuroimmunology and neuroplasticity; modern psychology uses relaxation for systematic desensitization and for facilitating healing of post-traumatic stress conditions.
4. Jon Kabat-Zinn includes relaxation breathing and body scanning as mindfulness-based stress reduction practice for pain and depression.[3]
5. Dean Ornish includes relaxation, meditation, breathing, and yoga in a cardiac rehab program to reverse heart disease.[4]
6. Dolores Krieger and Dora Kunz guided nurses to perform sustained centering and presencing, a practice of meditative inner connection and relaxed awareness, before entering into Therapeutic Touch practice with their clients.[5]

Caring for Ourselves, Caring for Others: A Spiritual Journey in Time of Continual Change and Global Uncertainty

1. Finding and cultivating a personal relaxation practice can help nurses restore, renew, deepen professional self-development, avoid burnout, and model a personal wellness path for their clients.
2. Living this path and sharing by example give nurses an important refuge, an inner understanding, and appreciation of the benefits and challenges their clients face as they start to integrate complementary practice into their everyday lives.
3. Whether individuals are being with themselves and with "all that is" in meditation, exploring their own past issues, traumas, or painful life experiences in counseling and psychotherapy, or expanding

their awareness in intuitive practices and energy healing, a foundation of deep relaxation of the body-mind-spirit is a fundamental step on the path

4. See Exhibit 16-3, Benefits of Relaxation, in *Holistic Nursing: A Handbook for Practice.*

5. This intensity and competitiveness of life can be our undoing, especially if we forget the importance to our body-mind-spirit of nondoing, which is different from "doing nothing."

6. The following are the generalized stress responses of the body, mind, and energy field: constriction of blood flow to the hands and feet (cool extremities); tightening of the muscles; constriction of one's energy field (closing down or blocking flow); increased heart rate; increased oxygen consumption; increased brain wave activity; increased sweat gland activity; increased blood pressure; increased anxiety.

The Stress Response

1. The last decade has brought new awareness to what constitutes an emergency response, both for individuals and for society. Whether we are dealing with a national or international tragedy or disaster or the everyday intense internal reactions we experience when faced with a truck cutting in front of us on the highway, a "code blue" coming over the loudspeaker, or a child darting into the street, we experience what some researchers refer to as an "adrenaline rush," the familiar fight-or-flight response. This response is a complex series of psychophysiologic processes that prepare us to deal with real or perceived emergencies.

2. See the relaxation exercise in Chapter 16 of *Holistic Nursing: A Handbook for Practice.*

■ MEDITATION

Relaxation Response Meditation

1. The phrase *relaxation response* originated with Herbert Benson and his colleagues at Harvard University; they used this nonreligious form of meditation to produce the opposite of the fight-or-flight response.

2. Its efficacy has been demonstrated in treating hypertension and anxiety.[6] The changes that occur when an individual reaches a

deep level of relaxation are exactly the opposite of those that occur in the fight-or-flight response.

3. Alterations take place in the automatic, endocrine, immune, and neuropeptide systems as follows: deep relaxation increases: peripheral blood flow (warm extremities); electrical resistance of skin (dry palms); production of slow alpha waves; activity of natural killer cells (improved immune function).

4. Deep relaxation decreases the following functions in the body: oxygen consumption; carbon dioxide elimination; blood lactate levels; respiratory rate and volume; heart rate; skeletal muscle tension; epinephrine level; gastric acidity and motility; sweat gland activity; blood pressure, especially in hypertensive individuals.[7]

5. Benson calls the relaxation response meditation "a very simple technique" and cites four basic elements common to the relaxation response: a quiet environment, a mental device (repeating silently a single-syllable word or sound), a passive attitude (not forcing the relaxation), and a comfortable position.

Breathing In and Breathing Out

1. Conscious awareness of breathing—whether the slow, deep, diaphragmatic breaths of hatha yoga or the mindful awareness of breathing in and out in mindfulness meditation—can be practiced in formal sessions of 20 to 45 minutes once or twice a day.

2. Conscious awareness of breathing also can be practiced informally by breathing with mindfulness during everyday activities.

3. Jon Kabat-Zinn developed an 8-week mindfulness-based stress-reduction program that demonstrates how conscious awareness of breathing can help to relieve chronic pain, depression, and anxiety. Several studies in clinics, communities, and prisons have demonstrated that Kabat-Zinn's program, as well as other modern forms of meditation, can improve quality of life and reduce symptoms.

4. See Table 16-1, Research-Based Outcomes of Meditation, in *Holistic Nursing: A Handbook for Practice.*

Breathing and Energy Healing Practice

1. The breath or life force, called *prana* in yoga and *qi* (or *chi* or *ki*) in Chinese energy practice, is the vital force or energy that animates life.
2. Nurses practicing Therapeutic Touch center themselves and use their breathing practice to help enhance this sustained centeredness and their openness to this healing life force.

Other Forms of Meditation

1. Hundreds of practices can be listed under the heading of meditation, for example, relaxation response, mindfulness, insight, transcendental, vispassana, and centering prayer. Each practice cultivates a qualitative state of mind that can induce a deep experience of relaxation and calm.
2. Other meditation practices invite meditators to gaze at the flame of a candle, a sacred image, or a mandala; to chant aloud; or to concentrate on a nondualist or unanswerable question (or koan), as in Zen practice.
3. Janet Macrae calls Therapeutic Touch a moving meditation.[8] Sufi, Native American, and shamanic ritual dancing are other forms of moving meditation.
4. The purpose of spiritually focused meditation is to awaken to a higher consciousness, to be at one with the sacredness of "All," and to become one with the Divine. Individuals practice such meditation to open the body-mind-spirit to the qualities of compassion, wisdom, forgiveness, skillfulness, no fear, stillness, openness, and interconnectedness.
5. What would health care be like if nurses, physicians, and other healthcare practitioners began by cultivating a heart of compassion and service? What would the healthcare system be like? Would burnout exist? (See the section on loving kindness meditation later in this text.)

Meditation Practices

1. Mindful breathing during nursing practice
   a. Nurses who wish to be more present with their clients, to practice self-care, and to awaken to the simple sacredness of everyday nursing practice (e.g., hanging an intravenous bag, writing nursing notes, eating, walking down a hall, feeding a patient) might want to practice mindful breathing each moment, as in the following exercises.
   b. Begin with the breath, reminding oneself to offer self-care in each moment by consciously breathing with each activity. Breath is a gift of self-renewal, freshness, and aliveness that deepens with practice. It is a gift nurses can give to themselves every moment.
2. Mindful breathing meditations
   a. Exploring and practicing relaxation and meditation help the nurse gain insight into specific methods and issues that clients might face as they work to integrate these techniques into their daily lives.
   b. When choosing a meditation practice to explore, the nurse should commit to that practice for at least 4-6 weeks before trying another, while keeping a journal of his or her reflections along the way.
   c. Exercise: Mindfulness of the Breath Exercise I (Lying Down) can be found in Chapter 16 of *Holistic Nursing*.
   d. Exercise: Mindfulness of the Breath Exercise II (Sitting) can be found in Chapter 16 of *Holistic Nursing*.
3. Walking meditation
   a. Walking as if one were planting peace with each step—this is the essence of walking meditation.[3pp33-39] This practice can be especially helpful during times of trauma and crisis and can be done to center oneself in the most challenging and traumatic of circumstances.
   b. To practice, start with the left foot and begin walking slowly by synchronizing the in and out of the breathing meditation practice with each step. Sometimes you might take three steps to the inhale and three steps to the exhale. Play with your practice, exploring how carefully you can become aware of the subtle sensations of slowly lifting, moving, and placing each step as you continue to be aware of your breathing.
4. Cultivating the heart of compassion meditation
   a. Loving kindness meditation
      - This meditation for helping professionals is adapted from Thich Nhat

Hanh's loving kindness meditation in *Teachings on Love*.[9]

- Sitting peacefully, begin as in sitting meditation practice, and then plant each phrase like a healing seed within your heart, following your breath and focusing on your intention to cultivate compassion. Say each line to yourself in your mind, or ask a friend to read this meditation aloud to you, pausing after each line so that you can slowly repeat it silently to yourself.
- Scripts for Lovingkindness Meditations Parts I–III can be found in Chapter 16 of *Holistic Nursing*.
- For other heart-opening meditations, see the St. Francis prayer and www.Beliefnet.com.

b. Quiet heart prayer

- One of the most frequently used traditional nursing spiritual therapies is prayer.[10]
- Prayer is a way of eliciting the relaxation response in the context of one's deeply held
- personal, religious, or philosophic beliefs. Benson refers to this as incorporating the "faith factor" into relaxation.
- Many people are comfortable with prayer as meditation. In healthcare settings, nurses need to accommodate the client's spiritual needs, either by calling on his or her personal spiritual and religious background and resources or by enlisting the help of appropriate family of the client, clergy, or chaplaincy staff.

▪ MODERN RELAXATION METHODS

Progressive Muscle Relaxation

1. In 1935, Edmund Jacobson detailed a strategy leading to deep muscle relaxation. In progressive muscle relaxation, the individual deliberately tenses muscle groups, focusing on the tightening sensations, and then slowly releases that tension. In this way, the individual learns to manage levels of muscle tension and deepen the experience of comfort
2. Table 16-2, Research-Based Outcomes of Relaxation, can be found in *Holistic Nursing*.

3. Exercise: Progressive Muscle Relaxation—Sample Script can be found in Chapter 16 of *Holistic Nursing*.
4. If the client is experiencing pain or difficulty with a particular part of the body, the exercise should begin as far away from the involved area as possible and conclude with the primary area of difficulty.
5. Clients should be coached to breathe throughout the session, thereby avoiding the temptation to hold their breath as they tighten their muscles.
6. Clients can learn to exhale as they tighten muscle groups. Tension in muscles should be held short of true discomfort.
7. Progressive muscle relaxation is an active intervention; therefore, it should be used with caution for clients with ischemic myocardial disease, hypertension, and back pain.
8. Table 16-3, Hypothesized Effects of Relaxation Therapies, can be found in *Holistic Nursing*.

Autogenic Training

1. Similar to self-hypnosis, autogenic strategies are specific present-time-oriented self-healing phrases inducing self-change from within.
2. Developed by Johannes Schultz and his student Wolfgang Luthe in 1932, autogenic training has been found to be effective in managing disorders in which cognitive involvement is prominent.
3. Exercise: Autogenic Training—Sample Script can be found in Chapter 16 of *Holistic Nursing*.

Selecting Relaxation Interventions for Clients

1. No formula exists for determining which relaxation intervention is best for which client. The approach must be tailored to the individual based on his or her condition, personal preferences, and available time.
2. Audio and video relaxation CDs and DVDs or online versions of relaxation videos or audio instructions present relaxation in a nonthreatening, gentle manner. These can be offered over hospital closed-circuit television; downloaded from the Internet onto clients' electronic devices, iPods, or MP3

players; or become part of a nursing comfort cart on each floor.

3. The following are guidelines for the client in the use of relaxation audio or videos:
   a. Listen to an exercise at least once a day, preferably twice a day.
   b. Never listen to a relaxation exercise when you are driving or operating a vehicle.
   c. Arrange to have uninterrupted privacy while you listen to the practice.
   d. Listen with headphones or ear buds to help block out distracting noises from the environment.
   e. Listen or watch in a relaxing position in which your body is supported.

Holistic Nurse Learning Experiment I

1. One of the most effective tools for understanding relaxation is self-exploration and self-experimentation.
2. Within herself or himself, the nurse is a mini laboratory able to explore these various methods and do inner research; all that is needed is a journal and the commitment to inner exploration and personal and professional self-development.
3. Exhibit 16-4, Inner Laboratory Journal, can be found in *Holistic Nursing*.

Hypnosis and Self-Hypnosis

1. Most people misunderstand the use of trance and hypnosis and associate it with stage professionals and entertainment.
2. Hypnosis and trance have been used for healing and therapeutic purposes in ancient societies with priest–healers and native shamans.
3. In the late 1700s, Viennese physician Franz Mesmer offered "magnetic" treatments to his patients that included hypnosis. The word *mesmerized* is now part of our language.
4. Dorothy Larkin describes hypnosis as "a process of therapeutic communication, awareness, and behavior within the context of a therapeutic relationship" (personal communication, June 16, 2003).
5. In hypnosis, attention can be more focused or more mobile, and there is a tendency for greater responsiveness to suggestion.
6. When people are disoriented, frightened, unconscious, or very ill they may experience

a hypnotic state which promotes hypersuggestibility[11] This naturally occurring trance opens up the client to the influence of nurses' therapeutic presence and therapeutic suggestions.

7. Larkin and many other nurse experts in hypnosis have explored ways in which therapeutic suggestion can enhance patient cooperation and comfort.[13]
8. Nurses can recognize a hypnotic experience in clients who have a faraway stare, glazed eyes, or fixed attention. Larkin notes that nurses can utilize this receptive state by offering therapeutic suggestion, reassurance, and health-promoting education. Continual assessment will need to be implemented so that if the subject's attention suddenly shifts, the nurse can concurrently change the offered therapeutic strategy to meet the patient's needs and altered perceptions.[13]
9. Therapeutic suggestions and conversational induction are also vital accompaniments in disbursing medication. For example, the nurse might say, "This medication will help to quiet your nervous system so that you can relax more comfortably into sleep" rather than, "This pill is for your insomnia." The former emphasizes the possible comfort response, and the latter focuses on the problem.
10. All nurses can learn to use reframing, conversational inductions, and positive therapeutic suggestion and to recognize an everyday hypnotic trance process of clients in crisis.
11. Nurses can also practice self-hypnosis and therapeutic suggestion as part of their personal self-care in addition to teaching clients this practice so that they can continue self-care at home.

Biofeedback

1. To monitor body-mind-spirit changes biofeedback uses modern equipment that can be found in most health facilities and that most nurses employ daily.
2. Biofeedback combines ancient awareness practice and technology.
3. Clients learn how to self-regulate when the devices monitoring the unitary body-mind-spirit are turned so that clients can read their displays.

4. Recall what has just been explored with regard to therapeutic hypnotic suggestion and reframing, and imagine how this new knowledge and awareness might be used to empower clients as they encounter the monitors and other technical equipment in the healthcare setting. If you can imagine turning your monitors around and teaching clients the positive meaning of the monitor's signals so that they can understand how their bodies respond to thoughts and feelings, then you have already begun to understand the impact and usefulness of biofeedback.
5. Exhibit 16-5, Clinical Indicators for Biofeedback, can be found in *Holistic Nursing*.
6. Biofeedback has been practiced since the 1960s. Its focus is to teach clients to create "psychosomatic health" instead of psychosomatic illness.[14]

Holistic Nurse Learning Experiment II

1. Biofeedback can offer nurses the opportunity for independent professional practice, whether in private practice or in an institutional setting. Many nurses integrate biofeedback into relaxation therapy, stress management, health counseling, and teaching.
2. Exercise: Progressive Muscle Relaxation—Sample Script can be found in Chapter 16 of *Holistic Nursing*.
3. Exercise: Biofeedback can be found in Chapter 16 of *Holistic Nursing*.
4. Exhibit 16-6, Important Factors in Relaxation Practice, can be found in *Holistic Nursing*.
5. Exercise: Biofeedback: Variation A Client Practice can be found in Chapter 16 of *Holistic Nursing*.
6. Exercise: Biofeedback: Variation B Group Self-Care Experiment can be found in Chapter 16 of *Holistic Nursing*.

Special Issues for Groups

1. "I don't have time. I'm too busy. I could be/should be catching up on my work, not relaxing." Sandy O'Brien and Jeanne Anselmo developed a staff wellness project using the practices described previously. The answer they found to the challenge of "I don't have time to practice" (the work-and-hurry sickness) is that we cannot afford not to care for ourselves.
2. According to the Nurses' Health Study from Harvard, the more friends and social ties nurses had the less likely they were to develop physical ailments and the more joyous their lives would be.
3. Researchers from UCLA demonstrated that women's social ties reduce women's the risk of heart disease by lowering blood pressure, cholesterol, and heart rate.[15]

Cautions and Contraindications for Relaxation, Meditation, and Biofeedback

1. Medication
   a. Medications must be monitored and possibly titrated for clients taking insulin, thyroid replacement medication, antihypertensives, cardiac medications, antianxiety agents, sleep medication.
   b. Working closely with clients' prescribing providers, note and document any changes in their symptoms; medications might need to be titrated as clients learn to deepen their relaxation.
2. Education and information
   a. Discussing issues and experiences associated with relaxation before and after each session helps to involve clients, positively empower them, and reframe any of the anticipatory anxiety or questions they might have.
3. Mental health history
   a. Clients with a history of dissociative experiences, acute psychosis, borderline personality, and post-traumatic stress disorder are better cared for by nurses and professionals skilled in treating such clients. Check your client's mental health history before beginning relaxation practice.[16]
4. Cryptotrauma
   a. Many patients have experienced undiagnosed physical or psychological trauma. Many times patients are reluctant to disclose these problems, and often health professionals are unskilled in or uncomfortable with exploring these issues. Domino and Haber report that 66% of women with chronic headaches at a multidisciplinary pain center had a

prior history of physical or sexual abuse (61% had experienced physical abuse; 11%, sexual abuse; and 28%, both physical and sexual abuse).

b. The term *cryptotrauma* indicates that the trauma that is a cause of the patient's pain is HIDDEN hidden or has not been revealed. Signals to watch for in clients with post-traumatic stress disorder (PTSD) and/or cryptotrauma include the following: hypervigilance, difficulty falling or staying asleep, irritability or outbursts of rage, difficulty concentrating, exaggerated startle response, dissociation, addiction, flashbacks, numbing panic attacks, disturbed self-perception, denigration, isolation, inability to be comfortable with touch, nightmares.[17]

c. Even with the most sensitive and careful history taking and preparations, clients with such disorders can have flashbacks related to the underlying trauma. If this occurs:

- First, do not panic. Remember your intention to help and support, and trust your therapeutic bond with the client.
- Second, center and ground yourself. Clients in a panic state related to anxiety or flashback are supersensitive to people around them; centering, calming, and grounding yourself will deeply help them.
- Third, reassure the client; speak to the client in a calm, soothing voice, and use therapeutic suggestions. Have the client open his or her eyes, feel his or her feet on the floor, or touch the furniture; if possible, have the client tighten and release the hands and feet and be aware of the body and of being with you in the present. If appropriate, hold the client's hand; use your judgment.
- Fourth, remember that the information with which the client is getting in touch is important for the client's wholeness and healing. A simple, short statement explaining this to the client helps to reframe the situation and plant therapeutic suggestions during these most open and suggestible moments.

- Seek appropriate referrals for the client as needed.

5. PTSD, cryptotrauma, and working in times of trauma, natural disaster, or major crisis

a. Clients who suffer from cryptotrauma or who have sustained one or more major losses around the time of a disaster are at the greatest risk for developing PTSD.

b. Nurses and other helping professionals who are aware of the previously mentioned symptoms for cryptotrauma could be the first line of help for assessing, recognizing, and helping a client, colleague, child, or even a neighbor or family member suffering from traumatic grief or PTSD after any major community trauma or crisis.

c. In a time of tragedies, such as school shootings; soldiers and military families coping with their uncertainty or the return of traumatized or wounded soldiers from war; or environmental disasters such as hurricanes, earthquakes, floods, tornadoes, and tsunamis, understanding lessons learned from the lived experience of our colleagues in communities that have been affected can be a great service to all.

d. Everyone grieves differently, and most people recover without much intervention.

6. Evolution of PTSD after a community crisis or disaster

a. The antithetical dimension of PTSD is that, left untreated, with time the symptoms might not get better but actually might get worse.

b. According to a study published in 2007 by Canadian researchers, those with PTSD are significantly more apt to have numerous health conditions, including cardiovascular diseases, respiratory diseases, chronic pain, gastrointestinal illnesses, and cancer. Those with PTSD were also more prone to other disabilities (short- and long-term), suicide, and poor quality of life.[18]

c. If we allow it, experiences of profound trauma help enliven and enlarge our hearts as a human family, helping us grow our understanding, compassion, wisdom, and interconnectedness so that we can heal both locally and globally (Barrett's Theory of Power).

d. Recognizing that we are living in a very mobile society, nurses and helping professionals can be confronted with a client or patient who has moved away from a disaster area or who has friends or family in the disaster and thereby might also be at risk for unrecognized PTSD. Many people have delayed responses or might not be correctly diagnosed.

e. Trauma therapists working with persons with PTSD often hear "I thought I'd be over this by now." The more time that elapses from the time of the event, the more distressing the symptoms and reactions might become for persons with PTSD.

7. Caring for those with PTSD

a. PTSD is characterized by avoidance, numbness, and feelings of helplessness and hopelessness.

b. For those suffering from PTSD, conversational induction and therapeutic suggestion can be even more helpful and appropriate than any form of deep relaxation (D. Larkin, personal communication, June 16, 2003).

c. As in any clinical situation, professional experience, clinical judgment, and the client's comfort level with the intervention all help to determine what is the best approach for that client.

d. Because rescue or relief workers and professionals involved with trauma work of disaster victims have to continuously return to the disaster site and reexperience the crisis, they, too, can experience vicarious traumatization. They need personal, workplace, and community healing support as well.

■ HOLISTIC NURSING PERSPECTIVES FOR LIVING IN A TIME OF UNCERTAINTY

1. According to Elizabeth Barrett: Power, from a Rogerian perspective, is the capacity to participate knowingly in the nature of change characterizing the continuous patterning of the human and environmental field. The observable, measurable pattern

manifestations of power are awareness, choices, freedom to act intentionally, and involvement in creating change.[19]

2. So, what awareness, choices, intentions, and involvement do we want to offer, as holistic nurses, to foster community unitary well-being in times of helplessness or uncertainty?

a. Our own practices of self-healing, meditation, and relaxation support us during times of illness and stress by building inner skills and resiliency.

b. Communities also can cultivate their inner resiliency by building their own inner capacities and building and training a more connected interprofessional team.

Cultivating Wellness Preparedness for Professionals, Communities, and Organizations

1. As holistic nursing leaders, we can build in preparedness in which communities focus on self-care and community care as shared values.

2. Encourage each other's self-care practice to create positive healing patterns and build resiliency to cope with uncertainty, trauma, or disaster.

Restorative Practices

1. Yoga: Yoga is a philosophy of living that unites physical, mental, and spiritual health. When practiced for the purpose of relaxation, it involves breathing and stretching exercises and postures. Daily practice of restorative yoga—even 10 to 15 minutes a day—creates energy, restorative rest, spiritual renewal, and calm.[20,21]

2. Qi gong: Qi gong practices, a part of Chinese medicine, combine simple movements with breath and meditation to facilitate a flow with nature's healing *qi*. Restoration and healing come from daily practice.

3. Restorative gardens: "Nature alone heals" is one of Nightingale's most famous quotes.[2] Many hospitals and healthcare centers are creating healing gardens, restorative gardens, greenhouses, meditative gardens, and labyrinths in their plazas, lobbies, rooftops, and other inner and outer spaces to help

cultivate relaxation, renewal, and peace. It dates back to medieval monastic healing sanctuaries; the medieval architectural designs included low windows so that patients could look out at nature's beauty. Simply helping clients to be with nature amid the high-tech healthcare system can improve their well-being, reduce their anxiety, and calm their fears. Nurses can benefit from resting in a garden or creating natural spaces within the healthcare setting.[22]

4. The holistic nurse integrates relaxation interventions to support clients at all stages of health.

5. Holistic caring process is found in Chapter 16 of *Holistic Nursing: A Handbook for Practice*.

▪ NOTES

1. Moriconi, C., & Stabler-Haas, S. (2011, March 19). *Mindfulness-based stress reduction and its effect on test anxiety and focused attention with baccalaureate nursing students: A pilot study.* Paper presented at Mindfulness in Education Conference, American University, Washington, DC.

2. Nightingale, F. (1992). *Notes on nursing* (Commemorative ed.). Philadelphia, PA: Lippincott. (Original work published 1860).

3. Kabat-Zinn, J. (1990). *Full catastrophe living: Using the wisdom of your body and mind to face stress, pain, and illness.* New York, NY: Bantam Doubleday Dell.

4. Ornish, D. (1990). *Dr. Dean Ornish's program for reversing heart disease.* New York, NY: Random House.

5. Krieger, D. (1993). *Accepting your power to heal: The personal practice of therapeutic touch.* Santa Fe, NM: Bear and Co.

6. Benson, H., Alexander, S., & Feldman, C. (1975). Decreased premature ventricular contraction through the use of the relaxation response in patients with stable ischemic heart disease. *Lancet, 2*(7931), 380.

7. Benson, H. (1984). *Beyond the relaxation response.* New York, NY: Times Books.

8. Macrae, J. (1987). *Therapeutic touch: A practical guide.* New York, NY: Knopf.

9. Nhat Hanh, T. (1997). *Teachings on love.* Berkeley, CA: Parallax Press.

10. Barnum, B. (2003). *Spirituality in nursing: From traditional to new age* (2nd ed.). New York, NY: Springer.

11. Cheek, D. (1981). Hypnosis. In A. Hastings, J. Fadiman, & J. S. Gordon. (Eds.), *The complete guide to holistic medicine: Health for the whole person* (pp. 141–156). New York, NY: Bantam Books.

12. Rogers, B. (1972). Therapeutic conversation and posthypnotic suggestion. *American Journal of Nursing, 72,* 714–717.

13. Larkin, D. (1988). Therapeutic suggestion. In R. Zahourek (Ed.), *Relaxation and imagery: Tools for therapeutic communication and intervention.* Philadelphia, PA: W. B. Saunders.

14. Green, E., & Green, A. (1970). *Biofeedback: The yoga of the West.* Cos Cob, CT: Hartley Film Foundation.

15. Taylor, S. E., & Klein, L. C. (2000). Female responses to stress: Tend and befriend, not fight or flight. *Psychological Review, 107*(3), 41.

16. Schwartz, M., Schwartz, N., & Monastra, V. (2003). Problems with relaxation and biofeedback-assisted relaxation, and guidelines for management. In M. Schwartz and Andrasik, F. (Eds.), *Biofeedback* (3rd ed., pp. 251–265). New York, NY: Guilford Press.

17. Domino, J., & Haber, J. D. (1987). Prior physical and sexual abuse in women with chronic headaches: Clinical correlates. *Headache, 27,* 310–314.

18. Sareen, J., Cox, B. J., Stein, M. B., Afifi, T., Fleet, C., & Amundson, G. (2007). Physical and mental comorbidity, disability, and suicidal behavior associated with posttraumatic stress disorder in a large community sample. *Psychosomatic Medicine, 69*(3), 242–248.

19. Barrett, E. (2000). The theoretical matrix for a Rogerian nursing practice. *Theoria: Journal of Nursing Theory, 9,* 4.

20. Laster, J. (1995). *Relax, renew: Restful yoga for stressful living.* Berkeley, CA: Rodwell Press.

21. Tolse, S. C. F. (2007, January). A case report of the design and implementation of a hospital based therapeutic yoga rehabilitation program. Abstract presentation at International Association of Yoga Therapists, Los Angeles, CA.

22. Gerlach-Spriggs, N., Kaufman, R., & Warner, S. B. (1998). *Restorative gardens: The healing landscape.* New Haven, CT: Yale University Press.

▣ STUDY QUESTIONS

Basic Level

1. To whom is the phrase *relaxation response* attributed?
   a. Florence Nightingale
   b. Jon Kabat-Zinn
   c. Herbert Benson
   d. Dolores Krieger

2. Which of the following are associated with the generalized stress response? Select all that apply.
   a. Constriction of blood flow to the hands and feet
   b. Tightening of the muscles
   c. Decreased anxiety
   d. Increased blood pressure

3. What are sample forms of relaxation practices? Select all that apply.
   a. Autogenic training
   b. Cryptotrauma
   c. Biofeedback
   d. Yoga

4. What does the nurse assess prior to teaching patients relaxation techniques?
   a. Religious and cultural perspectives
   b. Current medications
   c. Mental health history
   d. All of the above

5. What is passive volition?
   a. Letting go and watching the process
   b. Wilfully making things happen
   c. Attending to the past
   d. Attending to the future

Advanced Level

6. Which of the following answer choices are associated with conversational inductions and purposeful use of therapeutic suggestions? Select all that apply.

   a. Can enhance patient cooperation and comfort
   b. Can involve reframing, or changing the meaning of an experience
   c. Can be used to convey the expected therapeutic benefits of medications
   d. Can be a disrespectful manipulation of the patient

7. Which of the following is *not* related to Elizabeth Barrett's power as knowing participation in change theory?
   a. Awareness
   b. Choices
   c. Control
   d. Freedom

8. The patterns, challenges, and needs that are compatible with relaxation interventions include which of the following? Select all that apply.
   a. Social isolation
   b. Activity intolerance
   c. Powerlessness
   d. Anxiety

9. Symptoms of cryptotrauma and prolonged PTSD can include which of the following? Select all that apply.
   a. Flashbacks
   b. Hypervigilance
   c. Comfort with touch
   d. Numbing and/or panic attacks

10. A nurse who is knowingly living the power theory and facilitating healing change on the unit might initiate which of the following? Select all that apply.
    a. Practice and model self-care by integrating relaxation practices into daily living
    b. Begin report with a group mindfulness practice
    c. Incorporate patterns that will reduce noise and increase access to nature
    d. Increase efficiency by decreasing contact with patients

Chapter 18

Imagery

Megan McInnis Burt and
Bonney Gulino Schaub

■ DEFINITIONS

Body–mind imagery The conscious formation of an image that is directed to a body area or activity that requires attention or increased energy.

Clinical imagery The conscious use of the power of the imagination with the intention of activating physiologic, psychological, or spiritual healing.

Correct biologic imagery Biologically accurate images that are visualized to send messages to physiologic processes.

End-state imagery Images that contain specified imagined hopes and goals (e.g., a healed wound).

Guided imagery A highly structured imagery technique.

Imagery process Internal experiences of memories, dreams, fantasies, inner perceptions, and visions, sometimes involving one, several, or all of the senses, serving as the bridge for connecting body, mind, and spirit.

Imagery rehearsal An imagery technique designed to rehearse behaviors or prepare for activities or procedures.

Impromptu imagery The nurse's introduction of his or her spontaneous, intuitive images or perceptions into the therapeutic intervention.

Packaged imagery Commercial tapes that have general images.

Relationship imagery Imagery designed to explore relationships with other people or with a part of oneself (e.g., the part that is always judgmental) or with a symptom or part of one's body (e.g., connecting with the heart).

Spontaneous imagery The unexpected reception of an image, as if it "bubbled up," entering the stream of consciousness.

Symbolic imagery Inner images that represent a person's deeper knowledge, occurring in the form of metaphors or symbols. The meaning of the image might be immediately translatable to rational verbal thought, or at other times this meaning might emerge slowly over time.

Transpersonal imagery Images that connect one to expanded (i.e., beyond personality) levels of consciousness, such as imagining one's body as a mountain and beginning to feel an inner quality of immovable strength and solidity.

Visualization The use of external images (e.g., religious paintings, written words, nature photography) to evoke internal imagery experiences that energize desired emotions, qualities, outcomes, or goals.

■ THEORY AND RESEARCH

1. The clinical value of imagery has been well documented in the treatment of a wide variety of conditions such as cancer,[1] migraine headaches, irritable bowel syndrome,[2,3] hypertension, anxiety and depression,[4] fibromyalgia,[5,6] post-traumatic stress disorder,[7-9] immune system disorders,[10,11] asthma,[12] and

improvements in cognitive, emotional, and physiologic performance.[13,14]

2. The research definition of imagery is the perception of a stimulus in the absence of that stimulus. For example, if a person imagines a lemon and begins to taste lemon juice, he or she is having a perception (tasting the juice) of a stimulus (lemon) that is not present.

3. Imagery is relevant to the crucial issue of the placebo effect, a phenomenon in which the patient thinks (imagines) he or she is receiving a potent medication and experiences the anticipated effects, both positive (placebo) and negative (nocebo), of that medication, when in fact a neutral substance was administered.

4. Imagery is the *conscious* use of the power of the imagination with the intention of activating physiologic, psychological, or spiritual healing and accessing inner wisdom. Imagery's clinical focus is to use the imagination to promote life-affirming behaviors and goals. It has shown value in improving quality of life through decreasing stress, increasing positive mood, and improving general health status.[15]

Clinical Effectiveness of Imagery

1. Research on the physiologic effects of imagery include increased internal blood flow, demonstrated by increased temperature in specific skin areas; increased heart rate resulting from imaging sexually or emotionally arousing situations; alterations in body chemistry, such as gastric secretions and salivary pH; muscle stimulation as shown in electromyography; immune system responses; wound healing; heart rate control in response to either relaxing or anxiety-producing images; systolic and diastolic blood pressure changes in response to images of fear and anger.

2. Hall studied the effect of hypnosis and imagery on immune modulation, noting increases in the number of lymphocytes and general increased immune system responsiveness.[1,16]

3. Guided imagery with progressive muscle relaxation was demonstrated to be effective in the alleviation of pain and mobility

difficulties in osteoarthritis.[17] Positive outcomes were found in the introduction of imagery interventions to manage pain in an elderly orthopedic population.[18] The effectiveness of imagery in the reduction of recurrent abdominal pain,[19] in the reduction of postoperative pain,[20] and in pediatric hospice pain management[21] is an area for additional nursing research. The richness of imagery as an intervention in working with children has been described in many clinical settings.[22]

Clinical Imagery and States of Consciousness

1. Assagioli's concept of the wholeness of human consciousness, or psychosynthesis, describes the aspect of each person that holds inner wisdom and connection with life purpose.[23,24] Assagioli used imagery in three forms:
   a. Inner images, to explore the various levels of human experience, including biologic, social, and transpersonal experience.
   b. Inner images, to represent the intentions and goals of the patient.
   c. External images to help encourage transpersonal feelings in his patients such as pictures in museums.[25]

2. Assagioli's principles of "psychological laws" describe the interactive effects among images, ideas, emotions, physical responses, behaviors, attitudes, and impulses that affect, the body–mind for healing and psychospiritual growth.[24pp51-52]

■ CLINICAL TECHNIQUES IN IMAGERY

1. Nurses can employ impromptu imagery techniques that are specific, highly structured, and guided to correct biological, and end-state imagery techniques during a clinical interaction. For example, an emergency room nurse unable to establish an intravenous (IV) line could suggest that the woman embrace her injured arm as if it were a tiny baby and suggest, "Hold your arm, and send it loving energy." Within moments, the woman could be calm, and the nurse can start the IV infusion.

Imagery in Integrative/Holistic Health Coaching

1. Imagery can tap a deep level of self-knowledge in the patient. Using relationship imagery, a patient was asked to describe his relationship with his father; he offered a few familiar comments. But when he was asked to get an image of his father, the patient suddenly got in touch with the feelings of sadness and hopelessness that his father stimulated in him. This deeper level of self-knowledge allowed the patient to appreciate why he struggled with hopelessness in himself.

2. Nurses work with patients and family members who are grieving past or imminent losses. Imagery is a valuable resource at this time because the connection with the loved one is alive in the imagination and creates feelings that they have communicated at an extremely deep, meaningful, and comforting way with internal imagery processes.[26,27] These experiences can be helpful in making decisions, in rehearsing new behaviors, in understanding relationships, in making life choices, and in experiencing equanimity in the face of painful challenges.

Values and Spirituality

1. Nurses care for patients at times when values and spirituality have become a central concern for patients. Illness, divorce, ethical dilemmas, deaths, or other life crises often cause people to slow down and ask basic questions and reassess their deepest values and their sense of spiritual purpose in life. Imagery allows someone to imagine the actual results of a decision. For example, a nurse counseling a 59-year-old elementary school teacher struggling with a decision about retirement suggested that she close her eyes, focus on her breath, and imagine herself retired. After a few moments, the woman experienced an image of herself at home, looking bored and unhappy, which made her frustrated. The nurse guided her back into the imagery, trying to imagine doing service work in the community. Suddenly, she felt a peace and an ease settle into her experience. Imagining pictures of the future helps a person to make specific behavioral and emotional changes.

Transpersonal Use of Imagery

1. Cultures throughout the world have used prayer, meditation, imagery, diet, physical training, contemplation and study, ritual, art, and many other methods to experience transpersonal states of consciousness. Holistic nurses motivated by their own development through such experiences desire to pass the potential of transpersonal experiences on to others. Holistic nurses use transpersonal imagery to introduce patients safely to the transpersonal level of consciousness.[28-31] Transpersonal imagery taps into an expanded experience of the self to connect deeply with the flow of life energy and creation. This connection, and the imagery that emerges from it, can be interpreted as a connection with something greater.

2. Working with metaphors and symbols of transcendent experiences (ascent, elevation, illumination, enlightenment, light, deepening, expansion, awakening, rebirth, liberation, and love) is an effective way to help a patient who is experiencing spiritual distress, hopelessness, and helplessness. The patient can choose the symbol that he or she wants to explore, or the nurse can create the journey based on information from the patient. In times of illness and crisis, people might have spontaneous spiritual experiences and images.

Imagery with Disease and Illness

1. Addressing the personal experience of illness, such as general state of being, anxiety level, state of hopefulness or despair, and the meaning attributed to the situation through imagery, can promote a sense of well-being in clients and help them change their perceptions about their disease, treatment, and their inner resources and innate healing ability. The use of an interactive approach to guided imagery with medical patients, which was designed to promote relaxation and cultivate healing intentions, has been significantly helpful in increasing patients' insights into their health problems.[31]

Concrete Objective Information

1. Research has been conducted on the use of imagery rehearsal to provide coping strategies and prepare patients for difficult procedures. This helps to prepare the mind, avoid fear of the unknown, and recover more quickly. The nurse would describe through imagery what the person will experience at each stage of the procedure, including what will be felt, heard, seen, smelled, or tasted before, during, and after the operation including the sensory experiences of the postsurgical healing incision.

Fears in Imagery Work

Three predictable and understandable fears are encountered in imagery work:

1. *Nothing will happen.* Patients fear that they will not be able to imagine anything in response to the nurse's imagery suggestion but should be encouraged to be curious about any experience that occurs. For example, if the patient reports that her breathing became faster as soon as she heard the nurse's suggestion to relax, the nurse should be curious about why the patient believes her breathing became faster. Relaxation can be frightening for someone who has experienced trauma in childhood and feels the importance of maintaining vigilance.
2. *Too much will happen.* Patients fear that the imagery will evoke difficult or even overwhelming thoughts and feelings. However, imagery does not take away a person's defenses. If the imagery suggestion is too evocative, the patient will simply fail to hear it, ignore it, change it into a suggestion that is easier to work with, or open his or her eyes, stopping the process. The nurse uses imagery to evoke what is already present in the patient and evoke a response if the patient is ready.
3. *It will be done wrong.* Patients fear they cannot do imagery the "right way." The processes of the imagination are unique to each person; thus, each imagery experience is unique. A nurse might use the same imagery suggestion twice, and the same patient can experience two totally different responses to the imagery. The patient's experience is the center of all imagery work. The nurse can suggest imaging a walk in an open field, and the patient might respond by imaging the atmosphere in a dark room. The meaning of the dark room becomes of primary importance replacing the open field.

■ HOLISTIC CARING PROCESS

Holistic Assessment

1. Nurses become aware of their own imagery process and the rich variety of possible imagery experiences.
2. Nurses become aware of the client's hopes in regard to the session: reason for seeking help, wants, needs, desires, or recurrent and dominant themes.
3. Nurses become aware of the client's anxiety/tension levels to determine which types of relaxation inductions will be most effective.
4. The client understands that it is not necessary to literally hear, see, feel, touch, or taste when working with imagery, that it is best to trust the inner experience, that imagery is a way in which we communicate with ourselves and bring ourselves into contact with our body and find out what it needs.
5. Nurses become aware of the client's sensory modalities, visual, auditory, kinesthetic, and so forth, during the experience.
6. Nurses become aware of the client's previous experiences with the imagery process and the preferences for the degree of guidance.
7. Nurses become aware of the client's emotional comfort level with closing eyes, bringing attention inside, and opening to states of internal awareness and trust that it is safe to relax.
8. Nurses become aware of the client's knowledge of relaxation skills, or the nurse explains the normal sensations and the time to shift to the "letting go" state.
9. Nurses become aware of the client's ability to maintain attention and not drowse off in the session.

Identification of Patterns/Challenges/Needs

1. The following are the patterns/challenges/needs compatible with imagery interventions:

a. Social isolation
b. Role performance
c. Caregiver role strain
d. Parental role strain
e. Spiritual well-being
f. Spiritual distress
g. Altered effective coping
h. Impaired adjustment
i. Ineffective denial
j. Potential for growth
k. Decision conflict
l. Health-seeking behaviors
m. Sleep pattern disturbance
n. Relocation stress syndrome
o. Altered self-concept
p. Disturbance in body image
q. Disturbance in self-image
r. Potential hopelessness
s. Potential powerlessness
t. Pain
u. Anxiety
v. Fear
w. Post trauma response
x. Grief

Outcome Identification

1. Exhibit 17-1, found in Chapter 17 of *Holistic Nursing: A Handbook for Practice*, guides the nurse in client outcomes, nursing prescriptions, and evaluations for the use of imagery as a nursing intervention.

Therapeutic Care Plan and Interventions

1. Facilitation and interpretation of the imagery process
   a. The nurse serves as a guide and deeply listens to the way a client tells his or her story to get a sense of the client's outlook on and orientation toward the world and to determine whether less structure and guidance are indicated for more intuitive patients. Does the client have a materialistic, concrete outlook on problem solving and life in general, or a more intuitive, spontaneous perspective? The nurse should encourage clients' exploration of the meaning of their images, through contemplation, writing, drawing, and dialogue.

2. Guided imagery scripts
   a. The guidelines that follow help the nurse in the effective implementation of imagery scripts as nursing interventions:
      - Start the session with an induction, a general relaxation—focusing on breath, shortened passive progressive relaxation, or body awareness.
      - Reaffirm that there is no right or wrong way for the client to do imagery, that whatever occurs is useful information, and that the client has complete control over the process.
      - Follow the induction instructions for yourself so that you communicate a calming presence.
      - Personalize the imagery by using the client's name or other specific references several times during the process.
      - Speak slowly and smoothly, allowing for pauses and silence after each suggestion.
      - Observe the client's body language and breathing rhythm to assess responses to suggestions.
      - If there are signs of tension such as shallow breathing, tightness of muscles, or tense facial muscles in response to an imagery suggestion, ask, "What are you experiencing now?"
      - If the client appears to be struggling to get into the imagery, pause in the script and suggest that the client reconnect with the breath and go more deeply into relaxation.
      - Avoid saying "yes" or "right" or other words that communicate evaluative reactions to the client's experience. A more supportive comment such as "stay with your experience" can be made.
      - Provide encouragement and guidance for those with less vivid imagery. Vivid imagers, on the other hand, prefer more silence: Words can be distracting or intrusive to them. Extremely vivid imagers might prefer to keep their eyes partially open to prevent feeling overwhelmed.
      - End the session by bringing the person's awareness back to the room. You can do this by encouraging the person to begin to transition back to

the room by becoming aware of his or her body in the chair or the bed, by bringing awareness to his or her breath, and then slowly opening his or her eyes. An example of another classic reintegration method is: "At the count of 5, you will be fully awake and alert...1...2...3...4...5."

3. Induction for imagery
   a. A simple breathing technique can be useful to focus the client's mind inward and induce imagery. Resting the hands on the lower abdomen and breathing into the belly is an effective calming posture. Effectiveness is determined by noting the slowing of breathing, relaxation of facial muscles, and changes in skin color. (Script can be found in Chapter 17, *Holistic Nursing: A Handbook for Practice*.)

4. Connecting with life energy imagery
   a. Life energy imagery focuses on a person's sense of his or her inner energy and that the body is not just sick. This awareness can reframe a person's attitude, bringing a connection with inner healing mechanisms and with what is functioning healthfully, as opposed to focusing on the disease process. (Script can be found in Chapter 17, *Holistic Nursing: A Handbook for Practice*.)

5. Special or safe place imagery
   a. Clients need to identify a special place that is a safe retreat. It takes 10 to 20 minutes. (Script can be found in Chapter 17, *Holistic Nursing: A Handbook for Practice*.)

6. Worry and fear imagery
   a. Some images can help clients change the internal experience of worry and fear. Clients should set aside 10 to 20 minutes a day to worry, preferably in the morning before they start their daily routines. This approach reassures the subconscious that it has worried, and the person has greater success at stopping the habitual worry during the rest of the day. (Script can be found in Chapter 17, *Holistic Nursing: A Handbook for Practice*.)

7. Inner guide imagery
   a. The nurse can assist the client in creating purposeful self-dialogue that gains access to inner wisdom and personal truth that naturally reside within each

of us. It is advisable to allow 10 to 20 minutes for this exercise.
   b. The script for inner guide imagery can be found in Chapter 17, *Holistic Nursing: A Handbook for Practice*. This script helps clients gain an awareness of their own inner wisdom. Word choices should take into account the client's dominant sense. If a client prefers the visual, for example, the nurse uses the word *see*; if the client prefers the auditory, the word *hear*; if the client prefers the kinesthetic, the word *feel*.

8. Pain reduction imagery
   a. The red ball of pain. To decrease psychophysiologic pain, clients can learn to use distraction. This kind of imagery is good for both acute and chronic pain, as well as for the discomfort or pain of procedures. It takes 10 to 20 minutes. (Script can be found in Chapter 17, *Holistic Nursing: A Handbook for Practice*.)

9. Pain assessment imagery
   a. Imagery helps access and control both acute and chronic psychophysiologic pain. The following exercise can be done in 10 to 20 minutes. (Script can be found in Chapter 17, *Holistic Nursing: A Handbook for Practice*.)

10. Correct biologic imagery scripts
    a. Bone healing imagery
       ■ An imagery exercise for bone healing can be done in 20 to 30 minutes.[32] Prior to biologic imagery of bone healing, the nurse can explain the basic biologic concepts of physical healing, and this can enhance the imagery experience. (Script can be found in Chapter 17, *Holistic Nursing: A Handbook for Practice*.)
    b. Immune system odyssey imagery
       ■ Patients can be taught correct biologic images of the normal processes of the immune system including the functions of neutrophils, macrophages, T cells, and B cells.[32pp317-328] (Script can be found in Chapter 17, *Holistic Nursing: A Handbook for Practice*.)

11. Imagery and drawing
    a. In the imagery process, drawing is an effective way to open communication with the self and others. The emphasis is on the client's ability to get in touch with

feelings and healing potential through drawing. Drawing is a way of externalizing inner images and deepening understanding of inner processes and might be a safer way to talk about difficult feelings. When clients are overwhelmed with emotions, drawing images of the feelings can be therapeutic. Drawing is especially helpful with children who are not verbally sophisticated.

b. Drawing after being guided through an imagery exercise can bring further insights. This creative process can also evoke transcendent experiences and healing energy. Drawing works well when a client is crying and is unable to talk easily but wants to express what he or she is experiencing. When introducing drawing, the nurse can make some of the following suggestions:

- Express yourself with a few images. There is no one correct way to draw. Drawings can be either realistic or symbolic. The most important thing is that you express yourself in a nonlogical way. This can bring new awareness and understanding into your life.

- If you find that you are too focused on the result of the drawing exercise, use your nondominant hand. With your eyes closed, allow yourself to get into the expressive quality of drawing.

- Do not judge your drawing. Allow your body, mind, and spirit to connect as you begin simply to be with the paper and crayons in the present moment.

- Notice the energy flow from you. Let your body energy resonate with your imagery and spirit energy. Let the energies slowly begin to resonate together. Do not try to control the process because this inner quality comes from being immersed in the imagery and drawing experience.

- On the blank piece of paper, allow an image to begin to form that represents your feelings and thoughts in this moment. Choose colors that speak to you. If you wish to change the color that you started working with, feel free to do so.

- After you have drawn, you might want to write some details of your images. Often, what you felt or heard during the imagery drawing might surface into conscious awareness and provide new insights about your important images.

Evaluation

1. With the client, the nurse determines whether the client outcomes for imagery were successful. To evaluate the session further, the nurse may again explore the subjective effects of the experience with the client (see Exhibit 17-1 in *Holistic Nursing: A Handbook for Practice*). If an imagery intervention does not prove to be helpful, instead use creativity and try other imagery approaches.

2. Imagery is a tool for connecting with the unlimited capabilities of consciousness to affect the body–mind. The client can experience more self-awareness, self-acceptance, self-love, and self-worth. Clients learn a skill for self-care and self-knowledge that will be useful throughout their life.

3. Exhibit 17-2, Evaluating the Client's Subjective Experience with Imagery, can be found in *Holistic Nursing: A Handbook for Practice*.

■ NOTES

1. Hall, H. (2003). Imagery and cancer. In A. A. Sheikh (Ed.), *Healing images: The role of imagination in health* (pp. 408–426). Amityville, NY: Baywood.

2. Miller, V., & Whorwell, P. J. (2009). Hypnotherapy for functional gastrointestinal disorders: A review. *International Journal of Clinical and Experimental Hypnosis, 57*(3), 279–292.

3. Shinozaki, M., Kanazawa, M., Kano, M., Endo, Y., Nakaya, N., Hongo, M., & Fukudo, S. (2010). Effect of autogenic training on general improvement in patients with irritable bowel syndrome: A randomized controlled trial. *Applied Psychophysiology and Biofeedback, 35*(3), 189–198.

4. Apóstolo, J. L., & Kolcaba, K. (2009). The effects of guided imagery on comfort, depression, anxiety, and stress of psychiatric inpatients with depressive disorders. *Archives of Psychiatric Nursing, 23*(6), 403–411.

5. Menzies, V., Taylor, A. G., & Bourguignon, C. (2006). Effects of guided imagery on outcomes of pain, functional status, and self-efficacy in

persons diagnosed with fibromyalgia. *Journal of Complementary Medicine, 12*(1), 23–30.

6. Menzies, V., & Kim, S. (2008). Relaxation and guided imagery in Hispanic persons diagnosed with fibromyalgia: A pilot study. *Family and Community Health, 31*(3), 204–212.

7. Gordon, J. S., Staples, J. K., Blyta, A., Bytyqi, M., & Wilson, A. T. (2008). Treatment of post-traumatic stress disorder in postwar Kosovar adolescents using mind–body skills groups: A randomized controlled trial. *Journal of Clinical Psychiatry, 69*(9), 1469–1476.

8. Weis, J. M., Smucker, M. R., & Dresser, J. G. (2003). Imagery: Its history and use in the treatment of posttraumatic stress disorder. In A. A. Sheikh (Ed.), *Healing images: The role of imagination in health* (pp. 381–395). Amityville, NY: Baywood.

9. Nappi, C. M., Drummond, S. P., Thorp, S. R., & McQuaid, J. R. (2010). Effectiveness of imagery rehearsal therapy for the treatment of combat-related nightmares in veterans. *Behavioral Therapy, 41*(2), 237–244.

10. Trakhtenberg, E. C. (2008). The effects of guided imagery on the immune system: A critical review. *International Journal of Neuroscience, 118*(6), 839–855.

11. Eremin, O., Walker, M. B., Simpson, E., Heys, S.D., Ah-See, A. K., Hutcheon, A. W.,...Walker, L. G. (2008). Immunomodulatory effects of relaxation training and guided imagery in women with locally advanced breast cancer undergoing multimodality therapy: A randomised controlled trial. *Breast, 18*(1), 17–25.

12. Lahmann, C., Henningsen, P., Schulz, C., Schuster, T., Sauer, N., Noll-Hussong, M., & Loew, T. (2010). Effects of functional relaxation and guided imagery on IgE in dust-mite allergic adult asthmatics: A randomized, controlled clinical trial. *Journal of Nervous and Mental Disorders, 198*(2), 125–130.

13. McCraty, R., & Tomasino, D. (2006). Emotional stress, positive emotions, and psychophysiological coherence. In B. B. Arnetz and R. Ekman (Eds.), *Stress in health and disease* (pp. 342–365). Weinheim, Germany: Wiley-VCH. Retrieved from http://www.heartmath.org/research/research-publications/emotional-stress-positive-emotions-and-psychophysiological-coherence.html

14. Rein, G., Atkinson, M., & McCraty, R. (1995). The physiological and psychological effects of compassion and anger. *Journal of Advancement in Medicine, 8*(2), 87–105. Retrieved from http://www.heartmath.org/research/research-publications/physiological-and-psychological-effects-of-compassion-and-anger.html

15. Watanabe, E., Fukuda, S., & Shirakawa. T. (2005). Effects among healthy subjects of the duration of regularly practicing a guided imagery program.

BMC Complementary and Alternative Medicine, 5(21), 1–13.

16. Hall, H. (1990). Imagery, PNI and the psychology of healing. In R. Kunzendorf & A. Sheikh (Eds.) The Psychophysiology of Mental Imagery: Theory, Research and Application (Imagery and Human Development Series, (3). Amityville, NY: Baywood.

17. Baird, C. L., & Sands, L. (2004). A pilot study of the effectiveness of guided imagery with progressive muscle relaxation to reduce chronic pain and mobility difficulties of osteoarthritis. *Pain Management Nursing, 5*(3), 97–104.

18. Antall, G. F., & Kresevic, D. (2004). The use of guided imagery to manage pain in an elderly orthopaedic population. *Orthopaedic Nursing, 23*(5), 335–340.

19. Weydert, J. A., Shapiro, D. E., Acra, S. A., Monheim, C. J., Chambers, A. S., & Ball, T. M. (2006). Evaluation of guided imagery as a treatment for recurrent abdominal pain in children: A randomized controlled trial. *BMC Pediatrics, 6*, 29. Retrieved from http://www.ncbi.nlm.nih.gov/pmc/articles/PMC1660537

20. Huth, M. M., Broome, M. E., & Good, M. (2004). Imagery reduces children's post-operative pain. *Pain, 110*(1–2), 439–448.

21. Russell, C., & Smart, S. (2007). Guided imagery and distraction therapy in paediatric hospice care. *Paediatric Nursing, 19*(2), 24–25.

22. Huth, M. M., Van Kuiken, D. M., & Broome, M. E. (2006). Playing in the park: What school-age children tell us about imagery. *Journal of Pediatric Nursing, 21*(2), 115–125.

23. Assagioli, R. (1965). *Psychosynthesis: A manual of principles and techniques.* New York, NY: Hobbs, Dorman.

24. Assagioli, R. (1973). *Act of will.* New York, NY: Viking.

25. Schaub, B. G., & Schaub, R. (2003). *Dante's path: A practical approach to achieving inner wisdom.* New York, NY: Gotham Books.

26. Morrison, J. K. (2007). The dynamic, clinical use of imagery to promote psychotherapeutic grieving. In A. A. Sheikh & K. S. Sheikh (Eds.), *Healing with death imagery* (pp. 139–164). Amityville, NY: Baywood.

27. Kunzendorf, R. G. (2007). Confronting death through mental and artistic imagery. In A. A. Sheikh & K. S. Sheikh (Eds.), *Healing with death imagery* (pp. 47–65). Amityville, NY: Baywood.

28. Lane, M. R. (2005). Spirit body healing—a hermeneutic, phenomenological study examining the lived experience of art and healing. *Cancer Nursing, 28*(4), 285–291.

29. Schaub, B. G., & Schaub, R. (2003). Imagery and spiritual development. In A. A. Sheikh (Ed.),

Healing images: The role of imagination in health (pp. 489–498). Amityville, NY: Baywood.

30. Schaub, B. G., & Schaub, R. (1999). Spirituality and clinical practice. *Alternative Health Practitioner, 5*(2), 145–150.

31. Scherwitz, L. W., McHenry, P., & Herrero, R. (2005). Interactive guided imagery therapy with medical patients: Predictors of health outcomes. *Journal of Alternative and Complementary Medicine, 11*(1), 69–83.

32. Achterberg, J., & Dossey, B. (1994). *Rituals of healing.* New York, NY: Bantam Books.

■ STUDY QUESTIONS

Basic Level

1. Which of the following best describes the therapeutic intention for educating clients about the imagery process?
   a. Engaging the imagination in a guided prescriptive way can effect physical outcomes.
   b. Helping patients control their thoughts.
   c. Strengthening the mind–body connection.
   d. Empowering others by introducing them to a way to access a dormant deep resource of wisdom and healing that is already within them.

2. What should the holistic nurse do if the client is troubled by distracting thoughts during the imagery session?
   a. Shorten the length of the imagery session.
   b. Analyze the distracting thoughts.
   c. Lengthen the relaxation induction time before the session.
   d. Obtain orders for an anxiolytic agent.

3. Which of the following is the best way to characterize skilled imagery guides?
   a. To use long phrases.
   b. To avoid the use of metaphors.
   c. To offer the client choices.
   d. To focus on one sensory modality at a time.

4. What should the nurse do before beginning an imagery session?
   a. Make sure that the client understands that a deep sleep is the ultimate goal.
   b. Tell the client to analyze all images that emerge.

   c. Tell the client that uncomfortable images are sometimes the most revealing.
   d. Have the client develop a positive expectation of the experience.

5. During a nurse–patient caring moment, the nurse identifies an opportunity to offer imagery as a means to manage postsurgical pain. The nurse suggests to the patient that they might try something together that could be helpful, and the patient indicates a willingness to explore imagery. What would the nurse assess next?
   a. Determine the patient's preferred sensory modes (visual, auditory, kinaesthetic, emotional, etc.).
   b. Ask the patient what forms of relaxation had been helpful in the past.
   c. Educate the patient about the imagery process.
   d. Tell the patient that imagery will greatly reduce the pain.

6. In the nursing process, when using imagery, which statement best describes the evaluation of the patient outcomes?
   a. The outcomes should be predictable, measurable, and easily replicated.
   b. If an imagery intervention does not prove to be helpful, instead use creativity and try other imagery approaches.
   c. If the patient reports no relief from the problem, the nurse should determine that imagery is not helpful for this client.
   d. Patient responses are highly individualized, and once the patient has had a positive experience, this experience can often be duplicated.

7. Which statement best describes the imagery process?
   a. Imagery is a guided mind–body modality utilized to pattern physiologic responses.
   b. Imagery is a spontaneous inner resource experienced directly through visual images.
   c. Imagery taps a deep level of self-knowledge, wisdom, and healing that is already present in the individual.
   d. Not all individuals can benefit from the resource of their imagination.

Advanced Level

8. A nurse is working in a coaching role with a client in an outpatient clinic. The nurse recognizes that the patient is having difficulty with self-care and self-management of her diabetes. The nurse senses that exploring the patient's obstacles to self-care through an imagery experience might bring some insights to the patient. The nurse has some fear in offering this modality. Which of the following is a common fear for the nurse in offering imagery?

   a. The nurse fears that there could be reprimand by the supervisor for offering an intervention that is not evidence based.
   b. The nurse fears that the patient might react negatively by rejecting the modality as "silly."
   c. The nurse fears that the imagery method might be too evocative and have negative consequences for the patient.
   d. The nurse fears she will be distracted by interruptions, so it is not worth initiating the intervention.

9. While facilitating an imagery experience focused on "going to a safe place," the nurse notices that the client begins to breathe deeply and then begins to cry. What would be the best intervention?

   a. Gently guide the patient back to the room and encourage the opening of eyes.
   b. Encourage the client to stay with the inner experience and to describe the experience
   c. Ask the patient, "Why are you crying?"
   d. Stop the imagery experience and apologize for upsetting the client.

10. In an imagery intervention , the client describes being unable to visualize anything in the experience. Upon further exploration of the patient's experience, the patient states, "I couldn't do the imagery. I just felt very relaxed and I kept hearing in my mind the words 'let go.' " In evaluating the outcome of the client's imagery intervention, the holistic nurse concludes which of the following conclusions?

   a. Imagery might not be a holistic modality that can work for this patient.
   b. The patient might be psychotic and hearing voices, so imagery is contraindicated.
   c. The imagery process engages all the senses, so this client might not have been visual but might have used a different sensory mode to experience the resource of his imagination.
   d. The nurse probably did not offer the imagery intervention skillfully, so the patient was unable to visualize the imagery suggestions.

Chapter 19

Music: A Caring–Healing Modality

Shannon S. Spies Ingersoll
and Ana Schaper

■ DEFINITIONS

Caring consciousness A "deeper" level where the nurse is mindful, intentional, and present and chooses how he or she portrays "being" in the interaction (achieved through centering).

Caring–healing modality Auditory, visual, olfactory, tactile, gustatory, cognitive, and kinesthetic in nature and essential for holistic caring, healing practices, and health in the twenty-first century.

Caring moment(s) Influencing both individuals through a relationship and by being together in that given moment in time.

Centering A mind-body-spirit activity (breathing exercises, meditation) to prepare the body to enter into, prepare for, and begin caring consciousness in a relationship.

Entrainment Synchronization where the vibrations of one object cause the vibrations of another object (usually the less powerful one) to oscillate at the same rate.

Genre Category of artistic works of all kinds can be divided by form, style, or subject matter.

Intentionality Deliberately focusing consciousness on something, for example, a belief, will, expectation, attention, or action.

Transpersonal nursing Human-to-human interaction that entails wholeness, caring consciousness, and intentionality.[1]

Wholeness The inner sense of unity with all life on Earth (universal oneness and connectedness of all).[2]

■ THEORY AND RESEARCH

1. Music has been used throughout history as a caring–healing modality. Florence Nightingale advocated the use of music to aid healing.[3]
2. With the advent of pharmaceuticals, less attention was paid to the use of music in nurse caring.
3. Jean Watson's Theory of Human Caring defined the nurse as the intervention and music as a caring–healing modality.
4. There is a growing body of evidence supporting music as an effective healing modality, but nurses must critically review the evidence and consciously ask new research questions.

■ THE CAPACITY OF MUSIC TO PRODUCE A CLINICAL CHANGE

1. Several Cochrane Reviews have been conducted on the effectiveness of music.[4] However, the reviews report limited support for the use of music in clinical practice.
2. Historically, research on the effectiveness of music to produce a positive clinical outcome has been of low quality with small sample sizes and high risk for bias. Research design has improved greatly in more recently reported studies.
3. Reviews make a clear distinction between research in which the interventions are delivered by a certified music therapist (music therapy) and music interventions delivered by a health provider (also referred to as music medicine).[5]
4. Overall, music therapy interventions demonstrate greater effectiveness than music

delivered by a health provider. Strengths of music therapy research include:

   a. Use of theoretical framework to guide the research.

   b. Use of multiple modalities including active music participation.

   c. An individualized music therapy regime adapted over time.

   d. Direct interactions between the patient and the music therapist.

5. Music therapy[6] as delivered by a music therapist includes:

   a. Listening to live, improvised, or prerecorded music.

   b. Performing music on an instrument.

   c. Improvising music spontaneously using voice and/or instruments.

   d. Composing music.

   e. Music combined with other modalities.

6. When considering using music as a caring–healing modality, collaboration with a music therapist can enhance patients' music experience.

Effectiveness of Music Therapy Delivered by a Music Therapist

1. Music therapy research frequently involves patients dealing with chronic health issues.

2. Music therapy delivered over a course of 6–10 weeks for adults with depression reduced symptoms and improved cognitive function.[7]

3. Music therapy delivered in 20 or more sessions improved general functioning for patients with depression.[7,8]

4. Music therapy for brain-injured adults and patients with Parkinson's disease demonstrates its effectiveness in support of walking and other gate-related activities.[9–11]

5. Music therapy for people with schizophrenia or schizophrenia-like illness resulted in improved global state, mental state, and functioning.[12]

6. Music therapy can decrease the need for physical and chemical restraints in older adults with dementia or Alzheimer's disease living in assisted care or nursing homes.[13,14]

7. A systematic review of home-based music therapy for older adults with cancer concluded that music improves outcomes related to pain, depression, quality of life, and family/caregiver relationships.[15]

8. Researchers using a qualitative design to explore the impact of music therapy at a cancer care center identified four overarching spirituality themes: transcendence, connectedness, search for meaning, and faith and hope.[16]

9. A qualitative study on the impact of group improvisational music therapy in cancer patients identified the benefits as facilitating peer support, increasing self-confidence, relaxation, generation of positive feelings, stress relief, and enhanced communication through music.[17]

10. Qualitative data in a study of a home-based music therapy program for children in palliative care suggest that music provided both comfort and stimulation for the child during a time of diminished quality of life in cognitive and activity domains.[18]

11. A quantitative study on the impact of group music therapy sessions for mothers who have a child with a disability reported improved parent mental health, child communication, parental sensitivity, parental engagement with the child and acceptance of the child, child responsiveness to the parent, and child participation in program activities.[19]

12. Multiple studies suggest that family members also benefit from the music therapy designed for the patient.[11,15,18,19]

13. Playing musical instruments provides a unique opportunity for patients with depression symptoms to experience and express their emotions on a nonverbal level.[8]

Effectiveness of Music Delivered by a Health Provider

1. Research utilizing music medicine focuses primarily on the short-term management of pain, anxiety, and distress with outcome measurements taken at the end of the intervention.

2. A Cochrane Review on studies involving cardiac patients reported that music had a moderate effect on anxiety.[5] Anxiety reduction was highest in patients experiencing a myocardial infarction. There was no evidence for the anxiety-reducing effects of music for patients undergoing a cardiac procedure (intracardiac catheterization, coronary angiography, coronary artery bypass

grafting). When two or more music listening sessions were used for anxiety reduction, patients reported less pain.

3. A more recent study demonstrated that anxiety was reduced in patients undergoing coronary angiography who listened to music compared with controls.[20]

4. Women undergoing coronary angiography, who listened to music, reported a more positive impression of their environment and less discomfort associated with lying still. However, no effect in relaxation was demonstrated among women with high anxiety.[21]

5. A Cochrane Review of music interventions for mechanically ventilated patients supports a small effect in reducing patient anxiety.[22] These finding were supported in a recent study that included evidence of improvement in both subjective and physiologic measures.[23]

6. Another Cochrane Review concluded that the use of music reduced postoperative pain, increased the number of patients who reported at least 50% pain relief, and lowered morphine-like analgesic use.[24] However, the magnitude of the music effect was very small.

7. A systematic review of patients who underwent surgery concluded that patients listening to music reported less pain, a decrease in blood pressure and respiratory rates, and lower anxiety.[25] There were no differences in the effectiveness of music selected by the researchers compared with self-selected music.

8. A review of studies evaluating the effectiveness of music listening in the operating room during monitored anesthesia care demonstrated a reduction in sedation requirements during anesthesia, faster recovery, and decreased likelihood for converting to a general anesthetic.[26]

9. A study of patients' well-being after listening to music during early postoperative care determined that patients experiencing two or more music listening sessions had a positive response to the music and an awareness that music helped them refocus attention on a more pleasing, soothing stimulus.[27]

10. A combination of jaw relaxation techniques while listening to music resulted in less pain distress for patients on day 1 and day 2 after surgery compared with a patient teaching comparison group and a usual care control group.[28]

11. Patients who listened to 30 minutes of pre-selected music the night before spinal surgery, 1 hour before surgery, and on day 1 and day 2 after surgery had lower mean anxiety and pain scores and lower blood pressure measurements compared to controls.[29]

12. A Cochrane Review on the effectiveness of music on preoperative anxiety is in progress.[30]

13. In a study of music used by women undergoing same-day gynecological surgery, listening to music through headphones resulted in significantly lower anxiety compared to women using noise-blocking headphones without music and the usual care control group.[31]

14. Similarly, the cohort of same-day surgery patients undergoing general elective procedures who listened to music experienced a greater decrease in anxiety compared with controls.[32]

15. Among patients hospitalized for the management of chronic pain, patients listening to music two or more times a day reported a decrease in anxiety and depression symptoms and lower pain compared to controls.[33]
    a. There was lower use of anxiolytic agents in patients listening to music.
    b. The positive effects were sustained at 3 months.

16. Cancer patients who received 30 minutes of relaxing music reported significantly less pain compared with patients provided with a 30-minute rest period.[34]

17. Music had a greater effect on postchemotherapy anxiety compared to verbal relaxation and usual care. Patients with high-state anxiety experienced the most benefit from music listening.[35]

18. Patients listening to music delivered through headphones during interventional radiographic procedures required less sedation, but there was no change in anxiety levels.[36]

19. A Cochrane Review of music for improving psychological and physical outcomes in the care of cancer patients concluded that music interventions might decrease anxiety and improve mood and quality of life in cancer patients.[37]

20. Older adults on hemodialysis benefited from listening to self-selected music during treatment with fewer adverse reactions, a lower severity of reactions, and lower stress.[38]

21. There were lower levels of confusion in a cohort of older adults who received music listening sessions for 3 days following hip or knee surgery compared with controls.[39]

22. Music listening has also been evaluated in infants and children.

    a. An integrative review of preterm infants' response to music concluded that music appears to increase oxygen saturation levels, lower heart rates, reduce behavioral stress responses, improve weight gain, shorten length of hospitalization, and increase levels of quiet awake and quiet sleep states.[40]

    b. In a cohort of children aged 7 to 12 years undergoing a lumbar puncture, the music group reported lower anxiety, had less pain, and lower heart and respiration rates.[41]

    c. Among adolescents receiving immunizations, music listening groups reported less pain compared to the control group.[42]

23. In contrast to relative positive outcomes of the preceding studies, other research demonstrated no differences between music listening groups and controls.

    a. No differences were reported in pain or anxiety levels in a music group compared to a rest-only control group of patients undergoing cardiac surgery.[43]

    b. There was no difference in sleep quality among older adults listening to music over a 4-week period compared to controls.[44]

24. Music might not always be the best caring-healing modality for a patient. Nurses must specifically assess a patient's interest in music and the patient's care needs.

    a. In a qualitative review of music experiences of terminally ill patients, the reviewers provide examples of patients rejecting the use of music and suggest that music listening might not be a positive experience.[45]

    b. Music might not enhance positive outcomes when the music is unfamiliar, is experienced as unpleasant, or is associated with loss.[45,46]

    c. Not all patients find music relaxing or are interested in listening to music. Instead the patient might want to stay attuned to what is happening in the environment or prefers a different healing modality to meet his or her goal(s).[47]

    d. Four percent of the general population suffers from "amusia," or tone-deafness. This is usually inherited but might be a consequence of brain damage.[48]

25. Music might also contribute to disease processes. A critical review of music and epilepsy reported both proconvulsant and anticonvulsant effects of music. Surgical interventions and medications for managing epilepsy can affect a patient's perception of music.[49]

26. Although music cannot be used for every situation, the data suggest that the use of music increases patients' satisfaction with their care and contributes to their well-being.[20,27,41]

27. Few qualitative studies have been conducted outside of music therapy research. One study identified three themes capturing the effectiveness of listening to music postoperatively: feeling comfort in a discomforting and frightening situation, distraction from pain, and a feeling of being at home.[50] The last theme reflects patients' statements indicating that music transported them out of the hospital to their own homes, a familiar, comforting environment.

28. Only two studies were identified in which the nurse was considered an active component of the intervention.

    a. One study evaluating the effect of a music intervention for the management of chronic pain highlighted the role of nurse in developing a strong therapeutic relationship with patients in the intervention group.[33] The nurse–patient interaction was credited with the patients' sustained use of music after hospital discharge and long-term outcomes of lower depression and anxiety levels.

    b. A cross-over study evaluated the effectiveness of nurse presence compared with recorded music on anxiety, depression, and sleep in family caregivers.[51] Depression and anxiety levels significantly decreased for both interventions. Music played by the nurse was more effective in lowering anxiety and helping participants fall asleep easily. Other sleep parameters were not affected by the interventions.

Summary of Research Evidence

1. The results of music effectiveness research continue to be mixed. Therefore, the results of studies showing positive outcomes need to be applied with caution.
2. The vast majority of research has been conducted using Caucasian and Asian population samples. Identifying culturally appropriate music for patients is a key element.
3. There has been no reported research on the effectiveness of music related to gender.
4. Music is effective in reducing anxiety for patients, in particular, for patients with a high level of anxiety. Music might also reduce physiologic measures of anxiety including respiratory rate, heart rate, and blood pressure.
5. Music is effective in reducing pain, but only to a limited extent.
6. A highly variable response to music is likely among patients. Different effects of music might result from a combination of internal and external factors.
7. Delivery of two or more music listening sessions increases the likelihood of a positive outcome, including pain reduction. Listening to music before and after an invasive procedure can enhance effectiveness.
8. Music in combination with other healing modalities can enhance effectiveness.
9. Time duration for a listening session does not make a difference, but almost all research focused on anxiety and pain reduction is based on listening to music for an uninterrupted time period of 20 to 30 minutes.
10. Music genre might not make a difference, although the majority of studies used classical music.
11. Music tempo does make a difference. Chaotic music might not be healing to human cells. Music with a slower tempo that is described as calming and soothing appears

to be the most important element in enhancing music effectiveness to reduce pain and anxiety. In several studies by Nilsson, a selection of "genreless" music was used for music listening groups, available from MusiCure (www.musicure.com).[52]
12. Self-selected music not limited to slower tempos should be used when the goal is to motivate and/or communicate emotions.
13. Decision making on the choice of music selection is important. A key component to positive outcomes might be the determination of an intended goal with specific music chosen to meet that goal.
14. Music has meaning beyond its function in producing clinical outcomes.
15. Little attention, outside of structured music therapy interventions, has been given to gaining insight on music as a means for people to relate and share a health-related experience. Few research studies explore how music contributes to a person's development of the capacity to strive, endure, recover, heal, live, or die.
16. More research is needed using holistic nursing theories to guide the development and testing of music as a caring–healing modality.[53]

■ THEORETICAL BASIS FOR THE CAPACITY OF MUSIC TO PRODUCE A CLINICAL CHANGE

1. The goal of laboratory research addressing the functionality of music is to understand the mechanisms of action on a cellular or molecular level.
   a. Music can reduce the stress hormone cortisol.[43,48,54,55]
   b. Music, which elicits a strong pleasurable response, can lead to a release of endogenous dopamine.[56]
   c. Music can increase oxytocin, which has been shown to create a sense of calmness and diminish the sensation of pain.[57,58]
2. Neuroimagery has provided for rapid developments of theory on the functional neuroanatomy of music.[59,60] Complex musical compositions often elicit mixed feelings and perceptions.
3. Typically, a nurse healer can expect that music perceived as happy or sad or relaxing

will create a parallel emotional response.[61,62] However, this emotional response might be subtle.

   a. Emotional responses can be enhanced with the consistent delivery of happy (major key) or sad (minor key) music.

   b. Faster tempo of major key music results in higher happy ratings.

   c. Slower tempo of minor key music is associated with higher sad ratings.

   d. Mixed music cues (fast-pace minor key) resulted in feelings of ambivalence.

   e. Music combined with another congruent stimulus, such as art or external imagery, can reduce the possibility of mixed effects resulting in feelings of ambivalence.

4. When selecting music for the goal of reducing anxiety or for pain management, use music with a smooth melody and simple harmonic or chord progression:[63]

   a. A consistent tempo of 60–80 beats per minute.

   b. Delivered at low volume.

   c. With limited instrumentation.

   d. Without harsh contrasts (not harmonic) and/or percussive or accented rhythms.

5. When selecting music for the goal of improving gross motor movements or exercise, patient musical preference can be the most important element influencing good outcomes.[64]

6. Entrainment theory helps to illustrate the importance of making a best choice in the self-selection of music for a specific goal.[65,66] Entrainment theory is a physics theory used to understand the body's response to music. Entrainment is the synchronization process whereby the vibrations of one object cause the vibrations of another object (usually the less powerful) to oscillate at the same tempo or rate. Finger tapping, toe tapping, swaying to the music, and even head nodding reflect the human body's response to the rhythm and tempo of music.

7. Movement to music is the basis for a novel midrange nursing theory of music, mood, and movement (MMM Theory), which can guide the nurse–patient interaction in the selection of music for promoting exercise for wellness.[67] An in-home music program for older adults, based on the MMM Theory, significantly reduced depression scores over an 8-week trial compared to controls.[68]

8. Less than half of all oncology research on the effectiveness of music reports a theoretical framework.[69] In a review by Burns, 75% of studies using a theoretical framework demonstrated positive outcomes compared with 58% of studies without a theoretical framework. Theoretical frameworks:

   a. Provide congruency between the selection of the music and the intervention design.

   b. Frame both the positive and negative outcomes of the research.

Music: A Caring–Healing Modality

1. Consciousness and purposeful decision making are significant in the selection and evaluation of music listening.

   a. The nurse–patient interaction can be the key to effective music listening.

   b. Presently, no nursing theories capture the nurse–patient interaction and music.

2. Caring–healing modalities go back to the roots of the nursing profession and began with our founder Florence Nightingale.

   a. Nightingale viewed the nurse–patient relationship as a sacred pledge in which the nurse and patient become one, in body and soul.

   b. Watson's transpersonal nursing encompasses Nightingale's views and brings this work to the twenty-first century.

   c. Watson points out how Nightingale used basic needs along with one's environment to create an inner body to soul connection promoting healing.

   d. Presently, health care has become consumed with "task"-orientated care and has drifted away from deeper human-to-human connections using caring–healing modalities that promote health and caring.

   e. Watson's work brings forth this deeper human-to-human connection (nurse–patient interaction) through caring consciousness and intentionality using caring–healing modalities.

3. Watson uses caring–healing modalities (one being music) to connect with patients on a deeper level and change a difficult moment into a "caring moment."

4. Watson believes that caring–healing modalities promote inner wholeness, harmony, beauty, integrity, dignity, and humanity.

5. Caring consciousness and intentionality are key concepts of transpersonal nursing.[70]
   a. Caring consciousness is a deeper interaction of spiritual awareness that is reciprocal (transpersonal) between the nurse and patient.
   b. By engaging in caring consciousness, the nurse and patient experience life changes that affect their "being" and a "caring moment" is created.
6. Intentionality is direct purpose and effectiveness toward a belief, will, expectation, attention, or an action.
7. Intentionality entails "clearing of the mind" so that the nurse can focus on the "present moment" in time.
8. Applying caring consciousness and intentionality creates a "caring moment." This is a way nurses can heal their patients and themselves through a deeper understanding of one's self-promoting quality caring experiences.[54]
9. Music listening is one type of caring-healing modality that is used in establishing a "caring moment" between the nurse and patient.
10. Music listening can be as effective as music therapy.
    a. The nurse uses caring consciousness and intentionality to enhance the patient's experiences with music.
    b. Using music listening in the nurse–patient interaction, the nurse can encourage a meaningful and intentional dialogue with the patient while both are consciously attentive to the music.
11. By exploring music's healing effects through the interaction, life-changing experiences emerge that influence one's being.
12. Caring moments are minutes in time that influence the patient and nurse.[72] These moments exemplify value for human life and promote quality caring-healing experiences.
13. Other forms of artistic expression (paintings, sculptures, pottery) can be paired with music listening, thus supporting a greater sense of healing.[73] The sum of caring-healing modalities is greater than each one alone in creating a body-mind-spirit escape to "a place" viewed in the imagery or in the imagination.

Individual Musical Preferences

1. Music is a subjective phenomenon. Many genres are available for individuals to connect with on a personal level.
   a. Music listening can affect an individual's mind, mood, feelings, and actions.
2. The International Organization for Standardization (ISO), according to Morris, focuses on matching different genres of music to individuals' mood states.[65]
3. The ISO principle is two-sided: As moods are altered by the music, a "state of consciousness" is achieved. The "state of consciousness" attained through the ISO resembles caring consciousness in the nurse–patient interaction.
4. The individual is mindful, intentional, and present at that moment and chooses how to act through the music interaction compared to expressing one's self.
5. As individuals grow to appreciate how music affects their well-being possibly through journaling, the potential of music as a healing modality is empowered.
   a. Journaling consists of writing down specific genres and how and why these selections of music have affected emotions, actions, and overall life experiences.
6. Nurses' can use journaling as a way to start using music as a healing power in their own lives.
7. Future research and evidence-based practice will pave new directions in individual musical preferences and in using music as a caring-healing modality.

Holistic Caring Process

1. Music listening as a caring-healing modality is integrated into the patient's plan of care.

Holistic Assessment

1. During the assessment phase, the nurse healer assesses the individual's interest in music, genres the person enjoys, history with using music, and hearing ability.
   a. Nurses can engage patients in how music can be used as an effective healing modality in itself along with being an adjunct with other pharmacologic and nonpharmacologic therapies.

b. The nurse, patient, and family can then explore various types of music that might fit the context of the situation (consciousness) and the purpose for using music (intentionality).

c. Music listening goals frequently involve relaxing, reducing anxiety, or mediating pain responses.

d. Other goals can be achieved with music listening and consist of supporting deep breathing, promoting active and passive exercises, and establishing a caring–healing relationship with each other.

Identification of Patterns/ Challenges/Needs

1. The following are patterns, challenges, and needs that are compatible with music therapy:
   a. Hard of hearing
   b. Deaf
   c. Confusion
   d. Anxiety
   e. Pain
   f. Relaxation
   g. Depression
   h. Loss of memory
   i. Loneliness
   j. Spiritual distress
   k. Stress
   l. Motivational
   m. Fear
   n. Fatigue
   o. Hopelessness
   p. Outcomes
   q. Self-selected music from home can be used as downloads on an MP3 player/iPod. Music can also be selected from a music library specifically developed for a floor or an institution.
   r. Preventing infection when using headphones is attained with individual ear buds and music pillows. Changing cases on the music pillows is another option.

Holistic Care Plan and Interventions[73]

1. At the beginning of the session:
   a. If in a clinical or hospital setting, inform others of the need for minimal noise and disruptions (post a sign on the patient door requesting no interruptions for 30 minutes).
   b. If the patient has a hearing loss, consider a variety of methods for delivering music.
      - Headphones provide for individual control of sound level. Music pillows are available, or the nurse might find the most effective placement of the music player.
   c. Discuss how listening to music can help the patient reach intended goals (relaxation, anxiety reduction, pain mediation).
   d. Discuss the length of the session, usually 20 to 30 minutes.
   e. Ask the person to empty his or her bladder, if needed.
   f. Ask the person to remove eyeglasses.
   g. Minimize stimuli from the environment, such as by lowering the light level, closing a curtain or door.
   h. Assist the patient in finding a comfortable position, and offer an extra pillow or blanket if needed.
   i. Have the patient begin playing the music to make sure the equipment is functioning properly.
2. Evaluation: At the end of the session:
   a. Assess the patient's response and tolerance to the session.
   b. Create a caring moment by connecting with the person during a 5- to 10-minute interaction.
   c. Use the following script to begin this caring moment:[53]
      - What did you listen to today?
      - Tell me what you thought of when you listened to this music (memories)?
      - How does listening to (specific music selection) music make you feel?
      - Share a personal experience of how listening to music makes you feel.
      - In what ways did listening to the music help you? Did the music help you reach your goal?
      - What are your thoughts about having music listening available during your time here?
      - What would be helpful to make this a better experience for you?
      - If appropriate, schedule a follow-up session.

3. Documentation of session and plan of care
   a. Record the following information:
      - Person's goal or intention for listening to music.
      - Song or genre the person selects.
      - Time and tolerance of the listening session.
      - Outcome of the music listening experience.
      - An update of the plan to use music listening in the future.
   b. Today, nurse healers are challenged to define best practice for documentation of music as a caring–healing modality in their current and future record systems. With a move to electronic medical records, nurses have the opportunity to document how music listening is used and the patient's responses to inform not only the next nurse caring for the patient, but also future nursing care, when another procedure, treatment, or hospitalization takes place. The nurse healer's message to others can define the nature of patient-centered care in a future care context.

■ NOTES

1. Watson, J. (1999). *Postmodern nursing and beyond.* Philadelphia, PA: Churchill Livingstone.

2. Cowling, W. R., 3rd , Smith, M. C., & Watson, J. (2008). The power of wholeness, consciousness, and caring: A dialogue on nursing science, art, and healing. *Advances in Nursing Science, 31*(1), E41–E51.

3. Nightingale, F. (2010). *Notes on nursing: What it is and what it is not.* New York, NY: Cambridge University Press. (Original work published 1860.)

4. Cochrane Collaboration. (n.d.). Homepage. Retrieved from http://www.cochrane.org/

5. Bradt, J., & Dileo, C. (2009). Music for stress and anxiety reduction in coronary heart disease patients. *Cochrane Database of Systematic Reviews,* 2.

6. American Music Therapy Association. (n.d.). What is music therapy? Retrieved from http ://www.musictherapy.org/faq/#38

7. Maratos, A., Gold, C., Wang, X., & Crawford M. (2008). Music therapy for depression. *Cochrane Database of Systematic Reviews,* 1.

8. Erkkilia, J., Punkanen, M., Fachner, J., Ala-Ruona, E., Pöntiö, I., Tervaniemi, M.,...Gold, C. (2011). Individual music therapy for depression: Randomized controlled trial. *British Journal of Psychiatry, 199,* 132–139.

9. Bradt, J., Magee, W. L., Dileo, C., Wheeler, B. L., & McGilloway, E. (2010). Music therapy for acquired brain injury. *Cochrane Database of Systematic Reviews,* 10.

10. Weller, C. M., & Baker, F. A. (2011). The role of music therapy in physical rehabilitation: A systematic literature review. *Nordic Journal of Music Therapy, 20*(1), 43–61.

11. de Dreu, M. J., van der Wilk, A. S., Poppe, E., Kwakkel, G., & van Wegen, E. E. (2012). Rehabilitation, exercise therapy and music in patients with Parkinson's disease: A meta-analysis of the effects of music-based movement therapy on walking ability, balance and quality of life. *Parkinsonism & Related Disorders, 18*(Suppl. 1), S114–119.

12. Mossler, K., Chen, X., Heldal, O. T., & Gold, C. (2011). Music therapy for people with schizophrenia and schizophrenia-like disorders. *Cochrane Database of Systematic Reviews,* 12.

13. Vink, A. C., Birks, J. S., Bruinsma, M. S., & Scholten, R. J. (2009). Music therapy for people with dementia. *Cochrane Database of Systematic Reviews,* 1.

14. Witzke, J., Rhone, R. A., Backhaus, D., & Shaver, N. A. (2008). How sweet the sound: Research evidence for the use of music in Alzheimer's dementia. *Journal of Gerontological Nursing, 34*(10), 45–52.

15. Schmid, W., & Ostermann, T. (2010). Home-based music therapy—a systematic overview of settings and conditions for an innovative service in healthcare. *BMC Health Services Research, 10,* 291.

16. McClean, S., Bunt, L., & Daykin, N. (2012). The healing and spiritual properties of music therapy at a cancer care center. *Journal of Alternative & Complementary Medicine, 18*(4), 402–407.

17. Pothoulaki, M., MacDonald, R., & Flowers, P. (2012). An interpretative phenomenological analysis of an improvisational music therapy program for cancer patients. *Journal of Music Therapy, 49*(4), 45–67.

18. Lindenfelser, K. J., Hense, C., & McFerran, K. (2012). Music therapy in pediatric palliative care: Family-centered care to enhance quality of life. *American Journal of Hospice & Palliative Medicine, 29*(3), 219–226.

19. Williams, K. E., Berthelsen, D., Nicholson, J. M., Walker, S., & Abad, V. (2012). The effectiveness of a short-term group music therapy intervention for parents who have a child with a disability. *Journal of Music Therapy, 49*(1), 23–44.

20. Weeks, P. B., & Nilsson, U. (2011). Music interventions in patients during coronary angiographic procedures: A randomized controlled study of the effect on patients' anxiety and well-being. *European Journal of Cardiovascular Nursing, 10*(2), 88–93.

21. Nilsson, U. (2012). Effectiveness of music interventions for women with high anxiety during coronary angiographic procedures: A randomized controlled trial. *Journal of Cardiovascular Nursing, 11*(2), 150–153.

22. Bradt, J., Dileo, C., & Grocke, D. (2010). Music interventions for mechanically ventilated patients. *Cochrane Database of Systematic Reviews,* 12.

23. Davis, T., & Jones, P. (2012). Music therapy: Decreasing anxiety in the ventilated patient: A review of the literature. *DCCN—Dimensions of Critical Care Nursing, 3*(3), 159–166.

24. Cepeda, S. M., Carr, D. B., Lau, J., & Alvarez, H. (2010). Music for pain relief. *Cochrane Database of Systematic Reviews,* 8.

25. Nilsson, U. (2008). The anxiety- and pain-reducing effects of music interventions: A systematic review. *AORN Journal, 87*(4), 780.

26. Newman, A., Boyd, C., Meyers, D., & Bonanno, L. (2010). Implementation of music as an anesthetic adjunct during monitored anesthesia care. *Journal of PeriAnesthesia Nursing, 25*(6), 387–391.

27. Fredriksson, A., Hellström, L., & Nilsson, U. (2009). Patients' perception of music versus ordinary sound in a postanaesthesia care unit: A randomized crossover trial. *Intensive and Critical Care Nursing, 25*(4), 208–213.

28. Good, M., Albert, J. M., Anderson, G. C., Wotman, S., Cong, X., Lane, D., & Ahn, S. (2010). Supplementing relaxation and music for pain after surgery. *Nursing Research, 59*(4), 259–269.

29. Lin, P., Lin, M. L., Huang, L. C., Hsu, H. C., & Lin, C. C. (2011). Music therapy for patients receiving spine surgery. *Journal of Clinical Nursing, 20*(7), 960–968.

30. Dileo, C., Bradt, J., & Murphy, K. (2010). Music for preoperative anxiety. *Cochrane Database of Systematic Reviews,* 4.

31. Johnson, B., Raymond, S., & Goss, J. (2012). Perioperative music or headsets to decrease anxiety. *Journal of PeriAnesthesia Nursing, 27*(2), 146–154.

32. Ni, C. H., Tsai, W. H., Lee, L. M., Kao, C. C., & Chen, Y. C. (2011). Minimizing preoperative anxiety with music for day surgery patients—a randomized trial. *Journal of Clinical Nursing, 21,* 620–625.

33. Guetin, S., Ginies, P., Siou, D. K., Picot, M. C., Pommie, C., Guldner, E.,...Touchon, J. (2012). The effects of music intervention in the management of chronic pain: A single-blind, randomized controlled trial. *Clinical Journal of Pain, 28*(4), 328–337.

34. Huang, S., Good, M., & Zauszniewski, J. A. (2010). The effectiveness of music in relieving pain in cancer patients: A randomized controlled trial. *International Journal of Nursing Studies, 47*(11), 1354–1362.

35. Lin, M., Hsieh, Y. J., Hsu, Y. Y., Fetzer, S., & Hsu, M. C. (2011). A randomized controlled trial of the effect of music therapy and verbal relaxation on chemotherapy-induced anxiety. *Journal of Clinical Nursing, 20*(7), 988–999.

36. Kulkarni, S., Johnson, P. C., Kettles, S., & Kasthuri, R. S. (2012). Music during interventional radiological procedures, effect on sedation, pain and anxiety: A randomized controlled trial. *British Journal of Radiology, 85*(1016), 1059–1063.

37. Bradt, J., Dileo, C., Grocke, D., & Magill, L. (2011). Music interventions for improving psychological and physical outcomes in cancer patients. *Cochrane Database of Systematic Reviews,* 10 (8).

38. Lin, Y., Lu, K. C., Chen, C. M., & Chang, C. (2012). The effects of music as therapy on the overall well-being of elderly patients on maintenance hemodialysis. *Biological Research for Nursing, 14*(3), 277–285.

39. McCaffrey, R. (2009). The effect of music on acute confusion in older adults after hip or knee surgery. *Applied Nursing Research, 22*(2), 107–112.

40. Hodges, A. L., & Wilson, L. L. (2010). Preterm infants' responses to music: An integrative literature review. *Southern Online Journal of Nursing Research, 10*(3). Retrieved March 17, 2013, from http://www.resourcenter.net/images/SNRS/Files/SOJNR_articles2/Vol10Num03Art05.html

41. Nguyen, T. N., et al. (2010). Music therapy to reduce pain and anxiety in children with cancer undergoing lumbar puncture: A randomized clinical trial. *Journal of Pediatric Oncology Nursing, 27*(3), 146–155.

42. Kristjánsdóttir, O., & Kristjánsdóttir, G. (2011). Randomized clinical trial of musical distraction with and without headphones for adolescents' immunization pain. *Scandinavian Journal of Caring Sciences, 25*(1), 19–26.

43. Nilsson, U. (2009). The effect of music intervention in stress response to cardiac surgery in a randomized clinical trial. *Heart & Lung, 38*(3), 201–207.

44. Chan, M. F. (2011). A randomized controlled study of the effects of music on sleep quality in older people. *Journal of Clinical Nursing, 20*(7), 979–987.

45. Leow, Q. M., Drury, V. B., & Poon, W. (2010). Experience of terminally ill patients with music therapy: A literature review. *Singapore Nursing Journal, 37*(3), 48–52.

46. Austin, D. (2010). The psychophysiological effects of music therapy in intensive care units. *Pediatric Nursing, 22*(3), 14–20.

47. Beccaloni, A. M. (2011). The medicine of music: A systematic approach for adoption into perianesthesia practice. *Journal of PeriAnesthesia Nursing, 26*(5), 323–330.

48. Mrázová, M., & Celec, P. (2010). A systematic review of randomized controlled trials using music therapy for children. *Journal of Alternative and Complementary Medicine, 16*(10), 1089–1095.

49. Maguire, M. J. (2012). Music and epilepsy: A critical review. *Epilepsia, 53*(6), 947–961.

50. McCaffrey, R. (2008). Music listening: Its effects in creating a healing environment. *Journal of Psychosocial Nursing and Mental Health Services, 46*(10), 39–44.

51. Lai, H., Li, Y., & Lee, L. (2011). Effects of music intervention with nursing presence and recorded music on pyscho-physiological indices of cancer patient caregivers. *Journal of Clinical Nursing, 21,* 745–756.

52. MusiCure Music as Medicine. (n.d.). Homepage. Retrieved from http://www.musicure.com/

53. Spies Ingersoll, S., & Schaper, A. (2011). Therapeutic music pilot in the context of human caring theory. In J. Nelson & J. Watson (Eds.), *Measuring caring: International research on caritas as healing* (pp. 257–268). New York, NY: Spring Publishing.

54. Suda, M., Morimoto, K., Obata, A., Koizumi, H., & Maki, A. (2008). Emotional responses to music: Toward scientific perspectives on music therapy. *Brain Imaging, 19*(1), 75–78.

55. Ventura, T., Gomes, M. C., & Carreira, T. (2012). Cortisol and anxiety response to a relaxing intervention on pregnant women awaiting amniocentesis. *Psychoneuroendocrinology, 37*(1), 148–156.

56. Salimpoor, V. N., Benovoy, M., Larcher, K., Dagher, A., & Zatorre, R. J. (2011). Anatomically distinct dopamine release during anticipation and experience of peak emotion to music. *Nature Neuroscience, 14*(2), 257–262.

57. Nilsson, U. (2009). Soothing music can increase oxytocin levels during bed rest after open-heart surgery: A randomized control trial. *Journal of Clinical Nursing, 18*(15), 2153–2161.

58. Whitaker, M. H. (2010). Controlling pain sounds soothing: Music therapy for postoperative pain. *Nursing, 40*(12), 53–54.

59. Levitin, D. J., & Tirovolas, A. K. (2009). Current advances in the cognitive neuroscience of music. *Annals of the New York Academy of Sciences, 1156,* 211–231.

60. Altenmuller, E., Demorest, S. M., Fujioka, T., Halpern, A. R., Hannon, E. E., Loui, P.,...Zatore, R. J. (2012). Introduction to the neurosciences and music IV: Learning and memory. *Annals of the New York Academy of Sciences, 1252,* 1–16.

61. Hunter, P. G., Schellenberg, E. G., & Schimmack, U. (2010). Feelings and perceptions of happiness and sadness induced by music: Similarities, differences, and mixed emotions. *Psychology of Aesthetics, Creativity, and the Arts, 4*(1), 47–56.

62. Jeong, J. W., Diwadkar, V. A., Chugani, C. D., Sinsoongsud, P., Muzik, O.,...Chugani, D. C. (2011). Congruence of happy and sad emotion in music and faces modifies cortical audiovisual activation. *NeuroImage, 54*(4), 2973–2982.

63. Gooding, L., Swezey, S., & Zwischenberger, J. B. (2012). Using music interventions in perioperative care. *Southern Medical Journal, 105*(9), 486–490.

64. Altenmulller, E., Demorest, S. M., Fujioka, T., Halpern, A. R., Hannon, E. E., Loui, P.,...Zatorre, R. J. (2012). Introduction to the neurosciences and music IV: Learning and memory. *Annals of the New York Academy of Sciences, 1252,* 1–16.

65. Morris, D. L. (2009). Music therapy. In D. M. Dossey & L. Keegan (Eds.), *Holistic nursing: A handbook for practice* (5th ed., pp. 327–346.). Sudbury, MA: Jones and Bartlett.

66. Sand-Jecklin, K., & Emerson, H. (2010). The impact of a live therapeutic music intervention on patients' experience of pain, anxiety, and muscle tension. *Holistic Nursing Practice, 24*(1), 7–15.

67. Murrock, C. J., & Higgins, P. A. (2009). The theory of music, mood and movement to improve health outcomes. *Journal of Advanced Nursing, 65*(10), 2249–2257.

68. Chan, M. F., Wong, Z. Y., Onishi, H., & Thayala, N. V. (2011). Effects of music on depression in older people: A randomized controlled trial. *Journal of Clinical Nursing, 21,* 776–783.

69. Burns, D. (2012). Theoretical rationale for music selection in oncology intervention research: An integrative review. *Journal of Music Therapy, 49*(1), 7–22.

70. Watson, J. (2008). *Nursing: The philosophy and science of caring* (Rev. ed.). Boulder, CO: University Press of Colorado.

71. Watson, J. (2006). Caring theory as an ethical guide to administrative and clinical practices. *Nursing Administration Quarterly, 30*(1), 48–55.

72. Stein, T. R., Olivo, E. L., Grand, S. H., Namerow, P. B., Costa, J., & Oz, M. C. (2010). A pilot study to assess the effects of a guided imagery audiotape intervention on psychological outcomes in patients undergoing coronary artery bypass graft surgery. *Holistic Nursing Practice, 24*(4), 213–222.

73. The Joanna Briggs Institute best practice information sheet: Music as an intervention in hospitals. (March 2011). *Nursing and Health Sciences, 13*(1), 99–102.

74. Robb, S. L., Carpenter, J. S., & Burns, D. S. (2011). Reporting guidelines for music-based interventions. *Journal of Health Psychology, 16*(2), 342–352.

■ STUDY QUESTIONS:

Basic Level

1. Which of the following does the International Organization for Standardization (ISO) principle focus on?
   a. Matching different genres to individuals' preferences.
   b. Matching different genres to individuals' moods.
   c. Creating different genres to individuals' preferences.
   d. Creating different genres to individuals' moods.

2. Which of the following is true about music listening selections?
   a. They should be upbeat and have lyrics.
   b. They should be played for 15 minutes and be classical.
   c. They should be familiar genres and have no lyrics.
   d. They should be played for 30 minutes and be personal selections.

3. While a person is hospitalized, what can listening to music for two or more sessions do?
   a. Increase the family's satisfaction with nursing care.
   b. Decrease patient anxiety.
   c. Decrease patient anxiety and support a patient's pain management.
   d. Be easily integrated into a patient's care plan.

4. Which of the following is true about holistic music therapy delivered in the home?
   a. It can be used to decrease symptoms of depression.
   b. It supports patient- and family-centered care.
   c. It is less effective than group music therapy sessions.
   d. It is more expensive than music therapy provided in the clinical setting.

5. Research has shown that music can be effective in reducing anxiety in patients undergoing a same-day surgical experience. Using music as a caring–healing modality in this context is important for which of the following reasons?
   a. All patients are highly anxious about surgery.
   b. Patients might have to accommodate long waiting times.
   c. It is difficult to lie still while waiting.
   d. Patients cannot drink liquids at this time.

Advanced Level

6. What are two key concepts in developing a deeper human-to-human connection (caring moment) in the nurse–patient interaction?
   a. Caring and presence
   b. Honesty and respect
   c. Consciousness and intentionality
   d. Compassion and trust

7. Mr. L, a patient with epilepsy, has met with his physician to discuss a surgical intervention to manage his epilepsy. As the nurse meeting with the patient to begin his preoperative education, you discover that he is an avid guitar player and occasionally plays with a local band. In a surgical team meeting to develop a patient-centered plan of care for Mr. L, you discover that none of the team is aware of Mr. L's love of music. Which of the following questions should you bring to the team for discussion?
   a. How does music affect Mr. L's epilepsy?
   b. Is there evidence that the planned surgical procedure might affect Mr. L's perception of music?
   c. Should tests on music perceptions be included in Mr. L's neuropsychological workup?
   d. Should the team ask Mr. L to play for their next Christmas party?

8. As the nurse was assessing his patient, the patient shared her history with playing the clarinet in high school and her love of singing in the car. Which of the following approaches should the nurse use to conduct a holistic assessment?

   a. "I see music is important to you. Tell me more. What specific music do you like?"

   b. "I also love to sing in the car. Are you still playing the clarinet?"

   c. "Thank you for sharing. Any other musical experiences you would like to share?"

   d. "I also played an instrument in high school. Were you in the marching band as well?"

9. The quality nurse is conducting a chart review to assess the effectiveness of a new music program for patients. What data would be the best measure of music as a caring–healing modality?

   a. The type of music selected by the patient.

   b. A patient's subjective report of his response to the music.

   c. Length of time that the patient listened to music without interruptions.

   d. The number of times patients listened to their musical selections.

10. Research has shown that music therapy interventions demonstrate more effectiveness than music delivered by a health provider. The nurse can accomplish effective music listening with patients by taking which of the following steps?

    a. Sharing the nurse's music memories and dialoguing with the patient.

    b. Establishing a concrete genre of music and discussing the patient's experiences.

    c. Establishing an individualized music listening plan and having direct interaction with the patient.

    d. Sharing the patient's music memories and providing quiet music listening sessions.

Chapter 20

Touch and Hand-Mediated Therapies

Karen Avino

Original Authors: Christina Bergh Jackson
and Corinne Latini

■ DEFINITIONS

Acupressure (shiatsu) The application of finger and/or thumb pressure to specific sites along the body's energy meridians for the purpose of relieving tension, reestablishing the flow of energy along the meridian lines, and restoring balance to the human energy system.

Body therapy and/or touch therapy The broad range of techniques that a practitioner uses in which the hands are on or near the body to assist the recipient toward optimal function.

Centering A calm and focused sense of self-relatedness that can be thought of as a place of inner being, a place of quietude within oneself where one feels integrated and focused.

Chakra or energy center Specific center of consciousness in the human energy system that allows for the inflow and directing of energy from outside, as well as for outflow from the individual's energy field. There are seven major energy centers in relation to the spine and many minor centers at bone articulations in the palms of the hands and the soles of the feet.

Energy meridian An energy circuit or line of force. Eastern theories describe meridian lines flowing vertically through the body, culminating at points on the feet, hands, and ears.

Foot reflexology The application of pressure to points on the feet thought to correspond to other structures and organs throughout the body. Access to the entire nervous system is accomplished through the proprioceptive network of the feet.

Grounding The process of connecting to the Earth and the Earth's energy field, to calm the mind and focus one's inner flow of energy as a means to enhance healing endeavors.

Healing Touch A specific system of techniques that make use of the human energy system for healing.

Human energy system The entire interactive, dynamic system of human subtle energies, consisting of the energy centers, the multidimensional field, the meridians, and acupuncture points.

Intention The motivation or reason for touching; the direction of one's inner awareness and focus for healing.

M Technique A registered method of gentle, structured touch suitable for the very fragile or actively dying, or when the giver is not trained in massage. Simple to learn, the M Technique is profoundly relaxing to both the giver and receiver. Essential oils are used in specific ways with this technique.

Procedural touch Touch performed to diagnose, monitor, or treat an illness; touch that focuses on the end result of curing the illness or preventing further complications.

Reiki A form of energy healing in which the practitioner uses light touch through a series of hand positions over chakras to channel energy. *Reiki* means "universal life force energy" and is composed of two Japanese words, *rei* meaning universal and *ki* meaning life force.

Therapeutic massage The use of the hands to apply pressure and motion to the recipient's skin and underlying muscle to promote physical and psychological relaxation, improve circulation, relieve sore muscles, and accomplish other therapeutic effects.

Therapeutic touch A specific technique of centering intention while the practitioner moves the hands through a recipient's energy field for the purpose of assessing and treating energy field imbalance.

■ THEORY AND RESEARCH

1. Touch is unique in that we cannot touch another without being touched ourselves.

Touch in Ancient Times

1. Healing through touch is practiced in all cultures and is considered instinctive.
2. The Egyptians used bandages, poultices, touch, and manipulation.
   a. The Pyramids show illustrations of one person holding hands near another, with waves of energy depicted moving from the hands of the healer to the body nearby.
3. The oldest written documentation of the use of body touch to enhance healing comes from Asia.
   a. The *Huang Ti Nei Ching* is a classic work of internal medicine that was written 5,000 years ago.
   b. The *Nei Ching*, a 3,000- to 4,000-year-old Chinese book of health and medicine, records a system of touch based on acupuncture points and energy circuits.
4. The ancient Indian Vedas also described healing massage, as did the Polynesian Lomi practice and the traditions of Native Americans.
5. During the height of classical Greek civilization, Hippocrates wrote of the therapeutic effects and instructions for massage and manipulation.
   a. Hippocrates wrote of the great Aesculapian healing centers, at which many

whole-body therapies included touch for individuals to make the transition to a higher level of functioning.
   b. A significant part of therapy in the healing rites was massage used as a mode for dream work.
6. A Roman historian Plutarch wrote that Julius Caesar was treated for epilepsy by being pinched over his entire body every day.
7. Biblical accounts of the healings performed by Jesus of Nazareth include the use of touch in the form of laying hands on the body.
8. In two New Testament passages (using the new revised standard version [NRSV]), the human energy field is described.
   a. In Mark 5:25–34, a woman who had been bleeding for 12 years touched the back hem of Jesus' garment with an inner sense of knowing that this would heal her. Jesus felt that "power had gone forth from him" and turned around quickly, asking who had touched his clothing.
   b. Luke 6:18–19 tells of a crowd that had come to be healed of their diseases and demons through Jesus' touch, for "power came out from him and healed all of them."
9. Both shamans and traditional practitioners used touch widely until the rise of the Puritan culture during the 1600s, including the shift from primitive healing practices to modern scientific medicine.
   a. Puritan culture equated touch with sex, which was associated with original sin.
10. During the late nineteenth and early twentieth centuries, health care moved away from anything associated with superstition and primitive healing and was directed toward scientific medicine.
   a. All unnecessary touch was discouraged because of the association of touch with primitive healing, and because of the prevailing Puritan ethic.
11. Consequently, touch as a therapeutic intervention remained undeveloped in U.S. health care until research into its benefits began in the 1950s.

Cultural Variations

1. The fact that many cultures, both ancient and modern, have developed some form of touch therapy indicates that rubbing,

pressing, massaging, and holding are natural manifestations of the desire to heal and care for one another.

2. Attitudes toward touch vary among cultures, from necessary to forbidden.
3. The nurse must be aware of personal and cultural views and reactions to touch in addition to particular gender prohibitions within cultures.
4. Philosophic and cultural differences have influenced the development of touch in various areas of the world.
   a. The Eastern worldview is founded on energy, whereas the Western worldview is based on reductionism of matter.
   b. This basic cultural difference has led to the evolution of widely differing approaches to touch.
   c. The Eastern worldview holds that *qi* (or *chi*), also described as energy or vital force, is the center of body function.
   d. A meridian is an energy circuit or line of force that runs vertically through the body.
   e. Magnetic or bioelectrical patterns flow through the microcosm of the body in the same way that magnetic patterns flow through the planet and the universe.
   f. Meridian lines and zones are influenced by pressure placed on points along those lines.
5. Expert practitioners in acupuncture and acupressure purport to send healing energy to the recipient by an energy flow that moves through the body and out through their hands.
6. The Western worldview focuses on the physical effect of cellular changes occurring during touch that influences healing.
   a. For example, massage stimulates the cells and aids in waste discharge, promotes the dilation of the vascular system, and encourages lymphatic drainage.[1]
   b. Swedish and therapeutic massage techniques were developed to produce these physical changes.
7. A blending of Eastern and Western techniques has resulted in an explosion of new and widely practiced modalities.

Modern Concepts of Touch

1. Some studies led to the development of the concept of touch deprivation.
   a. In the 1950s, Harlow documented the significance of touch in normal animal growth and development through caging one group of infant monkeys with a monkey-shaped wire form that served as a surrogate mother and a second group with a soft cloth mother surrogate.[2]
   b. In 1958, a study examining abandoned infants and infants whose mothers were in prison found that infants whom the nurses held and cuddled thrived, whereas those who were left alone became ill and died.[3]
2. One study found significantly accelerated healing rates of the mice and seeds when treated with therapeutic touch by well-known healer Oskar Estebany.[4]
3. In 1973, an enzymologist replicated Grad's study as double-blinded using the enzyme trysin and found significantly increased healing.[5]
4. Both the American Nurses Association and the National League for Nursing endorse the use of biofield and touch therapies.
5. The North American Nursing Diagnosis Association includes the diagnosis *Disturbed Energy Field*, defined as a disruption of energy flow surrounding a person that disrupts harmony of body, mind, and/or spirit.
6. Nurses are using hand-mediated therapies with increasing frequency as they seek ways to help or heal those for whom they care.

Touching Styles

1. The touching process is more than skin-to-skin contact; it involves entering the patient's space, connecting, talking, following nonverbal cues, and eventually touching.
2. There are distinct characteristics that touch is: gestural, impactful, and reciprocal.
3. Practitioners also experience three responses from the touch experience: Emotions, past experiences, and receptivity to healing can emerge.
4. Relaxation of the muscles might be felt and a change in the breathing pattern might be observed.
5. An openness for the healing power of touch is necessary between the practitioner and the patient, which constitutes the "I–Thou relationship."[6]

6. One study found significantly higher compliance rates of antibiotics when general practitioners used touch to emphasize and anchor a particular message with patients, although it was cautioned that touch could be used as a coercive method or to facilitate hierarchical relationships.[7]

Body–Mind Communication

1. Touch is the first sense to develop in the human embryo and the one most vital to survival.
2. Touch can vary from subtle fleeting brush strokes to violent physical attacks.
3. Touch evokes the full range of emotions from hatred to the most intimate love.
4. Figurative references to touch in our daily language such as "That speech really touched me" or "This conversation helped me get in touch with my feelings" attest to its deep importance and value to us.
5. As the largest and most ancient sense organ of the body, the skin enables us to experience and learn about the environment.
6. A piece of skin the size of a quarter contains more than 3 million cells, 12 feet of nerves, 100 sweat glands, 50 nerve endings, and 3 feet of blood vessels.
7. There are estimated to be approximately 50 receptors per 100 square centimeters—a total of 900,000 sensory receptors over the human body.[8]
8. The skin is a giant communication system that brings messages from the external environment to the attention of the internal body-mind-spirit through touch.
9. The geriatric population is often a touch-deprived group.
10. Nurses must take into account social contexts and cultural differences before engaging in efforts to provide touch therapy.
11. Nurses should never assume that a patient will find touch comforting and should always ask before touching and observe the patient's response carefully.
12. To be truly effective, touch must be given authentically by a warm, genuine, caring individual to another who is willing to receive it.
13. A few key questions (e.g., "Would a back massage help you relax?" or "Would it help if I held your hand?") can help the patient clarify his or her own beliefs, values, and desires regarding different types, locations, and intensities of touch.
14. Holding hands with patients who have dementia to advanced stages of Alzheimer's disease[9] has been noted as a form of communication by volunteers in a nursing home.
15. Touch therapies are used to advocate and teach healthy lifestyle behavior patterns to patients to augment well-being during the course of the touch therapy treatments.
16. Guided imagery and/or music before and during treatment can heighten the relaxation response elicited during touch therapies.

Overview of Selected Touch Interventions and Techniques

1. Touch therapies can be classified into several categories: somatic and musculoskeletal therapies; Eastern, meridian-based, and point therapies; energy-based therapies; emotional bodywork; manipulative therapies; and other holistic touch therapies.
2. Except for therapeutic touch, Healing Touch, and Reiki, most body therapies involve actual physical contact.
3. The contact usually consists of the practitioner's touching, pushing, kneading, or rubbing the recipient's skin and the underlying fascia.
4. Each of the therapies has an explanatory theory, body of knowledge, history, and techniques.
5. Some methods require special licensure or certification, and others can be incorporated into a nurse's practice after minimal instruction through audiovisual media, conference, or classroom presentation.

Somatic and Musculoskeletal Therapies

1. Somatic and musculoskeletal therapies encompass therapeutic massage.
2. As a nursing intervention, therapeutic massage is effective in stimulating circulation of blood and lymph, dispersing nutrients, removing metabolic wastes, and enhancing relaxation.
   a. Several basic strokes are involved, including long smooth strokes (i.e., effleurage), kneading motions (i.e., petrissage),

vibration, compression, and tapping (i.e., tapotement).

3. Therapeutic massage has also been referred to as "soft massage" and has been associated with helping the recipient reestablish balance and as a means to draw attention away from suffering.[10]

4. Nurses have performed therapeutic massage primarily on the backs and sometimes on the hands and feet of their patients.

5. Back care has been incorporated into the standard bathing and evening care routine of most hospitals.

6. Massage licensure laws vary from state to state; some states require that even registered nurses take an additional course to become certified prior to practicing massage therapy.

7. Massage for the hands, feet, or neck and shoulders can have beneficial results in short time periods.

8. One study found massage therapy can be a beneficial tool for reducing psychological stress levels or anxiety in nurses over a 5-week period versus increased anxiety in the control group.[11]

9. Evidence supports the use of somatic and musculoskeletal therapies to enhance mood, cardiac health, immune function, pain relief, and treatment of patients with cancer; relieve chronic lower back pain, cancer pain, and migraine headache; enhance natural killer cell function; and help relieve depression and anxiety.[12]

10. One study found that the type of massage technique, length of session, and degree of pressure affected blood pressure (BP).
    a. Swedish massage was correlated with the greatest reduction in BP, while potentially painful styles of massage such as trigger point therapy and sport massage were associated with elevations in BP.[13]

11. One study in patients with advanced cancer emphasized the effectiveness of massage therapy in palliative care and included improved lymph drainage, increased relaxation, and improved attitude by the recipients toward touch.[14]

12. Women with breast cancer receiving massage therapy while undergoing chemotherapy reported reductions in nausea when compared to the control group.[15]

13. Adults with osteoarthritis of the knee showed significant improvement in the areas of pain, stiffness, range of motion, and physical function domains when compared to the control group.[16]

14. Aromatherapy is frequently used in conjunction with massage through the use of essential oils, scented creams, and fragrant candles.

15. Cancer patients who received aromatherapy massage reported significant improvement in clinical depression and/or anxiety when compared with control group participants.[17]

16. A meta-analysis of literature examining potential benefits of massage for children with cystic fibrosis reported that massage made children more comfortable, more relaxed, and able to move more freely.[18]

17. Children receiving massage therapy without antiviral medication had significant improvements in CD4 and CD8 cell counts as well as CD41CD251 cells, and an increase in natural killer cells, particularly in the younger children.[19]

18. Infants in Ecuador received massage therapy and demonstrated statistically significant differences in incidence of diarrhea.[20]

19. Low-birth-weight (LBW) babies who received gentle rubbing, stroking, and passive movements of the limbs massage had better quality of sleep with greater daytime alertness than control group infants did.[21]

20. In preterm babies, the moderate massage therapy group versus light pressure massage therapy group gained significantly more weight per day with greater relaxation and reduced arousability.[22]

21. The Care Through Touch Institute in San Francisco offers foot, neck, and shoulder massages to the homeless and provides a sense of being cared for that has had a profound effect on many of their lives.[23]

Eastern, Meridian-Based, and Point Therapies

1. The category of Eastern, meridian-based, and point therapies includes understanding meridians, pressure points, reflex points, imbalances in the energy system, and Eastern healing philosophy.

2. New programs and modalities are being created regularly in this rapidly growing field of energy-based interventions.

3. Several instruments have been used to measure the human energy field, including Kirlian photography and the superconducting quantum interference device.

4. Some of the studied healing methods used by nurses include therapeutic touch, Healing Touch, Reiki, acupressure, and reflexology.

5. Energetic touch therapies typically involve four phases:
   a. Centering oneself physically and psychologically.
   b. Exercising the natural sensitivity of the hand to assess the energy field and/or chakras of the patient for clues to understand the quality and balance of energy flow.
   c. Use the hands and intention to mobilize areas in the patient's energy field that appear to be nonflowing (e.g., sluggish, congested, or static), smooth and harmonize areas that seem perturbed, or work with balance and flow within chakras and along meridians.
   d. Allow energy flow and exchange to assist the patient to repattern and balance his or her energies.

6. The energetic healing process stops when there are no longer any differences in body symmetry relative to density or temperature variation, or when balance is perceived.

7. Four commonly observed responses are
   a. Flushed skin
   b. Deep sighs
   c. Physical relaxation
   d. Verbalized relaxation

8. Time should be limited when working with the young, the old, and the infirm.

9. Nurses should monitor patients for physical and emotional responses.

10. Healing modalities that use touch to help heal (therapeutic touch [TT], Healing Touch [HT], and Reiki) decrease anxiety, relieve pain, and facilitate the healing process.

11. Nurses can become increasingly involved in the use of energy-based modalities for reducing anxiety and pain, inspiring balance, and bringing the body–mind connection into focus.

12. They can be used in any type of environment, and interest in using these low-tech interventions in high-tech environments such as critical care is growing.[24]

13. Over the past three decades, Krieger, Hover-Kramer, Quinn, and others have documented the importance of therapeutic touch.[25-28]

Therapeutic Touch

1. A study that examined the effects of TT on hemoglobin (Hgb) and hematocrit (Hct) levels in anemic women found that both TT and sham TT groups exhibited significant increases in Hgb and Hct, whereas the control group receiving no treatment had no changes in Hgb or Hct.[29]

2. A descriptive study examined the effects of TT on adult tension headache pain and found that one session of TT was useful in reducing headache pain in all subjects receiving TT.[30]

Healing Touch

1. The Healing Touch Program curriculum is endorsed by the American Nurses Credentialing Center (ANCC) and American Holistic Nurses Association (AHNA) for continuing education credits.

2. A mixed method study assessed the role of HT in modulating chronic neuropathic pain and associated psychological stress after a spinal cord injury and found a reduction in pain, fatigue, and confusion and increased well-being when compared to the control group,[31] although the study was cited by others for lack of concrete measures.[32]

3. A pilot study investigating the effects of HT on patients with dementia found those who received HT were significantly less agitated.[33]

4. A pilot study of children who were diagnosed with acute lymphoblastic leukemia and were pediatric clinic oncology outpatients showed a significant decrease in stress and heart rate variability (HRV) when HT was compared with rest.[34]

Reiki

1. Reiki (*rei* meaning universal and *ki* meaning life force) is an ancient form of healing,

---

more than 3,000 years old, rediscovered in the 1900s in Japan by Dr. Mikao Usui.

2. Research has shown a decrease in pain, alleviation of anxiety, reduction in depression, and improved well-being of the mind, body, and spirit.[35]
3. In one study, Reiki was found to provide relaxation with the effects lasting longer after the second session. Participants also reported decreased back spasms, decreased shoulder and neck pain, and improved sleep patterns.[36]
4. A study found heightened levels of spirituality and greater attention to self-care, healing presence with patients, and increased personal awareness in nurses following Reiki treatments.[37]
5. Medical students showed significant improvements in confidence, practice, feelings and practice of compassion, and sense of personal achievement after learning TT and HT.[38]
6. A pilot study found pain at 24 hours post surgery was significantly less following Reiki treatments, yet was not significantly less at 48 and 72 hours post surgery with use of medication. Anxiety levels were significantly less in the Reiki group.[39]
7. A systematic review of the literature concluded that although many Reiki studies have been done, there are "serious methodological and reporting limitations which preclude a definitive conclusion on its effectiveness."[40]

Energy Field Disturbance

1. The North American Nursing Diagnosis Association (NANDA) defines energy field disturbance as a disruption of the flow of energy surrounding a person's being that results in a dis-harmony of the body, mind, and/or spirit. Defining characteristics include temperature changes (warmth/coolness); visual changes (image/color); disruption of the field (vacant/hold/spike/bulge); movement (wave/spike/tingling/dense/flowing); and sounds (tonewords).[41]

Nursing Intervention Classifications

1. The nursing interventions classification system, which lists therapeutic touch, also

specifies simple massage and touch as means to enhance the effects of these modalities.[42]

Acupressure and Shiatzu (Shiatsu)

1. Acupressure and shiatzu is the 4,000-year-old Eastern medicine system with 12 meridian lines and 657 points as the foundation.
2. *Shiatzu* comes from the Japanese words *shi* (finger) and *atzu* (pressure) and is practiced in Japan.
3. The practitioner applies pressure on these points with the thumbs, fingers, and heel of the hand to release congestion and allow energy to flow.
4. A difference between acupuncture and shiatzu is that the main function of shiatzu is to maintain health and well-being (prevention), rather than to treat imbalance, as often occurs in acupuncture.[43]

Reflexology

1. In the early 1900s, it was noted that application of pressure to certain points on the hands caused anesthesia in other parts of the body.
2. Reflexology theorizes that 10 equal longitudinal zones run the length of the body from the top of the head to the tips of the toes.
3. Pressure on specific areas stimulates the proprioceptive reflexes in the feet, thereby triggering a corresponding release that affects the endocrine, immune, and neuropeptide systems.
4. In a study comparing anxiety levels of oncology patients undergoing chemotherapy, the reflexology recipients reported significantly less anxiety both immediately and 24 hours post intervention.[44]
5. A pilot study indicated that women with severe menopausal symptoms experienced relaxation and enhanced sleep following reflexology treatments.[45]

Deep Tissue Techniques

1. Bodywork aims to affect structure by releasing chronic patterns of muscle tension and held trauma or restriction in connective tissue.
2. Deep finger pressure is used to penetrate through layers of muscle, fascia, and tendons

crossing or following the direction of muscle fibers.

3. Sports massage, myofascial release, somatic neuromuscular integration (i.e., soma), Aston-Patterning, Zentherapy, Rolfing, and Hellerwork are examples of this type of massage.[46]

Emotional Bodywork

1. Emotional bodywork combines psychotherapy and bodywork.
2. Techniques include Lomi, Rosen Method, somatic experiencing, Trager, and psychoenergetic balancing.
3. These methods derive from ancient traditions; others come from established health fields, such as chiropractic care.
4. All touch therapies can trigger memories, physical and emotional release, and catharsis related to the assumption of a body position that triggers state-dependent memory or cellular memory stimulation.[1]
5. Occasionally, individuals who have experienced abuse or trauma will release long-held emotional or physical tension as laughter, tears, uncontrollable twitching, shaking, deep sighs, anger, or a variety of other expressions.
6. Displaying calm acceptance, touching a neutral area of the body, and allowing the patient time to release emotion are all therapeutic responses to this type of occurrence.[47]

Manipulative Therapies

1. Manipulative therapies involve invasive bodywork and require a specific program of education.
2. Manipulative therapies include chiropractic and osteopathy (which involve manipulation of bones, ligaments, and soft tissue areas, including work on the head and dura). A similar, related field of practice is physical therapy.

Other Holistic Therapies and Programs Related to Touch

1. A sampling of bodywork, somatic therapies, and touch-related programs are noted in Table 19-1 in *Holistic Nursing: A Handbook for Practice* (6th edition).

2. Individualized massage and therapy techniques have been developed for those with specific needs such as, chair massage, geriatric massage, prenatal and perinatal massage, and infant massage.

■ HOLISTIC CARING PROCESS

Holistic Assessment

1. In preparing to use touch interventions, the nurse assesses the following parameters:
   a. The patient's perception of his or her body–mind situation.
   b. The patient's potential physical problems that might require referral to a physician for evaluation.
   c. The patient's history of emotional and psychiatric disorders.
      ▪ The nurse must modify the approach with patients who have present or past psychiatric disorders.
      ▪ Touch itself can present a problem, and the deeply relaxed, semihypnotic state that a balanced person finds enjoyable can actually frighten or alarm an unbalanced individual.
   d. The patient's values and cultural beliefs about touch and energy therapies.
   e. The patient's past experience with body therapies.

Identification of Patterns/Challenges/Needs

1. The following patterns/challenges/needs are compatible with the interventions for touch:
   a. Altered circulation
   b. Impairment in skin integrity
   c. Social isolation
   d. Altered spiritual state
   e. Impaired physical mobility
   f. Altered meaningfulness
   g. Altered comfort
   h. Anxiety
   i. Grieving
   j. Fear

Outcome Identification

1. Exhibit 19-1, Nursing Interventions: Touch, in Chapter 19 of *Holistic Nursing: A Handbook for Practice*, guides the nurse in patient

outcomes, nursing prescriptions, and evaluation for the use of touch as a nursing intervention.

Therapeutic Care Plan and Interventions

1. Before the session:
   a. Wash your hands.
   b. Have the patient empty his or her bladder to reduce muscle tension.
   c. Prepare the hospital bed, therapy table, or surface on which you will be working.
   d. Have small pillows, bolsters, or towel rolls available for supporting the head, back, or lower legs.
   e. Control the environment so that the room is warm, dimly lit, and quiet.
   f. Use relaxation and breathing techniques, imagery, or music to elicit the relaxation response.
   g. After you have talked with the patient, spend a few moments to quiet and center yourself, focus on your healing intention, and then begin.
2. At the beginning of the session:
   a. Explain to the patient the steps and ask permission to use touch.
   b. Explain what you are about to do before you actually begin and request feedback on concerns or discomfort.
   c. Position the head comfortably, adjusting the hair of the patient.
   d. For massage, have the patient disrobe to his or her level of comfort.
   e. Uncover only the body area that is being massaged or pressed or covered during energetic treatments.
   f. Typically begin with the patient lying on his or her back.
   g. Encourage the patient to take slow, deep, releasing breaths.
   h. Ensure that the patient will not be exposed during turning.
3. During the session:
   a. Be attuned to the patient's responses to therapy to build trust and achieve optimal relaxation.
   b. Be prepared for an emotional or physical release and provide support as necessary.
   c. Explain what you are about to do before you actually begin and request feedback on concerns or discomfort.

d. Use the patient outcomes that were established before the session and the patient's subjective experience to evaluate the session. (See Exhibit 19-1 and Exhibit 19-2 in *Holistic Nursing: A Handbook for Practice*.)

▌NOTES

1. Fontaine, K. (2010). *Complementary and alternative therapies for nursing practice* (3rd ed.). Upper Saddle River, NJ: Prentice Hall.
2. Harlow, H. (1958). Love in infant monkeys. *Scientific American, 200,* 68–74.
3. Spitz, R. (1965). *The first year of life.* New York, NY: International Universities Press.
4. Grad, B. (1965). Some biological effects of the laying on of hands: A review of experiments with animals and plants. *Journal of the American Society for Psychical Research, 59,* 95–127.
5. Smith, M. J. (1973). Enzymes are activated by the laying on of hands. *Human Dimensions, 3,* 46–48.
6. Leder, D., & Krucoff, M. W. (2008). The touch that heals: The uses and meanings of touch in the clinical encounter. *Journal of Alternative and Complementary Medicine, 14*(3), 321–327.
7. Gueguen, N., & Vion, M. (2009). The effect of a practitioner's touch on a patient's medication compliance. *Psychology, Health, & Medicine, 14*(6), 689–694.
8. Montagu, A., & Matson, F. (1979). *The human connection.* New York, NY: McGraw-Hill.
9. Ellis, J. (2010). The touch that means so much. *Nursing Older People, 22*(8), 10.
10. Beck, I., Runeson, I., & Blomqvist, K. (2009). To find inner peace: Soft massage as an established and integrated part of palliative care. *International Journal of Palliative Care, 15*(11), 541–545.
11. Bost, N. (2006). The effectiveness of a 15-minute weekly massage in reducing physical and psychologic stress in nurses. *Australian Journal of Advanced Nursing, 23*(4), 28–33.
12. Cuellar, N. (2006). *Conversations in complementary and alternative medicine: Insights and perspectives from leading practitioners.* Sudbury, MA: Jones and Bartlett.
13. Cambron, J. A. (2006). Changes in blood pressure after various forms of therapeutic massage: A preliminary study. *Journal of Alternative and Complementary Medicine, 12*(1), 65–70.
14. Smith, M. C., Yamashita, T. E., Bryant, L. L., Hemphill, L., & Kutner, J. S. (2009). Providing massage therapy for people with advanced cancer: What to expect. *Journal of Alternative and Complementary Medicine, 14*(4), 367–371.

15. Billhult, A., Bergbom, I., & Stener-Victorin, E. (2007). Massage relieves nausea in women with breast cancer who are undergoing chemotherapy. *Journal of Alternative and Complementary Medicine, 13*(1), 53–58.

16. Perlman, A. I., Sabina, A., Williams, A. L., Njike, V. Y., & Katz, D. L. (2006). Massage therapy for osteoarthritis of the knee: A randomized controlled trial. *Archives Internal Medicine, 166*(22), 2533–2538.

17. Wilkinson, S. M., Love, S. B., Westcombe, A. M., Gambles, M. A., Burgess, C. C., Cargill, A.,... Ramirez, A. J. (2007). Effectiveness of aromatherapy massage in the management of anxiety and depression in patients with cancer: A multicenter randomized controlled trial. *Journal of Clinical Oncology, 25*(5), 532–539.

18. Huth, M., Zink, K., & Van Horn, N. (2005). The effects of massage therapy in improving outcomes for youth with cystic fibrosis: An evidence review. *Pediatric Nursing, 31*(4), 44–52.

19. Shor-Posner, G., Hernandez-Reif, M., Miguez, M. J., Fletcher, M., Quintero, N., Baez, J.,...Zhang, G. (2006). Impact of a massage therapy clinical trial on immune status in young Dominican children infected with HIV-1. *Journal of Alternative and Complementary Medicine, 12*(6), 511–516.

20. Jump, V., Fargo, J., & Akers, J. (2006). Impact of massage therapy on health outcomes among orphaned infants in Ecuador. *Family and Community Health, 29*(4), 314–319.

21. Kelmanson, A., & Adulas, E. (2005). Massage therapy and sleep behavior in infants born with low birth weight. *Complementary Therapies in Clinical Practice, 12*(3), 200–205.

22. Field, T., Diego, M. A., Hernandez-Reif, M., Deeds, O., & Figuereido, B. et al. (2006). Moderate versus light pressure massage therapy leads to greater weight gain in preterm infants. *Infant Behavior Development, 29*(4), 574–578.

23. Jones, R. (2008, September/October). Touch for homeless patients: San Francisco's Care Through Touch Institute. *Massage & Bodywork,* 71–79.

24. Eschiti, V. S. (2007). Healing Touch: A low-tech intervention in high-tech settings. *Dimensions of Critical Care Nursing, 26*(1), 9–14.

25. Hover-Kramer, D. (2001). *Healing Touch: A guidebook for practitioners* (2nd ed.). Albany, NY: Thomson Delmar Learning.

26. Bruce, D. F., & Krieger, D. (2003). *Miracle touch: A complete guide to hands-on therapies that have the amazing ability to heal.* New York, NY: Three Rivers Press.

27. Krieger, D. (1993). *Accepting your power to heal: The personal practice of therapeutic touch.* Santa Fe, NM: Bear and Co.

28. Quinn, J. F., & Strelkauskas, A. J. (1993). Psychoimmunologic effects of therapeutic touch on practitioners and recently bereaved recipients: A pilot study. *Advances in Nursing Science, 15*(4), 13–26.

29. Movaffaghi, Z., Hasanpoor, M,. Farsi, M., Hooshmand, P, Abrishami, F. (2006). Effects of therapeutic touch on blood hemoglobin and hematocrit level. *Journal of Holistic Nursing, 24*(1), 41–48.

30. MacNeil, M. (2006). Therapeutic touch, pain, and caring: Implications for nursing practice. *International Journal for Human Caring, 10*(1), 40–48.

31. Wardell, D., Wardell, D. W., Rintala, D. H., Duan, Z., Tan, G. (2006). A pilot study of Healing Touch and progressive relaxation for chronic neuropathic pain in persons with spinal cord injury. *Journal of Holistic Nursing, 24*(4), 231–240.

32. Bowman, K. (2006). Commentary on "A Pilot Study of Healing Touch and Progressive Relaxation for Chronic Neuropathic Pain in Persons with Spinal Cord Injury." *Journal of Holistic Nursing, 24*(4), 241–242.

33. Wang, K. (2006). Pilot study to test the effectiveness of Healing Touch on agitation in people with dementia. *Geriatric Nursing, 27*(1), 34–40.

34. Kemper, K. J., Fletcher, N. B., Hamilton, C. A., & McLean, T. W. (2009). Impact of Healing Touch on pediatric oncology outpatients: Pilot study. *Journal of the Society for Integrative Oncology, 7*(1), 12–18.

35. Bourne, L. (2009). The art of Reiki and its uses in general. *Practicing Nursing, 20*(2), 11–14.

36. Richeson, N. E., Spross, J. A., Lutz, K., & Peng, C. (2010). Effects of Reiki on anxiety, depression, pain, and physiological factors in community-dwelling older adults. *Research in Gerontological Nursing, 3*(3), 187–199.

37. Brathovda, A. (2006). Reiki for self-care of nurses and healthcare providers. *Holistic Nursing Practice, 20*(2), 95–101.

38. Kemper, K., Larrimore, D., & Woods, C. (2006). Impact of a medical school elective in cultivating compassion through touch therapies. *Complementary Health Practice Review, 11*(1), 54.

39. Vitale, A., & O'Connor, P. (2006). The effect of Reiki on pain and anxiety in women with abdominal hysterectomies: A quasi-experimental pilot study. *Holistic Nursing Practice, 20*(6), 263–272.

40. vanderVaart, S., Gijsen, V. M., de Wildt, S. N., & Koren, G. (2009). A systematic review of the therapeutic effects of Reiki. *Journal of Alternative and Complementary Medicine, 15*(11), 1157–1169.

41. North American Nursing Diagnosis Association. (1994). *Nursing diagnoses: Definitions and classification 1995–1996.* Philadelphia, PA: Author.

42. Doenges, M. E., Moorhouse, M. F., & Murr, A. C. (2008). *Nursing diagnosis manual: Planning,*

individualizing, and documenting patient care (6th ed.). Philadelphia, PA: F. A. Davis.

43. Micozzi, M. (2006). *Fundamentals of complementary and integrative medicine* (3rd ed.). St. Louis, MO: Saunders Elsevier.

44. Quattrin, R., et al. (2006). Use of reflexology foot massage to reduce anxiety in hospitalized cancer patients in chemotherapy treatment: Methodology and outcomes. *Journal of Nursing Management, 14*, 96–105.

45. Morris, D. (2006). Pilot study using reflexology. *Beginnings, 26*(5), 28–29.

46. Rakel, D., & Faass, N. (2006). *Complementary medicine in clinical practice.* Sudbury, MA: Jones and Bartlett.

47. Hover-Kramer, D., & Shames, K. H. (1997). *Energetic approaches to emotional healing.* Albany, NY: Delmar.

■ STUDY QUESTIONS

Basic Level

1. The nurse intends to provide an energetic touch therapy session. Which is not a common phrase associated with energy therapies?
   a. Centering
   b. Using the hand to assess and balance the energy field
   c. Assisting the patient to repattern energies
   d. Directing the outcomes of the session

2. In determining whether touch is appropriate for a particular patient, which is most important to consider?
   a. Personal, gender, and cultural views
   b. Temperature of the environment
   c. Availability of table for use
   d. If there is a doctor's order on the chart

3. Which of the following statements is most accurate about touch?
   a. Nurses must be certified to provide touch therapies.
   b. All touch therapies can trigger memories and physical and emotional release.
   c. Touch therapies are not provided in the hospital.
   d. Relaxation in not an outcome of touch.

4. In an energy healing session, when does the nurse stop treatment?
   a. The energy is pulling her toward the body.
   b. An assessment reveals that the energy field is balanced.
   c. An emotional response occurs from the patient.
   d. The nurse experiences a vision about the patient.

5. Which of the following choices describes how NANDA defines an energy field disturbance?
   a. Blockage of the meridians, causing disease.
   b. Disregulation of the environmental airwaves.
   c. Disruption of flow, causing disharmony of body, mind, and/or spirit.
   d. Irregular flow of energy in the universe.

Advanced Level

6. The patient is unable to fall sleep because of anxiety about the following day's surgery. In this situation, what does the nurse consider?
   a. Touch therapy is one effective way to reduce anxiety.
   b. She should call the physician to get an order for sleeping medication.
   c. This is a normal response to surgery that will go away.
   d. The nurse can help the patient sleep by turning off the lights and closing the door.

7. Which of the following statements is most accurate?
   a. Nurses touch all patients frequently.
   b. Less-mobile patients respond less positively to touch.
   c. Poverty of touch is acute among elderly persons.
   d. It is commonly known that touch can be used as a comfort measure.

8. What are therapeutic massage techniques involving the use of effleurage, petrissage, and tapotement designed to do?
   a. Enhance circulation of blood and lymph.
   b. Apply deep pressure to the muscles.
   c. Increase heart rate and blood pressure.
   d. Provide energy and stimulate the patient.

9. A nurse working in a long-term care facility is considering activities to do with the volunteers and patients. Based on research, which of the following is true?
   a. Touching can decrease mobility in patients.
   b. Holding hands increases communication for dementia and Alzheimer's disease patients.
   c. Touch in dementia patients can cause agitation.
   d. Touch can impair communication.

10. Which is not a response to therapeutic touch?
    a. Flushed skin
    b. Deep sighs
    c. Increased respirations
    d. Verbalized relaxation

Chapter 21

Relationships

Mary Helming

■ DEFINITIONS

Archetype Name given by Jung and Arrien to specific patterns of human collective awareness that symbolically represent human potentials, such as the Healer, the Warrior, the Mother, or the Wise Person.

Boundaries Artificial separations between people that define the perimeters of the relationship.

Complementary transaction An interaction in which the ego states match (e.g., adult-to-adult communication). Complementary transactions support and strengthen relationships.

Defense patterns Protective mechanisms that justify individual action while detracting from relationship building.

Emotional intelligence Awareness and attention to personal emotional needs that allow individuals to be in a position of equality with others, rather than seeking power and control or becoming overly passive.

Forgiveness A willingness to acknowledge one's own mistakes and shortcomings and to allow others room to acknowledge their shortcomings as well.

■ THEORY AND RESEARCH

1. Relationship: Refers to kinship, passionate attachment, or a connection between those having relations or dealings. A relationship refers to two or more persons or things working together, belonging together, or being part of a whole, as in relatives within a family.

2. Interconnectedness: Implies that people can share the "universal reciprocity of love and responsibility" without regard to their culture, politics, or religion, according to Keegan and Drick.[1]

■ RELATIONSHIP THEORIES

1. The Theory of Human Relatedness (Hagerty and Patusky): People are "relational beings who experience some degree of involvement with external referents, including people, objects, groups, and natural environments."[2,p.440]

2. Four stages of human relatedness:
   a. *Connection* means there is active involvement with another, associated with enhanced comfort and wellness.
   b. *Disconnection* involves lack of involvement and is associated with lack of wellness and distress.
   c. *Parallelism* implies disengagement, or the lack of involvement with others. This can have a positive effect of creating solitude with associated physical and psychological replenishment.
   d. *Enmeshment* often describes negative, overinvolved relationships, fraught with anxiety, distress, and functional disability.

3. Four social competencies vital for relationships:
   a. Sense of belonging means there is an appropriate "fit" with the environment, group, or individual. There is a sense of being valued and needed in the relationship.
   b. Reciprocity is a positive aspect of relationship in which there is a perceived equal exchange between parties.

c. Mutuality represents how people tend to join with those they believe share similarities to them, or with whom they share an acceptance of differences.

d. Synchrony is a person's perception of congruent feelings or behaviors with another with whom the individual shares a relationship.

4. Existence of a subtle web of life that connects all human beings, their environment, and spirituality. Each person's actions can directly and indirectly affect others and can create a healing or toxic response or energy.

5. Koloroutis (2004) in *Relationship-Based Care: A Model for Transforming Practice*,[3] shows seven values that include relationship relevant to holistic nurses:

a. The meaning and essence of care are experienced in the moment when one human being connects with another.

b. Feeling connected to one another creates harmony and healing; feeling isolated destroys spirit.

c. The relationship between patients and their families and members of the clinical team belongs at the heart of care delivery.

d. Care providers' knowledge of self and self-care is a fundamental requirement for high-quality care and healthy interpersonal relationships.

e. Healthy relationships among members of the healthcare team lead to the delivery of high-quality care and result in high patient, physician, and staff satisfaction.

f. The value of relationship in patient care must be understood, valued, and agreed to by all members of the healthcare organization.

g. A therapeutic relationship between a patient's family and a professional nurse is essential to high-quality patient care.

▪ THERAPEUTIC RELATIONSHIPS IN HOLISTIC NURSING

1. Definition: A therapeutic relationship is a professional alliance between the nurse and the client or patient, who work together for a defined period of time to accomplish specific health-related goals.

2. Being therapeutic: Using oneself as an agent of healing in the dynamic relationship between provider and patient or client

3. Nine primary components explain the therapeutic relationship:

a. Demonstrating respect

b. Being genuine

c. Being there/being available

d. Accepting individuality

e. Having self-awareness

f. Maintaining boundaries

g. Demonstrating understanding and empathy

h. Providing support

i. Promoting equality[4]

4. Important areas for therapeutic relationships in nursing: Palliative care; critical care; public health; psychotherapy

5. Healing relationship: The act of relating to another human being within a healing environment.

a. Nightingale characterized the healing relationship as that which puts the patient in the best position for Nature to act on him or her. She spoke of the healing nurse–patient relationship.

b. Dossey describes Nightingale as a mystic, visionary, and healer.[5]

c. The greatest healing can occur when patients and clients can place their trust in the abilities of other healthcare professionals.

d. Holistic nurses can create healing relationships by a return to the ideals of patient-centered care.

6. Patient-centered care: Holistic nurses create healing relationships that provide dignity and respect; honor patient and family choices; incorporate cultural background, values, and beliefs of the patient/family into health care; and encourage patients and families to participate in decision making about their healthcare needs.

▪ PSYCHOLOGISTS: THEORY AND APPLICATIONS

Selected psychological theorists whose work encourages the use of the therapeutic relationship

1. Pavlov: Behavioral psychology, with the belief that most human actions are conditioned behaviors.

2. Freud: Psychoanalytical psychology, which looks at the subconscious as the key motivator for human behavior,

3. Humanistic psychology: Concept that caring, trust, and understanding of human complexity are key; human beings are not just controlled by subconscious forces or their environments, but are people of free will who maintain the ability to reach for their highest potential. Key concepts of humanistic psychology include self-actualization, creativity, intrinsic nature, individuality, becoming, and meaningfulness.[6]

4. Positive psychology: Developed based on human psychology.

5. Transactional analysis (TA): Eric Berne: Three ego states, people move among states; unconscious games played between people might be a substitute for true intimacy. Three ego states are Adult (rational, objective), Parent (authoritative figure), and Child (playful, curious, stubborn). All human beings need social interaction, even if it is negative interaction. Book: *Games People Play: The Psychology of Human Relationships* (1964)

6. Erik Erikson: Tasks of each age group must be completed; youth often develop identity crises in their 20s after completing higher education. Book: *Identity, Youth, and Crisis* (1968)
   a. Eight psychosocial stages of life; psychoanalytic approach:
      - Trust vs. mistrust (infancy)
      - Autonomy vs. shame (early childhood)
      - Initiative vs. doubt (preschool)
      - Competence vs. incompetence (elementary school)
      - Identity vs. role confusion (middle/high school)
      - Intimacy vs. isolation (college)
      - Generativity vs. stagnation (adult)
      - Ego integrity vs. ego despair (older age)

7. Carl Jung: Freudian psychoanalytic psychology. Concepts: Collective unconscious as the inherited human unconscious composed of universal mental images and thoughts, which are archetypes. Book: *Development of Personality* (1981)
   a. Archetypes: Concepts of personality expressed in myths and fairy tales; people fit into these roles interchangeably.
   b. Mother archetype: Most important, role of nurse, Mother of God, grandmothers, church, Earth, and Nature.
   c. Crone archetype: The wise old woman who is a visionary, who at the crossroads of life chooses the path of the soul rather than the ego, and she speaks the truth always.

8. Angeles Arrien: Transpersonal psychology; views life holistically. Concepts: Evolved Jungian archetypes, four primary archetypes identified. Book: *The Four-Fold Way* (1993)
   a. Healer archetype: Holistic nursing professionals manifest this archetype by relating to others compassionately and with love, bringing caring to human relationships, viewing others in a positive light, and bringing emotional comfort.
   b. Teacher archetype: Represents the mental quality in relationships, helping learners to achieve new knowledge, wisdom, and insight. Holistic nurses often exhibit the teacher quality.
   c. Warrior archetype: Symbolizes physical qualities of relationship building, uses courage to help improve behaviors of self and others, is firm, and uses knowledge, especially facts, effectively. Holistic nurses are very interested in helping patients improve their health and wellness behaviors and can use facts and their knowledge very effectively in this endeavor.
   d. Visionary archetype: Symbolizes the spiritual aspect of relationship. The Visionary is nonjudgmental and assists in conflict resolution and exemplifies sound intuitive knowing to assist others in achieving their highest good. Holistic nurses need to focus on the spiritual aspect of relationship, which tends to move others toward their highest potential.

9. Isabel Briggs Myers: Concept: Jungian based. Myers-Briggs Type Indicator (MBTI) test widely used to identify personality types. Basis of much psychometric testing; often used to gauge appropriate career choices for individuals, to describe marriage compatibility, and for personal development. Sensing type, feeling type, intuiting type, feeling type, extravert, introvert, judgment, perception personality types.

10. Abraham Maslow: Father of human psychology. Concept: Hierarchy of needs. People move from lowest physiologic needs

(food, water, oxygen) to safety and security, to love and belonging, to esteem and respect, to the highest level, self-actualization (need to do and be the person one is meant to be). Book: *Toward a Psychology of Being* (1968)

11. Carl Rogers: Humanistic psychologist. Concept: Patient-centered or client-centered therapy; some people have experienced being in open, trusting dialogue with another, without being judged, and having felt a sense of healing from this relationship. Based on Buber's I–Thou philosophy of treating the other as a person, not object.

12. Carl Rogers: Rogerian therapy: Preferable to listen to what clients were saying, rather than trying to "fix" them. Therapist does not need to remain detached and objective; could respond emotionally to the client. Book: *On Becoming a Person: A Therapist's View of Psychotherapy* (1995)

13. Daniel Goleman: Concept: Began new movement looking at significance of emotional versus intellectual intelligence. Qualities such as optimism, empathy toward others, resilience (the ability to recover from adversity), and ability to adapt to change are considered part of emotional intelligence. Also conscientiousness, goal orientation with delayed gratification to achieve goals, awareness of one's own shortcomings, confidence in being able to handle most problems, having ability to interact well with others, be cooperative, and manage close personal relationships. Book: *Emotional Intelligence* (1995)

14. Martin Seligman: Father of Positive Psychology. The study of emotions that are positive; traits that are positive, including virtues, intelligence, strength, and athleticism. Concepts: Positive emotions such as trust, hope, and confidence help us most in times of distress. Optimistic people interpret problems as controllable, transient, and limited to one situation. Pessimistic people believe troubles last forever, are uncontrollable, and undermine them. Learned helplessness: Concept that studied human and animal responses to uncontrollable events. Linked to passivity in emotionally stressed and traumatized human beings. Book: *Authentic Happiness: Using the New Positive Psychology to Realize Your Potential for Lasting Fulfillment* (2002)[7]

■ THE NURSE–PATIENT RELATIONSHIP

1. Role of holistic nurse: Assist patients on their *healing journeys*. Create healing relationships using patient-centered care.
2. Holistic nurses utilize *authentic relationships*, which represent true sharing of self and a willingness to be open and genuine.
3. Patient-centered care has been represented as a key means to achieve a healing relationship.
4. Nurse–patient relationship (NPR) is foundational to good nursing care. This relationship is traditionally defined as having three distinct phases: a beginning phase involving the development of trust; a middle phase, which is the active working phase; and the ending phase, in which the relationship might be terminated.
5. Types of nurse–patient relationships (Halldorsdottir):[3]
   a. The biocidic relationship is considered toxic.
   b. The biostatic relationship in considered cold.
   c. The biopassive relationship is considered detached and apathetic.
   d. The ideal relationship is bioactive. The bioactive relationship is described as concerned, kind, and life sustaining, as well as being the classic ideal nurse–patient relationship.
   e. Biogenic relationships are described as loving, full of compassion, fostering of spiritual growth and freedom, and restoring of dignity and well-being. These are high-level interactions and are likely the most supportive of healing.
6. Relationship theories
   a. Barbara Dossey's Theory of Integral Nursing: A grand theory, transcends holistic nursing theory and includes multiple dimensions of interrelationships. Within the theory are four quadrants demonstrating how human beings experience their world through relationships. The "I" quadrant represents the individual; the "We" quadrant demonstrates relationship to others within the context of culture, values, and vision, for example; the "It" quadrant represents the physical body; and the "Its" quadrant represents

relationships to environment and social systems. Further, integral nursing values the patient–practitioner relationship, the community–practitioner relationship, and the practitioner–practitioner relationship. The patient–practitioner relationship is an ideal combination of psychosocial spiritual care along with biotechnological care that favors holistic ideals. The community–practitioner relationship involves working with families, coworkers, companions, community, hospital, and religious organizations within the sphere of the practitioner. The practitioner–practitioner relationship involves collaborative and interdisciplinary work with the goal of improving patient care.[8]

b. Nurse theorists Paterson and Zderad describe the importance of person-to-person relationships in their humanistic nursing theory. Believe relating with other persons as presences; presence is the gift of self.[9]

c. Nurse theorist Jean Watson has developed a science of caring over the past three decades, drawing from the work of Florence Nightingale and Martha Rogers, and this science is said to be the hallmark of nursing practice. One of the major concepts of Caring Science is that it is *transpersonal*, defined as a subjective human-to-human relationship in which the nurse affects and is affected by the person of the other. Both are fully present in the moment and feel a union with the other, and thus share a phenomenal field that becomes part of the life history of both. The Ten Caritas Processes affiliated with Caring Science describe values in the ideal nurse–patient relationship and transcend to describe other life relationship ideals.[10]

d. Erickson, Swain, and Tomlin use the work of Maslow, Erikson, Piaget, Selye (Adaptation Response), Seligman (Positive Psychology), and Bowlby (Attachment Theory) to develop their theory titled Modeling and Role-Modeling.[11] This theory posits that the nurse-client relationship is the essence of nursing and that it should be interactive and interpersonal. Concepts integral to

Modeling and Role Modeling include assisting patients to adapt to adversity and maintain their biopsychosocial functioning, as well as promoting self-care among nurses. Five significant goals of nursing interventions include creating trust, assisting the client to maintain control, encouraging a positive orientation, promoting client strength, and assisting the client to set goals as well as promoting needs such as love, belonging, self-esteem, safety, and biophysical wellness.

■ RELATIONSHIP TO OTHER LIVING BEINGS

1. Relationships with animals are as important as relationships with other people, providing love, affection, companionship, and fidelity in an unconditional manner.
2. Animal-assisted therapy has shown remarkable health benefits in such areas as palliative care, geriatrics, Alzheimer's units, pediatrics, physical therapy, and correctional facilities. Animal-assisted therapy can help patients with psychological disorders, multiple sclerosis, spinal cord injuries, developmental disabilities, post myocardial infarction, and veterans with post-traumatic stress disorder.
3. Relationship to Nature is yet another means to interact with living things. Demonstrates relationship to living plants, living waters, and living ecosystems.
4. Embrace altruistic values and practice loving kindness with self and others.

■ SPIRITUALITY AND RELATIONSHIP TO A HIGHER POWER

1. Physician Herbert Benson: Human beings are "wired" for God.[12] Implies no human being can achieve true happiness without a relationship with a Higher Power or Source
2. Maslow's hierarchy of needs suggests those moving closer to self-actualization move closer in their search for the Source.
3. Burkhardt and Nagai-Jacobson: Prayer is considered the most fundamental and primordial language human beings use; simple conversation with God forms increasingly intimate relationships with the Divine.[13]

4. Helming: Describes lived experience of being healed through prayer.[14] Sixteen of 20 participants who attributed most of their healing to prayer, even if they utilized allopathic and integrative modalities, described the essence of this healing as *spiritually transformative.*

5. Some religions assist people to find spirituality in themselves; through other inspirational readings; through Nature, art, and music; and through silent times spent in meditation or contemplative prayer. Some feel that people never reach their potential without having a right relationship with the Divine. Some people believe that "Higher Power" does not need to be God but can be Nature or a sense of spirituality outside of oneself, a power larger than oneself.

■ QUALITIES THAT ENHANCE RELATIONSHIPS

1. Concepts in healthy relationships
   a. Trust: Ideal nurse–patient relationship requires the development of trust before patients can open up and engage in active problem resolution. Trust is an essential element of the therapeutic and healing relationship as well.
   b. Trust is "the glue or cement of relationships."
   c. Believers develop an intrinsic trust that God is ever present and caring. The popular phrase "Let go and let God" implies a willingness to trust the Higher Power's direction, assistance, and concern.
   d. Trust in the essential goodness of humankind.
   e. Building trust involves ability to risk being vulnerable, implying risking hurt from others through self-revelation of one's weaknesses as well as one's strengths.

■ ROADBLOCKS TO BUILDING TRUST

1. Excessive hurt in the past, creating fear of being hurt again
2. Being hurt by loved ones
3. A belief that people cannot be trusted
4. A belief that people manipulate others and use them

5. A history of physical, sexual, or emotional abuse or neglect
6. Having been put down repeatedly for one's beliefs or feelings
7. Unresolved grief, leading to fear of opening up to others because of the possibility of abandonment
8. Being the victim of a hostile or violent relationship, or of an acrimonious divorce
9. Being raised in an unpredictable and often volatile environment
10. Having such low self-esteem that one believes he or she is not worthy of trust or love
11. A fear that being vulnerable (opening up and revealing one's true self) is dangerous and can be used against you[15]

■ FORGIVENESS

1. Forgiveness: A significant hallmark of a healing relationship is forgiveness. To be empowered to forgive, it is necessary to release the anger and struggle that is part of resentment. Dincalci believes that forgiveness is transformative.[16]
2. Forgiveness therapy: Some clients who learn to forgive encounter a religious experience, develop a deeper understanding of life, and discover that all of their relationships tend to improve and are less subject to turmoil.

■ RELATIONSHIPS CONCEPTS

1. The patient–provider relationship: Assumes that the provider has power because the patient is seeking help from him or her. This is an asymmetrical relationship. The nurse or therapist is not intended to remain totally neutral, and emotion can be expressed, but neither the nurse or therapist should reveal significant personal information to the patient. This is a healthy boundary issue, with attempts to keep the relationship objective and helpful.
2. Therapeutic relationships: Relationships between a provider and patient are often considered a dyad of two, but in reality, they are really a triad because the family is always the third aspect of the relationship triangle, even if they are not physically present. Family therapy allows the nurse or therapist to view family interactions, but

this dynamic can be just as visible in a hospital setting or home care visit where the patient is observed interacting with family members in front of the nurse.

3. Boundaries: Boundaries are artificial separations between people that can be either healthy or unhealthy. They define the perimeter of a relationship. In psychotherapeutic work and in the therapeutic nurse–patient relationship, it is vital to recall that the nurse or therapist should have therapeutic neutrality, that he or she should not give directives about major life decisions to the patient or client.

   a. Boundaries can be considered rigid, permeable, or semipermeable. A formal relationship can be seen as more rigid and family relationships as more permeable.

   b. Nurses are constantly faced with boundary issues. In hospital and home situations, nurses see very personal sides of their patients and their families. Nurses must maintain professional boundaries, not revealing too much personal information, and keeping safety always in mind.

   c. Signs of ignored boundaries include the following:

      ▪ Disassociation: "Blanking out" during a stressful circumstance keeps a person out of touch with his or her feelings and can impair memories of the circumstance.

      ▪ Excessive detachment: People in families or groups operate too independently and there are no common goals or identities. The union is not healthy.

      ▪ Chip on the shoulder: As a result of anger over past emotional or physical violations or one's rights being ignored, the person creates distance.

      ▪ Over-enmeshment: Everyone must follow the same rules and think the same way; uniqueness is not permitted.

      ▪ Martyrdom or victim state: Victims isolate themselves defensively to avoid further hurt or allow themselves to continue to be victimized by others in the martyr state.

      ▪ Distant and cold: Barriers are set up to prevent others from entering one's

emotional or physical space. These are usually related to avoidance of past hurt or rejection.[17]

■ DISORDERS IN RELATIONSHIPS

1. Defense mechanisms: According to Freud, defense mechanisms are thought processes that protect the ego and help us to deal with stress. Nurses frequently encounter the six most commonly used defense mechanisms. Defense mechanisms can interfere with healthy relationships. They can create distance from the truth and block honest dialogue.[18]

   a. Denial is used to distance oneself from a perceived threat. It often appears that the person in denial is ignoring or denying reality. This mechanism can be helpful, as in the case of a family who gives a loved one the gift of a good death by laughing with the dying person and living life as fully as possible despite the knowledge that this loved one will likely not live for much longer. It can be harmful, as in the case of an addicted person who does not address his or her addiction.

   b. Rationalization is a process of filtering or reframing reality to make that reality more acceptable. It can involve not taking full responsibility for one's actions, and it can sometimes lessen the emotional impact of one's circumstances.

   c. Projection is used when one does not want to take responsibility for one's own thoughts and feelings. With this mechanism one ascribes one's own intentions, feelings, or motives to another person and does not take ownership of the thoughts or feelings.

   d. Displacement involves transferring unpleasant emotional pain from the direct source of the pain to another, less threatening person or thing.

   e. Repression is the unconscious denial of painful thoughts or feelings.

   f. Humor is frequently used to share otherwise unpleasant, unacceptable, or unwelcome thoughts and feelings. Laughter can provide physiologic benefit and assist in coping with difficult circumstances.

2. Anger: Anger is a transient but forceful emotion arising out of a threat. It can be expressed openly, or it might be suppressed quietly and persist as chronic resentment. Resentment is the long-term persistence of the pain of anger, long after the initial situation that sparked the anger has subsided. Anger can serve the following functions:
   a. It can give a sense of power, strength, and pride.
   b. It can be a motivator of change, but it generates fear and opposition as well.
   c. It can control others by manipulating them or making them feel guilty.
   d. It can keep others away so that the angry person feels less vulnerable and safer.
   e. It can be used as a defense mechanism to avoid communicating about painful or difficult topics, including the situation that caused the anger.
   f. It can keep a person in the role of victim, and there is sometimes secondary gain to feeling the victim or the martyr.[19]
3. Passive-aggressive: People remain passive and quiet externally, but they are repressing anger internally. The anger seeps out in small ways, such as going behind another's back to gossip about him or her in a spiteful way, while remaining superficially pleasant to the other.
   a. Helping patients to comprehend their anger, particularly when it is repressed, and assisting them to move toward forgiveness are essential aspects of the therapeutic nurse–patient relationship.
4. Power and control issues
   a. Dominant personality patterns can cause relationship conflicts. Controlling people tend to assert themselves over others and exert power over them. Although there are people who are willing to be subservient to controlling personalities, others reject this and power battles ensue.
   b. Obsessive-compulsive personality disorder tends toward highly controlling, rigid, and perfectionist behavior. They often fail to allow others to participate in projects or discussions, feeling that their way is the only right way. There is a preoccupation with inflexible rules, details, and lists.
5. Attachment disorders and inability to form relationships
   a. Reactive attachment disorder (RAD) is essentially a form of early post-traumatic stress disorder. The *DSM-IV* essentially defines two subtypes of RAD:
   b. Inhibited RAD: Children fail to initiate or respond to social relationships as appropriate for their age. Theoretically, the etiology of this abnormal attachment is the loss of the primary attachment figure and the inability of the child (usually the infant) to attach to a new primary caregiver.
      - Typical signs and symptoms of inhibited RAD include failure to thrive; blank expression; lifeless eyes; avoidance of eye contact; avoidance of closeness, hugs, and touch of others; lack of awareness of body language; lack of focus; and lack of ability to note others' facial expressions.
   c. Disinhibited RAD: The child is indiscriminate in relationships, overly familiar with strangers, and has diffuse attachments, rather than a primary attachment figure.
      - Typical signs and symptoms of disinhibited RAD include overfriendly approaches to strangers without normal stranger anxiety, hugging people who approach them, and asking strangers to give them food, toys, or comfort. This child is typically exposed to multiple caregivers simultaneously, and there is no ability to develop trust in just one person.[20]

■ HEALING THE HEALER

1. Carl Jung first wrote about the concept of the *wounded healer*.[21] The concept is that all healers (physicians, nurses, etc.) are "wounded" in some ways in their own life histories, and this wounding enables them to care for their patients in a more collegial fashion than with a supervisory style. Wounded healers might also react negatively to patients, without being aware of their subconscious motivations, for example, when a nurse whose father was an alcoholic cannot tolerate alcoholic patients and displays no empathy toward them.

2. Conti describes two types of wounded healers:[22,p.459]
   a. Walking wounded: "An individual who remains physically, emotionally and spiritually bound to past trauma. This wounding can be reflected in the nursing practice of the individual in many ways. The walking wounded have limited consciousness related to how their pain is manifested in their lives."
   b. Wounded healer: "Through self reflection and spiritual growth, the individual achieves expanded consciousness, through which the trauma is processed, converted and healed."

■ NOTES

1. Keegan, L., & Drick, C. (2011). *End of life: Nursing solutions for death with dignity.* New York, NY: Springer.

2. Hagerty, B. M.,& Patusky, K. L. (2003). Reconceptualizing the nurse–patient relationship. *Journal of Nursing Scholarship, 35,* 145–150.

3. Jackson, C. (2010, July–August). Using loving relationships to transform health care. *Holistic Nursing Practice,* 181–186.

4. Dziopa, F., & Ahern, K. (2009). What makes a quality therapeutic relationship in psychiatric/mental health nursing: A review of the research literature. *Internet Journal of Advanced Nursing Practice, 10*(1), 11–19.

5. Dossey, B. M. (2010). *Florence Nightingale: Mystic, visionary, healer* (Centennial ed.). Springhouse, PA: Springhouse.

6. Association for Humanistic Psychology. (n.d.). Humanistic psychology overview. Retrieved from http://www.ahpweb.org/index.php?option=com_k2&view=item&id=14:history&Itemid=24

7. Butler-Bowdon, T. (2007). *50 psychology classics: Who we are, how we think, what we do.* Boston, MA: Nicholas Brealey.

8. Dossey, B. M. (2013). Nursing: Integral, integrative, and holistic—local to global. In B. M. Dossey & L. Keegan (Eds.), *Holistic nursing: A handbook for practice* (6th ed., pp. 3–55). Burlington, MA: Jones & Bartlett Learning.

9. O'Connor, N. (1993). *Paterson and Zderad: Humanistic nursing theory.* Newbury Park, CA: Sage.

10. Watson, J. (2010). Florence Nightingale and the enduring legacy of transpersonal human caring-healing. *Journal of Holistic Nursing, 28*(1), 107–108.

11. Erickson, H. (2006). *Modeling and Role-Modeling: A view from the client's world.* Austin, TX: Unicorns Unlimited.

12. Benson, H. (1996). *Timeless healing: The power and biology of belief.* New York, NY: Simon and Schuster.

13. Burkhardt, M. A., & Nagai-Jacobson, M. G. (2009). Spirituality and health. In B. M. Dossey & L. Keegan (Eds.), *Holistic nursing: A handbook for practice* (5th ed., pp. 617–645). Sudbury, MA: Jones and Bartlett.

14. Helming, M. (2011). The lived experience of healing through prayer: A qualitative study. *Holistic Nursing Practice, 25*(1), 33–44.

15. Messina, J. J., & Messina, C. M. (n.d.). Building trust. Retrieved from http://jamesjmessina.com/toolsforpersonalgrowth/buildingtrust.html

16. Dinalci, J. (n.d.). Forgiveness transforms!" Retrieved from http://howtoforgivewhenyoucant.com/whyforgive.php

17. Messina, J. J., & Messina, C. G. (n.d.). Establishing healthy boundaries. Retrieved from http://jamesjmessina.com/growingdowninnerchild/healthyboundaries.html

18. Seaward, B. L. (2006). *Managing stress: Principles and strategies for health and well-being.* Sudbury, MA: Jones and Bartlett.

19. Casarjian, R. (1993). *Forgiveness: A bold choice for a peaceful heart.* New York, NY: Bantam.

20. Lubit, R. (n.d.). Child abuse and neglect: Reactive attachment disorder. Retrieved from http://www.emedicine.com/ped/topic2646.htm

21. Daneault, S. (2008). The wounded healer: Can this idea be of use to family physicians? *Canadian Family Physician, 54*(9), 1218–1219.

22. Conti, M. (n.d.). The theory of the nurse as wounded healer: Finding the essence of the therapeutic self. Retrieved from http://www.drconti-online.com/theory.html

■ STUDY QUESTIONS

Basic Level

1. Which of the following answer choices is the best definition of *relationship*?
   a. People can share the reciprocity of love and responsibility without regard to their culture, politics, or religion.
   b. Two or more persons or things working together, belonging together, or being part of a whole, as in relatives within a family
   c. Human-to-human relationship in which the nurse affects and is affected by the person of the other
   d. Using oneself as an agent of healing in the dynamic relationship

2. Which of the following describes the *ideal* nurse–patient relationship?
   a. Biocidic
   b. Biopassive
   c. Biogenic
   d. Bioactive

3. Which of the following is best description of boundaries?
   a. Having therapeutic neutrality and protecting one's privacy
   b. Thought processes that protect the ego
   c. Artificial separations between people that can be either healthy or unhealthy
   d. People in families or groups operating independently without common identities

4. Which of the following qualities exemplifies a good nurse–patient relationship?
   a. Maintaining distance for professionalism
   b. Demonstrating respect and empathy
   c. Doing everything for the patient
   d. Giving hope when the situation is hopeless

5. Which one of the following is a road block to building trust in relationships?
   a. Forgiving everything
   b. A history of physical, sexual, or emotional abuse
   c. A history of being adopted
   d. Having high self-esteem

Advanced Level

6. Which of the following statements about defense mechanisms is true?
   a. *Projection* is a process of filtering or reframing reality to make that reality more acceptable.
   b. *Repression* is the unconscious denial of painful thoughts or feelings.
   c. *Rationalization* is used to distance oneself from a perceived threat.
   d. *Humor* involves transferring unpleasant emotional pain from the direct source of the pain to another, less threatening person or thing.

7. The holistic nurse comprehends which of the following holistic theories correctly?
   a. Dossey's Integral Nursing Theory explains how human beings experience their world through relationships.
   b. Paterson and Zderdad's theory describes how role modeling helps adapt to adversity and maintain biopsychosocial functioning.
   c. Roger's Ten Caritas Processes describe values in the ideal nurse–patient relationship.
   d. Hagerty and Patusky describe three ego states among which people move.

8. Which of the following scenarios represents the Theory of Human Relatedness concept of enmeshment?
   a. Thirty-eight-year-old Joan works from home, lives with two cats, and rarely socializes.
   b. Forty-two-year-old Russ is happily married and active in his children's activities.
   c. Fifty-eight-year-old Irene allows her drug-addict daughter to live at home, not working, while she pays all her daughter's debts because she is afraid of consequences.
   d. Twenty-four-year-old Jacob blames his parents for his ruined relationships with his girlfriends.

9. The holistic nurse who understands that empathy toward others, resilience, and ability to adapt to change are key factors in helping her patients meet the challenges of overcoming illness is using which concept?
   a. Emotional intelligence by Goleman
   b. Hierarchy of needs by Maslow
   c. Importance of listening to patient by Rogers
   d. Feeler personality by Briggs-Myers

10. The psychiatric holistic nurse who uses courage to help improve behaviors of others while being firm and using factual knowledge is exhibiting which archetype?
    a. Crone
    b. Visionary
    c. Warrior
    d. Mother

Chapter 22

Dying in Peace

Deborah Shields and David Shields

Original Authors: Melodie Olson
and Lynn Keegan

■ DEFINITIONS

Culture Socially transmitted ways of life including but not limited to language, arts and sciences, thought, spirituality, social activity, and interaction.[1]

Death A moment in time.

Dying A stage of life that fits into a broader philosophy, giving both death and life meaning.

Grief A response to loss, characterized as dynamic, pervasive, individual, yet normative.

Hospice Hospice supports the patient through the dying process and the surviving family through the dying and bereavement processes. Hospice provides comprehensive medical and supportive services across a variety of settings and is based on the idea that dying is a part of the normal life cycle. Hospice provides care in the home, residential facilities, hospitals, and nursing facilities.

Loss The absence (or anticipated absence) of someone or something of real or symbolic meaning.

Mourning The expression of a sadness or sorrow resulting from a loss.

Myth Story lines created by individuals and cultures about meaning and journeying in life.

Nearing death awareness The dying person's knowledge of death and attempts to describe this experience to healthcare providers, family, and friends.

Palliative care An approach to care that improves quality of life of patients and their families facing life-threatening illnesses through the prevention, assessment, and treatment of pain and other physical, psychological, and spiritual problems.

Perideath The last hours of life, the actual death, and the care of the body after death.

Self-transcendence A spiritual concept referring to moving one's self into a wider sense of consciousness and understanding.[2]

Spirituality "The essence of our being."

■ THEORY AND RESEARCH

1. To die peacefully, to die with the knowledge that life has had meaning and that one is connected through time and space to others, to God, and to the universe, is to die well.
2. Helping people to die well requires knowledge and skill, as well as a willingness to be intensely involved in the most intimate phases of another's life.
3. Physical, spiritual, psychological, and social distress must be addressed with concern and compassion.
4. The nurse, in being present "in the moment" with the patient and family, inevitably confronts her or his own mortality.
5. Care for the caregiver (professional and family) is a requirement, a part of the care of the dying; the patient and the family are the unit of care.
6. Watson's Theory of Caring is one approach to easing the burden for those who are caring for the terminally ill.[3]
   a. The Theory of Human Caring focuses on the relationship between the whole

person of the caregiver (nurse) and the whole self of the client/family as it protects and preserves the humanity and dignity of the client.

b. In this partnership or relationship between caregiver and client and family, the burden becomes shared; each can ease the other's burden.

7. Developing theories to guide end-of-life care are based on standards of care, such as those identified by professional associations, state laws, and culture.

Grief and Loss

1. Grief theory links concepts of loss, bereavement, and mourning into a fabric of ideas that help decide action on the part of caregivers, family members, and patients.

2. Grief is not only normative, but dynamic, pervasive, and individual.

3. Each individual moves through bereavement at a different pace and copes in a different manner, depending on inner resources, support, and relationships.

4. Society might think that the period of mourning has been long enough (a normative statement), but the individual might need more (or less) time before beginning to take charge of a changed life.[4]

5. Grief is a necessary process for both the dying person and his or her significant others; the more bonded and intimate two people have been, the more intense the grief.

6. Grief is pervasive, affecting every area of life—relationships, physical symptoms, feelings, spirituality, and one's sense of meaning in life and schedules of care.

a. The person who is dying integrates care (e.g., regular laboratory tests, visits to the healthcare providers, various therapies) into a full schedule.

b. As death grows closer, visits by family and friends might be welcome; there comes a time when the one who is dying needs time to become introspective, to consider life's messages and meanings.

c. At any of these stages, caregivers can feel excluded from the dying one's life, wanting to be present yet having difficulty "reaching" the loved one.

7. Hope is a basic construct of spirituality and has been recognized as having both physiologic and psychological value.

8. Hope increases as death approaches, but the nature of hope changes. Hope for less pain, for example, is common, when hope for a cure has been abandoned.

9. Families and staff caregivers share in hope as it relates to spirituality and the end of life. The whole team grieves, and the whole team helps each other through the process.[5,6]

10. Spiritual development is related to the phases of grief originally identified by Kübler-Ross.[7]

11. Nursing care during each of the phases takes into account the spiritual maturity of the griever, whether it is the dying person or those who love that person:

a. A person who is in the early stages of spiritual maturity, whether a child or an adult, needs much external help, information, communication, and developing trust. This person might not achieve acceptance (and transcendence) without moving to a higher level of spiritual development.

b. Persons who have a more formal spiritual practice might use rituals, rites, symbols, and activities that incorporate them; thus, they might find comfort in planning their own funeral.

c. Skeptics might build on the comfort found in the formal structures but often add intellectual processes, such as bargaining with medical science (e.g., becoming part of experimental studies), reading books on death and dying, considering their contributions in this life, yet acknowledging a fear of the final moments—fear of pain and loss.

d. Those in the final spiritual stage believe in a common bond uniting humanity, the world, and the universe. They are attracted to the mystery of faith.[8] Therefore, the dying person in this stage might worry more about others, become angry about the effect the disease or the dying has on loved ones, choose humanitarian goals, become introspective and prayerful, and contact family and friends to say goodbye.

12. Nursing care requires assessment of a dying person's spiritual resources to assist with peaceful death.

13. The nurse's own developing spiritual maturity can be a useful support, as when one

accompanies an acquaintance for a while along a road.

14. The nurse maintains an attitude of being open, listening, and assessing the client's path even when his or her own journey changes directions.

15. Successfully dealing with grief allows the dying client to achieve peace and allows the family and significant others to move on with a changed life, cherishing memories while creating new ones.

Self-Transcendence

1. Self-transcendence: The sense of a temporal integration of self, the feeling that past and future enhance the present.

2. Frankl discovered that those who survived in the concentration camps seemed to transcend (beyond self) either toward other people or toward meaning.[9]

3. Transcendence might occur through creativity, the family, or works of art; through receptivity toward others; or through acceptance of a situation that cannot be changed.

4. People who can be identified as self-transcendent at the end of life tend to have less depression, less self-neglect, and less hopelessness:[10]

   a. They have a greater sense of well-being and a greater ability to cope with grief.

   b. The self-transcendent person lives in the present and usually sees death as a normal part of life.

5. Encouraging people to seek meaning and connections, either in the present or through the ages, helps people move toward self-transcendence to achieve peace.

6. Measures to support one's movement toward self-transcendence build on the need to look inward for connectedness and a sense of timelessness.

   a. Life review—the systematic review of one's life to see that it was meaningful, to remember those who are loved, and to know one's own place in history—is one example of a useful process.[11]

   b. Life review is the story of this life, of living in this space on this Earth in this time.

   c. Studies show that systematic life review helps reduce depression and anxiety, and it promotes a feeling of "This was my life, no one else would have done it this way, and I have a unique place in this universe."[12]

Myths and Beliefs

1. Myths are our story lines, values, beliefs, and images; they are our personal manual about the meaning and the journeys of the human spirit.[13]

2. Myths help us seek the unfolding mystery in life. In seeking life's meaning and purpose, personal myths help us manifest hope, learn to accept daily struggles and challenges, and deal with ambiguity and uncertainty.

3. Myths help us recognize strengths, choices, goals, and faith; they also help us to assess our perception of our world, recognize our capacity to pursue personal interests, and demonstrate love of self and self-forgiveness.

4. Myths provide a sense of connection and of oneness with all of life and nature.

5. Throughout life, we create many myths: Some serve us well, while others hinder our healing journey.

6. With healthier lifestyles, most people can add a vital 30 or more years to their life span; there is also more time to practice a new way of living so that dying in peace is a clear choice for each person.

Nearing Death Awareness

1. When people become aware that they are approaching death, they often talk about two things:

   a. They might attempt to describe what they are experiencing while dying.

   b. They might request something that they need for a peaceful death.

2. This awareness is not to be confused with near-death experiences that happen as a result of cardiac arrest, drowning, or trauma in which a person feels the self suddenly leave this life but quickly return.

3. In a state of nearing death awareness, a person's dying is slower, often because of a progressive illness such as acquired immunodeficiency syndrome (AIDS), cancer, or heart or lung disease.

4. The person becomes aware of a dimension that lies beyond, a drifting between

this world and another, perhaps a space of transcendence, yet not one that touches "an Ultimate."

5. The slower dying process allows the dying person to have more time to assess his or her life and to determine what remains to be finished before death.

6. Some dying patients try to describe being in two places at once or somewhere in between.

7. It is a time for a caregiver to respond to the dying person's wishes and needs and to listen to what dying is like for that person.

8. It is at this time that discussions about the patient's wishes about cardiopulmonary resuscitation should be learned if this topic has not been discussed prior to this time.[14]

9. This can be a period of challenge for many caregivers, and yet it can help each of us to prepare for what might happen in our dying.

10. Those individuals who are tired of living but who do not believe that it is time to die describe the dying process differently from those who are truly ready to depart.

   a. Statements of those who are truly ready are different in the clarity with which the words are spoken, the look in their eyes, or their touch; their statements, looks, or touches are like no others that have been made before or during the dying process.

■ HOLISTIC CARING PROCESS

Holistic Assessment

1. In preparing to use interventions for promoting peaceful dying, the nurse assesses both the dying person and the family or significant others in the following areas:

   a. Emotions that might surface during the process:

      ▪ Guilt: Blame of self and others over management of the dying person; distress over inability to decrease pain

      ▪ Anger: Toward God, disease, family or significant others, doctors, or survivors; over inability to fix things physically, emotionally, and spiritually

      ▪ Ability to laugh: The shortest distance between two people; relationship between comedy and tragedy (joy and sadness pathways cannot operate simultaneously)

      ▪ Love: An essential element in living and in dying; a state of self-giving and presence of being a person, where openness and willingness exist for self or another; the network that brings and weaves families and significant others together to work through the dying process and move into total acceptance of death

      ▪ Fear: Often evocation of separateness and aloneness, but can become a path leading deeper into the present moment; useful in that it reveals areas of resistance; return to unconditional love and a sense of equanimity after release of fear

      ▪ Forgiveness: Essential element for inner peace; an exercise in compassion that is both a process and an attitude; not necessarily reconciliation

      ▪ Faith: The larger vision of existence, which is different for each person; helps to harness energy to evoke healing resources and power

      ▪ Hope: Support of patient or family and significant others during death's darkness; an inner moment that perceives lightness when in the midst of darkness and has the potential for leading to deeper love; hope for decreased pain and increased physical and spiritual comfort, for a miracle, for peace of mind, for a remission, for peaceful death transition, and for acceptance of a shorter life than expected or the death of a loved one

   b. The patient's interactions with others and the effect of the patient's emotions on these interactions

   c. Need for education about what will happen and what can be done to help (for both patient and family)

   d. Comfort needs, assessed according to the patient's culture and wishes for: pain control and symptom management, hydration, nutrition, respiratory assistance, movement, touch

   e. Signs of psychiatric illness, under- or overmedication that can interfere with a patient's ability to cope with dying: hallucinations, delusions, depression, denial that interferes with the ability to move toward comfort and peace, excessive anxiety, confusion, agitation, or memory loss (especially in older adults), dementia.

Identification of Patterns/ Challenges/Needs

1. The following patterns/challenges/needs are compatible with dying in peace interventions:
   a. Altered circulation
   b. Altered oxygenation
   c. Altered body systems
   d. Altered communication
   e. Effective communication
   f. Spiritual distress
   g. Spiritual well-being
   h. Ineffective individual or family coping
   i. Self-care deficit
   j. Body image disturbance
   k. Powerlessness
   l. Hopelessness
   m. Pain
   n. Anxiety
   o. Death anxiety
   p. Grieving
   q. Fear

Outcome Identification

1. Guides the development and evaluation of nursing interventions for assisting patients and their families and significant others during the dying process
2. Exhibit 21-1, Nursing Interventions: Dying in Peace, can be found in *Holistic Nursing: A Handbook for Practice* (6th edition).

Therapeutic Care Plan and Interventions

1. Guidelines for the dying person and all of the caregivers, which are helpful in all settings, apply from the first awareness of a coming interaction with a patient and family who are moving through the dying process, through dying, and afterward
2. Before the interaction:
   a. Spend a few moments centering yourself to recognize and honor your presence there. Become a healing presence; be in the present moment with the client/family honoring the dignity and wholeness of all.
   b. Begin the session with intention to facilitate healing and peaceful dying.
3. At the beginning of the interaction:
   a. Encourage the patient and the family and significant others as the caregiver(s) to:
      - Set realistic goals.
      - Identify different behaviors that have surfaced in their interactions with each other during this period.
      - Gather a healing team and honor the patient's personal needs and feelings to avoid more suffering.
      - Accept current circumstances, and release things that are beyond their control.
      - Accept the fact that release might not be possible at this time, but they can work toward it.
      - Take frequent breaks, at least 20 minutes daily, to evoke high-quality quiet time with relaxation, imagery, music, meditation, prayer, journal keeping, or dream work to assist in the process of letting go.
      - Exercise, take long hot baths or showers, eat nutritious foods, eliminate excess caffeine or junk food, and ask other people for relief.
   b. Encourage the patient and caregivers to tell themselves over and over what a good job they are doing and that it is the best job that they can do. Repeating it helps in releasing guilt, anger, and frustration.
4. During the dying process:
   a. Recognize the one who is dying as the person who is usually the best teacher about what is right. The place of death is not as important as the care, trust, compassion, acceptance, and love that was provided and shared in the perideath interactions.
   b. Determine the care needed; include the patient and family in discussing this.
   c. Explore the advantages and disadvantages of dying at home (or alternative sites).
   d. When available, inpatient hospice units can help blend some of the advantages of care in the home with the additional support an individual might need that significant others cannot provide.

e. Integrate therapies as appropriate for the dying person, considering the person's beliefs, motivations, resources.

f. Incorporate the senses in rituals:

- Touching: Lovingly, freely, and joyfully convey through your hands what your heart is feeling. Touching is a powerful way to break the illusion of separateness, loneliness, and fear; it can evoke laughter, calmness, or tears. Create times to give and get hugs and hold hands. Avoid touching if it is not welcome.

- Smelling: Use lotions and colognes with mild fragrances, remembering that illness will probably change the types of fragrances that can be tolerated. Use caution because some odors cause nausea and unpleasant feelings. Try light, natural scents such as rosemary or vanilla, perhaps as a plant growing in the room or a candle in the bathroom.

- Tasting: Remember that taste varies with degrees of illness but stays with us until the end of life. Tasting and eating have social and symbolic meaning to patients and family. Explain what will happen if the patient stops eating within the progression of terminal illness and that it can be normal and might not cause undue suffering. Provide tastes and foods that are desired.

- Seeing: Arrange healing objects and different touchstones that have special meaning and symbolize people, places, and events in the patient's life. A room that receives soft, subdued rays from the sun can bring balance to surroundings. Sitting out on the patio in good weather allows the patient to feel the sun as well as see the sunlight. Light colors are usually more soothing than dark colors.

- Hearing: Remember that the sense of hearing is often sharp to the end of life, so special words at death can be heard. Be present in silence also, sitting or holding one another. Music can be nice, but not all the time.

g. Practice sitting quietly with relaxation, meditation, or prayer. Gentle sounds from wind chimes or environmental recordings of ocean waves, wind, rain, birds, and music can offer a sense of peace.

h. Music thanatology, referred to as sung prayer, uses the human voice when chanting or singing to bring balance to the dying, dissolving fears and lessening the burden, sorrows, and wounds.[15]

i. Use words ending in *ing* such as *releasing, letting, floating, softening* or words ending in *ness* such as *openness, beingness, awareness, vastness* to help the patient to relax.

j. Recognize the patient's going in and out of awareness. The moment of death itself has no pain but is a reflex last breath. It opens up very special exchanges of intention, intimacy, and bonding where the patient can share the dying spaces. The patient's eyes can take on a staring, a glazing, a spaciousness so different that the patient appears to be going to another realm of knowing or to be focusing on something that the caregiver cannot see; the dying person can return with a smile and possibly share that he or she was in a space of peace.

k. Knowing what body changes to expect as death approaches helps the family anticipate personal healing rituals and removes the fear, shock, and mystery from the moment of death.

l. Understand and accept the body's shutting down. The conscious dying person knows that it is time to leave the physical body and can choose to shut down physical life. The caregiver and family journey with the dying person as far as possible, and then tell the person it is all right to leave; this can evoke the purest, most special moments for all involved. For those people who wish to experience every morsel of life, even if that morsel is physical agony, respect the choice. For them, it might be inappropriate to suggest that they leave. Tell them that you love them and will stay with them as long as they need you.

5. At the moment of death:

a. Prepare rituals for the moment of death. The dying person usually has serenity and inner calm, particularly if healing rituals have been carried out prior to death. Before the dying person's eyes close, tight brow muscles can become relaxed; the peace in the face or within the room is often palpable. Trust your inner wisdom for how to touch, hold, talk, and be with the dying one in ways that deepen hope and faith for a peaceful crossing into death and beyond.

b. Surround yourself and the dying person with the peace and the light of love, taking the energy of love and light in with each breath; imagine and experience literally going inside the breath, flowing inside the breath with comeditation into the death of each moment.

c. Continue to communicate with family caregivers and those there to support the dying patient. Talk to the dying loved one as restlessness or agitation moves to unresponsiveness; give gentle love squeezes, touches, and hugs; play favorite music; read poems; or say mantras and prayers. Shut the half-closed eyes, stroke and hug the physical body, and adjust the loved one's head on the pillow for the last time. Give permission for this special person to be free, to soar, to meet God and others who have died before, if this is appropriate. Say all you need to say, and share your own kind of blessings for the smooth transition.

d. If appropriate, when the person has taken a last breath, carry out additional rituals that can be helpful to those present. Holding hands around the bed, saying a blessing or prayer, or anointing with healing oil, for example, can be planned ahead of time for this moment.

e. Schedule a follow-up session or visit with family and significant others, if appropriate. If grief support groups are available, a referral can be helpful.

f. Take care of yourself. Adequate rest, relaxation, exercise, and nutrition are always important; the person who cares for dying people needs to "go apart for a little while." Center, meditate, celebrate, or plan your own self-renewal times.

6. Specific interventions

a. Planning an ideal death: To help patients and families experience peace in the dying process, it is important to engage them in planning; to be of maximum assistance to someone else on the journey toward his or her own death, it is helpful for the nurse to explore this journey as well.

- Reflective discussion provides enormous insight about death myths, beliefs, problem solving, loving, and forgiving; these discussions can illuminate the patients' ideas about how they perceive an ideal death.

- Part of confronting death is deciding how to use medical care and technology; as part of their right to die individuals can decide whether they want medical treatment; what kind of treatment; and under what circumstances to start, continue, or stop treatment.

- A power of attorney for health care records the appointment of someone to make medical decisions for the individual, should that become necessary.

- An individual can record his or her wishes as a living will for four different life situations: (1) mental incompetence, (2) terminal illness, (3) irreversible coma, or (4) persistent vegetative state.

- Recording information about the individual's wishes regarding organ donation is also important.

- Most hospital and hospice organizations have available documents called advance directives. These documents can be changed by the dying person as long as he or she is competent.

- States vary in the legislative details of such documents. Specific information about the details to include in such a document can be found in the office of the state attorney general or by consulting an attorney.

- These wishes often reflect philosophic, personal, religious, and spiritual desires. Individuals should discuss these matters with the family and friends who will function on their behalf should they become incompetent. It is important for those who will be asked to make decisions to understand fully the nature of the request and about the effects of these choices. Those who cannot do what the patient asks of them should have the choice of withdrawing from the decision-making role.

b. Learning forgiveness
- Forgiveness is important because it helps us get on with life.
- Many people are "stuck" in feeling guilt or assigning blame.
- Self-guilt leads to depression, and blaming others leads to anger.
- Both of these conditions steal energy and focus, reduce coping ability, and rob a person of precious time that could be used in establishing a positive relationship and attending to end-of-life goals.
- Dunn compares forgiveness to removing a thorn (the hurt that needs forgiveness) so that healing can commence.[16]
- Many authors have described steps to forgiving self: (1) take responsibility for what we have done; (2) confess the nature of the wrongs to ourselves, another human being, or God;
- (3) atone, or being willing to make amends where possible, as long as we can do this without harm to ourselves or other people;
- (4) ask for forgiveness, if that is possible;
- (5) look to God for help;
- (6) receive or accept forgiveness.
- Steps to forgiving others are as follows: (1) acknowledging that a wrong has occurred; (2) recognizing that we are responsible for what we are holding on to; (3) confessing our story to ourselves, another person, and God; (4) receiving atonement, or considering whether any specific action needs to be taken; (5) looking to God for help; and (6) offering forgiveness.[17,18]
- These steps take time to complete. As the awareness of forgiving self and others is developed, we recognize unconditional love. Because it helps us connect more with our source of joy, not focusing on loss, sadness, or pain, unconditional love helps release us from fear

c. Becoming peaceful

- To learn how to let go of attachments, what is right and wrong, and what is good and bad, commitment and practice.
- Nurses encourage patients to hear their inner voice of judging and to release the judging.
- Nurses encourage patients just to listen, be ready for the next moment of listening, and to be in the present moment.
- Centering, meditation, and contemplative prayer are helpful in learning to listen to the inner self.
- The skill of opening and releasing ordinary fears allows a person to emerge with awareness in the healing moment and to be fully present when assisting another during death.
- Patients who are dying and their caregivers can set aside 20 minutes or more several times a day to practice opening to the moment.
- Breathing, relaxation, imagery, and music scripts are important experiential exercises to help learn the letting-go experience of calming the mind and creating a sense of spaciousness within the body.
- It can be helpful to create a special relaxation and imagery tape as part of a personal ritual to practice releasing and letting go; recording one or several of these scripts, after a 5- to 10-minute relaxation exercise, enables the dying patient and caregivers to use them repeatedly, even when professionals are not present.
- While consciously living, it is possible to experience conscious dying.
- Learning to confront our own death helps us be more present to assist others in facing their death. It reaffirms that we really need to do nothing but be present with another and speak with our hearts in dying time.

d. The pain process
- In 90–99% of cases, pain can be managed; pain medication response patterns should be evaluated at least every 72 hours, as well as after each administration.

- When giving the medication, the nurse reminds the patient that the pain medication is in the body and working.
- Nurses should understand and use the most current pain management strategies and treatments.
- Although the physical body can experience pain, the mind's fear of the pain is often more intense.
- Acute pain has qualities of suddenness and surprise that can evoke anxiety and fear; the best thing to do with this suddenness is to encourage the dying person to breathe rhythmically and soften into the pain to decrease the resistance to the experience.
- Even the worst of pain can be shifted in many ways. For example, shifting the pain experience by calling it sensations rather than pain often reduces discomfort.
- It also helps to encourage the person to make decisions over which he or she has control, such as decisions about medications, treatments, and daily routines.
- When guiding the person in pain, the nurse might suggest allowing pain images and the different felt experiences to emerge. Each person enters pain in a way that opens in the moment, and each person will know how far to go in exploring the pain.
- Common expressions an individual might have about the pain (e.g., pain attacks, it has a grip on me and takes my breath away, it has a loud and deafening pulsation, it is violent and unrelenting) and creates negative images that can interfere with the emergence of healing images.
- These negative images can become positive if the person focuses on the grip of pain being released, a deep belly breath coming forth evenly and effortlessly, or the pulsating sound becoming like the falling of gentle raindrops or snowflakes.
- Different relaxation and imagery exercises help the person practice letting go of the perception of the physical body; this letting-go helps ease both physical pain, such as difficult procedures, and emotional pain, such as conflicts, and allows the person to experience death with peace and dignity.
- With continued gentle exploration of opening and releasing into the pain, the person can begin to experience the pain as floating and diminishing; this is also a way of expanding one's sense of time.
- Another suggestion is to have the patient step aside in the mind and watch the pain to see how it might be changed to release some of the pressure, resistance, and holding on to the pain. Such guidance and presence over time will help the person to stay with a focused attention, opening and softening and expanding into the pain.

e. Blending breaths and comeditation

- The simple release of the breath and the *ah-h-h-h* sound is an ancient ritual for dying into peace.
- Comeditation is based on the principle that respiration evokes a particular state of mind and serves as a direct link to the nervous system. There is a direct correlation between breathing and thinking. At first, the *ah-h-h-h* sound might be like an echoing of words, but staying with the sound allows the release of tension, fears, and pain.
- Following are the steps for comeditation:
  - Position yourself comfortably close to the patient. A session may last 20 to 30 minutes or longer.
  - Suggest to the person that watching the breath is an ancient method of calming the body and the mind. Let the person first begin noticing the rise and fall of his or her abdomen with each breath in and each breath out.
  - Sitting at the person's midsection, focus on the rise and fall of the abdomen with each inhalation and each exhalation. Focus your

attention on the person's lower chest area, and observe closely for the natural flow of the exhalation from the person. With this focused attention, you can begin breathing in unison with the person. At the beginning of the exhalation, begin softly and out loud to make the sound *ah-h-h-h*, matching the respiration of the person.

- ◆ Occasionally, say simple, powerful phrases, such as *peaceful heart* or *releasing into the breath*. The fewer words spoken, however, the more powerful the breath work. If the person should fall asleep, you might wish to sit with the person for a while or sit until he or she awakes.

f. Mantras and prayers
  - A mantra is the repetition of a word or sound, either aloud or silently. The word can be given by another or discovered. It has meaning to the individual. Repetition moves one toward peace.
  - A prayer might be special phrases or repeated words, or it can be a unique and spontaneous communication with God.
  - There is considerable evidence for the effectiveness of at least two forms of prayer: directed (toward a specific goal or outcome) and nondirected (open-ended, nonspecific, non-goal-oriented approach).
  - In one form of contemplative prayer, *Lectio Divina*, one listens for the word of the Divine following a meditative focus on a few words of scripture.[19,20]
  - In centering prayer, individuals seek a place deep inside themselves, where they live in rich harmony and connection with other people and with God and in the place of wisdom.
  - Every faith group has prayers of the faithful that provide comfort and joy in the last moments.
  - Saying mantras and prayers can decrease the number of lonely hours at home, as well as in the hospital, although this is not the main reason for the practice. They serve as an affirmation of a deeper faith.

- In asking the dying person about wishes for prayers or repeated phrases, encourage the selection of phrases that are short, easy to remember, and rhythmic; personal selection of focus words enhances the faith factor.
- It can be helpful to pray for the highest good for the dying one or ourselves rather than for what we want.
- If we are praying for another, we need to hold the person for whom we are praying in our conscious thought, not ourselves. If we are totally focused on the patient, we cause ourselves less grief, frustration, and fear, recognizing that we are not responsible for outcomes.
- The nurse and the patient should agree on what to pray for before the prayer begins, and the nurse must be sensitive to the individual's formal system of belief.

g. Reminiscing and life review
  - A process basic to human existence is reminiscing and recounting past events, either alone or with friends.
  - We spend much of our time talking, thinking, or writing about plans, goals, resources, successes, disappointments, and failures; this is especially true when facing death.
  - A formal life review process can include six to eight sessions, each approximately 45 minutes in length.
  - During each session, the patient tells the story of that phase of life; the first session is primarily an introduction; the last session is a summing up or discussion of the meanings of the story.
  - The patient might feel emotions of all kinds during any session of the life review process, reflecting the emotions that he or she felt during the stage of life being discussed.
  - It is the acknowledgment of emotional content, in part, that facilitates integration.
  - As an individual begins to feel a sense of integration with the past and present, a kind of wholeness to life emerges. Unfinished business becomes finished. This is helpful in achieving peace. [12]

h. Where we die
- The environment in which people die, by choice or not, affects the ability of the person to achieve peace.
- Hospice and palliative care have evolved and helped to change the way and places where people die.
- Nurses seek to continue to look for ways to help people die with dignity and without needless suffering.
- As a culture, we are still debating when to stop life-prolonging interventions when one has reached the definitive time to die; however, even as these discussions continue, when it is time to die, where we die becomes a most important consideration.
- Many people are alone at their time of death. Countless hundreds come to their end in the nursing homes that permeate every state in the nation. And of these hundreds, many are alone without living or able-bodied family members.
- Still others face death at home, many hopefully with hospice care nearby.
- Unfortunately, many more are surrounded by machines and invaded with tubes in ICU.[21] Interventions to help them last a few more hours or a day are still in force, and thus they die wrapped in technology and seldom in the arms of caring people.[22]
- The Golden Room is a place that offers a new and expanded way to provide care for the terminally ill; the new concept of the Golden Room removes the dying patient from the acute care setting into a cluster of rooms separated from the regular patients in the general hospital and/or the nursing home. Another place for Golden Rooms is a free-standing building entirely dedicated to caring for the dying. These rooms are similar to contemporary hospice care but offer expanded facilities and personnel.

i. Death bed ritual (basic)
- Easing the transition from life to a peaceful death can be helped by integration of planned ritual.
- Ritual can occur at the moment of death or immediately after.
- If anointing has not already been done, it can be done at this time.
- Family, special friends, care staff, and clergy might choose to hold hands, surround the bed of the deceased, and share a moment of silence, a prayer, a song, or hugs. They might choose to touch the body, prepare the body according to rituals within the faith community involved, and say goodbye. It is important to allow as much time as needed.

j. Leave-taking rituals (basic)
- A nurse who works with survivors must remember that their grief period is unique for them; grief has no timetable.
- Healing grief requires a commitment to imagine a fulfilling life without a loved one.
- Action steps toward continued self-discovery after the death of a loved one can include dream work, meditation, movement, drawing, journal keeping, crying, sighing, drumming, chanting, singing, and music, as well as the following:[23]
  - Celebrating holidays.
  - Rearranging and giving away loved one's possessions.
  - Letting grief be present: There are periods after death when a person appears brave, in control, or strong to others. Grief will come, however. It is important to share with the grieving person that there is no special way to grieve. When pain, fear, and anger can dissipate, the body-mind-spirit knows the best way to grieve. Grieving allows love to heal the loss one feels for self and the person who has died.
  - Sustaining faith and hope: There are many ways to sustain faith and awareness toward life, meaning, and purpose during grieving time. For example, survivors sometimes have a sense of talking to deceased loved ones, being enveloped in their love, and feeling their presence.
  - Releasing anger and tears: The release of anger, sadness, and tears is a cleansing process of the

human spirit that makes a person more open to experience living in the moment. Holding grief in increases the suffering, fear, and separation.

♦ Healing memories: It is not necessary to stop thinking about the person who has died. Often, a grieving person who feels that the grief process is over finds that a memory, a song, or a meal suddenly evokes a sense of loss so deep that it seems as though it will never heal. The person needs to stay with the pain, sadness, guilt, anger, fear, or loneliness. Love and joy will begin to fill the heart again. The wisdom is to let pain in and to stay open to it, to let the pain penetrate every cell in your body, to trust pain, to know that what emerges from the pain is a new level of healing awareness.

♦ Getting unstuck: Grieving can bring on suffering; therefore, it can be helpful for survivors to ask for assistance from friends, family, or a healthcare professional to help them move past the blocks.

Evaluation

1. With the patient (family and significant others), the nurse evaluates whether the patient outcomes for planning and implementing a peaceful death were successfully achieved.

2. To evaluate the interventions further, the nurse can explore the subjective effects of the experience with the patient (family and significant others), using questions such as those shown in Exhibit 21-2, Evaluation of the Client's (Family's and Significant Others) Subjective Experience with Perideath Nursing Interventions, found in *Holistic Nursing: A Handbook for Practice*.

3. Like peaceful living and dying, the care of a dying person and the family and significant others is an art.

4. Preparing for death can be a series of conscious, spirit-filled, light-filled moments that lead to the ultimate peaceful moment of death. It is different for each person.

5. True healing and dying in peace come from integrating the creative process and the art of healing into our daily lives.

6. The paradox is that, although this healing awareness might appear at first to be rare, it is a very ordinary and natural event that is available to each of us at all times.

7. As each of us seeks to understand and integrate our spirit-filled lives as meaningful and connected with others throughout the ages, we learn about life and death.

8. The more we integrate solitude, inward-focused practice, and conscious awareness into daily life, the more peaceful are dying and the moment of death.

■ NOTES

1. Roshan Cultural Heritage Institute. (n.d.). Definition of culture. Retrieved from http://www.roshan-institute.org/474552

2. Keegan, L., & Drick, C. A. (2011). Theoretical frameworks. In L. Keegan & C. A. Drick (Eds.), *End of life: Nursing solutions for death with dignity* (pp. 101–124). New York, NY: Springer.

3. Watson, J. (2011). *The philosophy and science of caring* (Rev. ed.). Boulder, CO: University Press of Colorado.

4. Davies, B., & Steele, R. (2011). Supporting families in palliative care. In B. F. Ferrell & N. Coyle (Eds.), *Textbook of palliative care nursing* (pp. 613–629). New York, NY: Oxford University Press.

5. Erseck, M., & Cotter, V. T. (2011). The meaning of hope in the dying. In B. F. Ferrell & N. Coyle (Eds.), *Textbook of palliative care nursing* (pp. 579–597). New York, NY: Oxford University Press.

6. Lynn, J., Schuster, J. L., Wilkinson, A., & Simon, L. N. (eds.) (2008). Supporting people in difficult times: Relationships, spirituality, and bereavement. In *Improving care for the end of life: A sourcebook for health care managers and clinicians* (pp. 133–162). New York, NY: Oxford University Press.

7. Kübler-Ross, E. (1969). *On death and dying.* New York, NY: Macmillan.

8. Fowler, J. W. (1981). *Stages of faith: The psychology of human development and the quest for meaning.* New York, NY: Harper & Row.

9. Frankl, V. (1963). *Man's search for meaning* (3rd ed.). New York, NY: Simon & Schuster.

10. Reed, P. (2008). Self-transcendence theory. In M. Smith & P. Liehr (Eds.), *Middle range theory for nursing* (p. 105). New York, NY: Springer.

11. Haight, B. K., & Haight, B. S. (2007). *The handbook for the structured life review.* Baltimore, MD: Health Professions Press.

12. Growth House. (n.d.). Life review and reminiscence therapy. Retrieved from http://www.growthhouse.org/lifereview.html

13. Burns, P. (n.d.). Myth and legend from ancient times to the space age. Retrieved from http://www.pibburns.com/myth.htm

14. ELNEC (End-of-Life Consortium). (2010). *Graduate curriculum: Faculty guide*. Washington, DC: City of Hope and American Association of Colleges of Nursing.

15. Hollis, J. L. (2010). *Music at the end of life: Easing the pain and preparing the passage*. Santa Barbara, CA: Praeger.

16. Dunn, L. L. (2009). Spiritual needs: Focus on forgiveness [Editorial]. *Online Journal of Rural Nursing and Health Care*. Retrieved from http://www.rno.org/journal/index.php/online-journal/article/viewFile/188/235

17. Reik, B. M. (2010). Transgressions, guilt and forgiveness: A model of seeking forgiveness. *Journal of Psychology and Theology, 38*(4), 246–254. Retrieved from http://sccn612final.wikispaces.com/file/view/Transgressions,+Guilt+and+Forgiveness.pdf

18. Rahman, I. (2009). The seven steps to genuine forgiveness. *Free Online Library*. Retrieved from http://www.thefreelibrary.com/The+Seven+Steps+to+Genuine+Forgiveness-a01073981047

19. Gray, T. (2009). *Praying scripture for a change: An introduction to Lectio Divina*. Westchester, PA: Ascension Press.

20. Keating, T. (2008). *Spirituality, contemplation and transformation: Writings on centering prayer*. Brooklyn, NY: Lantern Books.

21. O'Mahony, S., McHenry, J., Blank, A., Snow, D., Karakas, S. E., Santoro, G.,...Kvetan, V. (2010). Preliminary report of the integration of a palliative care team into an intensive care unit. *Palliative Medicine, 24*(2), 154–165.

22. Keegan, L., & Drick, C. A. (2011). *End of life: Nursing solutions for death with dignity*. New York, NY: Springer.

23. Hammerschlag, C. (2011). *Healing ceremonies* (Kindle ed.). Amazon Digital Services.

■ STUDY QUESTIONS
Basic Level

1. Self-care for the nurse before caring for the dying individual most importantly begins with which of the following activities?
   a. Centering, to be in a focused and caring state
   b. Exercising daily for good health
   c. Setting limits for involvement with people
   d. Prioritizing care according to the nursing process

2. The holistic nurse understands that his or her most important skill in providing comfort to the dying person and the family is which of the following?
   a. Knowledge of pain control
   b. Communication
   c. Presence
   d. Compassion

3. Which of the following is a potential outcome for the self-transcendant person?
   a. New connections to people
   b. Ability to meditate and have less fear of death
   c. Ability to find creative solutions to pain control
   d. Less hopelessness and self-neglect

4. Mr. Jones is dying from advanced lung cancer and decides to register in a new clinical drug trial. The holistic nurse caring for him understands that this action might be a reflection of which of the following in Mr. Jones?
   a. Spiritual development
   b. Intellectual strength
   c. Denial of death
   d. Attraction to mystery

5. Assessment of spiritual concerns most importantly requires assessment of which of the following for a client?
   a. Attendance at religious events or services
   b. Method of prayer or meditation
   c. Concept of God or deity
   d. Religious denominational affiliation

6. Which of the following characterizes grief that follows the death of a loved one?
   a. A diagnosis requiring intervention
   b. Pervasive, affecting all aspects of life
   c. A set of well-defined stages people go through in order
   d. A precursor to clinical depression in most people

7. A professional nurse evaluates care for a dying client to determine whether it has met the client's goals for comfort and which other goal?
   a. Progress toward cure
   b. Communication with the doctor
   c. Increased wisdom during the dying process
   d. Participation in care for as long as possible

8. Assessment of pain most importantly depends on which of the following factors?
   a. The person's description of pain
   b. The person's history of pain management patterns
   c. The characteristics of the analgesic chosen
   d. The use of a culturally sensitive pain scale

Advanced Level

9. Miss Hall, a home hospice patient, is very anxious and says that her discomfort is like a ball of fire in her chest. The AHN-BC determines that which of the following is a priority intervention for this client?
   a. Increasing her antianxiety medication
   b. Repositioning her
   c. Exploring images that could release the grip of the pain
   d. Placing a cool cloth on her chest

10. The AHN-BC is facilitating a life review with Mr. Sun. In her planning, which of the following factors is the nurse aware of?
    a. Life review is reminiscing.
    b. The first session is when his life meaning will be revealed.
    c. He should be well rested because the process lasts 2–3 hours.
    d. The outcome might be an integration of life wholeness.

11. Mrs. Hill's son died 6 years ago; each year she celebrates his birthday. Which course of action should the holistic nurse take with Mrs. Hill?
    a. Mrs. Hill should be assessed for suicide risk.
    b. Mrs. Hill should be encouraged to do so if it helps her with her grief.
    c. Mrs. Hill should be taught a variety of coping skills.
    d. Mrs. Hill should be distracted by her friends to help her move beyond her grief.

12. The AHN-BC knows that for caregivers to be at least somewhat peaceful during the death of a loved one they must have knowledge of which of the following factors?
    a. The nature of the afterlife
    b. What the care team thinks should be done
    c. How to complete funeral arrangements
    d. The changes in the body during the death process

13. What does the AHN-BC know about near death experiences?
    a. They are proof of life after death.
    b. They are often comforting to people.
    c. They are the result of medication.
    d. They do not happen to people who are dying from a terminal illness.

14. Mrs. King has a living will and has decided that she wants no further medical treatment. When she loses consciousness, her son decides he wants his beloved mother placed on life support. The AHN-BC can best support him by doing which of the following actions?
    a. Telling him that he does not have the right to override his mother's wishes
    b. Having the social worker explain the legal implications of living wills
    c. Arranging with the physician to have Mrs. King intubated
    d. Listening to the reasons that he has made this decision

15. The AHN-BC notes that the nurses working in hospice are argumentative and short-tempered. She determines that a priority intervention is to convene a meeting. After an opening meditation, which activity might be most helpful to these nurses?
    a. Discuss the schedule and caseload
    b. Explore the nurses' feelings about a good death
    c. Participate in gentle yoga
    d. Determine a regular meeting schedule

Chapter 23

Weight Management Counseling

Sue Popkess-Vawter

▪ DEFINITIONS

Body mass index (BMI) Weight in kilograms divided by height squared (m²), with healthy weight less than or equal to 24.9.

Obesity Body mass index greater than or equal to 30.

Overeating Eating when not hungry or eating more than is required to satisfy hunger.

Overfat Percentage of body fat greater than recommended for a client's gender and age (e.g., 28% for women and 20% for men).

Overweight Body mass index of 25–29.9.

Self-talk Mental verbalizations that elicit emotional responses.

Weight cycling/yo-yo dieting Repeated weight loss and regain of more than 10 pounds in a repetitive pattern three or more times over the past 2 years.

Weight management Holistic, long-term lifestyle adjustments in clients' bio-psycho-socio-cultural-spiritual dimensions to promote a high level of individual wellness; caring for and assisting clients to reach sufficient self-acceptance, self-love, and self-responsibility to adjust their lifestyles to support eating for hunger, exercising regularly, and esteem.

▪ THEORY AND RESEARCH

Weight Gain Epidemic

1. Two-thirds of adults in the United States are overweight or obese despite initiatives to abate this unchecked problem.[1,2]

a. Weight management failures result from lack of practical, long-term interventions to address holistic influences of weight gain (e.g., biological, psychological, sociocultural, and spiritual).[3]

b. Experts agree that environmental influences, rather than biological reasons, explain the obesity epidemic of the past three decades.

c. Four key factors can explain the environmental stimulus–response nature of the rise in obesity in the United States: (1) fast-paced eating style of fatty, glycemic "fast foods" and super sizing; (2) excessive calorie intake; (3) reduced physical activity and greater use of high-tech devices; and (4) heightened sensitivity to food as a stimulant from the media.

2. Weight management approaches need to account for energy in (food), energy out (exercise), psychological aspects such as self-esteem and stress management, "toxic environments" that do not support healthy eating and exercise, comorbidity and obesogenic medications, and family–job influences.

a. Feelings of deprivation and preoccupation with food and dieting yielded a rise in eating disorders and weight cycling.

b. Long-term habits of overeating without hunger and little or no physical exercise in a fast-paced society can explain the U.S. weight crisis. To date, most weight loss interventions in the United States have not contributed to long-term weight loss and probably have exacerbated the overweight problem.

c. Comorbid conditions associated with overweight and obesity include heart disease and hypertension, stroke, gall-bladder disease, osteoarthritis, sleep apnea, respiratory problems, and cancers (e.g., endometrial, breast, prostate, colon); the most dramatically rising overweight comorbidity is type 2 diabetes.[4]

Approaches to Weight Management

1. Most weight management approaches are based on at least one of four categories of theories—biological, behavioral, psychological, and cognitive.
   a. Four biological theories explain excess weight gain from genetic and energy balance perspectives.
   b. Two genetic theories explain that individuals have a genetic predisposition to an excessive accumulation of fat, either by hypertrophy (enlarged size) or hyperplasia (excessive numbers) of fat cells.
   c. Set Point Theory, another popular theory, gained attention in the 1980s and 1990s. Nesbitt, who introduced this theory in 1972, claims that individuals have but one body weight at which their energy expenditure is normal.[5]
   d. Energy Balance Theory holds that an excessive number of calories ingested, but not required for metabolic needs, results in an excessive body weight. Conversely, fewer calories with demanding exercise and work create a deficit that allows weight loss to occur.
2. Behavioral theories are based on the premise that behaviors such as overeating are learned responses; behavior modification techniques (based on Skinner's Stimulus–Response Theory) aim to control stimuli that result in actions that perpetuate overeating.[6]
   a. Stimulus control strategies are designed to control eating by restricting calories, choices, locations, and timing.
   b. Many calorie-restricted diets and food supplements are a type of stimulus control strategy that concentrate on controlling antecedent stimuli (i.e., controlling what, when, where, and how much to eat).
   c. Stimulus-controlled diets focus on avoiding or eliminating hunger, thus minimizing the body's natural, physiologic,

internal signals of hunger so that individuals are forced to focus on external cues to tell them when they need to eat.
3. Behavioral change theory, such as Prochaska and DiClemente's Stages of Change or the Transtheoretical Model (TTM),[7] posit that health behavior change involves progress through five stages of change: precontemplation, contemplation, preparation, action, and maintenance.
4. The Holistic Self-Care Model (HSCM) for long-term weight management is based on the premise that stimulus control addresses only part of the reasons for weight gain—the external reasons. The other reasons for weight gain are internal.
   a. HSCM emphasizes healthy eating for hunger rather than the elimination of hunger.
   b. HSCM includes calculating calories to meet basic metabolic and exercise metabolic needs, based on Academy of Nutrition and Dietetics guidelines (daily calories greater or equal to 1,200).
   c. HSCM includes health-promoting behavioral techniques to monitor and record compliance with prescribed dietary restrictions.
   d. HSCM places greater emphasis on internal indicators of progress, such as changes in thinking and feelings, versus external indicators, such as weight, body shape, and body size.
   e. Behavioral therapy is effective on a short-term basis but is less effective for helping obese individuals address disturbed thinking, emotions, and body image related to overeating and poor self-esteem.
5. Psychological theories usually are directed toward decreasing stress-induced eating and helping to find ways to control eating in the presence of stressful situations.
   a. Negative body image, poor self-esteem, depression, and issues of social discrimination become the major focus of psychotherapy.
   b. Binge eating disorder, bulimia, and compulsive overeating are treated as relationship disorders.
   c. Individuals with eating disorders are encouraged to focus on related issues of abandonment and verbal, sexual, and

physical abuse rather than the eating problem per se.

d. Depression and obesity as related concerns are on the rise in the United States, chiefly among younger ages.[8]

6. Beck explains how unrealistic, negative thinking triggers unpleasant emotional responses, such as overeating and not exercising.[9]

a. Cognitive interventions are aimed at providing rapid symptomatic improvement, understanding mood changes, coping strategies for self-management when upset, and guiding personal growth.

b. Individuals are assisted in assessing basic values and attitudes that lead to negative feelings and reevaluating and challenging basic assumptions about self-worth.

c. Problem-solving and coping techniques help clients deal effectively with major, realistic problems (e.g., low self-esteem, guilt) and minor vague irritations (e.g., frustration, apathy) that seem to have no obvious external cause.

d. Cognitive restructuring techniques help identify and eliminate cognitive distortions that elicit irrational emotional responses by: (1) identifying automatic thoughts that are self-critical, (2) identifying cognitive distortions and unrealistic beliefs underlying thoughts, and (3) providing rational responses that defend the self.

e. Cognitive restructuring aims to substitute objective rational thoughts for illogical, harsh self-criticisms in response to negative events.

f. Clients learn how beliefs relate to thinking, thinking relates to feelings, and feelings relate to actions.

Failure of Traditional Weight Management Interventions

1. In 1994, failure rates for most weight reduction programs were estimated to be as high as 90–95%.[10]

a. Overweight adults comprised 47% of the population in 1976, 56% in 1988, and 65% in 1999, and prevalence of obese adults rose from 15% in 1976, to 23% in 1988, and to 31% in 1999.[11]

b. Weight gain trends appeared to reach a relatively steady state from 1999 to 2008. The National Health and Nutrition Examination Survey (NHANES) report for 2007–2008 showed overall prevalence of overweight and obesity for adults was 68% (approximately 72% among men and 64% among women).[1]

c. Obesity prevalence for women was 35.5% and 32.2% for men. Class 3 obesity was reported to have increased at greater rates than any other class of obesity in the United States.[12]

d. Over the past three decades, childhood obesity has more than doubled among children ages 2–5 years, has tripled among youth ages 6–11 years, and has more than tripled among adolescents ages 12–19 years. About 17% of American children ages 2–19 years were obese—a 1 in 6 incidence rate.

e. Overweight and obesity have greater effects on minorities; blacks had 51% and Hispanics had 21% higher obesity prevalence compared with whites.

2. Interventions that fail to promote long-term weight management are: (1) restrictive in calories, choices, and times to eat; (2) unidimensional, using only one major means to achieve weight loss, and do not include regular exercise; (3) do not permit individuals to tailor weight management to their preferences, lifestyles, and humanness; and (4) do not focus on internal motivations for overeating and not exercising regularly.

a. Interventions that restrict calories, choices, and times to eat offer temporary and artificial modification that is unrealistic for the long term.

b. Despite increasing dieting attempts, the prevalence of overweight Americans increased from 25% to 33% between 1980 and 1991. Although Americans were trying to eat less fat, they were getting fatter.

c. Responses to dietary restrictions and deprivation ultimately resulted in overeating, which might have led to weight gain reflected in the current 68% incidence of overweight and obesity.

d. National weight management guidelines were adjusted to be less restrictive for human fallibility.

3. Unidimensional medical weight loss interventions often fail in the long term, such as surgical reduction of the gastrointestinal tract, stomach expansion devices and lap band restriction devices to produce a full feeling, and drugs to suppress the appetite and block fat absorption.
   a. Often dramatic weight regain occurs when surgical procedures fail and medications are withdrawn because clients lack insight into why they overeat and do not exercise.
   b. Clients need to learn healthy eating, exercise, and self-esteem before or concurrently with other weight management treatments. Perhaps equally disconcerting about use of surgery and pharmacologic agents are the detrimental side effects.
   c. Dietary, pharmacologic, and surgical treatments that reduce intake and restrict calories, choices, and when to eat offer temporary modifications that are unrealistic for long term and often have rebound weight gain and damaging psychological consequences.[13]
4. Regular exercise as part of weight management plays a vital role in weight loss.
   a. Exercise can prevent a reduction in the resting metabolic rate, either by elevating it following the exercise or by maintaining or increasing fat-free mass (lean body mass).
   b. Research supports both aerobic and strength (i.e., resistance) exercises to promote healthy weight, including short 10-minute bouts of exercise throughout the day, three to five times per day.[14]
   c. Insulin resistance syndrome, or metabolic syndrome, is associated with a cluster of abnormalities typical for type 2 diabetes and its comorbidities,[15] including hypertension, overweight, glucose intolerance, lipid abnormalities, and high risk for cardiovascular disease.
5. Non-insulin-dependent diabetes mellitus (adult-onset diabetes, type 2 diabetes) accounts for almost 95% of all diagnosed cases of diabetes.[16]
   a. As overweight increases, so does type 2 diabetes risk with visceral adiposity—greater waist circumference, or an "apple shape."
   b. Waist measurements greater than 35 inches for women and 40 inches for men suggest higher risk than smaller waist measurements.
   c. Central obesity among Americans might be related to greater intake of high glycemic index foods (e.g., high sugar and starch, low fiber, refined and processed foods), in addition to recognized overindulgence of fatty, fast foods.
   d. High sugar and starch content in low-fiber, refined foods might be directly related to the growing incidence of insulin resistance; modest weight loss of 5% to 10% of initial body weight can improve glucose tolerance and reduce blood pressure, lipids, and mortality.[17]
6. Interventions that do not permit individuals to tailor weight management to their preferences, lifestyles, and humanness do not last.
   a. Weight loss programs fail when directives are too stringent for gaining ownership and accepting strategies as a way of life.
   b. Individuals will fail "the program" when not viewed as a long-term lifestyle change and do not address their individual preferences (e.g., dislike for certain foods and types of exercise), way of life (e.g., working nights, family versus single), and "being human" along the way (e.g., not feeling guilty or dropping out when they deviate from the plan).
   c. The Academy of Nutrition and Dietetics states long-term weight management takes a lifelong commitment to healthy lifestyle changes.[18]
   d. Daily physical activity and eating should be sustainable and enjoyable using personal tailoring of healthy, yet livable lifetime habits.
7. Interventions not focused on internal motivations for overeating and skipping exercise do not uncover underlying reasons for being overweight.
   a. Weight management should include biological, psychological, and social interventions to separate physical from emotional hunger.
   b. Toxic stress is the uncontrollable, chronic type of stress that causes sustained high levels of serum cortisol, the powerful

stress hormone necessary for fueling stressful events.[19]

c. Sustained high cortisol levels can lead to fatigue, impaired immune response, lower mental sharpness, and stimulated appetite, all of which can contribute to metabolic syndrome.

d. Attempts to lower stress usually include relaxation exercises and physical exercise; techniques to prevent a toxic stress response involve seeking a different, healthier perception of troublesome stressors through healthy self-esteem.

Multidimensional Weight Management Interventions

1. Successful weight management focuses on internal motivations for overeating and skipping exercise and are multidimensional and flexible.

   a. Suggested cognitive-behavioral strategies are self-monitoring, stress management, stimulus control, problem solving, contingency management, cognitive restructuring, and social support.

   b. Behavioral strategies and cognitive-behavioral strategies differ; behavioral strategies, or behavior modification, focus on changing individuals' behaviors with little or no concern for underlying reasons for overeating, not exercising, and unhealthy coping behaviors.

   c. Cognitive-behavioral strategies usually include cognitive restructuring designed to reprogram negative, derogatory self-talk to positive, constructive self-talk; self-talk is automatic thoughts in one's mind, often imparted by parents, authority figures, and religious teachings.

   d. Cognitive restructuring is defined for clients as reprogramming of negative, derogatory self-talk to positive, constructive self-talk.

   e. Cognitive-behavioral strategies directly address how negative beliefs and negative self-talk shortcomings and human interactions can repeatedly increase tension, distort attitudes, and lead to negative behaviors, such as overeating and skipping exercise.

f. Cognitive therapy based on Reversal Theory is the basis of the Holistic Self-Care Model (HSCM).

2. Reversal Theory defines *tension stress* as the discrepancy between where individuals are and where they want to be and is reviewed as the foundation for cognitive strategies used in HSCM.[20]

   a. Apter's Reversal Theory, a phenomenologic theory of arousal, motivation, action, posits that personality is inherently inconsistent.

   b. Individuals reverse between four opposing, paired states called metamotivational states: telic and paratelic, conformist and negativistic, mastery and sympathy, and alloic and autic.

   c. Telic is serious minded, goal oriented while paratelic is playful and spontaneous; conformist follows rules while negativistic is rebellious; mastery is being in control while sympathy is being tender; alloic is thinking of others while autic is thinking of oneself.

   d. Healthy individuals reverse between states easily and often daily, whereas some individuals become "stuck" in certain states.

   e. Each metamotivational state has associated pleasant and unpleasant feelings and responses to give rise to tension stress as a discrepancy between desired and actual feelings.

   f. Self-report questionnaires based on Reversal Theory were developed and tested for assessing overeating and skipping exercise.[21]

Holistic Self-Care Model

1. The Holistic Self-Care Model (HSCM) is designed to assist overweight clients with individualized nutritional, exercise, and psycho-social-spiritual strategies for a long-term pursuit of healthier and happier lifestyles.

   a. Holistic self-care emphasizes concurrent work in nutritional, exercise, and psycho-social-spiritual dimensions to reduce the percentage of body fat and increase physical fitness.

   b. HSCM takes an internal perspective to seek insight about negative self-talk that obstructs long-term guidance from the body's natural hunger and satiety signals and positive benefits of regular exercise.

c. HSCM provides a unique plan of face-to-face counseling appointments to continually support, guide, individualize, and adjust lifelong strategies; principles include using continual feedback among the eating, physical exercise, and esteem, as integration among mind, body, and spirit.

d. Clients are in charge of redesigning lifestyle patterns, consistent with self-care tenets.

e. Old habits can be changed through small, steady efforts that lead to greater success, as opposed to drastic changes that lead to feelings of deprivation, burnout, relapse, and eventual failure.

2. Spirituality can reunite parts of individuals so that they become whole based on belief in a higher power—a higher authority and guiding spirit, and existential beliefs of positive values, meanings, and sense of purpose.

a. When spirituality is part of caregiving, clients gain personal meaning, dignity, worth, and identity.

b. Cognitive restructuring called BIO strategies are part of the HSCM—the glue that can hold together bio-psycho-social-spiritual beings to make long-lasting, healthy lifestyle changes.

c. BIO strategies are defined as spiritually based, cognitive strategies designed to expand and maximize people's ability to manage healthy weight with long-term results: BIO is Balance from the Inside Out.

d. Spiritually based cognitive strategies promote internal self-awareness to guide self-care from moment to moment and change negative self-talk that blocks natural signals of hunger and satiety, need for regular exercise, and inner voice of guidance for healthy self-care.

3. BIO strategies use mnemonics such as EAT for Hunger, Exercise for LIFE, and ESTEEM for Self and Others.

a. EAT for Hunger promotes awareness for eating in response to hunger and satiety cues instead of emotional eating: Eat only when hunger occurs, Ask the body

what it needs, and Tell the self to stop when hunger is satisfied, not full.

b. Exercise for LIFE supports daily exercise and physical activity: Learn the habit, I am important, Friends, and Enjoy myself.

c. ESTEEM for Self and Others is a cognitive strategy to support self-esteem and coping through daily meditation, spiritual reading, and personal creativity: ESTEEM stands for Energy, Spirit, Time, Eating, Exercise, Meditation.

▮ HOLISTIC CARING PROCESS

Holistic Assessment

1. Before implementing weight management interventions, the nurse should assess the following parameters:

a. Body composition (baseline and every 6 months) and body mass index

b. Resting heart rate and blood pressure

c. Blood profile (baseline and every 6 months), including lipid profile, blood glucose, thyroid function, hemoglobin, and hematocrit

d. Physical fitness (exercise testing using submaximal bicycle ergometer or maximal treadmill)

e. Strength testing using repetition maximum for chest press and leg press (or comparable exercises)

2. Additionally, developing a psychological profile for each client should include the following:

a. Life review and dieting history, from clients' life stories and the evolution of their weight problem; identifying lifestyle patterns

b. BULIT (bulimia test) scale or other scale to screen for bulimia[22]

c. Body image according to a 10-point visual analog scale (1 being the best)

d. Overeating, exercise, feelings, tension stress questionnaires[23]

Nursing Diagnoses

1. The patterns/challenges/needs compatible with weight management interventions are as follows:

a. Altered nutrition (more than body requires)

b. Spiritual distress

c. Ineffective individual coping

d. Decreased physical mobility

e. Disturbance in body image

f. Disturbance in self-esteem

g. Hopelessness

h. Knowledge deficit

i. Anxiety

2. Specific patterns/challenges/needs related to the Holistic Self-Care Model and BIO strategies include the following:

a. Overeating related to increased tension stress

b. Decreased aerobic and resistance exercise related to a poor body image and a feeling of being unworthy to take time for exercise

c. Infrequent episodes of play and creativity related to early modeling and values that consider work to be more important than play

d. Lack of skills to express anger and disagreement, related to a belief that it is unacceptable behavior

e. Lack of skills to express feelings, related to early suppression of feelings to self-protect

f. Inability to put self first, related to early teaching that others have greater value and worth

Client Outcomes According to Stages of Change

1. Prochaska and DiClemente developed the Transtheoretical Therapy Model (TTM) to describe how individuals can move through five stages of motivational readiness for lifestyle changes: (1) precontemplation, (2) contemplation, (3) preparation, (4) action, and (5) maintenance.

a. Precontemplation (no intention of changing in the next 6 months): The client will verbalize reasons for not wanting to reduce weight and fat and perform regular exercise.

b. Contemplation (considering changing in the next 6 months, but not active yet): The client will report fewer overeating episodes and less tension stress during daily eating.

c. Preparation (making some changes, but not at goal): The client will report exercising more frequently, resulting in greater muscle strength, less fatigue, and more energy.

d. Action (6 months of active behavior change): The client will have lower levels of total cholesterol and low-density lipoproteins, a higher level of high-density lipoproteins, and blood glucose levels within normal limits.

e. Maintenance (sustained change past 6 months): The client will have a lower percentage of body fat, lower weight, lower resting heart rate, and lower blood pressure.

Plan and Interventions

1. Before the session spend a few moments centering yourself to recognize your presence and to begin the session with the intention to facilitate healing.

2. Create an environment in which the client is encouraged to share his or her story.

3. At the beginning of the session show a listing of the stages of change to the client and have him or her explain any differences between his or her stage at the last session and now. Proceed accordingly with the HSCM.

4. At the end of the session ask the client to review what he or she gained from the session and answer any questions. Give the client a copy of any relevant support materials, and ask him or her to explain how to use them. Ask him or her to complete a copy of the BIO Eating-Exercise-Esteem worksheet and verbalize what he or she has written and the times allotted for the behaviors.

5. Specific interventions used in the HSCM are listed and interpreted according to the five stages of change:

a. Clients in precontemplation are not ready to make lifestyle changes; a nurse cannot "motivate" or manipulate them to do so but should inform them about lifestyle assessment, risks, and options to raise consciousness without demands.

b. Clients in contemplation still believe that the reasons for not changing their behaviors (e.g., too tired, too hungry, too busy, don't have enough money) overbalance reasons that they should; past dieters often view future dietary restrictions, past failures very negatively.

c. Clients in preparation begin to make lifestyle changes, but they perform new behaviors sporadically and have not yet incorporated them as a permanent part of their lifestyles.

d. Around 3 to 6 months, clients progress to the action state when eating and exercise habits start to become well established and they experience pride and satisfaction in their lifestyle changes.

e. Maintenance usually occurs after 6 months of clients practicing and refining lifestyle changes. They should be encouraged to stay in touch with the nurse and continue to examine patterns when they overeat and do not exercise to discover ways to reinforce and strengthen areas of deficit.

Evaluation

1. The client received a clinic weight management brochure with a written report of physical and psychological findings and verbalized understanding of the report, implied risks, and invitation to learn more about the clinic weight program.

2. The client verbalized the three steps of the EAT for Hunger strategy, shared one difficulty with the strategy to work on in the next 6 months, and expressed satisfaction about eating for hunger.

3. The client described aerobic and strength exercises that are a good lifestyle fit, shared one difficulty with the strategy to work on in the next 6 months, and reported lower tension stress.

4. The client verbalized acceptance of a changed lifestyle, shared one difficulty with a BIO strategy on which to concentrate efforts in the next 6 months, and expressed satisfaction with improved lipid levels, weight, and blood pressure.

■ NOTES

1. Flegal, K. M., Carroll, M. D., Kit, B. K., & Ogden, C. L. (2010). Prevalence and trends in obesity among U.S. adults, 1999–2008. *Journal of the American Medical Association, 303,* 235–241.

2. Sondik, E. J., Huang, D. T., Klein, R. J., & Satcher, D. (2010). Progress toward the *Healthy People 2010* goals and objectives. *Annual Review of Public Health, 31,* 271–281.

3. U.S. Department of Health and Human Services. (2010). *The surgeon general's vision for a healthy and fit nation.* Rockville, MD: U.S. DHHS, Office of the Surgeon General.

4. Centers for Disease Control and Prevention. (2010). Obesity: Halting the epidemic by making health easier: At a glance 2010. Retrieved from http://www.cdc.gov/chronicdisease/resources/publications/aag/obesity.htm

5. Reiff, D. W., & Reiff, K. K. (1992). *Eating disorders.* Gaithersburg, MD: Aspen Publishers.

6. Skinner, B. F. (1974). *About behaviorism.* New York, NY: Random House.

7. Prochaska, J. O., & DiClemente, C. C. (1992). In search of how people change. *American Psychologist, 47,* 1102.

8. Centers for Disease Control and Prevention. (2011). An estimated 1 in 10 U.S. adults report depression. Retrieved from http://www.cdc.gov/Features/dsDepression

9. Beck, A. T. (1976). *Cognitive therapy and the emotional disorders.* New York, NY: International Universities Press.

10. Brownell, K. D., & Rodin, J. (1994). The dieting maelstrom: Is it possible and advisable to lose weight?" *American Psychologist, 49,* 781–791.

11. Centers for Disease Control and Prevention. (2011). Obesity trends among U.S. adults between 1985 and 2010. Retrieved from http://www.cdc.gov/obesity/downloads/obesity_trends_2010.pdf

12. Blackburn, G. L., Wollner, S., & Heymsfield, S. B. (2010). Lifestyle interventions for the treatment of class III obesity: A primary target for nutrition medicine in the obesity epidemic. *American Journal of Clinical Nutrition, 9,* 289S–292S.

13. Popkess-Vawter, S., Yoder, E., & Gajewski, B. (2005). The role of spirituality in holistic weight management. *Clinical Nursing Research, 14,* 158–174.

14. Goto, K., Tanaka, K., Ishii, N., Ichida, S., & Takamatsu, K. (2011). A single versus multiple bouts of moderate-intensity exercise for fat metabolism. *Clinical Physiology and Functional Imaging, 31,* 215–220.

15. National Heart, Lung, and Blood Institute. (2011). What is metabolic syndrome? Retrieved from http://www.nhlbi.nih.gov/health/dci/Diseases/ms/ms_diagnosis.html

16. National Institute of Diabetes and Digestive and Kidney Diseases. (2011). Fast facts on diabetes. Retrieved from http://diabetes.niddk.nih.gov/dm/pubs/statistics/#fast

17. National Heart, Lung, and Blood Institute. (2011). Facts about healthy weight. Retrieved from http://www.nhlbi.nih.gov/health/prof/heart/obesity/aim_kit/healthy_wt_facts.htm

18. American Dietetic Association. (2009). Position on weight management. *Journal of the American Diabetic Association, 109,* 330–346.

19. Peeke, P. (2007). *Fit to live*. London, England: Pan Macmillan.

20. Apter, M. (1989). *Reversal Theory: Motivation, emotion, and personality*. London, England: Routledge.

21. Popkess-Vawter, S., Gerkovich, M. M., & Wendel, S. (2000). Reliability and validity of the Overeating Tension Scale. *Journal of Nursing Measurement, 8*, 145–160.

22. Kramer-Jackman, K., & Popkess-Vawter, S. (2011). Method for technology-delivered healthcare measures. *Computers, Informatics, Nursing, 29*, 730–740.

23. Popkess-Vawter, S., & Owens, V. (1999). Use of the BULIT bulimia screening questionnaire to assess risk and progress in weight management for overweight women who weight cycle. *Addictive Behaviors, 24*, 497–507.

■ STUDY QUESTIONS

Basic Level

1. Which of the following is the most dramatically rising overweight comorbidity?
   a. Neurological deficits
   b. Type 2 diabetes
   c. Cirrhosis of the liver
   d. Hypothyroidism

2. Which theory has accurately and consistently explained the etiology of weight gain?
   a. Set Point Theory
   b. Adipocyte Hyperplasia Theory
   c. Adipocyte Hypertrophy Theory
   d. Energy Balance Theory

3. The Holistic Self-Care Model (HSCM) mainly focuses on which of the following areas?
   a. Internal reasons for weight gain
   b. External reasons for weight gain
   c. Internal and external reasons for weight gain
   d. Stimulus–control reasons for weight gain

4. Cognitive restructuring techniques focus on which of the following?
   a. Identifying cognitive distortions and unrealistic beliefs underlying thoughts
   b. Controlling antecedent stimuli that lead to overeating and skipping planned exercise
   c. Altering learned responses and cognitions using behavior modification
   d. Decreasing depression related to being overweight

5. Toxic stress is a chronic type of stress that causes which of the following conditions?
   a. Excessive energy and nervousness
   b. Heightened beta-wave brain activity
   c. Chronic loss of appetite
   d. Sustained high serum cortisol

Advanced Level

6. Reversal Theory is an important basis in cognitive-behavioral strategies for which of the following reasons?
   a. Individuals learn to reverse their thinking before overeating or skipping planned exercise.
   b. Metamotivational states can be matched with eating and exercise prescriptions.
   c. Tension stress, discrepancies between the way we feel and the way we want to feel, explains overeating and skipping exercise.
   d. Toxic stress prevention can add to the success of weight management protocols for healthy eating and exercise.

7. Which of the following descriptions best describes the HSCM principle of holism?
   a. Feedback among eating, exercise, and esteem is continual by integrating and supporting mind, body, and spirit.
   b. Religiosity and spirituality are individuals' private matters that should not be discussed.
   c. Mind, body, and spirit integration is possible usually after 4 to 6 months of cognitive-behavioral interventions.
   d. Clients should not be in charge of redesigning lifestyle patterns until they reach the TTM stage of action.

8. A nurse who uses the HSCM BIO strategies is most likely to make which of the following cluster diagnoses?
   a. Overeating, irregular exercise, depression, type 2 diabetes
   b. Overeating related to tension stress, decreased exercise related to poor body image, lacking skills in expression of anger
   c. Overeating evening meals, weight loss resistance resulting from habitual 20 to 30 minutes exercise without higher energy challenge
   d. Overeating carbohydrates, lack of exercise related to loneliness and shame about weight, family history of diabetes

9. Once individuals learn to use the EAT for Hunger strategy, what happens?
   a. They become aware of physical hunger, slowly eat smaller portions until hunger is gone, and eat again when hunger returns.
   b. They become aware of how smaller meals eaten on a regular schedule can keep them from getting overly hungry.
   c. They learn to drink water and exercise before eating three regular meals per day.
   d. They learn that hunger will not return for hours if they carefully listen to their feelings of being full.

10. A nurse who uses the ESTEEM for Self and Others strategy, helps individuals to do which of the following?

   a. Eat only when hungry, stand up for themselves, tell others what is on their mind, exercise at every opportunity, and meditate or pray.

   b. Use coping strategies to deal with anger, buy new clothes to feel good about their looks, and spend more time with those they love.

   c. Conserve energy on anaerobic exercise, do spiritual reading, spend more time with others, eat and exercise in a state of meditation.

   d. Learn to put themselves first more of the time and build self-esteem through daily meditation, spiritual time, and personal creativity.

Chapter 24

Smoking Cessation

Cynthia C. Barrere and
Christina Bergh Jackson

■ DEFINITIONS

Habit breakers New action behaviors that replace old "smoke signals" or triggers.

Quit line A telephone smoking cessation resource available 7 days a week to support tobacco cessation efforts.

Smoke signals/triggers Phenomena in the internal and external environment that create a desire to smoke.

■ THEORY AND RESEARCH

1. Smoking is best defined as inhalation of tobacco burned in cigarettes for nicotine absorption.
2. Nicotine is highly addictive for several reasons:
   a. It has powerful effects on brain function and the feel-good neurotransmitters dopamine, endorphins, and norepinephrine.
   b. It can both calm the user who is feeling anxious or stimulate the user who is feeling sluggish.
   c. It is legal and does not alter level of consciousness or ability to function.
   d. Smokers develop an emotional attachment to smoking as a default adaptation mechanism in lieu of other healthier coping mechanisms.
3. It is helpful to view tobacco use as a coping mechanism indicative of underlying issues in need of healing, rather than viewing smoking as the chief problem.
   a. Smokers often report starting at age 10 or 11 years to impress peers or cope with "stress."

b. Smoking is an indication of adverse childhood events and traumas from which children must recover and heal.
   c. Smoking as an attempt to handle stress and trauma provides a more complete picture of a holistic plan to support the cessation of tobacco use.

The Prevalence of Smoking and Its Health Consequences

1. Smoking continues to be the chief cause of preventable morbidity and mortality today.[1]
2. With an estimated 44.5 million smokers in the United States, it is thought that 430,000 premature deaths are caused annually because of smoking.[2] One out of every five adults is a smoker, and there is a disproportionately higher prevalence of smoking among adults with lower educational attainment.[1]
3. Less than half of smokers ever achieve long-term abstinence.[3]
4. These statistics are sobering and underscore the need to focus on smoking *prevention*.
5. Cigarette smoking (and secondhand smoke) contributes to four of the five leading causes of death per year in the United States, including lung cancer, coronary heart disease, chronic lung disease, and stroke.

Women and Smoking

1. Smoking during pregnancy harms both mother and baby and is a leading cause of morbidity and mortality during the intrauterine and early childhood stages of life.[4]

2. Marketing campaigns over the years have used glamorous imagery to promote cigarettes and offer "light" or low-tar alternatives that falsely claim safety advantages.
3. Chronic obstructive pulmonary disease (COPD), once thought of as a predominately male disease, now kills more women than breast cancer, and the number of new cases of COPD in women is increasing three times faster than in men.[5]
4. Smoking is a problem among nurses. Evidence suggests nurses often begin smoking in nursing school.[6]

Environmental Tobacco Smoke

1. Secondhand smoke or environmental tobacco smoke (ETS) also causes problems.
2. ETS is a combination of smoke from the burning end of a cigarette, cigar, or pipe and the smoke exhaled from a smoker's lungs. ETS also includes "thirdhand smoke," or the residual chemical contamination that remains in an environment (clinging to furniture, carpets, walls, etc.).[7]
3. Children of mothers who smoke more than 10 cigarettes per day are twice as likely to develop asthma as are children of nonsmokers.[8]

Physiologic Responses to Smoking

1. Smoking and tobacco contribute directly to death. Smoking strips the lungs of their normal defenses and completely paralyzes the natural cleansing processes. As exposure continues, the bronchi begin to thicken, which predisposes the person to bacterial and viral infections, asthma, emphysema, and cancer.[9]
2. The smoker's heart rate and blood pressure significantly elevate, increasing the risk of cardiac, stroke, and vascular disease.[8]
3. With each inhalation, irritating gases affect the eyes, nose, and throat; carbon monoxide enters the bloodstream, and its concentration eventually rises to a level 4 to 15 times as high as that of a nonsmoker.
4. The constriction of tiny blood vessels decreases the delivery of oxygen to the skin and contributes to "smoker's face," where deep lines appear around the mouth, eyes, and center of the brow. The muscular puffing action also contributes to lines around the mouth.
5. There is an established link between nicotine and erection problems in male smokers.
6. Smoking adversely affects fertility by decreasing sperm count and sperm motility. Female smokers are significantly more likely than nonsmoking females to be infertile.

Cultural Considerations and Special Populations

1. Resources must be linguistically appropriate, and accessible, including for those with sensory impairments such as deafness or blindness.
2. The Internet is a valuable resource for those with special needs of any kind.
3. Smokers diagnosed with mental illness (including schizophrenia, psychosis) can benefit from cessation counseling and resources accessible and tailored to accommodate special needs.[10]
4. Native American tobacco users often have difficulty with smoking cessation because tobacco use is part of sacred ceremony.

■ SMOKING CESSATION
Measuring Successful Cessation

1. Smoking cessation is not easy; success is measured in small increments.
2. Measures of smoking cessation success can be defined as point prevalence (a measure taken at one point in time) at the end of a cessation program or long-term abstinence lasting for 1 year or more.[11]

Self-Quitters, Healthcare Provider Counseling, and Nurse Follow-up Advice

1. The quitter must be motivated and ready to quit. Careful exploration of these factors with the client, and strategic support to bolster strengths and minimize challenges, can amplify chances of quitting.
2. Smokers who received nonsmoking advice from their healthcare providers were nearly twice as likely to quit smoking.
3. Heavy smokers (25 cigarettes a day) are more likely to participate in an organized cessation program.

4. Motivational interviewing (covered in Chapter 10 of *Holistic Nursing: A Handbook for Practice* [6th edition]) by primary care providers increases the success rate of quitting."[12]

5. The "5 As" behavioral approach has been adopted by the Tobacco Free Nurses.[13] Key elements of this approach include the following:

   a. Ask: Always ask about tobacco use during every patient encounter.
   b. Advise: Provide any and all tobacco users with strong verbal encouragement to quit.
   c. Assess: Determine motivation to quit and stage of readiness.
   d. Assist: Provide counseling, refer to cessation resources, and arrange support.
   e. Arrange: Plan follow-up visits to encourage ongoing abstinence or new attempts to quit.

6. Medical and nursing education need to integrate smoking cessation strategies into their curricula.

Quit Lines

1. Twenty-four-hour-a-day telephone quit lines are available to assist smokers who would like to quit.

2. Trained counselors are available to talk with callers to evaluate where they are in the smoking cessation process and assist with the development of a quit plan.

Pharmacologic Therapies in Support of Cessation

1. Nicotine replacement therapy decreases intensity of withdrawal symptoms and the urge to smoke.

2. Nicotine gum, lozenges, and the transdermal patch are available over the counter, and nicotine cartridge inhalers, nasal spray, and higher-dose patches are available by prescription.[14]

3. Nicotine replacement therapy does not release the client from the bad effects of nicotine including nausea, dyspepsia, altered cardiac rhythms, dizziness, headache, and local irritations of the nose, mouth, and skin that vary with mode of delivery[15] and should be discontinued as soon as possible.

Life Span Considerations

1. It is critical to identify teens in need of cessation counseling because this is when so many smokers become addicted.

2. Facilitators of smoking programs aimed at youth must be able to connect in nonjudgmental ways with teens to enhance trustworthiness, caring, and the ability to hold confidence.[16]

3. Teens are also at risk for trying smokeless tobacco (i.e. snuff, chewing tobacco), which is addictive and dangerous.

4. Nurses can promote self-efficacy and therefore successful smoking cessation by facilitating strategic support and growth.[17,18]

5. Cessation in older smokers can derive significant health and financial benefits.

Risks Associated with Quitting

1. Clients taking theophylline, clozapine, warfarin, insulin, or olanzapine while smoking might need to have dosage adjustments (reductions) once they abstain from tobacco.[19]

2. Psychoemotional risks of cessation include a tendency toward depression and risk of suicide, especially if other coping mechanisms and outlets for emotional issues are not facilitated and developed.

3. Smokers can experience flu-like symptoms and/or cough as they withdraw from smoking and the body detoxifies itself. Nutritious foods and appropriate supplements, fluids, and exercise can support healing and feelings of well-being.

The Transtheoretical Model of Change

1. The Transtheoretical Model of Change provides a theoretical basis for explaining when and how people change behaviors.[20] The model supports the notion that change occurs in a cyclic rather than linear fashion.[21] Five stages of change that provide a temporal structure for monitoring the change process include the following:

   a. Precontemplation: No intention of quitting within the next 6 months
   b. Contemplation: Seriously considering quitting within the next 6 months
   c. Preparation: Seriously planning to quit within the next 30 days and has made at least one quit attempt in past year

d. Action: Former smoker continuously quit for fewer than 6 months

e. Maintenance: Former smoker continuously quit for longer than 6 months

Behavioral and Lifestyle Approaches to Smoking Cessation

1. Smoking cessation is stressful to the body; careful planning and self-care can help a great deal.
2. The smoker might like the image of being "in training," as an athlete would be.
3. Using a variety of preferred strategies in combination can bolster the client's ability to be successful.
4. Smoking diary
   a. Clients might find it helpful to keep a smoking diary of when, where, how often, and what moods are associated with smoking.
   b. The client records the feelings associated with smoking and begins to think about new habits to replace these urges.
   c. Keeping such a record for several weeks before the quit date allows the client to identify patterns and smoking triggers upon which an action plan and strategies to quit can be developed.
5. Preparing for the quit date
   a. In preparation for quitting, the client should take the time to identify personal reasons for quitting.
   b. Once certain that it is time to quit, the client's goal is to be a nonsmoker in 5 days.
   c. The nurse can encourage the client to identify family members, friends, or a specific person who might want to join the effort as a quit-smoking partner.
6. Preparing for nicotine withdrawal
   a. Preparation for nicotine withdrawal facilitates the process of being a nonsmoker.
   b. There is no one best way to quit smoking.
   c. Some people are successful at just quitting "cold turkey" and going through the nicotine withdrawal, with the worst part usually lasting 5 days or fewer.
   d. Others require a gradual decrease of nicotine with the use of nicotine replacement therapy.

e. The client must decide which approach to try.

7. Preparing a smoke-free environment
   a. During the first few nonsmoking days, the client rids the body of toxic waste left from the cigarettes by bathing, brushing teeth, drinking water, exercising, relaxing, imaging, resting, and eating healthy.
   b. A fresh nonsmoking living environment can be accomplished by placing clean filters in heating and cooling units and cleaning carpets, drapes, clothes, office, and car.
   c. Signs can be placed on the office door or at home: "Thank you for not smoking."
   d. The client should become aware of how quickly the senses of smell and taste increase and how disgusting the smell and taste of cigarettes become.
8. Identifying smoking triggers and creating habit breakers
   a. Identification of personal smoking triggers and creating habit breakers can assist the process.
   b. Becoming smoke free is directly related to minor changes in daily routines, referred to as habit breakers.
   c. Many ex-smokers report that the first 5 days of being smoke free are the hardest. Minor or major changes in daily activities can be less stressful if accompanied by a healing state of awareness.
   d. Relapses can become learning situations.
   e. The client can identify negative self-talk or a stressful situation in which a new habit breaker might not have been used soon enough.
   f. The client can list selected events and times when smoking is most likely such as reading the newspaper, during a coffee break, and after eating a meal and create a habit breaker for each.
9. Nutritional counseling
   a. Nutritional counseling should encourage the client to choose nutrient-dense foods.
   b. In general, vegetables, fruits, whole grains, and high-quality protein are essential. Nuts, seeds, vegetable juices, lots of good water to maintain generous

hydration and flush out toxins, a high-potency multivitamin/mineral supplement with omega-3 fish oils, B supplement, vitamin C, and vitamin D are indicated.

10. Exercise
    a. Regular exercise has been shown to reduce stress in the body and improve mood.
    b. It is beneficial for the client to engage in a regular program of enjoyable movement at the highest level of vigor possible.
    c. Exercise reduces cravings and mood disturbance, improves self-esteem, promotes self-concept as a person who engages in healthy behaviors, and reduces weight gain.
    d. Yoga postures can be helpful for smoking cessation. The breathing, stretching, strengthening, and meditative aspects of yoga practice are of benefit to those seeking a release from addictive behaviors.

11. Client bill of rights
    a. Clients engaged in smoking cessation can develop and recite their bill of rights.
    b. The client can be creative and update/add to this list at any time.
    c. A sample client bill of rights is found in Chapter 23 of *Holistic Nursing: Handbook for Practice*.

12. Integration of rewards
    a. The client should plan a reward at least every 5 to 7 days for having a smoke-free lifestyle.
    b. These rewards should continue as long as the client needs to be aware of new lifestyle habits and/or prevent relapse.

13. Reinforcement of positive self-talk
    a. The client needs to learn to recognize the self-talk that sabotages his or her positive outlook.
    b. The nurse can teach the client positive affirmations such as "I am feeling more free," "I am feeling in control."
    c. The nurse can assist with cognitive restructuring of automatic negative thoughts and negative rationalization of those who are quitting and assist the patient to reframe negative statements.

14. Journaling and self-reflection
    a. Journal writing and self-reflection can help to get feelings up and out through the quit process.
    b. Self-reflection can lead to self-awareness, and journaling can assist the smoker to identify positive changes that can be made.

15. Breathing techniques
    a. Breathing is a powerful strategy to soothe, energize, and calm the client.
    b. The *4-2-8 count breath* can be very helpful, and the counts can be varied to meet the needs of the individual client because breathing rhythm mimics smoking behavior.
    c. Another useful breathing technique is the "Butt Kicking Breath" demonstrated online at www.sadienardini.com.
    d. Alternate-nostril breathing can soothe and shift mood in a positive direction, therefore enhancing quit efforts.

16. Guided imagery and hypnosis
    a. For an example of a smoking cessation guided imagery script, see Chapter 23, in *Holistic Nursing: Handbook for Practice*.
    b. Hypnosis, a process that includes relaxation techniques, guided imagery, and suggestion, is often used in behavioral approaches to smoking cessation.
    c. Guided imagery with suggestions (hypnosis) enhances the client's success at becoming smoke free.
    d. For additional nursing interventions, see Exhibit 23-1, Nursing Interventions: Smoking Cessation, in *Holistic Nursing: Handbook for Practice*.

■ NOTES

1. Centers for Disease Control and Prevention. (2009). Cigarette smoking among adults and trends in smoking cessation—United States, 2008. *Morbidity and Mortality Weekly Report, 58*(44), 1227–1233.

2. National Institutes of Health State-of-the-Science Panel. (2006). National Institutes of Health State-of-the-Science Conference statement: Tobacco use: Prevention, cessation, and control. *Annals of Internal Medicine, 145*(11), 839–844.

3. Shahab, L., & McEwen, A. (2009). Online support for smoking cessation: A systematic review of the literature. *Addiction, 104,* 1792–1804.

4. Karatay, G., Gulumser, K., & Emiroglu, O. (2010). The effect of motivational interviewing on smoking cessation in pregnant women. *Journal of Advanced Nursing, 66*(6), 1328–1337.

5. Rahmanian, S., Diaz, P. T., & Wewers, M. E. (2011). Tobacco use and cessation among women: Research and treatment-related issues. *Journal of Women's Health, 20*(3), 349–357.

6. Bialous, S., Sarna, L., Wells, M., Elashoff, D., Wewers, M. E., & Froelicher, E. S. (2009). Characteristics of nurses who used the Internet-based Nurses QuitNet for smoking cessation. *Public Health Nursing, 26*(4), 329–338.

7. Winickoff, J. P., Friebely, J., Tanski, S. E., Sherrod, C., Matt, G. E., Hovell, M., F.,...McMillen, R. C. (2009). Beliefs about the health effects of 'thirdhand' smoke and home smoking bans. *Pediatrics, 123*(1), 74–79.

8. Fagerstrom, K. (2002). The epidemiology of smoking: Health consequences and benefits of cessation. *Drugs, 62,* 1–9.

9. Grossman, J., Donaldson, S., Belton, L., & Oliver, R. H. (2008). 5 A's smoking cessation with recovering women in treatment. *Journal of Addictions Nursing, 19,* 1–8.

10. Morrison, K., & Naegle, M. (2010). An evidence-based protocol for smoking cessation for persons with psychotic disorders. *Journal of Addictions Nursing, 21,* 79–86.

11. West, R. (2007). The clinical significance of 'small' effects of smoking cessation treatments. *Addiction, 102,* 506–509.

12. Lai, D. T., Cahill, K., Qin, Y., & Tang, J. L. (2010). Motivational interviewing for smoking cessation, *Cochrane Database Systematic Review,* 1, CD006936.

13. U.S. Preventive Services Task Force. (2003, November). *Counseling to prevent tobacco use and tobacco-related diseases: Recommendation statement.* Rockville, MD: Agency for Healthcare Research and Quality.

14. Feigenbaum, J. (2010). Pharmacological aids to promote smoking cessation. *Journal of Addictions Nursing, 21,* 87–97.

15. Huber, G., & Mahajan, V. (2008). Successful smoking cessation. *Disease Management and Health Outcomes, 16*(5), 335–343.

16. Jarrett, T., Horn, K., & Zhang, J. (2009). Teen perceptions of facilitator characteristics in a school-based smoking cessation program. *Journal of School Health, 79*(7), 297–303.

17. Heale, R., & Griffin, M. (2009). Self-efficacy with application to adolescent smoking cessation: A concept analysis. *Journal of Advanced Nursing, 65*(4), 912–918.

18. Bricker, J. B., Liu, J., Comstock, B. A., & Peterson, A. V. (2010). Social cognitive mediators of adolescent smoking cessation: Results from a large randomized intervention trial. *Psychology of Addictive Behaviors, 24*(3), 436–445.

19. Schaffer, S., Yoon, S., & Zadezensky, I. (2009). A review of smoking cessation: Potentially risky effects on prescribed medications. *Journal of Clinical Nursing, 18,* 1533–1540.

20. Prochaska, J. O., Plumber, B. A., Velicer, W. F., Rossi, J. S., Redding, C. A., Greene, G. W.,... Laforge, R. (2004). Multiple risk expert systems interventions: Impact of simultaneous stage-matched expert systems for smoking, high-fat diet, and sun exposure in a population of parents. *Health Psychology, 23,* 503–516.

21. Prochaska, J. O., Velicer, W. F., Redding, C., Rossi, J. S., Goldstein, M., DePue, J.,...Brett, A. P. (2005). Stage-based expert systems to guide a population of primary care patients to quit smoking, eat healthier, prevent skin cancer, and receive regular mammograms. *Preventive Medicine, 41,* 406–416.

◼ STUDY QUESTIONS

Basic Level

1. **Which of the following answer choices best defines smoking?**
   a. The use of tobacco
   b. A natural means of reducing body weight
   c. Inhalation of tobacco burned in cigarettes for nicotine absorption
   d. Chewing tobacco leaves

2. **Which of the following answer choices best defines smoking cessation?**
   a. Stopping the use of cigarettes, cigars, pipes, and all continuous tobacco intake
   b. Ceasing the use of tobacco in social situations only
   c. Throwing out all smoking paraphernalia
   d. Getting rid of cigarettes in automobiles

3. **According to the Transtheoretical Model, what are the five stages of smoking cessation (behavioral change)?**
   a. Precontemplation, contemplation, preparation, action, and maintenance
   b. Precontemplation, contemplation, preparation, announcement, and maintenance
   c. Precontemplation, contemplation, programming, announcement, and maintenance
   d. Precontemplation, contemplation, programming, action, and maintenance

4. At a minimum, what should a smoking diary include?
   a. Date, time, activity, cigarette brand
   b. Date, time, activity, perception of cigarette
   c. Date, time, activity, social support groups
   d. Date, time, activity, perception of urgency of cigarette

5. When are smokers at the action stage of smoking cessation or behavioral change?
   a. They entertain thoughts about quitting.
   b. They actively endeavor to promote smoking cessation and abstinence for at least 6 months.
   c. They experience continued smoking abstinence beginning 6 months after cessation.
   d. They are ready and open to advice about smoking cessation.

Advanced Level

6. Mr. Conti, a 47-year-old man, seeks help with smoking cessation. He has thought about quitting cigarettes and has even made two attempts, but resumed smoking after only 2 days in each case. Which of the following interventions might the nurse suggest to Mr. Conti with more long term smoking cessation success?
   a. Encourage him to keep a smoking diary, rest, and stay away from his family and friends
   b. Encourage him to exercise, keep a smoking diary, and refrain from visiting family and friends
   c. Assess his knowledge about the health effects of smoking, have him do a self-assessment of why he smokes, have him list the reasons he wants to quit
   d. Assess his knowledge about the health effects of smoking, rest, and encourage him to seek support from family, friends, and coworkers

7. The nurse practitioner is doing a physical exam on Ms. Winters, a 22-year-old woman. She appears healthy. She has an odor of cigarette smoke about her person.

What kind of assessment questions does the nurse ask her?
   a. "Do you smoke? If so, how many cigarettes a day do you smoke? What are your reasons for smoking?"
   b. "Do you like smoking? How many cigarettes a day do you smoke? Why haven't you stopped smoking?"
   c. "How many cigarettes a day do you smoke? Do you know how dangerous cigarette smoking is? Why haven't you stopped smoking?"
   d. "Do you smoke? If so, how many cigarettes a day do you smoke? How many years have you been smoking?"

8. For Ms. Winters in question 7, how can the nurse begin to help her with smoking cessation?
   a. Tell her that when she smokes up to 1 pack a day, she needs to quit.
   b. Tell her that smoking can kill her and she needs to quit.
   c. Ask her if she would like to have some help with cessation.
   d. Ask her if she realizes the hazards of smoking.

9. John, a 19-year-old high school student, has no plans, interests, or hobbies. He likes to hang out with the guys (mostly younger). He appears to be healthy but needs a physical exam for a part-time job. The assessment of smoking status finds John to be a current, heavy smoker, smoking 2 packs per day. What is the nurse's assessment?
   a. Recognize that John is probably at the precontemplation stage and it will be a challenge to motivate him to quit.
   b. Recognize that John is probably at the precontemplation stage and will need support from the nurse to get started on cessation.
   c. Recognize that John is probably at the contemplation stage and will want to stop smoking to be a better role model for the younger guys.
   d. Recognize that John is probable at the contemplation stage and it will be a challenge to motivate him to quit.

10. Ms. Stowe, a 58-year-old woman, is afraid to stop smoking. She smokes 15 cigarettes per day "to keep her weight down." Smoking also helps her concentrate on her job as a realtor, reduces her stress, and boosts her self-confidence. She is in the contemplation stage for smoking cessation. The nurse working with Ms. Stowe can suggest which of the following interventions to help move her into the preparation stage of smoking cessation?

a. Persuade her to exercise actively, watch her diet to maintain her weight, and cut down to 10 cigarettes a day.

b. Persuade her to exercise actively, watch her diet to maintain her weight, and institute a stress reduction strategy such as breathing exercises.

c. Institute a stress reduction strategy such as breathing exercises, seek support from family and friends, and keep her feet elevated three times a day to rest.

d. Watch her diet to maintain her weight, institute a stress reduction strategy such as breathing exercises, and cut down to 12 cigarettes a day.

Chapter 25

Addiction and Recovery Counseling

Bonney Gulino Schaub and
Megan McInnis Burt

■ DEFINITIONS

Addiction A physiologic or psychological dependence on a substance (e.g., alcohol, cocaine) or behavior (e.g., gambling, sex, eating).

Denial A major dynamic in the process of addiction in which the person willfully refuses to accept the reality of his or her behavior and its effect on self and others.

Detoxification The physical process of withdrawing from using drugs or alcohol.

Dry drunk Referring to alcoholism (*dry* refers to not drinking) where a person has stopped drinking but has not extended this change to developing mentally, emotionally, and spiritually.

New consciousness A concept used in Alcoholics Anonymous (AA) that refers to a movement away from addictive thinking and toward an understanding of one's life purpose or spiritual purpose.

Recovery The mental, emotional, physical, and spiritual actions that support conscious living and freedom from addictive behaviors.

Relapse A return to addictive behavior.

Spiritual awakening An expansion of awareness that results in a realization that the isolated individual is, in fact, participating in a universe of divine intention and order.

■ THEORY AND RESEARCH

1. Addiction is a chronic, often relapsing brain disease that causes compulsive drug seeking and use, despite harmful consequences to the addicted individual and to those around him or her. Although the initial decision to take drugs is voluntary for most people, the brain changes that occur over time challenge a person's self-control and ability to resist intense impulses urging him or her to take drugs. Similar to other chronic, relapsing diseases, such as diabetes, asthma, or heart disease, drug addiction can be managed successfully. And as with other chronic diseases, it is not uncommon for a person to relapse and begin abusing drugs again. Relapse, however, does not signal treatment failure—rather, it indicates that treatment should be reinstated, adjusted, or that an alternative treatment is needed to help the individual. Treatment of chronic diseases involves changing deeply embedded behaviors.[1-3]

2. It can be wrongfully assumed that drug abusers lack moral principles or willpower and that they could stop using drugs simply by choosing to change their behavior. In reality, drug addiction is a complex disease, and quitting takes more than good intentions. In fact, because drugs change the brain in ways that foster compulsive drug abuse, quitting is difficult, even for those who are ready to do so.

3. Drugs of abuse such as cocaine trigger epigenetic changes in certain brain regions, affecting hundreds of genes at once. Some of these changes remain long after the drug has been cleared from the system. Research in this area suggests that some of the long-term effects of drug abuse and addiction might be written in epigenetic code.[4-6]

4. It is estimated that more than 28 million children are living in homes with adults who have alcohol use disorders.[7] Children raised in homes with substance-abusing parents are at increased risk for chronic anxiety disorders and social phobias as well as at increased risk for their own substance abuse.[8] In the United States in 2008, almost one-third of adolescents aged 12 to 17 years drank alcohol in the past year, around one-fifth used an illicit drug, and almost one-sixth smoked cigarettes. Caffeine is a widely used psychoactive substance that is legal, easy to obtain, and socially acceptable to consume. Although once relatively restricted to use among adults, caffeine-containing drinks are now consumed regularly by children. Children and adolescents are the fastest growing population of caffeine users with an increase of 70% in the past 30 years. Energy drinks sales have grown by more than 50% since 2005 and represent the fastest growing segment of the beverage industry.[9]

5. Because of the prevalence of alcoholism and other addictions, nurses in every practice setting inevitably will work with individuals who are addicted, who are in recovery, or whose lives are affected by the addiction of a friend or family member.

■ ADDICTION DEFINED

1. Alcoholics Anonymous (AA), in its basic book (referred to by people in AA as the Big Book), describes alcoholism as a "mental obsession and a physical compulsion."[10] This description of a pattern of thinking and behaving applies to many things besides alcohol, most obviously the use of other substances such as cocaine, heroin, methamphetamine, and marijuana. The elements of obsession and compulsion are evident in the actions of people with unhealthy relationships to food, exercise, work, gambling, Internet use, television viewing, shopping, sexual behaviors (including compulsive use of pornography), and other activities. A recent study suggests that the use of tanning beds can be addictive.[11,12]

2. Certain elements distinguish the process of addiction from other use of any of these substances or behaviors. The key difference is in the individual's relationship to the substance or behavior. In the addictive process, the element of choice is absent. A woman no longer chooses to relax with a glass of wine at a dinner party—she goes to the party because it is an opportunity to drink a great deal. A man no longer enjoys watching a sporting event—he watches it only because he has a bet on it. A young college student takes up running to lose weight and feels compelled to go for a run despite her knee injury because she will be depressed and obsessing about her weight without a run of at least 5 miles a day. The mental obsession has overruled the ability to reflect on behavior and has bypassed any self-awareness that could lead to alternative behaviors. These addictive behaviors often coexist with substance abuse. The addictive use of any of these activities serves the same purpose as alcohol or drugs: The person is seeking relief and distraction from painful, unsafe, and vulnerable feelings.

■ THE CYCLE OF ADDICTION

1. All addictions have a basic cycle. In the early stage of addiction, people use substances as a means of changing unsafe or vulnerable feelings. Some commonly heard descriptions of feelings are phrases such as, "Everything gets to me," and "Everything is just too much." Typically, there are physical signs of anxiety such as light-headedness, palpitations, painful self-consciousness, social discomfort, and heightened agitation or irritability.

2. Vulnerability is a normal human emotion that everyone has experienced, but the person vulnerable to addiction feels it more intensely and more frequently. Characteristics such as a low frustration tolerance, a low pain threshold, and a need for instant gratification go along with this vulnerability.

3. Most people who have become addicted to a substance have a vivid memory of their first experience of relief from the feelings of discomfort. This first encounter typically occurs in early adolescence, a time of normal emotional turmoil and struggle for social identity and acceptance. Getting high might have alleviated social anxiety or the pain of family conflicts. The incidence of substance abuse is high among young people in conflict about their sexual identity because they often lack support and positive role models in their life. Sharing drugs or alcohol becomes a way of being accepted into a peer group. The stage is set for dependence and progression to addiction. The process of building emotional and social skills, a major developmental task of adolescence, stops because an instant solution has been found. Picking up where they have left off in emotional and social skill building is one of the major challenges for people in recovery.

4. The early stage of the addictive cycle: In the early stage of addiction, a person has some awareness of seeking relief from discomfort. It might simply be an awareness of feeling stressed, anxious, or self-conscious. The following is a typical progression of feelings and responses in the early stage of addiction:
   a. Unsafe feelings
   b. Mental focus on the feelings
   c. A desire to get rid of the feelings
   d. The use of chemicals to get rid of the feelings
   e. Nervous system disturbance caused by the chemicals
   f. The return of unsafe feelings[13p5]

5. The middle stage of the addictive cycle: In the middle stage of addiction, the unsafe feeling is not experienced as a thought. It is experienced only as danger or discomfort. The person knows that immediate relief comes with use of the substance. The following is the typical progression and recurring pattern in the middle stage of addiction:
   a. Unsafe feelings
   b. The use of chemicals to get rid of the feelings
   c. Nervous system disturbance caused by the chemicals
   d. Unsafe feelings[13pp8,15]

6. The late stage of the addictive cycle: People in the depths of addiction rarely talk about feeling high. The need is more frequently described as a desire to feel normal. The impulse is to escape a feeling that is intolerable. At the late stage of addiction, physical instability replaces the emotional vulnerability. The addiction has come full circle. What was initially used as an answer to unsafe feelings has become the source of unsafe feelings. Mental instability and confusion, mental terrors and paranoia, and hallucinations or feelings of unreality are all possible results of the neurologic damage from the substances. The following is the recurring pattern of the late stage of addiction:
   a. Nervous system disturbance
   b. The use of chemicals
   c. The return of nervous system disturbance[13pp11,16]

■ MODELS OF ADDICTION

1. Many models have been put forth to explain why a person develops an addiction. Nurses working with addicted patients can recognize recurring themes such as familial and environmental patterns of addiction or early childhood trauma and loss. Each of these models offers a piece of a complex puzzle.

2. Medical model: In the medical model, the emphasis is on the physiologic effect of the substance itself. The body's tolerance for the drug leads to the need for greater and greater amounts to achieve the desired effect, which results in addiction. The absence of the drug leads to cravings, and then to a withdrawal or abstinence syndrome characterized by symptoms such as fever, nausea, seizures, chills, hallucinations, and delirium tremens. In this model, the progression toward addiction is a property of the drug's effect. Those in the media often demonstrate this attitude toward addiction when they describe a celebrity who has attended a 30-day alcohol or drug rehabilitation program as free of drugs. In fact, 30 days is just the beginning of treatment. Most drugs of abuse directly or indirectly target the brain's reward system by flooding the circuit with dopamine. Dopamine

is a neurotransmitter present in regions of the brain that regulate movement, emotion, cognition, motivation, and feelings of pleasure. The overstimulation of this system, which rewards our natural behaviors, produces the euphoric effects sought by people who abuse drugs and teaches them to repeat the behavior.

3. Genetic disease model: Research in genetics has focused primarily on alcoholism with strong patterns of alcoholism within families. People with close relatives who are alcoholic are at three to four times greater risk for alcoholism. The closer the genetic tie and the higher the number of affected relatives, the greater the risk. Adoption studies show a three times greater incidence of alcoholism in children of alcoholics, even if they have been raised in a nonalcoholic family.[14] There is evidence that alcohol and tobacco both act on a part of the brain that is involved in rewards, emotions, memory, and thinking. Both alcohol and tobacco have an impact on the neurons that release dopamine, binding at the receptor sites. The presence of a common mechanism of action might shed light on the interplay of alcohol and tobacco addiction.[15]

   a. The emerging field of epigenetics is advancing understanding of the role of genetics in addictions. Epigenetics is the study of changes in the regulation of gene expression and gene activity that are not dependent on DNA sequence. The field of epigenetics refers to the science that studies how the development, functioning, and evolution of biological systems are influenced by forces operating outside the DNA sequence, such as environmental and energetic influences. Studies indicate there is an alteration in gene expression by repeated substance abuse that can produce lasting changes in gene expression within the reward pathways of the brain. Epigenetic mechanisms are providing insight into how drugs alter genetic expression. Insights into the long-lasting adaptations that underlie chronic relapsing addiction are on the edge of research and have implications for new treatments.[16]

4. Dysfunctional family system model: The frequent appearance of addictions within the families of addicts might indicate that substance abuse can be a learned behavior. In effect, children learn by daily close observation of the adults in their environment that conflicts and stressors are to be dealt with using drugs and alcohol. Children usually do not have a conscious awareness of this message. They might not have a full understanding of the role that addiction played in their home life until they reach adulthood and begin their own recovery. It is important to acknowledge that many other people who have grown up in such an environment are aware of the damage done and make a conscious choice to abstain from alcohol or other substances.

5. Self-medication model: According to the self-medication model, the addict has an underlying psychiatric disorder and is, in effect, self-prescribing to alleviate symptoms. For example, in a Canadian survey of more than 14,000 residents ages 18 to 76 years, there was a significantly greater use of alcohol among those who were suffering from depression.[17] Addicts characteristically have tried a variety of substances and have found that they have a strong preference for a particular category of drug and drug effect. It is not unusual for addicts to say that their preferred substance makes them feel normal.

6. Psychosexual, psychoanalytic model: Emerging from Freud's conceptualization of psychosexual stages of development, addiction appears to be a fixation at the oral stage of development. In the psychosexual, psychoanalytic model, an infant or child whose basic needs are unmet becomes focused on seeking gratification of those unmet needs. Emotional development becomes fixated at the age of this early trauma.[13p23] Oral gratification is the most basic need of the infant, as shown in the way an infant receives nourishment and pleasure through sucking. In adulthood, people continue to seek comfort and pleasure from gratification of oral needs through behaviors such as eating, smoking, talking, touching their mouth, and various chewing behaviors. Whereas healthy human activity includes some limited seeking of oral gratification, the addict is fixated at this developmental phase. The

compelling need for comfort derived from oral gratification then becomes focused on the consuming of substances.

7. Ego psychology model: Also emerging from Freudian theory, ego psychology suggests that when an infant's or child's environment does not provide an adequate degree of nurturance and acknowledgment, the child grows into adulthood with an impaired sense of self. This results in feelings of emptiness and hypersensitivity that lead to a self-absorbed and narcissistic relationship with the world. The addict's behaviors are then seen as self-soothing attempts to relieve the basic feelings of emptiness.[13p24]

8. Cultural model: Our culture might be a contributing factor in addiction because it teaches us to seek materialistic answers outside ourselves to experience well-being. People in the United States are confronted with a relentless message of consumerism and quick fixes. This then leads to a society of consumers with impulse disorders who seek instant gratification and believe that there is a pill for every ill.

   a. In recent years, media advertising has bombarded people with messages about both over-the-counter (OTC) and prescription medications. In light of this, it is interesting to note the following information. The total number of drug-related emergency department (ED) visits increased 81% from 2004 (2.5 million) to 2009 (4.6 million). ED visits involving nonmedical use of pharmaceuticals increased 98.4% over the same period, from 627,291 visits to 1,244,679. The largest pharmaceutical increases were observed for oxycodone products (242.2% increase), alprazolam (148.3% increase), and hydrocodone products (124.5% increase). Among ED visits involving illicit drugs, only those involving Ecstasy increased more than 100% from 2004 to 2009 (123.2% increase). Among patients aged 21 years or older, there was an increase of 111.0%.[18,19]

   b. There is also an increased awareness of the abuse of substances among athletes. The primary abuse is of recreational drugs such as cocaine and alcohol. There is a significant increase in the use of performance-enhancing (i.e., ergogenic) drugs such as amphetamines, as well as designer stimulants such as Ecstasy (i.e., methylenedioxymethamphetamine, or MDMA). Two readily available drugs that are amphetamine mimicking when taken in high doses are pseudoephedrine, available in cold medications, and ephedrine marketed as a dietary supplement. Anabolic steroids and other drugs are taken in an attempt to enhance performance and build muscle mass. Additionally, human growth hormone (HGH) precursors are marketed in various forms, promising increased muscle mass, increased energy, and performance enhancement.[20]

9. Character defect model of AA: Alcoholics and other addicts are seen as having different characters and morals from nonaddicts in the character defect model of AA. Although the idea of a moral defect is not used extensively in addiction treatment settings, it is a concept that pervades the AA literature. A person in recovery might explain his or her "character defect" as the reason for his or her difficulty in making behavioral and attitudinal changes.

10. Trance model: Derived from learning theory and the principles of hypnosis, the trance model proposes that the memory of the intense pleasure experienced in response to a substance is never forgotten. The experience is recorded by the pleasure-seeking, pain-avoiding part of the brain and remains, in effect, a deeply planted, posthypnotic suggestion that repeatedly seeks expression. The addict essentially falls in love with the feelings that the addictive behaviors produce. The AA literature speaks to this idea in stating, "The urge to repeat the experience of becoming 'high' is so strong that we will forsake...our responsibilities and values,...our families, our jobs, our personal welfare, our respect, and our integrity...to satisfy the urge."[21p2]

11. Transpersonal intoxication model: According to the transpersonal intoxication model, the desire to break free of a limited, time-bound, socially defined sense of self as well as the desire to expand consciousness are the driving forces in addiction. Many people have experimented with lysergic acid

diethylamide (LSD), marijuana, psilocybin mushrooms, peyote cactus, and other psychedelic substances and have experienced expanded states of awareness that have resulted in spiritual and creative breakthroughs. The challenge then is to integrate these insights into daily life.

   a. There is a significant degree of substance abuse and addiction among artists, writers, performers, and musicians. This model suggests that their desire to break free of mental and emotional limitations is at the heart of their substance use. Artists often mention a fear of losing this creative capacity—of becoming ordinary—as they enter recovery. They have given creative power to the substance rather than trusting it resides within. The ability to practice their creative endeavor while sober becomes a major milestone in the recovery process.

12. Transpersonal–existential model: In the transpersonal–existential model, the human condition is such that humans are inherently anxious because they have knowledge of their mortality. Everyone finds ways to bypass or deny this awareness of reality. Becker wrote that a person has to protect himself against the world, and he can do this only as any other animal would—"by...shutting off experience and developing an obliviousness both to the terrors of the world and to his own anxieties. Otherwise he would be crippled for action...some people have more trouble with their lies than others. The world is too much for them."[22p178] This heightened awareness and sensitivity to the human condition can lead to addiction as a solution to the existential pain.

13. Vulnerability model of recovery from addiction: A holistic nursing model of the recovery process, the vulnerability model of recovery honors the biological, emotional, social, familial, neurochemical, and spiritual aspects of addiction. It focuses on the lived experience of the addict, which is that of essential vulnerability. The model points to specific ways that the holistic nurse can facilitate the healing journey of full bio-psycho-social-spiritual recovery. The basic points are presented in Exhibit 24-1 in *Holistic Nursing: A Handbook for Practice* (6th ed.).

■ RECOGNITION OF ADDICTION

1. Given the prevalence of alcoholism and other addictions, it can be assumed that nurses in every clinical area are working with people whose lives are affected by this problem and it is essential that all nurses become skilled in assessing addiction, as well as recognizing risk factors and behaviors suggestive of substance abuse. Nurses must first examine any preconceived notions that they might have about what an addict or alcoholic looks like. Addiction is a problem that occurs in every profession, in every educational and socioeconomic group, in every ethnic group, and in every age group. The most challenging, and potentially frustrating, aspect of working with people at the stage of active addiction is their pervasive denial of the problem, even when confronted with blatant evidence of their addiction. Alcoholics Anonymous uses the phrase "self-will run riot" in describing this behavior. It is the key obstacle to entering into the healing process of recovery. (For definitions of denial, see Exhibit 24-2 in *Holistic Nursing: A Handbook for Practice* (6th ed.).

2. The addict's loyalty to the substance is profound. It surpasses loyalty to family and friends and is the cause of the addict's manipulations. The nurse should not personalize these manipulations. Attempts to be of help often meet outright rejection or failure. The root of the addict's behaviors is an intense fear of living without the mood-altering effects of the alcohol or drugs. The behaviors are attempts to control the world and avoid painful feelings. The first step of recovery is relinquishing this control effort and admitting to oneself and others that the addictive process is not working, that it is actually making everything worse, that he or she does not know what to do, and that he or she must learn a new way to be in the world. This new way means a change in attitude to recognize that people who want to help stop the addictive behaviors are acting from a place of caring. (See Exhibit 24-2 in *Holistic Nursing: A Handbook for Practice*.)

■ DETOXIFICATION

1. The simplest, most straightforward aspect of the recovery process is detoxification. When medical management of detoxification is necessary, brief inpatient or outpatient treatment is available in many hospitals and addiction treatment centers.
2. Acupuncture has been successfully used in detoxifying many people from alcohol, heroin, nicotine, and other drugs. In recent years, it has gained wider acceptance and has been found to be a powerfully effective, natural treatment that is simple, safe, and inexpensive. Acupuncture can improve patient outcomes in terms of program retention and reductions in cravings, anxiety, sleep disturbance, and need for pharmaceuticals.[23,24]

■ ALCOHOLICS ANONYMOUS

1. With its 12-step, self-help treatment approach, AA offers one of the most important, effective, and widely accepted interventions in addiction treatment. The 12 steps of Alcoholics Anonymous put forth a systematic progression of actions that, when followed, assist the person in recovery to find a new way to be in the world. Ongoing peer support as well as support for spiritual development were cited as significant factors in the effectiveness of this program.[25-27]
2. An important element in AA is the practice of providing service to other members of the program by becoming a sponsor. Members who have achieved a strong recovery are encouraged to be available to newer participants to help them in their sobriety. They might attend meetings with the new participant, be available by phone on a regular basis, and generally serve as a role model and guide toward effective use of the program.

■ EARLY RECOVERY

1. Detoxification is the initial step in early recovery, and it is just the beginning of the addicted person's process of making new choices, moment by moment, hour by hour, and day by day.

2. The nurse can help the person in recovery to make healthy choices by intensive questioning about old patterns of substance abuse and other behaviors. This information can then be used to develop new ways of responding. Because behaviors associated with addiction are totally integrated into the person's life, he or she needs help in recognizing them and accepting the fact that they are no longer possible. The following are some important questions for the nurse to ask:
   a. Where did the addictive behavior take place? Some people stay isolated in their home or car when using drugs, while others prefer social settings such as bars, clubs, or the work environment.
   b. What special rituals were a part of the addictive behavior? People typically have a routine associated with their substance use. For example, a marijuana abuser might purchase her favorite foods before using the drug.
   c. What locations served as cues for the addictive behavior? The alcoholic might associate strong memories with particular liquor stores or bars, and these places can have strong pulls. A particular street sign or exit on the expressway can trigger the desire to go to the neighborhood where drugs were bought and shared.
   d. What people in the environment were associated with the addictive behavior? The person in recovery might come to realize that everyone he or she knows is associated with the drug use. People in recovery often cannot name a single person they can count on to be drug free. The feeling of loss of family and friends associated with this realization can be profound.

■ NUTRITIONAL FACTORS

1. Alcohol has high caloric content, but it is useless as a source of nutrients. Malnutrition is common in alcoholics because they often fail to consume adequate amounts of food. In addition, alcohol interferes with the absorption of vitamins and minerals. Alcoholics typically are deficient in B vitamins, especially thiamine, pyridoxine, vitamin B_{12}, and folate. There is also some

evidence that the B vitamin deficiency itself might increase alcohol cravings.

2. Some studies indicate that alcoholics who followed healthy dietary plans that included both nutritional and vitamin supplementation, along with nutrition education, were more successful at maintaining sobriety.[28] As stated earlier, recovery is a process of repeatedly choosing healthy, life-affirming actions.

3. For the recovering alcoholic or other addict, working with a holistic nurse to develop a nutritious eating plan can be an important first step on the path to health. As with any treatment plan, the key to its success depends on compliance. Having a variety of approaches helps to develop personalized care and increase the likelihood of acceptance.

■ BODY WORK AND ENERGY WORK

1. In the early phase of recovery, shortly after cessation of use and resolution of any primary withdrawal symptoms, the person in recovery might experience difficulty sleeping, general agitation, and irritability. Acupuncture has been found to be very effective in the reduction of withdrawal symptoms and in the overall rebalancing of the physical system. Other types of body work such as Reiki, therapeutic touch, massage, and reflexology can be of help in calming the body.

2. The energy-based approach of Healing Touch (HT) has been effectively used with patients in recovery from alcoholism.[29] Another innovative practitioner has introduced the use of drumming circles into recovery work. One aspect of this treatment's effectiveness is in creating a sense of connectedness with self and others.[30]

3. Avoiding caffeine, drinking plenty of water and soothing herbal teas, exercising, and taking warm baths or showers are all helpful during this period when the body is literally releasing and cleansing itself of toxins.

■ BODY–MIND RESPONSES

1. Benson and Wallace conducted a classic study on the application of meditation to the treatment of substance abuse. Their study found that those who used prescription and illicit drugs began reducing their intake of drugs as they learned to enter a deep state of relaxation and the more they meditated, the less they drank.[31]

2. In another study, addicts practicing Vipassana meditation (VM) showed significant reductions in alcohol, marijuana, and crack cocaine use.[32] Qi gong, which blends relaxation, breathing, guided imagery, inward attention, and mindfulness to elicit a tranquil, healing state, was introduced into a short-term residential treatment program. Participants reported greater reductions in craving, anxiety, and withdrawal symptoms.[33] Brain wave biofeedback also has been used successfully with people in recovery.[34]

■ RELAPSE

1. A person can achieve abstinence and still not make life changes at the level of emotions and spirit. A person can, in fact, stop drinking and continue to be hostile, rageful, blaming, and irresponsible. These people are controlling their behavior through force of will. Alcoholics Anonymous calls these individuals "dry drunks." The person functioning in recovery in this way is at greater risk for relapse.

2. Relapse is an ongoing issue in every stage of recovery. Many people stop completely without treatment, or with very brief intervention, but others relapse repeatedly. In AA, there is a saying, "The further you are from your last drink, the closer you are to your next." It is helpful to differentiate between someone who very briefly returns to drinking and then returns to abstinence versus someone who resumes heavy drinking. The brief episode is referred to as a lapse rather than a full relapse. This distinction is important to avoid the all-or-nothing, black-and-white thinking that can sabotage the process of recovery.

3. It is estimated that up to 75% of people in recovery relapse within the first year. It is significant to note that the figure is estimated to be up to 90% for women with sexual abuse and trauma history. This information points back to the vulnerability

model. If sexual abuse and trauma caused the unbearable feelings of vulnerability that led to addiction, abstaining from the substances that served as emotional anesthesia results in a return of these feelings. The painful feelings must be connected to the trauma rather than to the absence of the substance. This opens the door for a second recovery process—the treatment and recovery from trauma.[13p75]

4. Alcoholics Anonymous has a helpful acronym that identifies the times that a person in recovery might be most vulnerable to drinking: HALT. This is shorthand for hungry, angry, lonely, tired. If the person in recovery notices the impulse to drink, he or she must stop to determine whether any of these factors are creating this feeling. It is also advised to avoid letting these situations develop. This simple advice is very helpful in recovery.

■ DEEPENING OF THE RECOVERY PROCESS

1. Choosing to take new actions in response to vulnerability is the key to recovery. If the element of choice is absent in the obsession and compulsion of addiction, then reclaiming the ability to make life-affirming choices—reclaiming free will—is the essence of recovery. The use of will can be considered the use of one's life energy. "Willingness and willfulness become possibilities every time we truly engage life. There is only one other option—to avoid engagement entirely [will-lessness]."[35p104]

2. The energy of willfulness is reflected in behaviors of force, exertion, strain, contraction, constriction, violence, manipulation, controlling actions, and drive. It is the fight aspect of the fight-or-flight response to perceived danger. Will-lessness—the withdrawal of energy—is seen in behaviors reflecting withdrawal, escape, giving up, immobilization, collapse, and numbness. Will-lessness is the flight response to fear and vulnerability.

3. Every person tends to favor one of these patterns of behavior. Typically, a person who is predominantly willful eventually becomes exhausted and collapses into will-less behaviors. A person following a very restrictive and rigid weight loss diet ultimately binges. A person who has fallen into a pattern of total will-lessness (e.g., has gone on an extended alcohol binge) suddenly becomes scared, vows to stop drinking, and goes on a health kick. This grasp of control cannot be sustained because it is not grounded in any deeper changes. Consequently, the person swings back to the will-less behavior. The array of behaviors that can be identified as willful and will-less is shown in Figures 24-1 and 24-2 in *Holistic Nursing: A Handbook for Practice*.

4. These models are useful in teaching a person in recovery about patterns of behavior. People readily recognize these descriptions, and these behaviors can be observed in every aspect of a person's life.

5. The goal in recovery from addictions is to lead a life of balance, harmony, and increasing serenity. It can be likened to the ideal of many of the world's wisdom traditions. It is spoken of in the Buddhist path of the middle way, in the Taoist concept of the balance of yin and yang energies, in the Greek ideal of the golden mean, and in the common sense of moderation in all things. The qualities of life lived from this ideal are depicted in Figure 24-3 in *Holistic Nursing: A Handbook for Practice*.

■ SPIRITUAL DEVELOPMENT AND TRANSFORMATION

1. Spiritual development is an innate evolutionary capacity within all people. Spirituality is not a concept, but a process of learning about love, caring, empathy, and meaning in life. Participants in 12-step programs are encouraged to seek spiritual growth and connection with their own higher power. Studies have found that people in recovery who score higher in standardized spirituality measures are more successful in maintaining abstinence than those with lower scores. Spirituality in these studies was not equated with participation in religion. Rather, individuals in treatment spoke of experiencing a turning point in their life, feeling "protection and support from a higher power, guidance

of an inner voice, life meaning, gratitude, and an appreciation of service work."[36] These experiences point to the fact that long-term recovery is a process that goes beyond abstinence and can lead to deep healing and an enriched sense of meaning and purpose.[37,38]

2. Because of their compatibility with 12-step programs and AA philosophy, spiritually oriented therapies and psychotherapy are important components of care. Addiction treatment is one of few areas in health care where spiritual development and exploration are not only openly addressed, but are recognized as an integral aspect of care. It is genuinely difficult for spiritually repressed nurses or psychotherapists to assist clients who are working through AA's 12-step program. A person who feels alienated by the spiritual components of AA is unlikely to participate in meetings. Some individuals hear *God* or *Higher Power* in meetings and reject AA's "God talk." If so, nurses can find out if the person can facilitate a broader approach to spirituality. For some, the idea of a higher power can be translated into Mother Nature, or the healing energy and intention of the people in their AA group. Clients can seek out books on different spiritual philosophies or explore spiritual practices such as yoga, tai chi, or meditation to experience expanded awareness. (For more information on the psychophysiology of body–mind healing, see Chapter 31 in *Holistic Nursing: A Handbook for Practice*.) To evaluate the session further, the nurse can explore the subjective effects of the experience with the client (Exhibit 24-6 in *Holistic Nursing: A Handbook for Practice*).

■ NOTES

1. Office of National Drug Control Policy. (2004). *The economic costs of drug abuse in the United States, 1992–2002.* Publication No. 207303. Washington, DC: Executive Office of the President. Retrieved from http://www.ncjrs.gov/ondcppubs/publications/pdf/economic_costs.pdf

2. Centers for Disease Control and Prevention. (2007, October). *Best practices for comprehensive tobacco control programs.* Atlanta, GA: U.S. Department of Health and Human Services, Centers for Disease Control and Prevention, National Center for Chronic Disease Prevention and Health Promotion, Office on Smoking and Health. Retrieved from http://www.cdc.gov/tobacco/stateandcommunity/best_practices/pdfs/2007/bestpractices_complete.pdf

3. Rehm, J., Mathers, C., Popova, S., Thavorncharoensap, M., Teerawattananon, Y., & Patra, J. (2009). Global burden of disease and injury and economic cost attributable to alcohol use and alcohol-use disorders. *Lancet, 373*(9682), 2223–2233.

4. Kumar, A., Choi, K. H., Renthal, W., Tsankova, N. M., Theobald, D. E., Truong, H. T.,...Nestler, E. J. (2008). Chromatin remodeling is a key mechanism underlying cocaine-induced plasticity in striatum. *Neuron, 48*(2), 303–314.

5. Maze, I., & Nestler, E. J. (2011, January). Epigenetic landscape of addiction. *Annals of the New York Academy of Sciences, 1216,* 99–113. doi:10.1111/j.1749-6632.2010.05893.x

6. McQuown, S. C., & Wood, M. A. (2010). Epigenetic regulation in substance use disorders. *Current Psychiatry Report, 12*(2), 145–153.

7. Rice, C. E., Dandreaux, D., Handley, E. D., & Chassin, L. (2006). Children of alcoholics: Risk and resilience. *Prevention Researcher, 13*(4), 3–6.

8. Pagano, M., Rende, R., Rodriguez, B. F., Hargraves, E. L., Moskowitz, A. T., & Keller, M. B. (2007). Impact of parental history of substance use disorders on the clinical course of anxiety disorders. *Substance Abuse Treatment, Prevention, and Policy, 2*(13), 2–13.

9. Office of Applied Studies. (2009). *Results from the 2008 National Survey on Drug Use and Health: National findings.* HHS Publication No. SMA 09-4434, NSDUH Series H-36. Rockville, MD: Substance Abuse and Mental Health Services Administration. Retrieved from http://oas.samhsa.gov/nsduh/2k8nsduh2k8Results.cfm

10. Alcoholics Anonymous. (1976). *Alcoholics anonymous.* New York, NY: AA World Services.

11. Kaur, M., Liguori, A., Lang, W., Rapp, S. R., Fleischer, A. B. Jr., & Feldman, S. R. (2006). Induction of withdrawal-like symptoms in a small randomized, controlled trial of opioid blockade in frequent tanners. *Journal of the American Academy of Dermatology, 54*(4), 709–711.

12. Zeller, S., Lazovich, D., Forster, J., & Widome, R. (2006). Do adolescent tanners exhibit dependency?

Journal of the American Academy of Dermatology, 54(4), 589–596.

13. Schaub, B., & Schaub, R. (2000). *Healing addictions.* Albany, NY: Delmar.

14. American Psychiatric Association. (2000). *Diagnostic and statistical manual of mental disorders-TR.* Washington, DC: Author.

15. National Institute of Alcohol Abuse and Alcoholism. (2007, January). Alcohol and tobacco. *Alcohol Alert, 71.* Retrieved from http://www.niaaa.nih.gov /publications/journals-and-reports/alcohol-alert

16. McQuown, S. C., & Wood, M. A. (2010, April). Epigenetic regulation in substance use disorders. *Current Psychiatry Report, 12*(2), 145–153. doi:10.1007 /s11920-010-0099-5

17. Graham, K., & Massak, A. (2007). Alcohol consumption and the use of antidepressants. *Canadian Medical Association Journal, 176*(5), 633–637.

18. Substance Abuse and Mental Health Services Administration, Center for Behavioral Health Statistics and Quality (formerly the Office of Applied Studies). (2010, December 28). *The DAWN report: Highlights of the 2009 Drug Abuse Warning Network (DAWN) findings on drug-related emergency department visits.* Rockville, MD: SAMHSA. Retrieved from http://www.oas.samhsa.gov/2k10 /DAWN034/EDHighlights.htm

19. Substance Abuse and Mental Health Services Administration, Center for Behavioral Health Statistics and Quality, Drug Abuse Warning Network. (n.d.). DAWN 2010 emergency department Excel files—national tables. Retrieved from http ://www.samhsa.gov/data/DAWN.aspx#DAWN %202010%20ED%20Excel%20Files%20-%20 National%20Tables

20. Agostino, P. (April 25, 2005). Unsportsmanlike conduct. *Nurse Week.*

21. Hazelden Foundation. (1987). *The twelve steps of Alcoholics Anonymous.* New York, NY: Harper/ Hazelden.

22. Becker, E. (1973). *The denial of death.* New York, NY: Free Press.

23. NIH Consensus Conference. (1998). Acupuncture. *Journal of the American Medical Association, 280*(17), 1518–1524.

24. Liu, T.-T., Shi, J., Epstein, D. H., Bao, Y.-P., & Lu, L. (2009). A meta-analysis of acupuncture combined with opioid receptor agonists for treatment of opiate-withdrawal symptoms. *Cellular Molecular Neurobiology, 29,* 449–454.

25. Robinson, E. A., Krentzman, A. R., Webb, J. R., & Brower, K. J. (2011, July). Six-month changes in spirituality and religiousness in alcoholics predict drinking outcomes at nine months. *Journal of Studies on Alcohol and Drugs, 72*(4), 660–668.

26. Bradley, C. A. (2011). Women in AA: "Sharing experience, strength and hope" the relational nature of spirituality. *Journal of Religion and Spirituality in Social Work, 30*(2), 89–112.

27. Straussner, S. A., & Byrne, H. (2009). Alcoholics Anonymous: Key research findings from 2002– 2007. *Alcoholism Treatment Quarterly, 27*(4), 349–367.

28. Werbach, M. R. (1991). *Nutritional influences on mental illness.* Tarzana, CA: Third Line Press.

29. Brey, R. J. (2006, November 30). The role of Healing Touch in the treatment of persons in recovery from alcoholism. *Counselor: The Magazine for Addiction Professionals.*

30. Winkelman, M. (2003). Complementary therapy for addiction: Drumming out drugs. *American Journal of Public Health, 93*(4), 647–651.

31. Benson, H., & Wallace, R. K. (1972). Decreased drug abuse with transcendental meditation. In *Drug Abuse—Proceedings of the International Conference* (pp. 369–376). Philadelphia, PA: Lea & Febiger.

32. Bowen, S., Witkiewitz, K., Dillworth, T. M., Chawla, N., Simpson, T. L., Ostafin, B. D.,… Marlatt, G. A. (2006). Mindfulness meditation and substance use in an incarcerated population. *Psychology of Addictive Behavior, 20*(3), 343–347.

33. Chen, K. W., Comerford, A., Shinnick, P., & Ziedonis, D. M. (2010). Introducing qigong meditation into residential addiction treatment: A pilot study where gender makes a difference. *Journal of Alternative and Complementary Medicine, 16*(8), 875–882.

34. Sokhadze, T. M., Cannon, R. L., & Trudeau, D. L. (2008). EEG biofeedback as a treatment for substance use disorders: Review, rating of efficacy, and recommendations for further research. *Applied Psychophysiology and Biofeedback, 33*(1), 1–28.

35. May, G. (1991). *Addiction and grace.* San Francisco, CA: Harper.

36. White, W., & Laudet, A. (2006). Spirituality, science and addiction. *Counselor: The Magazine for Addiction Professionals, 7*(1), 56–59.

37. Laudet, A. B., Morgan, K., & White, W. (2006). The role of social supports, spirituality, religiousness, life meaning and affiliation with 12-step fellowships in quality-of-life satisfaction among individuals in recovery from alcohol and drug problems. *Alcohol Treatment Quarterly, 24*(1–2), 33–73.

38. Robinson, E. A., Cranford, J. A., Webb, J. R., & Brower, K. J. (2007). Six-month changes in spirituality, religiousness, and heavy drinking in a treatment seeking sample. *Journal of Studies on Alcohol and Drugs, 68*(2), 282–290.

◼ STUDY QUESTIONS

Basic Level

1. When a person has stopped drinking alcohol but has not extended this change to developing mentally, emotionally, and spiritually, what is this behavior pattern referred to as?
   a. Early recovery
   b. Sobriety
   c. Dry drunk
   d. Relapse

2. The following cycle: (a) Nervous system disturbance, (b) the use of chemicals, (c) the return of nervous system disturbance describes the recurring pattern of what stage of addiction?
   a. Early stage of the addictive cycle
   b. Middle stage of the addictive cycle
   c. Late stage of the addictive cycle
   d. Precontemplative stage of the addictive cycle

3. Addiction is a repetitive, maladaptive, avoidant, substitutive process of getting rid of vulnerability. This vulnerability is anxiety rooted in the human condition. This statement relates to which theoretical model of addiction?
   a. Character defect model of AA
   b. Transpersonal intoxication model
   c. Vulnerability model
   d. Psychoanalytic model

4. What is the defense mechanism most prevalent in the individual involved in addiction that can become a major obstacle for treatment?
   a. Sublimation
   b. Denial
   c. Repression
   d. Projection

5. What concept used in AA best refers to a movement away from addictive thinking and toward an understanding of one's life or spiritual purpose?
   a. Recovery
   b. Sobriety
   c. New consciousness
   d. The 12 steps

Advanced Level Questions

6. Certain elements distinguish the process of addiction from the recreational use of certain substances or behaviors. What key element is absent in the individual involved in the addictive process?
   a. Choice
   b. Self-discipline
   c. Responsibility
   d. Impaired serotonin reuptake

7. Which statement best describes why spiritual development is important to the recovery process?
   a. Religion provides a way for us to experience being taken care of by a deity.
   b. The existential truth that the human condition is vulnerable requires the experience of an expanded sense of self to find peace and wisdom in the face of that vulnerability.
   c. Religion provides a moral framework to guide right action, which is helpful for treating immorality in the person who is an addict.
   d. Spirituality has the capacity to help the addict dissociate from reality, which can often be difficult.

8. A nurse working on an intensive care unit is treating a patient who sustained multiple trauma after being in a car accident. His urine for toxicology results were positive for alcohol and cocaine. The nurse's personal history includes a father who died from alcoholism. Ordinarily a highly skilled, compassionate practitioner, the nurse became short tempered and irritable and tried to avoid this patient. She even made statements to her peers like, "I have other, more sick, patients to take care of." What statement best describes the nurse's reaction?
   a. ICU nurses often have to deal with addictions as a comorbidity and cause for hospitalization. This creates frustration for the nurse and compromises her capacity to care for the more ill patients.
   b. The nurse recognizes that she might be responding from a place of her own vulnerability and takes responsibility to do

her self-care and self-awareness practice to avoid transferring her wounded experience onto the patient.

c. The nurse is reacting to the increased demands and stress within the environment of care.

d. The nurse is expressing frustration related to a social and systematic problem in health care related to lack of appropriate treatment for people with addictions.

9. What statement best describes the process of relapsing into addiction?

a. Relapse is an ongoing issue in every stage of recovery and not unusual in the journey of recovery.

b. Relapse is a symptom of lack of motivation for sobriety.

c. Relapse can be avoided by regular attendance at 12-step meetings.

d. Avoiding triggers can prevent relapse.

10. How best might holistic nurses engage in self-care to provide for clients involved in addiction?

a. Practice meditation and deep breathing to center themselves prior to patient contact.

b. Use imagery and visualization techniques to energetically shield themselves from the manipulation and negative behaviors that often accompany people in the addictive process.

c. Engage in self-awareness practices that will help them recognize their own experiences, meanings, judgments, projections, and reactions to addiction and vulnerability that they might bring into the caring interaction.

d. Use autogenic suggestions to self-regulate.

Chapter 26

Aromatherapy

Marty Downey and Kamron Keep

Original Author: Jane Buckle

◼ DEFINITIONS

Aromatherapy The use of essential oils for therapeutic purposes.

Chemotype A cloned variety of a plant that always has the same chemistry.

Clinical aromatherapy The use of essential oils for specific, measurable health outcomes.

Essential oil The distillate from an aromatic plant, or the oil expressed from the peel of a citrus fruit.

Learned memory The ability of the mind to condition the response to an aroma based on previous experience.

Limbic system The oldest part of the brain; it contains the amygdala, hippocampus, thalamus, and hypothalamus.

M Technique A registered form of very gentle, structured touch suitable when the receiver is very fragile, actively dying, or the giver is not trained in massage. Recognized as part of holistic nursing care.[1-6]

◼ HISTORY[1]

1. Aromatherapy is often misunderstood and maligned because many people think aromatherapy is just about inhaling aromas. Aromatherapy is part of herbal medicine that dates back 6,000 years and has been used in many parts of the world. According to the World Health Organization, more than 85% of the world population still relies on herbal medicine, and many of the herbs are aromatic.

2. The renaissance of modern aromatherapy began in France just prior to World War II, at about the same time the first antibiotics were being introduced.

3. A medical doctor, Jean Valnet, a chemist, Maurice Gattefosse, and a surgical assistant, Marguerite Maury, were key figures in the rediscovery of this ancient art of healing.[7] They did not use aromatherapy for nice aromas or for stress reduction, two of the most popular ways aromatherapy is used today; they used aromatherapy clinically to help wounds heal, to fight infections, and to reduce skin problems, and they used essential oils topically.

4. This more clinical approach to aromatherapy has survived in France and Germany, where aromatherapy is seen as an extension of orthodox medicine. German doctors and nurses are tested in the use of essential oils to become licensed.

5. The clinical use of aromatherapy is easy to understand because many of today's drugs originally came from plants. For example, aspirin from willow bark and digoxin from foxglove. Even the contraceptive pill originally came from a plant—the humble yam—and the yew tree produces a cytotoxic drug to fight cancer.[1-3,8]

6. However, it should not be assumed that the essential oil will have the same therapeutic actions as the whole plant because some of the medicinally active substances are water soluble and can be lost in the distillation process.[9]

■ THEORY AND RESEARCH

1. Aromatherapy uses essential oils obtained from aromatic plants for the physical, psychological, and spiritual benefit of the patient.
2. Essential oils are powerful; they can be up to 100 times more concentrated than the herb itself. Approximately 300 essential oils are used by practitioners today with about 10 of these essential oils more commonly used by consumers.[8]
3. It is important to consider that although many essential oils are used by practitioners, only a handful have been formally tested on their use and safety for skin application. A practitioner should be familiar with the safety and efficacy of each essential oil prior to use.[1,9]
4. Many essential oils have familiar smells, such as lavender, rose, and rosemary. Essential oils are highly volatile droplets created by the plant to prevent (or treat) infection, regulate growth, and mend the plant's damaged tissue. These tiny droplets are stored in veins, glands, or sacs by the plant, and when they are crushed or rubbed, the essential oil and its aroma are released.
5. Some plants store large amounts of essential oil, some store very little. This, along with the difficulty of harvesting the essential oil, dictates the price of each type of oil. More than 220 pounds (100 kilograms) of fresh rose petals are needed to produce a little more than 2 ounces (60 grams) of essential oil, making rose one of the most expensive essential oils, and therefore one of the most frequently adulterated.[9]
6. There are a few important things to know about essential oils before they can be used safely: extraction, the botanical name (for clear identification), method of application, safety, storage, and contraindications. These topics are discussed in the following subsections as well as in Exhibit 25-2 in *Holistic Nursing: A Handbook for Practice* (6th ed.).

Extraction

1. Only steam-distilled or expressed extracts produce essential oils. These two methods give a product with no additional solvent or impurity.

2. However, many "essential oils" on the market are actually extracted with solvent, which can produce allergic or sensitive reactions in the user.
3. A bottle of essential oil should state that the contents are pure essential oils: steam distilled or expressed. (Only the peel from citrus plants such as mandarin, lime, or lemon produces an *expressed* oil.)

Identification by Botanical Name[1-10]

1. It is very important to know the botanical name of a plant because there can be many different species of the same plant, and using just the common name can lead to confusion. For example, there are three species of lavender and many hybrids, each with different chemistry and, therefore, very different therapeutic effects.
2. There are 400 different species of eucalyptus. Identification is simple if the full botanical name is given. This should include the genus, species, and where relevant, the chemotype.
3. The genus of lavender is *Lavandula*, and so all lavender plant names begin with *Lavandula*. The species is the second part of the name.
4. The chemotype, if there is one, comes last. See Table 25-1 in *Holistic Nursing: A Handbook for Practice* for a list of the botanical and common names for the essential oils mentioned in this chapter.
5. Do not buy just anything that is labeled "lavender oil" because there is no way of knowing which botanical type of lavender is in the bottle. One lavender, *Lavandula angustifolia*, is soothing, calming, and exceptional for burns, but another lavender, *Lavandula latifolia*, is a stimulant and expectorant (helps someone to cough up mucus). This second lavender will not promote sleep or soothe burns.

Methods of Application

1. Essential oils can be absorbed by the body in three ways: through ingestion, through olfaction, and through topical application.
   a. Touch in aromatherapy
      ■ Aromatherapy often is used with several touch therapies including

massage, and the M Technique.[1] This registered method of touch is suitable when massage is inappropriate, either because the receiver is too fragile or the giver is not trained in massage.[2]

- The M Technique is used in hospitals, hospices, and long-term care facilities in the United States, the United Kingdom, the Netherlands, and South Africa. It is simple to learn and produces a profound relaxation response in just a few minutes, reducing perceptions of chronic pain and agitation in dementia and at the end of life.[3,4]
- The M Technique appears to be more relaxing than conventional massage and to have an accumulative effect.[5] Gentle stroking enhances absorption of essential oils through the skin into the bloodstream. (For M Technique training programs, see www.ahna.org/Endorsedprograms and www.rjbuckle.com.)

b. Olfaction[6,8-11]
- The fastest effect from aromatherapy is through olfaction.
- Essential oils are composed of many different chemical components that travel via the nose to the olfactory bulb.
- There is debate as to whether the components are recognized by shape or vibration. Either way, they trigger responses in the limbic system of the brain—the oldest part of the brain—where the aroma is processed. The limbic part of the brain contains the amygdala, where fear and anger are analyzed; the thalamus, where pain is analyzed; and the hippocampus, which is involved in the formation and retrieval of explicit memories. This is why an aroma can trigger memories that have lain dormant for years.
- Smell is very important, beginning with the newborn baby's identification of its mother and continuing into old age, where studies show that the depression of residential older adults can be reduced with the aromas of familiar fruits and flowers.

- The effect of odors on the brain was "mapped" using computer-generated graphics.[11] Brain electrical activity mapping (BEAM) indicates how a subject, linked to an electroencephalogram (EEG), rates different odors even when the subject is asleep.[12] These maps indicate that aromas can have a psychological effect even when the aroma is subliminal (i.e., below the level of human awareness), and that, provided the olfactory nerve is intact, the aroma still has a measurable effect on the brain.

c. Topical applications[1-11]
- Components within essential oils are absorbed into, and through, the skin via diffusion.
- The two layers of the skin, the dermis and fat layer, together act as a reservoir before the components within the essential oils reach the bloodstream.
- There is some evidence that massage or hot water enhances absorption. Essential oils, because they are lipophilic (dissolve in fat), can be stored in the fatty areas of the body and can pass through the blood–brain barrier and into the brain itself.

Negative Reactions

1. Essential oils are commonly used in the pharmaceutical, perfume, and food industries.[8-11] Pure essential oils rarely produce an allergic effect, unlike synthetics.[10]
2. Today, increasingly more essential oils are being replaced with synthetic copies.
3. Some people, especially those with multiple allergies, eczema, asthma, skin sensitivities, or during hormonal changes and stress, can be more susceptible to various skin reactions and should be carefully monitored with the topical use of essential oils.[1,10,13]
4. Aromatherapy practitioners are most at risk for adverse skin reactions and scent overload and should use caution with repeated use.

Nursing Theory Related to Aromatherapy

1. Aromatherapy links into many of the most recognized nursing theories. Certainly, it

resonates with Watson's Theory of Caring because aromatherapy allows nurses a method of showing their care at a deep level.[14]

2. It resonates with Barrett's Theory of Power because it allows the patient to participate knowingly in change and offers a model for change through empowerment.[15]

3. Nightingale put forward the first theory of nursing—putting the patient in the best condition for Nature to act—and thus aromatherapy clearly fits here because it allows the patient to relax sufficiently for the healing process to occur from within.[16] Nightingale also suggested creating an environmental space conducive to healing—aromatherapy fits very well here as well, because essential oils create a safe environment at many levels.

4. Erickson's work led to the Modeling Theory, which requires building trust, promoting positive orientation, promoting strength, and setting mutual health-directed goals—these requirements also fit exceptionally well with aromatherapy.[17]

5. Rogers's theory suggests that human beings are more than just physical entities and have specific energy fields. Aromas clearly affect both the psyche and the human energy field.[15]

■ HOW AROMATHERAPY WORKS

1. The term *aromatherapy* refers to the therapeutic use of essential oils—the volatile organic constituents of plants.

2. Essential oils are thought to work at psychological, physiologic, and cellular levels.[1] This means that they can affect our body, our mind, and all the delicate links in between.

3. The effects of aroma can be rapid, and sometimes just thinking about a smell can be as powerful as the actual smell itself. Take a moment to think of your favorite flower. Then, think about a smell that makes you feel nauseated.

4. The effects of an aroma can be relaxing or stimulating depending on the previous experience of the individual (called the *learned memory*), as well as the actual chemical makeup of the essential oil used.[1,7]

■ WHO USES AROMATHERAPY?

1. Aromatherapy is used by nurses in the United Kingdom, France, Germany, Switzerland, Sweden, Australia, New Zealand, Korea, and Japan. In France and Germany, medical doctors and pharmacists also use aromatherapy as part of conventional medicine, often for the control of infection. Aromatherapy is the fastest growing therapy among nurses in the United States.[6]

2. Although essential oils are generally very safe to use, some guidelines need to be followed. Reference-backed, patient-centered clinical training is strongly recommended.

■ ADVERSE REACTIONS

1. There is some evidence of adverse skin reactions caused by sensitivity in rare instances. It is important to use properly diluted, pure essential oils safely and consider the client's medical history to help prevent this from occurring.[1,6,7,9,13]

2. Bergamot used in conjunction with sunshine or tanning beds can result in skin damage ranging from redness to full-thickness burns.[18]

3. It is recommended that essential oils should be used with caution during pregnancy, although the risk is extremely small when the essential oils are used only topically or inhaled; however, sage, pennyroyal, camphor, parsley, tarragon, wintergreen, juniper, hyssop, and basil should be avoided.[19] Tisserand and Balacs state that there is "no evidence that essential oils are abortifient in the amounts used in aromatherapy."[20]

4. In breastfeeding: Caution: Essential oils should not be used during breastfeeding because they could affect the infant's ability to detect the mother's scent.[1,6,10]

5. See Exhibit 25-2, Use of Aromatherapy Contraindications, Warnings, and Precautions, in *Holistic Nursing: A Handbook for Practice*.

■ ADMINISTRATION OF ESSENTIAL OILS

1. Essential oils can be used topically or inhaled.

2. A typical topical application uses a 1–5% mixture: 1–5 drops of essential oils diluted

in 5 cc (a teaspoon) of cold-pressed vegetable oil such as sweet almond oil.

3. Some wound infections might require higher concentrations—up to 20%. Certain essential oils, such as lavender and tea tree, can be topically applied undiluted for stings or bites. Others, such as clove and thyme, should never be used undiluted on the skin because their high phenol content would cause burning.

4. For insomnia, nausea, or depression, the client should inhale the correct oil for 5–10 minutes as necessary.

5. The nurse can use touch methods such as massage, the M Technique, or other comfort touch techniques where appropriate.

6. Simple stress management can be incorporated into an everyday regime with the use of baths and foot soaks, vaporizers, and sprays.

7. Oral intake of essential oils, although extremely effective for acute infection or gastrointestinal problems, is *not* recognized as part of holistic nursing care at this time.[7]

8. See Exhibit 25-3, Drug Interaction with Application of Essential Oils, in *Holistic Nursing: A Handbook for Practice*.

■ SELF-CARE APPLICATION OF AROMATHERAPY ESSENTIAL OILS[1,6,7]

1. Aromatherapy can be very useful when self-applied for stress management, insomnia, or depression because the oils are portable and can be used anywhere at any time.

2. A drop of peppermint can help clear your mind at the end of a busy day, or a drop of ylang ylang can help soothe nerves.

3. It is simple to choose an essential oil that is pleasing as well as efficacious.

■ CREDENTIALING AS AROMATHERAPIST

1. At the moment there is no recognized national certification for aromatherapy. The closest thing is the Aromatherapy Registration Council (ARC) exam set by the Aromatherapy Registration Board (ARB), a nonprofit entity that provides a national exam for lay people (www.aromatherapycouncil.org). Details of the exams are available from the website. The exam is open to anyone who has studied aromatherapy for 200 hours and meets the criteria. There is little, if any, clinical content in the exam.

2. There are two professional bodies: the National Association of Holistic Aromatherapy (NAHA) and Alliance of International Aromatherapists (AIA). At present, there are no requirements to become certified or accredited, and aromatherapy training can range from 1 day to several years.

3. However, because nurses are accountable, if a nurse wants to use aromatherapy in his or her nursing care, it is strongly recommended that he or she be able to show documented evidence of clinical training, preferably one that is nurse taught and patient centered. Please see the American Holistic Nurses Association website for endorsed and approved aromatherapy courses for nurses (www.ahna.org).

■ SPECIFIC USES OF ESSENTIAL OILS FOR HEALTH PROMOTION

1. Dementia
   a. Lin et al. conducted a cross-over randomized trial on 70 Chinese older adults with dementia.[21] Half the subjects were randomly assigned to the active group (lavender inhalation) for 3 weeks and then switched to the control group (sunflower inhalation) for another 3 weeks; the other half did the opposite. Also, Fowler shows aromatherapy could help crisis management during the night shift for adolescents in a residential treatment center.[22]
   b. An in vitro study by Huang et al. in 2008 demonstrates that lavender essential oil reversibly inhibited GABA-induced currents in a concentration-dependent manner whereas no inhibition of NMDA- or AMPA-induced currents was noted.[23] Lavender is commonly used to relax and soothe patients with dementia.

2. Pain management
   a. Previous studies using aromatherapy for pain suggest that both inhaled and topically applied essential oils can affect the perception of pain. More recent research indicates that some essential oils might

have analgesic properties. Also, aromatherapy uses touch, particularly the M Technique, and this technique has profound effects on chronic pain on its own, which are enhanced with essential oils.

b. In 2006, Han et al. found a mixture of essential oils topically applied to the abdomen of 67 nurses had a statistically significant effect on reducing menstrual pain.[24] The essential oils used were *Lavandula angustifolia*, *Salvia sclarea*, and *Rosa centifolia*. Subjects were nurses who rated their pain less than 6 on a 10-point visual analog scale and who did not use contraceptive drugs.

c. Kim et al. explored the use of 2% lavender oil inhaled immediately postoperatively in a randomized controlled study of 50 patients undergoing breast biopsy surgery.[25] It is strange that such a low percentage was used for inhalation (2%)—normally full-strength essential oil is used—and hardly surprising that pain scores were not affected. However, subjects did report a higher satisfaction with pain control rate in the lavender group. Perhaps it might have been simpler to have evaluated the difference in "comfort."

d. This was the outcome measure in a study by Nord looking at promoting comfort in pediatric perianesthesia.[26] She used lavender and ginger on 91 patients: The control group received a nonactive vegetable oil with a slight aroma (jojoba). The mean distress was lower for the experimental group.

3. Infection

a. There is considerable published research available on the in vitro antibacterial, antifungal, and antiviral effects of a great number of essential oils.

b. A search on Medline using the botanical name of the individual aromatic plant coupled with the term *essential oil* produces between 20 and 100 papers per essential oil.

c. The world is experiencing a soaring increase in resistant infections. Methicillin-resistant *Staphylococcus aureus* (MRSA) has become endemic.[27] Even vancomycin, often used to treat MRSA, has shown disappointing cure rates: 44% failure in

treating bacteria and 40% failure in treating lower respiratory tract infections.[28]

d. Some antifungal drugs are no longer working, and some antivirals are no longer effective.[29,30]

e. Warnke et al. tested tea tree against several *Staphylococcus* strains including MRSA, four *Streptococcus* strains, and three *Candida* strains including *Candida krusei*.[31] Tea tree showed considerable efficacy.

f. Bowler et al. used tea tree in conjunction with conventional antibiotics to control MRSA spread in residents of five nursing homes in Wisconsin.[32] After intervention and follow-up for 12 months or more, the prevalence of MRSA carriage at the nursing homes decreased by 67% ($p < .001$), and 120 of 147 (82%) nursing home residents and 111 of 125 (89%) clinic patients remained culture negative for MRSA.

g. Tea tree was one of the essential oils originally tested by Edwards-Jones et al. in a wound dressing pack.[33] They looked at both the vapor and topical effect of essential oils and found geranium and tea tree were the most effective against MRSA in a dressing.

h. In another study, Thomson et al. presented a research protocol for a randomized controlled trial of tea tree oil (5%) body wash versus standard body wash to prevent colonization with MRSA in critically ill adults.[34] Sherry and Warnke broke new ground when they applied essential oils directly into the bones of patients suffering from osteomyelitis (MRSA) and presented their findings at the American Academy of Orthopedic Surgeons.[35] Twenty-five patients with MRSA infections were treated: 16 involved bone, 6 a joint, and 3 soft tissue. Ten patients were diabetic. Following debridement, diluted essential oils were applied to the infected sites. In the case of bone, calcium (Osteoset) beads soaked in essential oils were used. In 22 cases, the infection was completely resolved either without antibiotics (19) or with antibiotics (3).

i. In Australia, 90% of hospital-acquired infections are MRSA. In vitro studies on tea tree and eucalyptus show that both were effective within 1 minute against 90% of the five multiple-resistant tuberculosis (TB) organisms tested. The paper concludes that essential oils could be a possible mass treatment for TB.[35]

j. Finally, three other studies that might be useful in nursing care include the following. An essential oil mixture of diluted tea tree, peppermint, and lemon reduced malodor and volatile sulfur compounds (VSC) in intensive care unit patients.[36]

k. Black pepper stimulated swallowing reflex in people with swallowing dysfunction following stroke. This Japanese study found inhalation of black pepper essential oil for 1 minute reduced the delay in swallowing, compared with lavender oil or distilled water ($p < .03$) ($n = 105$).[37]

l. A paper by Lesho suggests that essential oils would be useful to reduce the incidence of hospital-acquired and ventilator-associated pneumonia.[38]

m. The kind of application depends on whether a psychological or physiologic response is required. Nurses should remember to ask their patients if they like the aroma before beginning their aromatherapy treatment and make sure to have some clinical training. Essential oil companies used by author, Jane Buckle, are listed in Chapter 25 of *Holistic Nursing: A Handbook for Practice*.

■ CONCLUSION

1. There is tremendous emphasis on "doing" in the Western world, where we are judged (and tend to judge others) on what we "do" rather than our ability "to be." But illness takes away a patient's ability "to do" and forces him or her to address his or her "being" on a much broader scale. This can be quite frightening. However, it allows the nurse an opportunity to share with the patient a glimpse of a multidimensional world, which until then has remained hidden. Aromatherapy gives caring to the soul, the mind, and the body—a true holistic therapy. And it smells good!

2. Please refer to Exhibits 25-4, 25-5, 25-6, 25-7, 25-8 in *Holistic Nursing: A Handbook for Practice*.

3. Table 25-1 is a partial list of essential oils for use by holistic nurses trained in aromatherapy. The following list is modified from Chapter 25 in *Holistic Nursing: A Handbook for Practice*.

Common Name	Botanical Name
Basil	*Ocimum basilicum*
Chamomile, German	*Matricaria recutita*
Chamomile, Roman	*Chamaemelum nobile*
Clary sage	*Salvia sclarea*
Coriander seed	*Coriandrum sativum*
Eucalyptus	*Eucalyptus globulus*
Fennel	*Foeniculum vulgare var. dulce*
Geranium	*Pelargonium graveolens*
Ginger	*Zingiber officinale*
Hyssop	*Hyssopus officinalis*
Lavender, true	*Lavandula angustifolia*
Lemongrass	*Cymbopogon citratus*
Neroli	*Citrus aurantium var. amara*
Palmarosa	*Cymbopogon martinii*
Peppermint	*Mentha piperita*
Rose	*Rosa damascena*
Sandalwood	*Santalum album*

■ NOTES

1. Buckle, J. (2003). *Clinical aromatherapy: Essential oils in practice*. New York, NY: Churchill Livingstone.

2. Buckle, J. (2006). Take five and relax. *Nursing Spectrum* (New York & New Jersey edition), *18A*(11), 23–23.

3. Buckle, J. (2009). The M Technique for dementia, *Working with Older People, 13*(3), 22–24.

4. Buckle, J. (2008). The M Technique: Touch for the critically ill or actively dying. *Positive Health, 152*(1) Retrieved from http://www.positivehealth.com/article/bodywork/the-m-technique-touch-for-the-critically-ill-or-actively-dying

5. Buckle, J., Newberg, A., Wintering, N., Hutton, E., Lido, C., & Farrar, J. T. (2008). Measurement of regional cerebral blood flow associated with the M Technique—light massage therapy: A case series and longitudinal study using SPECT. *Journal of Alternative and Complementary Medicine, 14*(8), 903–910.

6. Buckle, J. (2006). Should nursing take aromatherapy more seriously?" *British Journal of Nursing, 16*(2), 116–120.

7. Buckle, J. (2013). Aromatherapy. In B. Dossey & L. Keegan (Eds.), *Holistic Nursing: A Handbook for Practice* (Chap. 25). Burlington, MA: Jones & Bartlett Learning.

8. Worwood, V. (2006). *Aromatherapy for the soul*. Publishers Group West.

9. Watt, M. (2001). *Plant aromatics*. Friendsville, Maryland: Appalachian Valley Natural Products.

10. Burr, C. (2003). *The emperor of scent*. New York, NY: Random House.

11. Brownlee, C. (2005). Mapping aroma: Smells light up distinct brain parts. *Science News, 167*(22), 340–341.

12. Goel, N., Kim, H., & Lao, R. (2005). The olfactory stimulus modifies nighttime sleep in young men and women. *Chronobiology International, 22*(5), 889–904.

13. Fu, Y., Zu, Y., Chen, L., Shi, X., Wang, Z., Sun, S., & Efferth, T. (2007). Antimicrobial activity of clove and rosemary essential oils alone and in combination. *Phytotherapy Research, 21*(10), 989–994.

14. Watson, J. (2005). *Caring science as sacred science*. (Philadelphia, PA: F. A. Davis.

15. Barrett, E. (2000). The theoretical matrix for a Rogerian nursing practice. *Theoria: Journal of Nursing Theory, 9*(4), 3–7.

16. Dossey, B. (2009). *Florence Nightingale: Mystic, visionary, healer*. Philadelphia, PA: F. A. Davis.

17. Erickson, H. (2007). Philosophy and theory of holism. *Nursing Clinics of North America, 42,* 139–163.

18. Kejlovia, K., Jirova, D., Bendova, H., Gajdos, P., & Kolarava, H. (2010). Phototoxicity of essential oils intended for cosmetic use. *Toxicology in Vitro, 24*(8), 2084–2089.

19. Bastard, J., & Tiran, D. (2006). Aromatherapy and massage for antenatal anxiety: Its effect on the fetus. *Complementary Therapies in Clinical Practice, 12*(1), 48–54.

20. Tisserand, R., & Balacs, T. (1995). *Essential oil safety*. London, England: Churchill Livingstone.

21. Lin, P., Chan, W., Ng, B., & Lam, L. (2007). Efficacy of aromatherapy (*Lavandula angustifolia*) as an intervention for agitated behaviors in Chinese older persons with dementia: A cross-over randomized trial. *International Journal of Geriatric Psychiatry, 22*(5), 405–410.

22. Fowler, N. (2005). Aromatherapy used as an integrative tool for crisis management by adolescents in a residential treatment center. *Journal of Child and Adolescent Psychiatric Nursing, 19*(2), 69–76.

23. Huang, L., Abuhamdah, S., Howes, M-J. R., Dixon, C. L., Elliot, M. S. J., Ballard, C.,...Francis, P. T. (2008). Both *Melissa officinalis* (Mo) and *Lavandula angustifolia* (La) essential oils have putative anti-agitation properties in humans, indicating common components with a depressant action in the central nervous system. *Journal of Pharmacy and Pharmacology, 60*(11), 1515–1522.

24. Han, S., Hur, H., Buckle, J., Choi, J., & Lee, M. (2006). Effects of aromatherapy on symptoms of dysmenorrhea in college students: A randomized, placebo-controlled clinical trial. *Journal of Complementary and Alternative Medicine, 12*(6), 38–41.

25. Kim, J., Wajda, M., & Cuff, G. (2006). Evaluation of aromatherapy in treating postoperative pain: Pilot study. *Pain Practice, 6*(4), 273–276.

26. Nord, D. (2009). Effectiveness of the essential oils lavender and ginger in promoting children's comfort in a perianesthesia setting. *Journal of Perianesthesia Nursing, 24*(5), 307–312.

27. Arias, C., & Murray, B. (2009). Antibiotic-resistant bugs in the 21st century: A clinical super challenge. *New England Journal of Medicine, 360,* 439–443.

28. Wegner, D. (2005, January). No mercy for MRSA: Treatment alternatives to vancomycin and linezolid. *Medical Laboratory Observer, 37*(1), 26–29.

29. Espnel-Ingroff, A. (2008). Mechanisms of resistance to antifungal agents: Yeasts and filamentous fungi. *Revista Iberoamericana de Micologia, 25*(2), 101–106.

30. Gilbert, C., & Bolvin, G. (2005). Human cytomegalovirus resistance to antiviral drugs. *Antimicrobial Agents and Chemotherapy, 49*(3), 873–883.

31. Warnke, P., Becker, S. T., Podschun, R., Sivananthan, S., Springer, I. N., & Russo, P. A. (2009). The battle against multi-resistant strains: Renaissance of antimicrobial essential oils as a promising force to fight hospital-acquired infections. *Journal of Craniomaxillofacial Surg*ery, *37*(7), 392–397.

32. Bowler, W., Bresnahan, J., Bradfish, A., & Fernandez, C. (2010). An integrated approach to methicillin-resistant *Staphylococcus aureus* control in a rural, regional-referral healthcare setting. *Infection Control and Hospital Epidemiology, 31*(3), 269–275.

33. Edwards-Jones, V., Buck, R., Shawcross, S., Dawson, M., & Dunn, K. (2004). The effect of essential oils on methicillin-resistant *Staphylococcus aureus* using a dressing model. *Burns, 30*(8), 772–777.

34. Thompson, G., Blackwood, B., McMullan, R., Alderdice, F. A., Trinder, T. J., Lavery, G. G., & McAuley, D. F. (2008). A randomized controlled trial of tea tree oil (5%) body wash versus standard body wash to prevent colonization with methicillin-resistant *Staphylococcus aureus* (MRSA) in critically ill adults: Research protocol. *BMC Infectious Disease, 28*(8), 161.

35. Sherry, E., & Warnke, P. (2002, February 13–17). *Alternative for MRSA and tuberculosis (TB): Eucalyptus and tea tree oils as new topical antibacterials.* Paper presented at Orthopedic Surgery Conference, Dallas, TX.

36. Hur, M., Park, J., Maddock-Jennings, W., Kim, D., & Lee, M. (2007). Reduction of mouth malodor and volatile sulphur compounds in intensive care patients using essential oil mouthwash. *Phytotherapy Research, 21*(7), 641–643.

37. Ebihara, T., Ebihara, S., Maruyama, M., Okazaki, T., & Takahashi, H. (2006). A randomized trial of olfactory stimulation using black pepper oil in older people with swallowing dysfunction. *Journal of the American Geriatric Society, 54*(9), 1410–1416.

38. Lesho, E. (2005). Role of inhaled antibacterials in hospital-acquired and ventilator-associated pneumonia. *Expert Review of Anti-Infective Therapy, 3*(3), 445–451.

■ STUDY QUESTIONS

Basic Level

1. Which of the following answer choices is the best definition of aromatherapy?
   a. The distillate from an aromatic plant
   b. A cloned variety of a plant that has the same chemistry
   c. The process of inhaling aromas
   d. The use of essential oils for therapeutic purposes

2. Which part of a plant produces an expressed oil?
   a. Flower petal
   b. The root
   c. Citrus peel
   d. The leaves

3. Through which method is the fastest effect of aromatherapy achieved?
   a. Inhalation
   b. Compress
   c. Bathing
   d. Massage

4. A patient tells the nurse that every time she smells lavender she is reminded of her grandmother and how they used to gather lavender flowers together so that they could make sachets. It was a very comforting, relaxing time for her. The patient is wondering why the aroma of lavender gives her the same feeling she had when she was with her grandmother, especially after all these years. What is the likely cause of this occurrence?
   a. Placebo memory
   b. Learned memory
   c. Subliminal memory
   d. Olfactory memory

5. When purchasing essential oils, what is important information to find on the label to avoid confusion?
   a. The part of plant distilled
   b. Where the plant was grown
   c. The botanical name of the plant
   d. How the plant was harvested

Advanced Level

6. A patient presents with nausea post surgery, despite medication intervention. The patient does not have any allergies or aversions to fragrance. The nurse aromatherapist determines aromatherapy would be appropriate. Based on the symptoms, which essential oil would be the most appropriate for the nurse to offer this patient for inhalation?
   a. Lavender (*Lavandula angustifolia*)
   b. Eucalyptus, Blue Gum (*Eucalyptus globulus*)
   c. Frankincense (*Boswellia carteri*)
   d. Peppermint (*Mentha piperita*)

7. A nurse from an outpatient medical clinic is working with a 55-year-old patient who is experiencing moderate anxiety and stress. The patient is otherwise healthy and the only medication she takes is for her high cholesterol, which is well managed. The patient works part-time at a landscaping nursery and spends a lot of time outside in the hot sun. The patient would prefer to try one of the clinic's complementary approaches to managing her stress. The nurse is trained in aromatherapy and offers to make a massage blend to help the client with her anxiety. Based on this information, which is the best essential oil blend and dilution for the patient?
   a. Lavender 1% and frankincense 1.5%, in sweet almond oil
   b. Bergamot 2% and lavender 1%, in sweet almond oil
   c. Tea tree 10% and lavender 10%, in sweet almond oil
   d. Red thyme 1% and rosemary 1%, in sweet almond oil

8. A nurse is considering training in aromatherapy. What is important for her to consider when choosing a program?
   a. The aromatherapy training is clinically based and patient centered.
   b. The aromatherapy training is offered through the NAHA or AIA.
   c. The aromatherapy training offers national certification for graduates.
   d. The aromatherapy training includes a kit with quality essential oils.

9. Which of the following actions does the nurse aromatherapist do when evaluating the effectiveness of an aromatherapy treatment?
   a. Determine the patient's like or dislikes of the essential oil used
   b. Determine the patient's physiologic outcomes, such as decreased pain
   c. Determine the patient's skin integrity following the session
   d. Determine the patient's home aromatherapy regimen

10. A patient presents to an outpatient clinic with redness and an apparent allergic reaction on her chest. The patient states she has been using an essential oil she purchased from a local body shop for relaxation. She likes to rub it on her chest so that she can breathe it in during her meditation practice. Upon assessment, you determine that the patient has been using a 2% dilution of frankincense in grapeseed oil. The patient described the bottle she purchased as clear and labeled as "Frankincense." What is a likely cause of this reaction?
   a. The frankincense used is a synthetic oil.
   b. The client used a dilution that was too high.
   c. Frankincense should be not be used topically.
   d. The patient has an unknown ragweed allergy.

Chapter 27

Evolving from Therapeutic to Holistic Communication

Lucia M. Thornton and Carla Mariano

■ DEFINITIONS

Energy field The fundamental unit of the living and nonliving. *Field* is a unifying concept. *Energy* signifies the dynamic nature of the field; a field is in continuous motion and is infinite.[1]

Holistic communication A caring–healing process that calls forth the full use of self in interacting with another. It incorporates the constructs and processes of therapeutic communication within a framework that acknowledges the infinite, spiritual, and energetic nature of Being, the centrality of being heart centered, and the importance of intention, self-knowledge, transcendent presence, and intuition in our interactions.[2]

Person An energy field that is infinite and spiritual in essence and is in continual mutual process with the environment. Each person manifests unique physical, mental, emotional, and social or relational patterns that are interrelated, inseparable, and continually evolving.[3]

Therapeutic communication A goal-directed form of communication used to achieve goals that promote client health and well-being.[2p15] Empathy, unconditional regard, genuineness, respect, concern, caring, and compassion are conveyed through active listening, active observing, focusing, restating, reflecting, and interpreting.[2p533]

■ THEORY AND RESEARCH

1. Pioneers in therapeutic communication: Therapeutic communication is a field of study that has been influenced by theorists,

researchers, and clinicians from a multitude of professions including nursing, psychology, sociology, and physics.
   a. Hildegard Peplau: Considered to be the "mother of psychiatric nursing," Peplau was the first to emphasize the nurse–client relationship as being the foundation of nursing practice. The concept of partnership between nurse and client originated in Peplau's interpersonal model. The essence of Peplau's work revolved around the concept of the shared experience. She shifted the focus of nursing practice from one that was based on medical intervention to an interpersonal model in which the nurse became the therapeutic agent.
   b. Martin Buber: Introduced the idea that the therapeutic process involves mutual discovery and emphasized the importance of mutual respect in the client–therapist interaction. He coined the term *I–Thou relationship*, which reflects a reverence in the client–therapist relationship. In this orientation, the therapist consciously creates a transcendent space in the relationship, fostering shared authenticity and compassion.
   c. Harry Stack Sullivan: A contemporary of Peplau and influenced the development of her interpersonal model. Sullivan introduced the idea of the therapeutic relationship and described it as being a human connection that heals.
   d. Carl Rogers: Perceived the therapist as an agent of healing. The hallmark characteristics that Rogers identified as being essential to the client-centered relationship were unconditional regard, empathy, and genuineness.

2. All of these therapists, and many others not mentioned, have contributed ideas that have significantly influenced the effectiveness of the therapeutic communication process. The concepts of partnership, healing, reverence, unconditional regard, empathy, genuineness, spirituality, and many more first found their place in therapeutic communication before being embraced by holistic nursing.

■ NURSING THEORY RELATED TO HOLISTIC COMMUNICATION

Martha Rogers's Theory

1. The term *unitary human being* is used in place of *person* and we are defined as "irreducible, indivisible, pan-dimensional energy fields identified by pattern and manifesting characteristics that are specific to the whole and which cannot be predicted from knowledge of the parts."[1p7]
2. *Energy field* is defined as "the fundamental unit of the living and the nonliving. Field is a unifying concept. Energy signifies the dynamic nature of the field; a field is in continuous motion and is infinite.[1p7]
3. The nature of therapeutic communication changes when Rogers's definitions are applied. Using Rogers's definitions:
   a. Communication shifts from being a linear or circular process to a pandimensional energetic process.
   b. Communication can be perceived as a field phenomenon.
   c. Communication can extend beyond the realm of this physical universe, beyond the space–time continuum, and into other dimensions.
4. Rogers describes person and environment as "open systems" and states that "man and environment are continuously exchanging matter and energy with one another."[4p54] This implies the following:
   a. All of our thoughts, behaviors, and emotions, both conscious and unconscious, interact and affect everything and everyone in our environment.
   b. If we are to act in a way that is therapeutic and healing, we ourselves must be whole and healed.

c. Self-awareness and self-knowledge are necessary for nurses to engage in effective therapeutic communication.

Margaret Newman's Theory

1. The task of nursing intervention, according to Newman, "is not to try to change another person's patterns but to recognize it as information that depicts the whole and relate to it as it unfolds."[5p13]
2. The nurse must first be able to recognize her own patterns before entering into this process with a patient.
3. Self-knowledge is paramount for the nurse to be effective in a caring–healing relationship.
4. The responsibility of the nurse is not to make people well or to prevent their getting sick, but to assist people in recognizing the power that is within them to move to higher levels of consciousness.
5. The nurse's awareness of being rather than doing is the primary mechanism for helping.
6. Newman illuminates the concepts of pattern recognition, being fully present, and the importance of self-awareness and transformation in the holistic communication process.

Jean Watson's Theory

1. Watson defines person as "an embodied spirit; a transpersonal, transcendent, evolving consciousness; unity of mind-body-spirit; person-nature-universe as oneness, connected."[6p129]
2. Watson is the first nursing theorist to address the concept of soul.
3. Watson introduces the transpersonal caring process as a means of communicating on a soul-to-soul level with another.
4. Engaging with another at the transpersonal level is not a technique that can be learned. Rather, it is the ability of the person to access the higher self and move from that place of higher consciousness in interactions with another.
5. This process calls for the "full use of the self."[7p69]
6. Watson's description of the art of transpersonal caring serves as a description of

the caring–healing process of holistic communication.

■ THERAPEUTIC COMMUNICATION SKILLS: A PREREQUISITE FOR HOLISTIC COMMUNICATION

1. Traditional models of therapeutic communication do the following:
   a. Define and prescribe various stages or phases
   b. Delineate various roles for the nurse or therapist
   c. Identify verbal and nonverbal communication skills
   d. Identify therapist characteristics that are essential to creating a therapeutic milieu
2. Foundations for therapeutic communication include empathy, unconditional regard, genuineness, respect, concern, caring, and compassion.
3. Developing and refining communication skills, including active listening, active observing, focusing, restating, reflecting, and interpreting, are also important in facilitating the therapeutic process.
4. Mastering these skills is a lifelong process that is facilitated by reflective practices, guidance, sage mentoring, and a commitment to self-knowledge and awareness.

■ DISTINGUISHING CHARACTERISTICS OF A HOLISTIC ORIENTATION TO COMMUNICATION

1. Preaccess and assessment phase
   a. The holistic communication process acknowledges the importance of being centered and creating an intention before engaging in a caring–healing interaction with another.
   b. These two processes, being centered and creating intention, constitute the preaccess phase involved in holistic interactions.
   c. This phase lays the foundation for caring–healing communication and occurs before any person-to-person interaction takes place. As the nurse stays present to the moment, to self, and to

the person, a healing environment is maintained. Consciously creating a healing environment, no matter where one is working, nurtures both the client and the self at a deep level.[2p537]
2. Acknowledgment of the infinite and sacred nature of being
   a. Holistic nursing acknowledges that people are infinite, sacred, and spiritual beings.
   b. Florence Nightingale spoke of human beings as a "reflection of the Divine with physical, metaphysical, and intellectual attributes."[8]
   c. Jean Watson teaches that we are sacred beings.
   d. Martha Rogers speaks of unitary human beings as "energy fields that are infinite in nature."[1p30]
   e. The Model of Whole-Person Caring combines these concepts to define person as "an energy field that is open, infinite, and spiritual in essence and in continual mutual process with the environment. Each person manifests unique physical, mental, emotional, and social or relational patterns that are interrelated, inseparable, and continually evolving."[9p15]
   f. Thus, from the perspective of holistic nursing theorists and models, people are infinite and sacred in nature.
   g. This orientation makes a difference in how we approach each other. It shifts how we speak, how we listen, how we relate, and how we interact. When we perceive human beings as sacred, our words, actions, and behaviors are significantly affected.
   h. When we view ourselves and others as spiritual, infinite beings with finite bodies, our relationship to illness, diseases, and death shifts dramatically.
   i. Communication can be oriented to soul's purpose in addition to symptom relief. This orientation creates a potential to explore and derive meaning from life's challenges and create a healing environment even in the face of death and terminal illness.
   j. When one understands that this physical life is a small part of the infinite journey, the stigma of death becomes

obsolete and the nurse can be fully present to persons with terminal illnesses and facing death.

3. Heart-centering, heart coherence, and the intuitive heart
   a. Heart-centering is one of the first processes the nurse engages in prior to any interaction. This process involves the nurse focusing her or his attention on the heart, setting aside concerns and thoughts, and connecting with feelings of love and compassion.
   b. Maintaining this heart-centeredness throughout interactions has many positive effects for the nurse. Research conducted at the Institute of HeartMath shows that this process:
      - Creates coherence in the electromagnetic energy field
      - Balances heart rhythms
      - Increases IgA (immunoglobulin A) levels and natural killer cell levels
      - Increases mental clarity and problem solving
      - Reduces sleeplessness, body aches, fatigue, anger, sadness, hypertension, and other chronic problems[10]
      - Might help to connect people with their intuitive inner guidance
   c. Research suggests that the heart's energy field (energetic heart) is coupled to a field of information that is not bound by the classic limits of time and space. This evidence comes from a rigorous experimental study that investigated the proposition that the body receives and processes information about a future event before the event actually happens.[11]
   d. McCraty and Childre explain that the intuitive heart or heart intelligence is coupled to a deeper part of oneself, what some may call their "higher power" or their "higher capacities."
   e. When we are heart-centered and coherent, we have a tighter coupling and closer alignment with our deeper source of intuitive intelligence.[12pp15-16]
   f. Research also shows that the positive mental and physiologic effects experienced by the nurse can be transmitted to the person.
      - It is believed that information about a person's emotional state is encoded in the heart's electromagnetic field and is communicated into the external environment.[12p20]
      - When the nurse becomes heart-centered a caring–healing field is created in which the person feels safe, nurtured, and loved and is in an optimal environment for healing communication to occur.

4. Grounding
   a. Grounding is the process of connecting to the Earth and the Earth's energy field to calm the mind and focus one's inner flow of energy as a means to enhance healing endeavors.[13]
   b. Centering and grounding can be considered a single continuous process because one flows into the other. As such, grounding can also be viewed as part of the preaccess phase of the holistic communication process.
   c. Communication can bring up many feelings and thoughts that are emotionally charged and difficult for the nurse to deal with.
   d. Grounding provides the nurse with a steady physical, psychological, and energetic platform on which to anchor the communication process.
   e. In physical terms, grounding provides a connection between an electric circuit and the Earth.
   f. In psychological terms, grounding helps establish a feeling of self-awareness and provides a connection to the consciousness of one's own self.
   g. Energetically, grounding establishes an awareness of the unity of body, mind, and spirit.

5. Creating intention
   a. Creating an intention ideally precedes interaction with a person and is part of the preaccess phase of the holistic nurse caring process. Intentionality is interpreted in different ways.
   b. Intention can be defined as "the conscious alignment with creative essence and divine purpose that allows the highest good to flow through a healing intervention or through life itself."[14]
   c. Creating an intention is a process that affects not only the mental and emotional realms, but also the physical world.

d. Physicists have demonstrated that conscious intent can be imprinted in materials that can be shipped to a distant laboratory, where they bring out the intentional effect that is imprinted on them. Recent advances in theoretical physics suggest that the space between atoms and molecules is not inert. Physicists speculate that "this 'vacuum' may be where the intent is imprinted."[15]

e. Creating an intention is a powerful way for the nurse to create an optimal environment for a caring–healing interaction.

6. Caring–healing, transcendent presence
   a. *Presence* has been defined as a way of being, a way of relating, a way of being with, and a way of being there.
   b. What distinguishes holistic communication from other types of communication is the depth and profound quality of presence.
   c. Watson speaks of the full use of self in the transpersonal caring process. When the nurse becomes heart-centered, she has the capacity to resonate with the person at a heart and soul level. At this level, the nurse connects with the person at a deep psychosocial, heart-felt, and spiritual level. This is a difficult concept to describe and remains more of a felt experience. The nurse must be able to access and rest in the depth of her own beingness before she can bring this caring, healing, transcendent presence into a relationship.
   d. Being able to communicate from more profound levels of presence is the result of experience and engaging in processes of deep reflection and inquiry.
   e. Cultivating this type of presence is something that also can be taught through experiential techniques and role modeling.
   f. Various self-reflective practices such as journaling, meditation, relaxation, contemplation, dream analysis, narrative, and storytelling in one's personal daily practice can help cultivate a deeper relationship with the essence of one's existence that can then be brought into a relationship with another.
   g. The nurse must be able to connect with her own heart, soul, and transcendent nature before she can establish that connection with others.

7. Intuition
   a. *Intuition* is defined as "a perceived inner knowing and insight into things and events without the conscious use of rational process; the ability to be present to another dimension of knowing."[14p722]
   b. The usefulness of intuition in the nursing process is well researched and documented.
   c. Although intuitive knowing is something that occurs more readily with the experienced nurse, it can be consciously cultivated through various practices.
   d. Ways to cultivate intuition are listening to music, engaging in relaxation techniques, and journal writing, which can be useful in increasing one's intuitive and spiritual development.
   e. Meditation also increases one's intuitive knowing. Regular meditation practice enables one to enter the intuitional state at will.[2p539]
   f. When the nurse utilizes intuition she engages the full use of self, which is essential in accessing and communicating with the whole person. Intuition allows the nurse to access the subtle energies and the conscious and unconscious fields that are not readily perceived.
   g. This process allows the nurse to sense the Being of another and communicate at levels where profound healing occurs.

■ TOOLS AND PRACTICES TO ENHANCE HOLISTIC COMMUNICATION

1. Knowing self
   a. Awareness and understanding of one's self and one's values, beliefs, motivations, goals, feelings, and actions are imperative in relating in a caring–healing manner.
   b. When we are aware of ourselves and understand who we are and the basis for our own attitudes, preconceptions, and reactions, we are in a much better position to empathize, appreciate other people's differences and uniqueness, and encourage their self-revelations.

   c. To nurture caring–healing communication and relationships, we need to conduct assessments of ourselves as individuals, as well as our communications, spirituality, and cultural beliefs and traditions.[16]

2. Meditation

   a. Meditation is a quiet turning inward—the practice of focusing one's attention internally to achieve clearer consciousness and inner stillness.

   b. Meditation is both a state of mind and a method. The state is one in which the mind is quiet, open, and receptive. The meditator is relaxed but alert. The method involves the focusing of attention on something such as the breath, an image, a word, or action such as tai chi or qi gong.

   c. Meditation allows a better understanding of the self and increased receptivity to insights arising from one's deeper being.

   d. There are numerous methods and schools of meditation. However, all methods believe in emptying the mind and letting go of the mind's chatter that preoccupies us.[17]

   e. Meditation is perhaps the single most useful reflective practice to help gain self-awareness and self-knowledge, increase intuition, and enhance one's spiritual development. Because self-awareness, self-knowledge, and intuition are foundational to creating a caring-healing presence, meditating regularly is an important practice to engage in.

3. Engaging your observer

   a. The nonjudgmental aspect of your self is called the Observer or Witness. Some perceive this aspect as our higher Self.

   b. The Witness is our ability to observe life without engaging our past patterns of reacting and becoming emotionally charged.

   c. The Observer acts as a third party who allows the nurse to separate from difficult emotions and feelings in situations so that communication occurs from a space of clarity and wisdom.

   d. Engaging your Observer is a process that is useful when confronting a situation or communication that is particularly difficult and emotionally charged.

   e. Utilizing this technique enhances self-knowledge and self-awareness because it provides constant feedback related to one's responses and reactions to situations.

   f. The Observer is able to transcend the ego while embracing the whole of the moment so that one responds with wisdom rather than reacting from conditioned response.[18]

   g. Engaging the Observer involves centering, being aware of internal reactions, gratefully acknowledging these reactions, and responding from the higher Self.

   h. This technique allows one to access the higher Self and move from that place of higher consciousness in interactions with another. This is central to the transpersonal caring process and communicating from a holistic perspective.[19]

4. Drawing out the person's story

   a. A cornerstone of holistic communication is assisting individuals to find meaning in their experience, meanings such as the person's concerns in relation to health and family economics, as well as to deeper meanings related to the person's purpose in life.

   b. Nurses need to ask clients, patients, and families to share what meaning something has for them (e.g., symptoms, illness, treatment, outlook, fears). Only then will we truly glean an understanding of the individual's experience as he or she sees it and shape our interventions to meet the person's needs.

   c. One of the best ways to understand what the person is most concerned about and the meaning something has for that person is through the use of narrative and story.

   d. Client narratives, whether they arise from individuals, families, or communities, provide the context of the experiences and are used as an important focus in understanding the person's situation.

   e. The nurse first ascertains what the individual thinks or believes is happening to him or her, and then assists the person to identify what will help the situation.

   f. The assessment begins from where the individual is. Space and time are allowed for exploration. Each person's health encounter is truly seen as unique.

g. This requires a perspective that the nurse is not "the expert" regarding another's health/illness experience. By simply asking, "What do you think is going on with you (or is happening to you)?" and "What do you think would help?" allows patients time to tell their story and give their perspective.[20]

h. The same principle applies to cultural competence. Asking, "What do I need to know about you culturally (or your culture) to care for you?" provides much more individualized and useful information about various cultures, their health beliefs and practices, and needs.[20]

i. Listening to the patient's story provides a holistic perspective and allows the nurse to get an overall sense of what the person is experiencing. This is more than simply using therapeutic techniques such as responding, reflecting, and summarizing.

j. This is deep listening or, as some say, "listening with the heart and not just the ears." It is done with conscious intention and without preconceptions, busyness, distractions, or analysis.

k. Through presence or "being with in the moment," nurses provide each person with an interpersonal encounter that is experienced as a connection with one who is giving undivided attention to the needs and concerns of the individual. Using unconditional positive regard, nurses convey to the individual receiving care the belief in his or her worth and value as a human being, not solely the recipient of medical and nursing interventions.[20p57]

■ CARING–HEALING RESPONSES TO FREQUENTLY ASKED QUESTIONS AND STATEMENTS

Following are some of the questions clients, patients, and families regularly ask nurses. A brief description of the underlying dynamic of the question or statement, ineffective responses, and caring–healing responses are identified.[21,22]

1. "Am I dying?"
   a. *Dynamic:* Request for information, reassurance.
   b. *Ineffective responses:* "I really am not able to discuss that. You should talk with your doctor" or "You always have to keep hope" or "Don't say that, look how you are improving every day."
   c. *Caring–healing response:* In a very gentle voice, "Do you think you are dying?" "Can you tell me why you think you are dying?" Follow up with, "What does death mean to you?"

2. "Why did God [or whomever one believes in] do this to me?" and "I don't want to go on living."
   a. *Dynamic:* Spiritual distress.
   b. *Ineffective responses:* "Sometimes in life, bad things happen to people who don't deserve them," or "Don't feel that way. God has not abandoned you," or "We can't always understand why things happen, but there is a reason."
   c. *Caring–healing response:* Be silent. If acceptable, hold the person's hand and let the person know by your full attention and presence that you are willing to bear witness to their deepest despair and sorrow. "This seems to be a very difficult time for you on many different levels." Wait for a response. If none, gently ask, "Can you explain that to me so that I can understand?"

3. "Don't tell anybody else what I am telling you."
   a. *Dynamic:* Can I trust you?
   b. *Ineffective responses:* "You can trust me not to tell anyone else" or "Your request makes me really uncomfortable."
   c. *Caring–healing response:* "Is there a particular reason why you do not want me to share this information?" Wait for a response. Depending on the answer, "I understand your wish to keep this between us, but others may need to know this information to provide you with [what you need, or the best care possible, or to help you make a decision, etc.]" or "If it is not imperative for anyone else to know, certainly I will keep it confidential."

4. Repeated requests for the nurse's personal information.
   a. *Dynamic:* A need to be connected.
   b. *Ineffective responses:* "I don't talk with clients or patients about my personal life" or answering every question that the individual asks.
   c. *Caring–healing response:* "Is there a reason why you would like to know about [the topic asked about]?"

5. Silence.
   a. *Dynamic:* Individual is thinking, processing, feeling, cannot put thoughts and feelings into words, or is physically or emotionally exhausted. Silence is a form of communication and has a great deal of meaning.
   b. *Ineffective responses:* Filling the silence with any words to keep conversation alive or "I can see that you do not want to talk now, so I will come back later."
   c. *Caring–healing response:* "You seem quiet." Wait for a response. "Would you like to talk or would you just like me to sit here with you for a while?" Get in touch with your own discomfort if this is an issue for you, relax into the silence, understanding that this is what the person needs at this time. Communicate through presence and intent that you are there for this person.

6. "What should I do? What would you do?"
   a. *Dynamic:* Insecurity about decision, lack of knowledge, second guessing, too much input.
   b. *Ineffective responses:* "Well, I would..." or "When this happened to [me, my brother/friend/another patient], I/she/he did..." or "I think you should discuss this with your doctor."
   c. *Caring–healing response:* "First, tell me what you understand about your illness and treatment." Wait for a response. Then, "Tell me what you think you should do or what you feel would be best or most helpful for you." The nurse is an option giver, not the prescriber. Discuss options, implications of each option, and the individual's thoughts, feelings, beliefs, and concerns about each option so that the person has sufficient information to make an informed decision with which he or she is comfortable.

7. Anger.
   a. *Dynamic:* Powerlessness.
   b. *Ineffective responses:* "Don't get angry at me, I am just trying to help you," or "I don't have to take this from [a patient, a colleague, a family, the doctor, etc.]," or "Call security."
   c. *Caring–healing response:* Stop and center, and then send peace. Visualize the person as he or she was as an innocent, precious baby. The energy tends to change immediately when we image babies because they connect with our joy. Wait calmly until the angry person completes the attack, and then begin the discussion.

8. Fear.
   a. *Dynamic:* Projection, misperception. Fear and worry are the most common form of imagery.
   b. *Ineffective response:* "Don't worry, everything will work out."
   c. *Caring–healing response:* "Can you share with me what your understanding is or what you think is going to happen?" Then, reality test by gently asking, "What do you think is the worst that can happen?" and "What might be a positive that can happen in this circumstance?"

9. Anxiety
   a. *Dynamic:* Projection, unknowing, too much input, inability to stay in the present or listen to and trust one's own inner wisdom.
   b. *Ineffective responses:* "Constantly thinking or worrying about this is not going to help; it will only make it worse" or "Try to get your mind off of it."
   c. *Caring–healing response:* "It sounds like a lot is going on, so let's see if we can focus on right now and deal with after that" or "What do you think is best or necessary for you? What is your body, mind, and gut telling you?"

10. "It's all my fault."
    a. *Dynamic:* Guilt often rooted in shame.
    b. *Ineffective responses:* "Of course you are not to blame" or "Well, it was going to happen some time or another, it's not your fault."

c. *Caring–healing response:* "Can you tell me why you think you are responsible for [or are to blame for]...?"

11. "I am such a burden [e.g., bothering you, having you see me like this, having to clean me up, can't do anything for myself]."

   a. *Dynamic:* Guilt as an assault on one's assumptions and beliefs about oneself and what one wants others to believe about him or her, creating vulnerability and exposure.

   b. *Ineffective response:* "Oh, I've seen [or dealt with] worse. You're not so bad."

   c. *Caring–healing response:* "It is a gift to care for you and share this part of your journey [your experience] with you" or "It is my pleasure."

CONCLUSION

1. Holistic communication is a caring–healing process that calls forth the full use of self in interacting with another.

2. The elements that distinguish holistic communication are:

   a. Acknowledgment of the infinite and sacred nature of Being

   b. The use of centering, grounding, intention, and intuition

   c. Caring–healing, transcendent presence

3. Holistic communication can be viewed as a field experience in which there is constant mutual exchange between the nurse's field and the patient's field.

4. Communication is constantly occurring on physical, mental, emotional, and energetic levels.

5. We are never not communicating.

6. Self-knowledge and self-awareness are foundational to the process of holistic communication. Tools and practices that help the nurse gain a greater understanding and awareness of self include journaling, dream analysis, relaxation techniques, self-reflective practices, and meditation.

7. Growing in self-knowledge and self-awareness increases the nurse's effectiveness as an instrument in the caring–healing process.

8. Holistic communication invites us to engage our higher Self as we meet another in that transcendent space where profound healing occurs.

9. When this happens, a "healing field of communication" is created in which both the nurse and person are enriched and nurtured.

NOTES

1. Rogers, M. (1990). Nursing: Science of unitary, irreducible, human beings: Update 1992. In E. A. M. Barrett (Ed.), *Visions of Rogers' science-based nursing*. New York, NY: National League for Nursing.

2. Thornton, L., & Mariano, C. (2009). Evolving from therapeutic to holistic communication. In B. Dossey & L. Keegan (Eds.), *Holistic nursing: A handbook for practice* (5th ed., p. 533). Sudbury, MA: Jones and Bartlett.

3. Thornton, L. (2011). Where heart and soul meet the bottom line: Using the model of whole-person caring to promote health and wellness in your organization. *LOHAS Journal, 12*(1), 31–33.

4. Rogers, M. (1977). *An introduction to the theoretical basis of nursing* (7th ed.). Philadelphia, PA: F. A. Davis.

5. Newman, M. (1994). *Health as expanding consciousness* (2nd ed.). New York, NY: National League for Nursing Press.

6. Watson, J. (1999). *Postmodern nursing and beyond*. New York, NY: Churchill Livingstone.

7. Watson, J. (19999). *Nursing: Human science and human care, a theory of nursing*. Sudbury, MA: NLN Press/Jones and Bartlett.

8. Macrae, J. (1995). Suggestions for thought from Florence Nightingale. AHNA Conference: Changing the face of healing: keynote speech. Phoenix, AZ.

9. Thornton, L. (2010). A spiritual and energetically-based model supporting the practice of Healing Touch. *Energy Magazine, 45*, 15.

10. McCraty, R., & Reese, R. (2009). *The central role of the heart in generating and sustaining positive emotions*. Institute of HeartMath, Publication No. 06-022. Boulder Creek, CA: HeartMath Research Center.

11. McCraty, R., Atkinson, M., & Bradley, R. T. (2004). Electrophysiological evidence of intuition: Part 1. The surprising role of the heart. *Journal of Alternative and Complementary Medicine, 10*(1), 133–143.

12. McCraty, R., & Childre, D. (2010). Coherence: Bridging personal, social, and global health. *Alternative Therapies, 16*(4), 12.

13. Jackson, C., & Keegan, L. (2009). Touch. In B. Dossey & L. Keegan (Eds.), *Holistic nursing: A handbook for practice* (5th ed., p. 348). Sudbury, MA: Jones and Bartlett.

14. McKivergin, M. (2009). The nurse as an instrument of healing. In B. Dossey & L. Keegan (Eds.), *Holistic nursing: A handbook for practice* (5th ed., p. 722). Sudbury, MA: Jones and Bartlett.

15. Tiller, W., & Dibble, W. (2009). A brief introduction to intention-host device research. White paper, William A. Tiller Foundation. Retrieved from http://www.tillerfoundation.com/White%20Paper%20I.pdf

16. Mariano, C. (2007). Holistic nursing as a specialty: Scope and standards of practice. *Clinics of North America, 42*(2), 165–188.

17. Mariano, C. (2010). Holistic integrative therapies in palliative care. In M. Matzo & D. Sherman (Eds.), *Palliative care: Quality care to the end of life* (3rd ed., pp. 44–45). New York, NY: Springer.

18. Thornton, L. (2011). Self-compassion: A prescription for well-being. *Imprint, 58*(2), 43.

19. Thornton, L. (2008). Transcending differences; a holistic approach. *Imprint, 55*(5), 47.

20. Mariano, C. (2009). Holistic nursing: Scope and standards of practice. In B. Dossey & L. Keegan (Eds.), *Holistic nursing: A handbook for practice* (5th ed., p. 54). Sudbury, MA: Jones and Bartlett.

21. Mariano, C. (2010). Why am I here? The koan of our journey. Keynote address, Birchtree Center for Healthcare, NJ.

22. Mariano, C. (2007, 2012). Therapeutic interactions. Adapted course materials, New York University and Pacific College of Oriental Medicine.

■ STUDY QUESTIONS

Basic Level

1. Which of the following is the best definition of therapeutic communication?
   a. Interaction occurring between a nurse and client that helps the client gain insight into his or her behavior and facilitates resolution of the client's problems.
   b. A goal-directed form of communication used to achieve goals that promote client health and well-being. Empathy, unconditional regard, genuineness, respect, concern, caring, and compassion are conveyed through active listening, active observing, focusing, restating, reflecting, and interpreting.
   c. Communication from which the nurse creates and establishes a plan of therapy based on the client's history and symptoms.
   d. A form of communication that creates a therapeutic milieu for the client.

2. Which of the following is the best definition of holistic communication?
   a. Communication that considers the whole person and addresses the body, mind, and spirit.
   b. A caring–healing process that calls forth the full use of self in interacting with another. It incorporates the constructs and processes of therapeutic communication within a framework that acknowledges the infinite, spiritual, and energetic nature of Being, the centrality of being heart-centered, and the importance of intention, self-knowledge, transcendent presence, and intuition in our interactions.
   c. A process in which the nurse is fully engaged in communication with the patient and assesses the patient's strengths in dealing with mental, physical, emotional, and relational challenges.
   d. Involves an equality of communication between the nurse and client. Holistic communication implies that both the client and nurse are teachers/learners in all interactions and that the nurse offers her expertise in behavioral and psychological tools and therapies if the client identifies these interventions as useful.

3. Which of the following is the best definition of person?
   a. An energy field that is infinite and spiritual in essence and is in continual mutual process with the environment. Each person manifests unique physical, mental, emotional, and social or relational patterns that are interrelated, inseparable, and continually evolving.
   b. An amalgamation of the spiritual, mental, emotional, relational, and cultural attributes of an individual.
   c. The sum of the experiences, feelings, physical reactions, and relationships of an individual and that individual's relationship with others and the environment.
   d. The totality of the cognitive, emotional, physical, and relational patterns that are manifested by each individual.

4. Therapeutic communication includes which of the following skills and interactions?
   1. Empathy and unconditional regard
   2. Active listening, active observing, focusing, and restating
   3. Genuineness, respect, concern, caring, and compassion
   4. Reflecting, interpreting, and assessing
      a. 1, 2, 3
      b. 1, 2
      c. 2, 3, 4
      d. All of the above

5. Which elements distinguish holistic communication?
   1. Acknowledgment of the infinite and sacred nature of Being
   2. Recognizing the primary importance of the nurse's relationship
   3. The use of centering, grounding, intention, and intuition
   4. Caring–healing, transcendent presence
      a. 1, 2, 3
      b. 1, 2, 4
      c. 1, 3, 4
      d. All of the above

6. Which of the following nurse leaders and theorists best acknowledge our infinite and sacred nature?
   a. Nightingale, King, and Levine
   b. Newman, Peplau, and Orem
   c. Rogers, Johnson, and Roy
   d. Nightingale, Rogers, and Watson

Advanced Level

7. Which is the dynamic underlying a client's requests for personal information from a nurse?
   a. Insecurity
   b. Powerlessness
   c. A need to be connected
   d. Fear and worry

8. Which processes constitute the preaccess phase of holistic interactions?
   1. Creating intention
   2. Interpreting
   3. Reflective technique
   4. Being centered
      a. 1 and 3
      b. 1 and 4
      c. 2 and 3
      d. 3 and 4

9. What does engaging the Observer allow the nurse to do?
   a. Change the topic when the client becomes upset
   b. Be aware of one's internal reactions and respond from a higher consciousness
   c. Fill silences to keep the conversation with the client alive
   d. Reassure the client that everything will work out for the best

10. Which of the following does meditation *not* involve?
    a. Focusing one's attention internally
    b. Increased receptivity to insights
    c. Reflection and self-knowledge
    d. Planning nursing interventions for the day

11. Which of the following is the most appropriate response a nurse can make when a client expresses insecurity about a treatment decision?
    a. Refer the client to his or her physician
    b. Explain what you would do in the situation
    c. Ascertain what the client understands about his or her illness and treatment
    d. Bring the client an article that discusses the specific illness and treatment

Chapter 28

Environmental Health

Karen Avino and Susan Luck

Original Authors: Susan Luck
and Lynn Keegan

■ DEFINITIONS

Ambience An environment or its distinct atmosphere; the totality of feeling that one experiences from a particular environment.

Anthropocentrism The worldview that places human beings as the central fact or final aim of the universe.

Bisphenol A (BPA) An organic compound with two phenol functional groups. It is used to make polycarbonate plastic and epoxy resins, along with other applications, and since the mid-1930s is known to be estrogenic.

Chaos Theory Sometimes called the "new science," this theory offers a way of seeing order and patterns where formerly only the random, the erratic, and the unpredictable had been observed.

Detoxification The metabolic process by which the toxic qualities of a poison or toxin are reduced or eliminated from the body.

Earth jurisprudence Earth law recognizes the Earth as the primary source of law that sets human law in a context that is wider than humanity

Ecology The scientific study of interrelationships between and among organisms, and among them and all aspects, living and non-living, of their environment.

Ecominnea The concept of an ecologically sound society.

Electromagnetic fields (EMFs) The field force in motion coupled with electric and magnetic fields that are generated by time-varying currents and accelerated charges.

Endocrine disruptors (xenoestrogens) Synthetic hormone-mimicking compounds found in many pesticides, drugs, plastics, and personal care products.

Environment Everything that surrounds an individual or group of people: physical, social, psychological, cultural, and spiritual characteristics; external and internal features; animate and inanimate objects; climate; seen and unseen vibrations, frequencies, and energy patterns not yet understood.

Environmental ethics A division of philosophy concerned with valuing the environment, primarily as it relates to humankind, secondarily as it relates to other creatures and to the land.

Environmental justice A subbranch of ethics examining the innate and relational value among organisms and all aspects of their environment.

Epistemology The branch of philosophy that addresses the origin, nature, methods, and limits of knowledge.

Ergonomics The study of and realization of the importance of human factors in engineering.

Permaculture An approach to designing human settlements and agricultural systems that are modeled on the relationships found in natural ecologies.

Persistent organic pollutants (POPs) Chemical substances that persist in the environment, bioaccumulate through the food web, and pose a risk of causing adverse effects to human health and the environment.

Personal space The area around an individual that should be under the control of that individual, including air, light, temperature, sound, scent, and color.

Phthalates Classified as "plasticizers," a group of industrial chemicals used to make plastics such as polyvinyl chloride (PVC) more flexible or resilient. They are also known to be endocrine disruptors.

Precautionary principle When an activity raises threats of harm to human health or the environment, precautionary measures shall be taken, even if some cause-and-effect relationships are not fully established scientifically.

Restorative justice An ethical perception that directs that environmental damages not only be curtailed, but also repaired and recompensed in some meaningful way.

Superfund sites Hazardous waste landfills or abandoned manufacturing sites, names of which appear on the Environmental Protection Agency's National Priorities List.

Sustainable future Meeting the needs of the present without compromising the needs of future generations.

Toxic substance A substance that can cause harm to a person through either short- or long-term exposure, as by (1) inhalation; (2) ingestion into the body in the form of vapors, gases, fumes, dusts, solids, liquids, or mists; or (3) skin absorption.

■ THEORY AND RESEARCH

1. Recognize that we are the microcosm of the macrocosm; a world of vast complexity and unpredictability; understanding that our health and the health of our planet are inextricably interwoven.
2. Engage in practices that create healing environments in our home, workplace, and community.
3. Reside in knowing that each individual makes a difference toward healing the global community beginning with individual actions.

Environmental Leadership in Holistic Nursing

1. The five themes of the constellation of environment:
   a. Sharing, listening, and learning through our personal and collective life stories.
   b. Increasing self-awareness and self-care when living in a toxic world.
   c. Choosing a sustainable future.
   d. Building communities that support learning and positive actions for creating change: *start local, think global.*
   e. Working from the inside out: healing our internal and external environments.

Telling Our Story: Local to Global

1. Holistic practice embraces the interconnectedness of body, mind, and spirit, knowing that when there is disharmony or disruption in our internal or external environment, we are out of balance. Holistic nurses are called to lead the way to heal our planet and all who dwell here today and for any foreseeable future.
2. As living beings, we are a reflection of our world, and any environmental assault directly affects our energetic patterns and well-being.
3. Florence Nightingale, through her 13 canons, gave the most basic instruction of all: "The art of nursing requires us to alter the environment safely."[1]
4. In *Notes on Nursing*, Florence Nightingale wrote, "No amount of medical knowledge will lessen the accountability for nurses to do what nurses do, that is, manage the environment to promote positive life processes."

Florence Nightingale as Environmentalist

1. Florence Nightingale, the founder of modern nursing, understood ecological

medicine and environmental health as involving the health of not only humans, but of all species and ecosystems with which we are connected physically, psychologically, and spiritually.

2. Dossey delineates many of Nightingale's tenets. One of these is the precautionary principle. The essence of the precautionary principle is if there is a suspicion about a harmful environment or exposure, even though all of the evidence is not in, remove the person from the situation or stop the use of suspected harmful exposures. It emphasizes that zero tolerance for the contamination of our environments is acceptable, not minimal or moderate contamination.[2,3]

3. Nightingale understood that nurses have an ethical and moral responsibility to take anticipatory actions to prevent harm.

4. Precautionary principle proponents and health policy analysts today advocate that it is incumbent on those introducing a new chemical or technology to demonstrate that it is safe, and not for the rest of us to prove it is harmful.[4]

5. The roots of the environmental movement in the United States can be attributed to Native American cultures and traditions deeply honoring the feminine nurturing Earth for sustaining life for present and future generations.

   a. Caring for our environment did not emerge until the 1960s and 1970s, when activists elucidated the dangers of DDT and other hazardous materials—polychlorinated biphenyls (PCBs), mercury, lead, and other heavy metals.

   b. In 1976, the Environmental Protection Agency was established and environmental legislation and protection agencies widened the focus from preservation to protection and banned the pesticide DDT, which would later be classified as a "hormonal disruptor" and a carcinogen, and removed lead from paint in 1978.[5]

   c. Since the 1970s, two federal agencies, the Environmental Protection Agency (EPA) and the Occupational Safety and Health Administration (OSHA), were formed to monitor environmental concerns.

   d. In the 1980s, several states enacted right-to-know laws that require employers to notify employees of health hazards, to provide formal education regarding the safe use of toxic substances, and to keep medical records of those workers routinely exposed to specific toxic substances.

   e. In the 1980s, *Healthy People 2020* was created as a set of health prevention goals that challenges health providers to strongly consider the environment's effect on several health indicators. The environment can influence several of the indicators being targeted, and these include asthma, work-related assaults, lead exposure, needlestick injuries, noise-induced hearing loss, and worksite stress.[6] These have implications for occupational risk exposure.

6. In the 1980s, the discovery of the hole in the ozone layer over Antarctica, along with escalating concern over global warming and climate change, introduced another phase of environmentalism.

7. The holistic outlook recognizes all systems as interacting. If one part is affected, change of a greater or lesser magnitude occurs everywhere, including the universe. Figure 29-1, Current Environmental Concerns, can be found in *Holistic Nursing: A Handbook for Practice* (6th ed.). Noise, lighting, air quality, space allocation, and workplace toxins have gained increasing attention as chronic stressors.

Living in a Toxic World

1. In 2006, the World Health Organization (WHO) issued a report titled *Preventing Disease Through Healthy Environments—Towards an Estimate of the Environmental Burden of Disease*, the most comprehensive and systematic study yet undertaken on how *preventable* environmental hazards contribute to a wide range of diseases and injuries. The estimate reflects how much death, illness, and disability could be realistically avoided every year as a result of better environmental management. The report stated that nearly one-quarter of global disease is caused by environmental exposures, and "well targeted interventions can prevent

much of the environmental risk," saving suffering and millions of lives every year.[7]

2. Today there are many by-products of waste from industrial and agricultural processes. Chemical compounds are in our food, air, and water. The bioaccumulation of chemicals in humans is fueling metabolic and systemic dysfunctions of the immune, neurological, and endocrine systems. This toxic burden can trigger autoimmune reactivity, asthma, allergies, cancers, cognitive deficits, mood changes, neurological illness, reproductive dysfunction, glucose dysregulation, and obesity.[7,8]

Our Environmental Story

1. In less than one lifetime, production of synthetic organic chemicals (e.g., dyes, plastics, pesticides, and solvents) has increased more than 1,000-fold in the United States alone.
2. According to the National Toxicology Program, more than 80,000 chemicals are registered for use in the United States. Others, such as pesticides and herbicides, are designed to be usefully lethal.
3. In addition, many chemicals are emitted as by-products of production or incineration (particularly relevant to the hospital industry).
4. PCBs were created in 1929 for use only in electrical wiring, lubricants, and liquid seals. Many chemicals, including DDT and PCBs, although banned by the Environmental Protection Agency can still be found in human blood samples today along with 250 other synthetic chemicals in the bodies of almost everyone in the industrial world.
5. A recent study by the Centers for Disease Control and Prevention conservatively estimates that Americans of all ages carry a body burden of at least 148 chemicals, some of them banned for decades.[9]
6. The new field of epigenetics studies how the expressions of our genes are influenced under environmental stress.
7. Environmental elements known to be hazardous include asbestos, lead, cigarette smoke, silica, benzene, mercury, chlorine, formaldehyde, poor lighting, stress, and noise. Studies show an increased risk of death resulting from leukemia, particularly

myeloid leukemia, among workers exposed to formaldehyde.[10]

Children's Health

1. Children are the most vulnerable to environmental exposures for the following reasons:
   a. Their bodily systems are still developing. They eat more, drink more, and breathe more in proportion to their body size. Their behaviors, such as crawling on the ground, can expose them more to chemicals and organisms
   b. Some peer-reviewed studies found children exposed in the womb to high levels of a class of pesticides known as organophosphates had lower average intelligence than other children by the time they reached age 7 years. Researchers found that exposure during pregnancy can impair a child's cognitive development.
2. Pesticide exposure in our food supply is associated with neurologic and learning disabilities and risk of cancer. Home pesticide and insecticide use is linked to brain cancer, leukemia from home and garden pesticides, and nonlymphocytic leukemia from extermination use. Positive disease associations have been found with exposures during pregnancy and childhood to pesticides, insecticides, and/or herbicides.[11]
3. The risk of childhood brain cancer increases with exposures received from either parent typically through lawn and garden care. Clothing washed immediately after exposure or wearing lowered risk.[12-14]

Endocrine Disruptors

1. Human beings and animals are most vulnerable to hormonal disruption during prenatal development. Other critical windows when the endocrine system is particularly sensitive to hormonal disruption include early life, puberty, pregnancy, and lactation.[15]
2. Endocrine disruptors are chemicals that interfere with the body's endocrine system and produce adverse developmental, reproductive, neurologic, and immune effects in humans and pose the greatest risk

during prenatal and early postnatal development when organ and neural systems are forming.

   a. Until 1971, diethylstilbesterol (DES) was administered to pregnant women to prevent miscarriages. As a result, female children of mothers who took DES during pregnancy have a higher incidence of certain forms of ovarian, cervical, and vaginal cancer.[16]

3. A wide range of substances, both natural and man-made, is thought to cause endocrine disruption, including pharmaceuticals, polychlorinated biphenyls, DDT, dieldrin, atrazine and other pesticides and herbicides, and plasticizers such as bisphenol A and phthalates.

4. Endocrine disruptors are found in many everyday products, including plastic bottles, metal food cans, detergents, flame retardants, food, toys, cosmetics, pesticides, and industrial chemicals and by-products such as polychlorinated biphenyls (PCBs), dioxins, and phenols. Many endocrine disruptors affect sex hormone function and reproduction.

5. Bisphenol A is widely used in the manufacturing of plastics including baby bottles, toys, metal cans, technology applications, paints and adhesives, and as a protective coating in many products. According to the U.S. Centers for Disease Control and Prevention, 95% of Americans have detectable levels of bisphenol A in their bodies at and above the concentrations known to cause adverse effects.

6. The mechanisms of action and the effects of endocrine-disrupting chemicals on male and female reproduction, thyroid function, metabolism, and obesity are well documented.[17]

Women's Health

1. The conception rates fell 44% in the United States between 1960 and 2002.[18] Hormone disruptors can affect both parents, and scientists have linked fertility problems to exposure to BPA, DDT, DES, cigarette smoke, and PCBs.[19]

2. In human studies, early puberty is linked to greater cumulative estrogenic exposure to multiple contaminants, such as phthalates,

BPA, and organochlorine pesticides among others.[20] Girls with early puberty have increased risk for depression, obesity, polycystic ovarian syndrome, breast cancer, and experimentation with sex and drugs at a younger age.

Pesticides Permeate Our World

1. Atrazine, an endocrine disruptor chemical, is a herbicide used globally. Atrazine has been banned by the European Union. Atrazine concerns include being found in drinking water and the pollutant's ability to emasculate amphibians and fish as well as cause birth defects, such as hypospadias, in male newborns.

2. In 2009, the National Resource Defense Council (NRDC) found contamination of watersheds and drinking water systems across the Midwest and southern United States.[21]

Early Child Development

1. Environmental factors during pregnancy might play a larger role than genetics in the development of autism spectrum disorders. Studies found that genetics account for about 38% of the risk of autism and that environmental factors account for about 62%. Another study found that children faced a higher risk of autism if their mothers took antidepressants during the year prior to giving birth.

2. One study links dietary pesticide exposure (organophosphates, OPs) to attention deficit disorders in children. Fruits with the highest concentration of pesticides included strawberries, raspberries, and blueberries that were grown with conventional agriculture techniques.[22]

Breast Cancer

1. Breast cancer in the United States increased more than 40% between 1973 and 1998. Breast cancer arises from genetic, lifestyle, and environmental causes, several of which relate to lifetime exposure to hormones.[23]

2. Only about 5% of women diagnosed with breast cancer have a link to the breast cancer gene. Contributing factors that increase

breast cancer risk include having children late in life, early onset of puberty, exposure to radiation from chest x-rays during child-hood, taking hormone replacement therapy, alcohol abuse, tobacco exposure, second-hand smoke exposure, and obesity disease.

3. According to the latest research, cumulative toxic exposures often beginning in utero show clear links to increased risks for breast cancer later in life.[24]

4. Research also links the role of the environment to the rise in testicular and prostate cancers in men.[25]

5. Our modern poor-quality diet, combined with agricultural pesticides and animals being raised on antibiotics, chemical feed, and growth hormones, can dispose many to a toxic body burden.

6. Up to 40% of cancers are avoidable: Eat a plant-based diet, maintain moderate weight, and get exercise.

7. Cancer can be reduced by lifestyle interventions that can lower exposures to toxicants and enhance innate immune systems, increasing cellular energy for healthy metabolism and improving detoxification pathways through nutrition, stress reduction, and exercise.[25,26]

8. Everyday products that contain endocrine disruptors that people can try to avoid or eliminate are as follows:
   a. Pesticides, herbicides, including pesticide residues in soil
   b. Dry cleaning chemicals
   c. Solvents: paints, varnishes, cleaning fluids
   d. Spermicidal contraceptives and treated condoms
   e. Perfume fragrances, air fresheners, cleaning fragrances
   f. Car exhaust, car interiors—especially that "new car smell" (off-gassing)
   g. Plastics, plastic baby bottles, plastic food storage containers, Styrofoam, tin cans (BPA lining)
   h. PVC plumbing pipes;
   i. Pharmaceutical runoff in the water supply
   j. BHA and BHT, common food preservatives, and FD&C Red No. 3, a common food dye
   k. Personal care products that contain parabens, phthalates

9. The precautionary principle should be used while demanding health policy actions and regulation of the chemical industry.

10. Following is a review of the prevention strategies that can be implemented:
    a. Choose your food wisely; eat organically grown and raised foods. Choose seasonal and local foods.
    b. Limit intake of animal fats because endocrine disruptors and heavy metals accumulate in the food and are stored in fat. Monitor fish consumption. Eat wild-caught salmon, sardines, and cod.
    c. Avoid pesticides. The Environmental Working Group database (www.ewg.org) offers guidelines on the fruits and vegetables containing both the highest pesticide residues and the lowest. Wash all produce before consuming, or peel them if they are not organically grown.
    d. Support your body's natural ability to detoxify by exercising, sweating, using saunas.
    e. Get regular sleep (you detoxify at night); drink plenty of clean or filtered water; eat fiber.
    f. Drink beverages such as green tea that contain antioxidants and phytonutrients that can detoxify.
    g. If planning a pregnancy or breastfeeding, eliminate as many chemicals as possible for 1 year prior to conception. Guidelines for pregnant women on eating fish are listed at www.americanpregnancy.org/pregnancyhealth/fishmercury.htm.
    h. Check for hormone-disrupting chemicals and heavy metals in your water supply. Drink purified water out of PBA-free bottles or bottles marked with codes 2, 4, and 5.
    i. Never let infants chew on soft plastic toys and never microwave food in a plastic bowl or covered in plastic wrap. A good rule of thumb is that the softer the plastic, the more chemicals it contains.

■ THE WATER WE DRINK

1. There is a global water shortage crisis. In the Western world, chemicals taint drinking water in wells and urban or rural water supplies. The EPA has identified more than 6,000 chemicals in water.[27]

a. In 2011, the EPA's Drinking Water Strategy (DWS) focused on carcinogenic volatile organic compounds (VOCs) as a group and identified four goals. Effective methods must meet the following standards:
  - Are sustainable and water and energy efficient
  - Are cost-effective for utilities and consumers
  - Address a broad array of contaminants
  - Improve public health protection

■ THE AIR WE BREATHE

1. Between 2001 and 2009, asthma rates in the United States grew by 4.3 million people.
2. Since 1970, the EPA has protected public health by setting and enforcing standards to protect the quality of the air and water. Many older power plants and industrial facilities employ loopholes in the current regulations to allow them to pollute at much higher levels than recommended.

■ CLIMATE CHANGE: REDUCING GLOBAL WARMING

1. The Clean Air Act states the pollution that causes global warming and climate change must be treated like any other air pollution.
2. In December 2009, the EPA responded to the Supreme Court by issuing an "endangerment finding" determining that carbon dioxide and five other greenhouse gases are dangerous to both health and welfare.
3. In April 2010, the EPA took its first steps to develop standards for vehicles, setting in motion standards for cars and light-duty trucks and separate standards for medium- and heavy-duty trucks.
   a. Improving emissions performance in cars and light trucks would reduce heat-trapping carbon pollution that causes global warming while saving consumers billions of dollars and cutting oil use.
   b. The first-ever standards to cut carbon dioxide emissions and improve fuel efficiency in medium- and heavy-duty trucks would reduce global warming pollution. Instituting standards to reduce global warming pollution from power plants would help reduce pollution that is increasing deaths and illnesses from heat waves, air pollution, infectious diseases, and severe weather events.[28]

■ INCREASING AWARENESS FOR CHANGE

1. In 1992, Al Gore raised awareness of environmental issues and stressed that only a radical rethinking of our relationship with nature can save the Earth's ecology for future generations.[29]

■ SUSTAINABLE HEALTH CARE

1. A nurse-inspired environmental health movement, Health Care Without Harm (HCWH), is at the forefront to transform the way hospitals are designed, built, and operated and to green health care. Issues to be addressed in environmentally responsible health care include waste management; elimination of toxic materials; safer cleaners, chemicals, and pesticides; healthy food systems; cleaner energy; and safe disposal of pharmaceuticals.[30]

■ CHOOSING A SUSTAINABLE FUTURE

1. In 1993 in the United States, the President's Council on Sustainable Development developed a vision statement.[31]
2. Sustainability demands a redefinition of consumption goals, such as use of renewable resources at a rate that does not exceed their rates of regeneration and use of nonrenewable resources at a rate that does not exceed the rate at which sustainable, renewable substitutes are developed.
3. The Leadership in Energy and Environmental Design (LEED) Council is an internationally recognized green building certification system that verifies that a building or community was designed and built using strategies intended to improve performance such as energy savings, water efficiency, CO_2 emissions reduction, improved indoor environmental air quality, and stewardship of resources.[32]

Green Buildings Are Eco-Friendly Structures

1. Green buildings evolved from an initial focus on building energy use to a broader focus on the full range of sustainable/green strategies. The Sustainable Industry Council is now moving to the next phase of this evolutionary process.
2. Green engineering advances the sustainability of manufacturing processes, construction, and infrastructure and supports research on environmentally benign manufacturing and chemical processes.
3. Ecological engineering focuses on the aspects of restoring ecological function to natural systems.
4. Earth Systems Engineering considers large-scale engineering projects that involve mitigation of greenhouse gas emissions, adaptation to climate change, and other global-scale concerns.

Cultivating Healing Environments

1. Molter suggests that the healing environment in the critical care setting is a synergistic integration of components of a holistic intention in care that includes complementary therapies, family and patient-centered interventions, and an aesthetic setting with administrative support of health professionals who value a body-mind-spirit approach. Multiple driving forces are leading the way to the development of healing environments, such as the increased utilization of complementary and alternative therapies by the general public and nurses, steady increases of persons living with chronic illness, and the holistic movement toward care versus cure.[33,34]
2. In 1990, the American Association of Critical Care Nurses established guidelines for creating a healing and humane environment. The *AACN Protocols for Practice: Creating Healing Environments* summarizes evidence-based interventions that focus on environmental design and strategies, family needs interventions and presence, family visitation and partnership, family pet visiting and animal-assisted therapy, spiritual and complementary therapies, and pain management.[33]

3. Nurses have modeled and evolved the Nightingale tenets for use in practice. For example, one hospital's use of a theoretical Model of Whole-Person Caring resulted in increased patient and employee satisfaction and decreased nursing turnover and now serves as the foundation for a comprehensive healing environment.[35]

Creating Optimal Healing Environments

1. Samueli Institute's Optimal Healing Environments (OHE) program seeks to build the knowledge base with research to influence the healing process through an approach that encompasses all of the social, psychological, organizational, behavioral, and physical conditions to demonstrate how healing translates directly into current healthcare practices.[36]
2. Optimal healing environments are created through eight domains that include the inner environment of the patient and caregiver, the interpersonal environment of relationships and healing practices, and the external environment of healing spaces and sustainable communities.[37]
   a. The eight domains of an optimal healing environment are the following:
      - Developing healing intention
      - Experiencing personal wholeness
      - Cultivating healing relationships
      - Creating healing organizations
      - Practicing healthy lifestyles
      - Applying integrative health care
      - Building healing spaces
      - Fostering ecological sustainability

Working from the Inside Out

1. Holistic nurses are role models to others in the way we live our lives, which emerges from our day-to-day choices. In holistic practice, nurses assist others in examining their options and encourage them to make life-affirming choices.
2. As nurses deepen environmental awareness, engagement in our self-grief work grows and fuels the commitment to "make it right" as we claim accountability and acknowledge our own vulnerability as planetary citizens

■ NOISE AND THE STRESS RESPONSE

1. There is a link between noise pollution and adverse mental and physical health.
2. Elevated workplace or other noise can cause hearing impairment, hypertension, ischemic heart disease, annoyance, and sleep disturbance. Changes in the immune system and birth defects have been attributed to noise exposure.
3. Studies show that noise causes changes in blood pressure, sleep patterns, and digestion, all signs of stress on the body. Science now shows that noise raises stress levels to the point of causing heart and immune system problems and can alter brain chemistry in harmful ways.
4. The Noise Control Act of 1972 in the United States was the direct result of early scientific studies showing the extreme havoc noise causes for humans.
5. A 1980 study examining the impact of airport noise on children's health found higher blood pressure in kids living near the Los Angeles LAX airport than in those living farther away.[38]
6. One study suggests that the quality of work performance and perceived annoyance might be influenced by a continuous exposure to low-frequency noise at commonly occurring noise levels. Subjects categorized as highly sensitive to low-frequency noise might be at highest risk.[39]
7. Noise causes the release of different stress hormones, such as corticotropin releasing hormone (CRH) and adrenocorticotropic hormone (ACTH), especially in sleeping persons during the vagotropic night/early morning phase. Advances in hospital technology have led to increased sound levels in the critical care unit. In one study, there was a causal relationship between critical care units and suppression of REM sleep.[40]

■ RADIATION EXPOSURES: LIVING IN THE MODERN WORLD

1. Radiation is part of our natural environment, from materials in the Earth itself and from the sun.

2. Estimates are that we receive up to 100,000 times more radiation than our great-grandparents did over a lifetime.

Radiation in Tobacco Leaves

1. Former U.S. Surgeon General Koop stated that tobacco radiation is probably responsible for 90% of tobacco-related cancer. Naturally occurring radioactive minerals accumulate on sticky surfaces of tobacco leaves.
2. Second-hand smoke is harmful to nearby nonsmokers, especially children.[41]

Microwave Cooking

1. Research shows that cooking food in a microwave can alter the physical makeup of the food by breaking up the molecular structure and creating a whole new set of chemicals, known as unique radiolytic products (URPs) through irradiation.

Food Irradiation

1. Food irradiation is a process whereby food is exposed to a controlled source of ionizing radiation to prolong shelf life and reduce food losses, improve microbiologic safety, and/or reduce the use of chemical fumigants and additives in controlling organisms. It is used on grain, dried spices, dried or fresh fruits and vegetables. It is used to inhibit sprouting in tubers and bulbs; retard postharvest ripening of fruits; inactivate parasites in meats and fish; eliminate spoilage microbes from fresh fruits and vegetables; extend shelf life in poultry, meats, fish, and shellfish; decontaminate poultry and beef; and sterilize foods and feeds.[42]
2. Nutritionally, irradiation can destroy 20–80% of several essential nutrients including vitamin A; thiamine; vitamins B_2, B_3, B_6, B_{12}; folic acid; and vitamins C, E, and K. Some essential fatty acids might also be affected.[43] Irradiation kills friendly bacteria and enzymes, effectively rendering the food "dead."[43]
3. In the United States, packaging must list that food is irradiated. (The symbol for

irradiation is a green flower-like graphic called the radura.)

4. Food irradiation has not been adequately tested on humans and more research is needed.[42]

Diagnostic Radiation

1. The average lifetime dose of diagnostic radiation has increased sevenfold since 1980. Increased exposure to x-rays can cause mutations in DNA that can lead to cancer.

2. CT scans: Two recent studies concerning radiation exposure associated with computed tomography (CT) scans in vascular and cardiac imaging have raised concerns about long-term cancer risks. One chest CT scan results in more than 100 times the radiation dose of a routine chest x-ray.

3. The highest doses of radiation are routinely used for coronary angiography.[44] The younger a patient is at the time of the scan, the higher is the risk of cancer eventually developing.[41]

Airport Scanners

1. Most airport scanners deliver less radiation than a passenger is likely to receive from atmospheric radiation while airborne.

2. Pregnant women and children should not be scanned.

3. A study of airline pilots and cabin crews found these groups to have a significant incidence of leukemia and skin and breast cancer as a result of chromosomal damage from ionizing cosmic radiation encountered during years of flying at high altitudes.

Cell Phones

1. Radiofrequency energy is a form of nonionizing electromagnetic radiation; exposure depends on the technology of the phone, distance between the phone's antenna and the user, the extent and type of use, and distance of the user from base stations. Studies have not shown a consistent link between cell phone use and cancer.

2. The Interphone Study that includes 13 countries found cell phone users are at risk for two of the most common types of brain tumor, glioma and meningioma, compared to nonusers.

Electromagnetic Fields

1. Electromagnetic fields (EMFs) can adversely affect health, and it is important to reduce exposure.

2. An important formula for EMF protection is to know how much to increase distance from the source depending on the type of EMF hazard. See the Radiation Dose Chart at the American Nuclear Society website: www.ans.org/pi/resources/dosechart.

■ SMOKING

1. The health effects of smoking for women are more serious than for men. Women face additional hazards in pregnancy, female-specific cancers such as cancer of the cervix, and exposure to passive smoking.

2. Breathing secondhand smoke (SHS) causes heart disease and lung cancer in adults and increased risks for sudden infant death syndrome, acute respiratory infections, middle ear disease, worsened asthma, respiratory symptoms, and slowed lung growth in children.

■ DETOXIFICATION

1. Internal biochemical processes combined with man-made chemicals can overwhelm the body's detoxification pathways and accumulate stored in tissues, particularly body fat. The lymphatic system, liver, bowels, kidneys, skin, and lungs rid the body of toxins.

2. Research in fields of human genomics, nutrition, and lifestyle choices provides new information to minimize exposures and prevent toxins from wreaking havoc on immune systems and overall health.

3. Blood carries toxins to the liver, which uses enzymes, amino acids, and phytonutrients to detoxify harmful substances by converting them into a water-soluble form to be eliminated via the urine or feces.

4. Carrying a large toxic body burden can stress the ability of this system, built for natural toxins and biochemical by-products, not the man-made ones people have to deal with in these modern times.

5. If detoxification pathways in the liver are impaired, the breakdown of toxins can form intermediary metabolites that are often more toxic than the original item.

6. Optimizing the body's ability to detoxify includes: maintaining good elimination patterns, consuming a whole-food diet, avoiding chemicals in food, and using fresh air, natural sunlight, and exercise.
7. Table 29-3, Nursing Interventions: Environment, in *Holistic Nursing: A Handbook for Practice* shows client outcomes, nursing prescriptions, and use of the environment as a nursing intervention.

■ NOTES

1. Dossey, B. M., et al. (2005). *Florence Nightingale today: Healing, leadership, global action.* Washington, DC: Nursebooks.org.
2. Nightingale, F. (1860). *Notes on nursing: What it is, and what it is not.* London, England: Harrison and Sons.
3. Frumkin, H. (Ed.). (2010). *Environmental health: From global to local* (2nd ed.). San Francisco, CA: Wiley.
4. Morello-Frosch, R. (2002). Integrating environmental justice and the precautionary principle in research and policy making: The case of ambient air toxics exposures and health risks among schoolchildren in Los Angeles. *Annals of the American Academy of Political and Social Science, 584*(1), 47–68.
5. Agency for Toxic Substances and Disease Registry. (2002, September). Toxicological profile for DDT, DDE, and DDD. Retrieved from http://www.atsdr.cdc.gov/toxprofiles/tp.asp?id=81&tid=20
6. Olszewski, K., Parks, C., & Chikotas, N. E. (2007). Occupational safety and health objectives of *Healthy People 2010*: A systematic approach for occupational health nurses, part II. *American Association of Occupational Health Nurses Journal, 5*(3), 115–125.
7. Luccio-Camelo, D. C., & Prins, G. S. (2011). Disruption of androgen receptor signaling in males by environmental chemicals. *Journal of Steroid Biochemistry and Molecular Biology, 127*(1–2), 74–82.
8. Jones, O. A. H., Maguire, M. L., & Griffin, J. L. (2008). Environmental pollution and diabetes: A neglected association. *Lancet, 371*(9609), 287–288.
9. U.S. Department of Health and Human Services, Centers for Disease Control and Prevention. (2009). *Fourth national report on human exposure to environmental chemicals 2009.* Atlanta, GA: CDC.
10. Beane Freeman, L., Blair, A., Lubin, J. H., et al. (2009). Mortality from lymphohematopoietic malignancies among workers in formaldehyde industries: The National Cancer Institute Cohort. *Journal of the National Cancer Institute, 101*(10), 751–761.
11. Van Maele-Fabry, G., Lantin, A. C., Hoet, P., & Lison, D. (2011). Review, residential exposure to pesticides and childhood leukaemia: A systematic review and meta-analysis. *Environmental International, 37*(1), 280–291.
12. Van Maele-Fabry, G., Lantin, A. C., Hoet, P., & Lison, D. (2010). Childhood leukemia and parental occupational exposure to pesticides: A systematic review and meta-analysis. *Cancer Causes and Control, 21*(6), 787–809.
13. Wigle, D. T., Turner, M. C., & Krewski, D. (2009). A systematic review and meta-analysis of childhood leukemia and parental occupational pesticide exposure. *Environmental Health Perspectives, 117*(10), 1505–1513.
14. Hernández-Morales, A. L., Zonana-Nacach, A., & Zaragoza-Sandoval, V. M. (2009). Associated risk factors in acute leukemia in children. A cases and controls study. *Revista Medica del Instituto Mexicano del Seguro Social, 47*(5), 497–503. (Spanish)
15. Crain, D. A., & Janssen, S. J. (2008). Female reproductive disorders: The roles of endocrine disrupting compounds and developmental timing. *Fertility and Sterility, 90,* 911–940.
16. Newbold, R. R., & Padilla-Banks, E. (2006). Adverse effects of the model environmental estrogen diethylstilbestrol are transmitted to subsequent generations. *Endocrinology, 147*(6), S11–S17.
17. Endocrine Society. (2009). *Endocrine-disrupting chemicals.* Chevy Chase, MD: Author. Retrieved from http://www.endo-society.org/journals/scientificstatements/upload/edc_scientific_statement.pdf
18. IBID.
19. Luccio-Camelo, D. C., & Prins, G. S. (2011). Disruption of androgen receptor signaling in males by environmental chemicals. *Journal of Steroid Biochemistry and Molecular Biology, 127*(1–2), 74–82.
20. Chakraborty, J. R., & Chakraborty, T. R. (2009). Estrogen-like endocrine disrupting chemicals affecting puberty in humans—a review. *Environmental Science and Technology, 43*(9), 2993.
21. Fack, F., et al. (2009). Effects of the endocrine disruptors atrazine and PCB 153 on the protein expression of MCF-7 human cells. *Journal of Proteome Research, 8*(12), 5485–5496.
22. Kuehn, B. M. (2010). Increased risk of ADHD associated with early exposure to pesticides, PCBs. *Journal of the American Medical Association, 304*(1), 27–28.
23. IBID.
24. Soto, A., Vandenberg, L., Maffini, M., & Sonnenschein, C. (2008). Does breast cancer start in the womb? *Basic and Clinical Pharmacology and Toxicology, 102*(2), 125–133.
25. World Cancer Research Fund & American Institute for Cancer Research. (2007). *Second expert report: Food, nutrition, physical activity, and the*

prevention of cancer: A global perspective. London, England: World Cancer Research Fund.

26. Sung, B., Prasad, S., Yadav, V. R., Lavasanifar, A., & Aggarwal, B. B. (2011). Cancer and diet: How are they related? *Free Radical Research, 45*(8), 864–879.

27. U.S. Government Accountability Office. (2011). *Safe Drinking Water Act: Improvements in implementation are needed to better assure the public of safe drinking water.* GAO-11-803T. Washington, DC: Author. Retrieved from http://www.gao.gov/new.items/d11803t.pdf

28. McKelvey, L. (2010). Background on national emission standards for industrial, commercial, and institutional boiler and process heaters; and commercial/industrial sold waste incineration (CISWI) units [Webinar]. Retrieved from http://www.epa.gov/ttn/atw/129/ciwi/20100609combustion.pdf

29. Gore, A. (2006). *An inconvenient truth.* New York, NY: Rodale Press.

30. Orr, D. (1998, March 4–8). *Transformation or irrelevance: The challenge of academic planning for environmental education in the 21st century.* Address to the North American Association for Environmental Education, Florida Gulf Coast University, FL.

31. *The President's Council on Sustainable Development, Sustainable America: A new consensus for prosperity, opportunity and a healthy environment.* (1996). Washington, DC: U.S. Government Printing Office.

32. Kats, G. H. (2003). *Green building costs and financial benefits.* Boston, MA: Massachusetts Technology Collaborative. Retrieved from http://www.dcaaia.com/images/firm/Kats-Green-Buildings-Cost.pdf

33. Lindquist, R., Tracy, M. F., & Savik, K. (2003). Personal use of complementary and alternative therapies by critical care nurses. *Critical Care Nursing Clinics of North America, 15*(3), 393–399.

34. Molter, N. C. (2003). Creating a healing environment for critical care. *Critical Care Nursing Clinics of North America, 15*(3), 295–304.

35. Thornton, L. (2005). The model of whole-person caring: Creating and sustaining a healing environment. *Holistic Nursing Practice, 19*(3), 106–115.

36. Firth, K., Smith, K., & Gourdin, K. (2010, Fall). The nature and prevalence of healing and wellness initiatives in American hospitals. *Wellness Management.* Retrieved from http://samueli.stage.bridgelinedigital.net/detail/detail-page?ContentId=bad22e22-cdff-483c-9945-2f37c2b5dbd6

37. IBID.

38. Passchier-Vermeer, W., & Passchier, W. F. (2000). Noise exposure and public health. *Environmental Health Perspectives, 108*(Suppl. 1), 123–131.

39. Babisch, W. (2005). Guest editorial: Noise and health. *Environmental Health Perspectives, 113,* A14–A15.

40. White, A., & Burgess, M. (1992–1993). Strategies for reduction of noise levels in ICUs. *Australian Journal of Advanced Nursing, 10*(2), 22–26.

41. Retrieved from http://www.usda.gov

42. Malmo-Levine, D. (2002). Radioactive tobacco. American Computer Science Association. Retrieved from http://www.acsa2000.net/HealthAlert/radioactive_tobacco.html

43. RadTown USA. (2010). Radiation in tobacco. Retrieved from http://www.epa.gov/radtown/tobacco.html

44. Smith-Bindman, R., et al. (2009). Radiation dose associated with common computed tomography examinations and the associated lifetime attributable risk of cancer [abstract]. *Archives of Internal Medicine, 169*(22), 2078–2086.

■ STUDY QUESTIONS

Basic Level

1. Which of the following statements characterizes environmental health in nursing practice?
   a. It is not relevant to professional nursing.
   b. It has no scientific basis and is fear based.
   c. It is unnecessary in a health assessment.
   d. It has its roots in Florence Nightingale's philosophy.

2. What is the precautionary principle intended to do?
   a. Promote the use of medication to prevent disease.
   b. Assist older adults in the decision-making process.
   c. Guard against unnecessary medical treatments.
   d. Demand health policy actions and regulation of the chemical industry.

3. What do chemicals in the home and workplace increase the risk of?
   a. Pain
   b. Digestive problems
   c. Asthma
   d. Tinnitus

4. Chemical exposures are ubiquitous and found in all of the following forms except which one?
   a. Municipal drinking water supply
   b. Foods consumed daily
   c. Personal care products
   d. Sun exposure

5. What does creating optimal external healing environments enable nurses to do?
   a. Become more efficient in their tasks.
   b. Be burdened with additional workload.
   c. Use a placebo in place of evidence-based practice.
   d. Enhance clients' healing potential.

Advanced Level

6. Which of the following statements characterizes small amounts of radiation and electromagnetic field exposure?
   a. They do not affect health.
   b. In the form of X-rays and scanners they are safe.
   c. They are cumulative and can increase the risk of cancer.
   d. They are not a concern in healthy individuals.

7. Effective interventions in the prevention of breast cancer include all of the following except which one?
   a. Avoid sun exposure.
   b. Limit pesticides in the home and food supply.
   c. Avoid bisphenol A (BPA) especially when pregnant.
   d. Increase intake of cruciferous vegetables.

8. The most effective way Nancy Nurse can become involved in environmental awareness in her workplace is by doing which of the following?

   a. Developing a healing intention.
   b. Becoming involved in Health Care Without Harm.
   c. Practicing self-care and a healthy lifestyle.
   d. Avoiding wearing perfume to work.

9. A young couple comes to the clinic with their new baby. The nurse identifies that the father is a farmworker and exposed to pesticides. What information would be most relevant to share with the new parents?
   a. After work and before handling the child, the father should change clothes and wash well.
   b. The family should eat only organic fruits and vegetables.
   c. They should use only BPA-free bottles.
   d. Many toys contain PCBs.

10. A female patient with breast cancer tells you that she has cleaned up her home environment by changing to safe cleaning products, has replaced all plastic products with PBA-free items, drinks clean water, and has improved her diet. What other information can you give her regarding endocrine disruptors?
    a. Avoid personal products that contain parabens and phthalates.
    b. Take her clothes to the dry cleaner to rid them of any residue.
    c. Eat fatty fish such as salmon frequently.
    d. All water filters adequately remove endocrine disruptors.

Chapter 29

Cultural Diversity and Care

Joan Engebretson

■ DEFINITIONS

Acculturation The process of the adaptation or accommodation of an individual immigrant or immigrant group to a new culture.

Culturally competent health care Health care delivered with knowledge of and sensitivity to cultural factors that influence the health and illness behaviors of an individual client, family, or community.

Culture The values, beliefs, customs, social structures, and patterns of human activity and the symbolic structures that provide meaning and significance to human behavior.

Ethnicity Designation of a population subgroup that shares a common social and cultural heritage.

Ethnocentrism A worldview that is based to a great extent on socialization of individuals within their own culture, to the extent that such individuals believe that all others see the world as they do.

Race A social classification that denotes a biological or genetically transmitted set of distinguishable physical characteristics.

Stereotyping Consigning cultural attributes to a group of people based on assumptions, opinions, or attitudes.

Xenophobia An inherent fear or hatred of cultural differences.

■ THEORY AND RESEARCH

Cultural Theories

1. Basic theoretical understanding of cultural values, beliefs, and behaviors: Basic value orientations and beliefs. Kluckholm identified five cultural categories addressing universal concerns of human nature:[1,2]
   a. Innate human nature
   b. Relationship to nature
   c. Time
   d. Purpose
   e. Other persons
2. Factors in the development of cultural patterns and behaviors:
   a. Geography and migration
   b. Religion
   c. Gender roles
   d. Communication
   e. Technology
3. Cultural diversity and disparities:
   a. Race and ethnicity
   b. Socioeconomic status
   c. Health disparities
   d. Common myths and errors
4. Cultural competency in health care:
   a. Cultural competency models
   b. Cultural competency and cultural competency in the era of evidence-based practice
5. Theories in the anthropology of healing and health care: Culture of biomedicine, Kleinman's sectors of health care and

explanatory models, and the Multiparadigm Model of Healing

a. General Cultural Theories: Basic theoretical understanding of cultural values, beliefs, and behaviors; core understanding of culture and its application to health care include the following:

- Culture is learned through language and socialization and is reflected in behaviors, both collective and individual. This fosters group identity.
- Although some underlying beliefs and values of a culture are stable, culture is dynamic and changes in response to history and environment, making it difficult to generalize to individuals, time, or situation.
- Culture is often tacit and not often described or expressed at the conscious level.
- Cultural beliefs and values regarding health affect behaviors of patients and providers.

b. Basic value orientations and beliefs. Kluckholm identified five universal categories of human nature that are reflected in cultures.[1,2] These values are fairly stable and are central to understanding political, economic, and social structures as well as human behavior.

- Innate human nature as being *good, evil,* or *mixed.* This has implications for the ways parenting and child education are oriented.
- Human relationship to the forces of nature as *being subjugated to the forces of nature, harmonious coexistence with nature,* or *using human abilities to master nature.* American culture generally is oriented toward a mastery over nature. Evident by drive to develop technology to enhance life, with implications for medicine development.
- Human relationship to time as *past oriented, present oriented,* or *future oriented.* Generally, U.S. culture is future oriented as opposed to other cultures that revere the past or are present oriented. The latter are not driven to have the clock direct their lives.
- The purpose of being seen as focused on *being (internally focused), being in becoming (develop and grow in personally valued areas),* or *doing (achievement valued by self and others).* Many have noted that American culture is oriented toward achievement, but counterculture movements advocate the becoming orientation.
- Human relationship to other persons as *individualistic, familial,* or *communal orientation.* U.S. culture is generally very individualist in its orientation. We might value our families and communities, but at heart the culture is highly individualistic.

■ FACTORS IN THE DEVELOPMENT OF CULTURAL PATTERNS AND BEHAVIORS

1. The following elements play important roles in the development of culture and cultural changes.

a. Geography and migrations have played a huge role in the development of culture. *Climate* and *geography* affect the type of food that is available and social, economic, and political organizations that evolve in a particular region. For example, the social structure of a nomadic hunting group differs from an agrarian or urban group.

- Climate changes as well as socioeconomic or political factors have influenced migration over the course of human history. *Migrations* force both the immigrants and the host culture to adapt and assimilate ideas and customs from each other. The process of acculturation as well as the reasons for migration (voluntary in search of better resources, political in search of safety, or involuntary such as by slavery) have a large impact on the cultural practices and beliefs as well as the acculturation process.

b. *Acculturation* is the process of adaptation, assimilation, or accommodation of immigrant groups to a new culture. This is sometimes called hybridization as when immigrants integrate the new culture into their lives yet retain heritage consistency. Social roles and gender roles can be in conflict in this process.

This is not a simple or uniform process and includes much variation.[3]

c. Religion, as distinct from spirituality, is an organized system of beliefs that unites a group in beliefs and practices. *Religion* stems from the root word meaning to bind together in common belief. Religious beliefs and values orient around meaning in life and appropriate behaviors. Religions form communities of like-minded peoples. Religions are foundational in human behavior and have huge impact on behavior.

d. Gender roles: Acceptable and appropriate social roles regarding gender are important elements of culture. Some religious beliefs reinforce these gendered roles; however, many are carried on without a true base in religion. In the United States and Europe, the social roles for women have been challenged and expanded through the feminist movement.

e. Communication and travel: One factor that promotes cultural change is communication. As cultures mix and begin to communicate with each other, ideas mix and have a great impact on culture. International travel and worldwide media have led to unprecedented exposure to different values and beliefs and practices.

f. Technology: Technological advances change the way people live their daily lives.[4] The development of the printing press changed culture from an oral culture to a written one. Now we have electronic media that are changing values and behaviors of contemporary society. Often these technological advances challenge values and beliefs and raise ethical question related to their use. This is particularly true in medicine and health care.

■ CULTURAL DIVERSITY AND DISPARITIES

1. Race and ethnicity: These terms are often used inappropriately. *Ethnicity* refers to a group or nationality that shares common social and cultural heritage. These categorizations are problematic; however, we must recognize that they are the primary classifications in demographic data in the United States.

a. Race refers to a biological genetically transmitted set of distinguishing characteristics. However, the concept of race that is often used in demographic categorization includes black, white, Native Hawaiian or American Indian, and Asian and is a social construction with little basis in biology. Black and white are colors, Hawaiian and Native American refer to indigenous groups in the United States with a great deal of heterogeneity, and Asian refers to peoples from half the globe. Additionally, groups of people have historically intermingled and moved, often making even biological categories inappropriate. Note: There are some genetic predispositions to diseases and responses to pharmaceuticals that are clinically important.[5]

b. Ethnicity refers to a group with shared cultural heritage that can include language. Again the common demographic categories are Hispanic or non-Hispanic. This refers to the Spanish language, which is European in origin. This designation has been applied to peoples from South and Central America and the Caribbean, areas that include a variety of indigenous peoples and immigrants with much heterogeneity.

2. Socioeconomic status (SES): Socioeconomic status includes educational level, which influences jobs and income level as well as health-related behavior. This underlies three major determinants of health: access to health care, health behaviors, and environmental exposure to health-related agents.[6,7]

3. Health disparities: Despite the fact that humans are 99.9% identical at the DNA level, there are differences in the prevalence of illness among groups. These can be explained by genetic differences; dietary, cultural, environmental, and socioeconomic factors; and a combination of these.[8,9]

4. Common myths and errors: Problems arise categorizing people into cultural groups.

a. Stereotyping: This is a common problem when attempting to apply cultural knowledge to individual patients. The heterogeneity of ethnic or religious groups is often underestimated. There can be greater disparity within one group on education and socioeconomic status than between two with similar SES but different ethnicities.

b. Ethnocentricity: Common views and practices stemming from lack of knowledge of other cultures and presumption that one's own behavior is not influenced by culture.

c. Xenophobia: An inherent fear of cultural differences, with the demeaning of other beliefs and values. This is often associated with prejudice or racism.

d. Cultural imposition: This is the perception that cultural adaptation involves an adherence to the beliefs of the dominant culture, which they believe is superior and should be imposed on others. Some relate this to colonialism.

e. Cultural blindness: This position comes from a belief in equality that ignores cultural differences. This is often a movement to contrast with xenophobia, in that the perspective sees everyone as equal. This ignores cultural heritage and the heterogeneity of cultural beliefs.

5. Cultural competency in health care: With increasing diversity in the population and recognition of health disparities, the Office of Minority Health developed standards that apply to both institutional and individual provider levels.[10]

a. Institutions: Healthcare institutions are mandated to provide adequate translation and encouraged to employ a culturally diverse workforce. Guidelines have been established by a number of organizations and agencies. Individual providers are encouraged to provide culturally appropriate care.[10-13]

b. Individual provider cultural competency: Cultural competency has been discussed in the literature and cultural sensitivity programs have been instituted in many healthcare settings. A number of organizations have developed resources for developing cultural sensitivity or competency. Cultural competency might be a misnomer because it implies that at some point the provider becomes competent as he or she develops a skill. Nonetheless that term is used commonly.[11-16]

- Models for cultural competency: Cultural Competency Continuum from the Center for Cultural Competency at Georgetown University is one of the most cited models.[17] This continuum positions cultural destructiveness at the lowest level and cultural proficiency as the highest. This model was expanded to incorporate the clinical base of evidence-based practice.[18]

- Cultural destructiveness: The willful harm or malfeasance that discriminates against a group. The Civil Rights Act makes this level illegal as well as unethical.

- Cultural incapacity: This refers to incompetence or unintentional behaviors that can be harmful to a patient. This results from ignorance, insensitive attitudes, or allocation of resources.

- Cultural blindness: This is exemplified by standardization and treating all patients alike without accommodating to or recognizing cultural differences. The push to standardize interventions without any concern for cultural issues exemplifies this level.

- Precompetence: This is the beginning of recognizing cultural differences and is demonstrated by involving translators, attempting to develop health education for specific cultural groups and some cultural sensitivity training. Having a nurse from a specific ethnic background develop patient materials is a good example of this level.

- Cultural competence: At this level the provider begins to accept, respect, appreciate, and accommodate cultural differences and begins to develop an appreciation of his or her own cultural background. The provider is committed to an ongoing learning process related to cultural diversity in patient care.

- Cultural proficiency: This is the highest level and is exemplified by incorporating an understanding of various cultures and understanding cultural diversity. At the clinical level this cultural understanding is combined with the understanding of heterogeneity within cultures, resulting in individualized patient-centered care.

c. Cultural competence and evidence-based practice:[18] This model uses the continuum and explores it with an ethical lens and the application of evidence-based practice. In the fervor to apply research evidence, many get stuck in the mindset of cultural blindness and work from a standardization perspective. Evidence-based practice, as described by some of the leading developers, must contain three aspects:

- Research evidence
- Patient's values, preferences, and circumstances
- Expertise of the clinician[19]

d. Therefore, to practice cultural competence/proficiency, the nurse must continue to understand and incorporate cultural knowledge and research and apply it in individualized patient-centered care that is holistic care. Betancourt identified the following skills:

- Assess cross-cultural issues
- Explore meaning to the patient
- Determine the social context in which the patient lives
- Engage in a negotiation process with the patient[20]

6. Theories in the anthropology of healing and health care: A subgroup of anthropology, medical anthropology studies different systems and practices of healing across cultures, such as Ayurveda, traditional Chinese medicine, and magicoreligious. It seeks to understand other approaches to health and healing. This perspective also views biomedicine as a unique cultural approach with distinct values, beliefs, understandings, dress, language, and so forth.[21-29]

a. Biomedicine and culture: Much has been written about the culture of biomedicine, sometimes referred to as academic medicine.[30] Although the limits of this model are beginning to be recognized in behavioral health care, health promotion, and complex phenomena, this model is still very pervasive in health care. This model is based on the scientific objective perspective and reflects the scientific method, mind–body dualism, and Western capitalism.[31,32] There are four main constructs:

- *Determinism*: A linear cause-and-effect relationship exists for all natural phenomena.
- *Mechanism*: The relationship of life to structure and function of machines suggests the possibility of control through mechanical or engineered interventions. These mechanisms might be at the cellular to the behavioral levels.
- *Reductionism*: The division of all life into isolated smaller parts, which facilitates the study of the whole.
- *Objective materialism*: That which is real can be observed and measured.

b. Kleinman's sectors of health care: Kleinman, a physician and an anthropologist who studied Chinese approaches to health, identified three sectors that are present in all healthcare systems: professional, popular, and folk.[33]

- Professional or academic sector: Sometimes referred to as orthodox medicine, this sector is the foundation for biomedicine and corresponds to the scientific paradigm. This has held a legal, political, and ideological monopoly and includes all healthcare professions, physicians, nurses, and so forth.
- Folk sector: This includes all secular and sacred healers who are generally outside the professional sector. Many of the complementary and alternative therapies originate from this sector. Many nurses and some physicians are incorporating or integrating these healing approaches or modalities into their clinical practice.
- Popular: This sector includes all the personal and social networks that laypeople use to understand and plan their health care and direct their health-related behaviors. This includes the patient and family in which the majority of health-related decisions are made and is the sector about which we know the least. With social media and the Internet, patients are able to access some

material from the professional and folk sectors; however, the information is largely interpreted in the popular sector.

c. Kleinman's explanatory models:[33] These explanatory models are notions that individuals or groups have about understanding the causes, symptoms, and treatments of illness. These reflect cultural interpretations of disease, treatment, and health. These models are used to recognize, interpret, respond to, cope with, and make sense of an illness experience. It is very important to patient care that the provider explores the explanatory model of the patient to promote better communication and culturally competent care. The provider can compare, contrast, and discuss the etiology, pathology, course of the disease, treatment, and possible outcome of the medical model with the patient's explanatory model.

d. Other cultural models of health and illness: Many other folk or cultural models of health and illness have been explored. A couple examples are noted here:

- Natural and unnatural illness: Giger and Davidhizar and other anthropologists describe folk medicine as classifying diseases as natural or unnatural.[27] In natural types, everything in nature is connected. A natural illness results from a disturbance with nature, and recovery requires a restoration of that relationship with nature. In contrast, unnatural illnesses are often attributed to punishment from a higher power for one's improper behavior or breaking a taboo.

- Multiparadigm model of healing:[34] This model of healing and health was developed to place biomedicine into a unified holistic model with diverse modalities. This model grouped various modalities into four paradigms, or underlying philosophies of healing, across the horizontal axis. As one moves across the model to the right, all healing is conceptualized as more holistic in that it might affect the entire human. The vertical axis includes healing activities: (1) physical manipulation (surgery, irrigations); (2) ingested or applied substances (pharmaceuticals, supplements); (3) uses of energy (laser, Healing Touch); (4) psychological modalities (mind–body techniques, imagery); and (5) spiritual modalities (attendance at church, prayer). As one moves from top to bottom on the vertical axis, the modalities move from more material to more ethereal. The modalities in the model serve as examples, and others can be added. In systems of healing, several modalities may be employed through a common perspective. The four paradigms are as follows:

  - The *mechanical paradigm* is based on disease as a disruption of structure and function, and the purpose of treatment is to restore or replace that function. This is most similar to biomedicine and is self-correcting and produces increasingly sophisticated understandings of the mechanisms of the human body.

  - The *purification paradigm* underlies many healing and religious practices and aims to cleanse and rid the body of polluting influences. This paradigm goes back to early Egyptians and has been prevalent in many cathartic treatments.

  - The *balance paradigm* is evident in multiple historical and contemporary cultures. It was the base of Hippocratic medicine of balancing the humors. It is also epitomized in many Eastern healing approaches in the balance of yin and yang and *chi*.

  - The *supranormal paradigm* corresponds to many of the magicoreligious healing practices and has been used to explain phenomena that current understanding of physical laws cannot explain, such as spontaneous healing, prayer, divine intervention, and vital energies.

■ BACKGROUND INFORMATION FOR UNDERSTANDING CULTURE AND CONTEXT

1. Contemporary Western cultural groups: In general, Western (European and North American) cultural bases were discussed previously. Since the 20th century, the rate of immigration, the communication from areas around the world, and the rate of technological development have affected Western culture dramatically. Exposure to different cultures and technological and scientific advances has led to cultural change in many areas pertaining to health care. One of the most important aspects is the need for nurses and healthcare providers to understand some of the cultural backgrounds of our many immigrants and other people around the world. Another of the more significant changes is an interest among the population and providers in different approaches to health.

2. Ethnic groups in North America: Although it is important not to stereotype from information about diverse cultures, it is important to have some background to better understand individuals. Following are the categories in which demographic and census data are kept in the United States; data are collected every 10 years.[35,36]

   a. American Indian and Alaska Natives: This group constitutes only 1% of the population and often has a high rate of poverty, with health issues associated with poverty. They cluster in tribal groups with considerable variation in language, beliefs, and customs among tribes. They value harmony with nature, present time orientation, and integration of rituals and religion into everyday life. Many adhere to folk healing, which often includes shamanic or supranormal approaches.

   b. European Americans: This is the largest ethnic group in North America and constitutes the dominant culture (65–80%, depending on how Hispanics are counted). However, the percentage is declining. The major migration from Europe occurred in the late 1700s through the 1800s, and many of the ideas of this group come from the European Age of Reason: dominance over nature, belief in progress and technological advancement, and individualism.

   c. African Americans: This group (around 14%) is rapidly growing, with the largest concentrations in the South and along the East Coast. Many are descendants of slaves, while others have more recently immigrated from Africa and the Caribbean. There is a strong matriarchal tradition with strong bonds to family, kinship, and church. There is some adherence to folk healers, but many have absorbed dominant culture.

   d. Asian Americans: This group from the Pacific Rim, including China, Japan, Korea, Thailand, Laos, Vietnam, Cambodia, the Philippines, and other Asian countries, accounts for around 5% of the population. Although there is wide diversity of language and customs, many adhere to a patriarchal social structure, revere their elders, and value achievement and honor. Incidence of tuberculosis, hepatitis, and some infectious diseases is high among new immigrants. Stress-related diseases and suicides are high because many do not seek mental health care as a result of stigma and a threat to their honor. Many use traditional healing practices to balance the *chi* as well as traditional herbal preparations. Some practice dermabrasion or coining, pinching or rubbing.

   e. Pacific Islanders and Native Hawaiians: This group constitutes less than 1% of the U.S. population, with Native Hawaiians the largest subgroup. Most live in the West including California and Hawaii. Many are socioeconomically disadvantaged and lack access to social and health services. They also have high rates of health-related risk behaviors such as smoking, heavy alcohol consumption, and high fat/caloric diet.

   f. Hispanic: This is the fastest growing ethnic group in the United States and constituted 12.5% of the population in 2001. Although the majority comes from Mexico, this group originates from Puerto Rico, Cuba, and other

Central and South American countries. Although Spanish is the common language, there is much diversity in dialects and customs. Some of the health beliefs include illness as punishment for sins as well as traditional humeral beliefs regarding hot and cold remedies and spiritual elements.

3. Factors in a cultural assessment: Giger and Davidhizar identified phenomena present in all cultural groups relevant to an assessment of cultural issues in provision of health care.[34]

   a. Communication: Cultural variations in expression include use of touch, body contact, gestures, and verbal and nonverbal communication. Language is an important expression of culture, and translation of individual words can miss important meanings.

   b. Personal space: This refers to the comfort level related to how close one can position oneself to another person in different situations. Western culture has zones of intimate (< 18 inches), personal (18–36 inches), and social (3–6 feet) space.

   c. Time: In addition to the general orientation to past, present, and future, cultures orient to social time and clock time.

   d. Social organization: This refers to family and other organizational structures, dynamics, and expected social roles.

   e. Environmental control: This relates to perceptions of ability of an individual to control nature, the environment, and personal relationships.

   f. Biological variations: It is important to distinguish between strictly biological factors and cultural and social adaptations.

■ APPLICATION OF CULTURAL CONCEPTS TO CLINICAL PRACTICE

1. Using the evidence-based practice triad to incorporate culture into clinical encounters: A model was developed for nurses to use a cultural negotiation model to reflect holistic values and incorporate cultural sensitivity.[37]

   a. The research evidence: Getting as much information about cultural variation and the research on various cultural groups, as well as a foundation in the understanding of the importance of culture in belief and behaviors, is an ongoing practice.

   b. The provider's expertise: This is an important part of developing cultural proficiency.
   - The nurse can expand cultural expertise by relationships with people from different cultures through travel, personal social relationships, and learning from patients.
   - Personal exploration of values clarification and beliefs can be very important in the nurse's development of cultural proficiency.
   - The medical system has its own culture, which some have likened to traveling in a foreign land with unique language, dress, customs, social roles, and behaviors. The nurse can function as a cultural broker with patients.

   c. Patient's values, beliefs, and circumstances: The nurse must develop good communication skills to understand the patient. In this process it is important to note:
   - The basic patient–provider relationship has an inherent inequality in that the provider is assumed to be higher based on medical knowledge.
   - Communication is often not planned and involves emotionally laden issues.
   - Both verbal and nonverbal communication is important.
   - Use of Kleinman's explanatory models can be useful to help focus on the patient's perspective of the health problem.
   - If needed, use of translators might be necessary. Trained interpreters are preferred over family members. Both patient and translator need to be oriented to the specific purpose. Sit so that the patient can see both the nurse and translator. Observe for nonverbal communication that does not match content. Slow the process and limit medical jargon. Consider the impact of differences in gender, educational level, age, or SES. Consider repeating information to increase accuracy.

■ NOTES

1. Kluckhohn, F. R. (1976). Dominant and variant value orientations. In P. J. Brink (Ed.), *Transcultural nursing: A book of readings* (pp. 63–81). Englewood Cliffs, NJ: Prentice Hall.

2. Hills, M. D. (2002). Kluckhohn and Strodtbeck's Values Orientation Theory. Online Readings in Psychology and Culture, Unit 4. Retrieved from http://scholarworks.gvsu.edu/orpc/vol4/iss4/3

3. Oetting, E. R., & Beauvais, F. (1990–1991). Orthogonal Cultural Identification Theory: The cultural identification of minority adolescents. *International Journal of Addiction*, 5A, 6A, 655–685.

4. Postman, N. (1993). *Technopoly*. New York, NY: Vintage Books.

5. Burroughs, V. J., Maxey, R. W., & Levy, R. A. (2002). Racial and ethnic differences in response to medicines: Towards individualized pharmaceutical treatment. *Journal of the National Medical Association*, 94(10), S1–S25.

6. Adler, N. E., & Newman, K. (2002). Socioeconomic disparities in health: Pathways and policies. And Inequality in education, income, and occupation exacerbates the gaps between the health "haves" and "have-nots." *Health Affairs, 21,* 60–76.

7. Marmor, T. R., Barer, M. L., & Evans, R. G. (1994). *Why are some people healthy and others not? The determinants of healthy populations.* New York, NY: Aldine de Gruyter.

8. Collins, F. S. (2003). Genomics and health disparities. In *Disparities in health in America: Working toward social justice*. Houston, TX: Summer Workshop.

9. Centers for Disease Control and Prevention. (2011). CDC health disparities and inequalities report—United States, 2011. *Morbidity and Mortality Weekly Report, 60*(Suppl.). Retrieved from http://www.cdc.gov/mmwr/pdf/other/su6001.pdf

10. Office of Minority Health. (2001, March). *National standards for culturally and linguistically appropriate services in health care.* Washington, DC: U.S. Department of Health and Human Services. Retrieved from http://minorityhealth.hhs.gov/assets/pdf/checked/executive.pdf

11. Agency for Healthcare Research and Quality. (n.d.). Cultural and linguistic competence. Retrieved from http://www.ahrq.gov/health-care-information/topics/topic-cultural-competence.html

12. Health Resources and Services Administration. (n.d.). Home page. Retrieved from http://www.hrsa.gov

13. Joint Commission. (2010). Advancing effective communication, cultural competence, and patient- and family-centered care: A roadmap for hospitals. Retrieved from http://www.jointcommission.org/Advancing_Effective_Communication/.

14. Giger, J., Davidhizar, R. E., Purnell, L., Harden, J. T., Phillips, J., & Strickland, O. (2007). American Academy of Nursing expert panel report: Developing cultural competence to eliminate health disparities in ethnic minorities and other vulnerable populations. *Journal of Transcultural Nursing, 18*(95), 95–102.

15. Sue, D. W., & Sue, D. (2003). *Counseling the culturally different: Theory and practice.* 4th ed. New York, NY: Wiley.

16. National Council on Interpreting in Health Care. (2005). *National standards of practice for interpreters in health care.* Washington, DC: Author. Retrieved from http://mchb.hrsa.gov/training/documents/pdf_library/National_Standards_of_Practice_for_Interpreters_in_Health_Care%20(12-05).pdf

17. Cross, T. (1989). *Toward a culturally competent system of care* (Vol. 1). Washington, DC: CASSP Technical Assistance Center, Georgetown University Child Development Center.

18. Engebretson, J., Mahoney, J., & Carlson, E. D (2008). Cultural competence in the era of evidence-based practice. *Journal of Professional Nursing, 24*(3), 172–178.

19. Strauss, S., Glasziou, P., Richardson, W. S., & Haynes, R. B. (2005). *Evidence-based medicine: How to practice and teach EBM* (2nd ed.). New York, NY: Elsevier Churchill Livingstone.

20. Betancourt, J. R. (2006). Cultural competency: Providing quality care to diverse populations. *Consultant Pharmacist, 21*(12), 988–995.

21. Campinha-Bacote, J. (2001). A model and instrument for addressing cultural competence in health care. *Journal of Nursing Education, 38,* 204–207.

22. Douglas, M. (2002). Developing frameworks for providing culturally competent health care. *Journal of Transcultural Nursing, 13,* 177.

23. Purnell, L., & Paulanka, B. (1998). *Transcultural health care: A culturally competent approach.* Philadelphia, PA: F. A. Davis.

24. Giger, J., & Davidhizar, R. (2007). *Transcultural nursing: Assessment and intervention* (5th ed.). St. Louis, MO: Mosby.

25. Spector, R. E. (2000). *Cultural diversity in health and illness* (5th ed.). Upper Saddle River, NJ: Prentice Hall.

26. Leininger, M. (2001). *Culture care diversity and universality: A theory of nursing.* Sudbury, MA: Jones and Bartlett.

27. Lipson, J. G., & Desantis, L. A. (2007). Current approaches to integrating elements of cultural competence in nursing education. *Journal of Transcultural Nursing, 18*(1), 10S–20S.

28. Beach, M. C., Price, E. G., Gary, T. L., Robinson, K. A., Gozu, A., Palacio, A.,...Cooper, L. A. (2005). Cultural competence: A systematic review of health care provider educational interventions. *Medical Care, 43*(4), 356–373.

29. Dreher, M., & MacNaughton, N. (2002). Cultural competence in nursing: Foundation or fallacy? *Nursing Outlook, 50*(5), 181–186.

30. Loustaunau, M. O., & Sobo, E. J. (1997). *The cultural context of health, illness, and medicine.* Westport, CT: Bergin & Garvey Press.

31. Lock, M., & Gordon, D. (1988). *Biomedicine examined.* Dordrecht, Netherlands: Kluwer Academic.

32. Gregg, G. R., & Saha, S. (2006). Losing culture on the way to competence: The use and misuse of culture in medical education. *Academic Medicine, 41,* 1–8.

33. Kleinman, A. (1980). *Patients and healers in the context of culture: An exploration of the borderland between anthropology, medicine and psychiatry.* Berkeley, CA: University of California Press.

34. Giger, J., & Davidhizar, R. (1999). *Transcultural nursing: Assessment and intervention* (3rd ed.). St. Louis, MO: Mosby.

35. Engebretson, J. (1997). A multiparadigm approach to nursing. *Advances in Nursing Science, 20,* 22–34.

36. U.S. Census Bureau. (2010). 2010 Census briefs: The black population 2010. Retrieved from http://www.census.gov/prod/cen2010/briefs /c2010br-06.pdf

37. Engebretson, J., & Littleton, L. (2001). Cultural negotiation: A constructivist-based model for nursing practice. *Nursing Outlook, 49,* 223–230.

■ STUDY QUESTIONS

Basic Level

1. Which of the following answer choices describes the best understanding of culture for healthcare providers?
   a. The practices, histories, and beliefs of a racial group
   b. The behaviors of an ethnic group related to seeking health care
   c. The shared beliefs, values, customs, and social structures of a group
   d. The customs and beliefs of minorities

2. A nurse who advocates that all patients should be treated alike using the same research-based treatments exemplifies which level of cultural competence?
   a. Cultural incompetence
   b. Cultural blindness
   c. Cultural precompetence
   d. Cultural competence

3. In regard to culture, which of the following answer choices characterizes evidence-based practice?
   a. Denies cultural variation
   b. Requires application of standardized medical treatment
   c. Focuses only on individualized treatment
   d. Incorporates understanding of the individual patient's culture along with research

4. Which of the following answer choices best describes xenophobia?
   a. Fear of cultural differences and demeaning others' values
   b. Applying some aspect of cultural practices to all members of an ethnic group
   c. Advocating for equality of all people regardless of their background or ethnicity
   d. Assisting groups from other cultures to adopt the dominant beliefs and values

5. Which of the following is one of the three sectors of health care described by Kleinman?
   a. The folk sector, which includes all sacred and secular healers
   b. Third-party payers sector
   c. The media coverage of health and medicine
   d. Board-certified physicians sector

Advanced Level

6. Which of the following is true of biomedicine?
   a. It is culturally neutral because it is founded on science and objectivity.
   b. It is culturally destructive because it limits services based on minority cultures.
   c. It is culturally competent because many cultural and ethnic groups are providers.
   d. It has its own culture that both providers and patients acculturate toward.

7. In the Multiparadigm Model of Healing, which paradigm is most distant from the biomedical paradigm?
   a. Mechanical
   b. Purification
   c. Balance
   d. Supranormal

8. What are healthcare institutions required to do?
   a. Provide culturally competent care
   b. Hire minorities
   c. Provide adequate translation services
   d. Provide cultural competency training for all employees

9. According to the value orientations described by Kluckholm, which of the following answer choices best characterizes U.S. culture?

   a. Past oriented, coexistence with nature, and individualistic
   b. Future oriented, subjugation of nature, and individualistic
   c. Present oriented, achievement focused, and familial
   d. Future oriented, achievement focused

10. Which of the following is the best example of cultural proficiency in an organization?
    a. Cultural matching in which the African American nurse sees all the African American patients
    b. Providing the same care for all the patients
    c. A commitment to continual learning about cultural variation and providing individualized patient cared.
    d. Including cultural sensitivity sessions led by staff members of various ethnic groups

Chapter 30

The Psychophysiology of Body–Mind Healing

Kimberley A. Evans

Original Authors: Genevieve M. Bartol
and Nancy F. Courts

■ DEFINITIONS

Allostasis The adaptation process to maintain homeostasis and well-being.

Allostatic load When one experiences overwhelming stress or has inadequate coping skills.

Autopoiesis The self-organizing force in living systems.

Bifurcation A point at which transformational change occurs in a complex system; a fork in the road of life.

Body–mind A state of integration that includes body, mind, and spirit.

Chaos The stable and orderly but irregular, unpredictable behavior of a complex system.

Cycles One of the simplest nonlinear behaviors that is periodic and recurrent.

Epigenetics The study of how genes produce their effect on the phenotype of the organism.

Information Theory A mathematical model that helps explain the connections between consciousness and body–mind healing.

Limbic-hypothalamic system The major anatomic modulating link connecting the brain/mind and the autonomic, endocrine, immune, and neuropeptide systems.

Mind modulation The bidirectional interrelationships of thoughts and feelings with neurohormonal messengers of the nervous, endocrine, immune, and neuropeptide systems that support body–mind connections.

Network Interconnected and interrelated system.

Neuropeptides Messenger molecules produced at various sites throughout the body to transmit body–mind patterns of communication.

Neuroplasticity The ability of the nervous system to respond to intrinsic and/or extrinsic stimuli by reorganizing its structure, function, and connections.

Neurotransmitters Chemicals that facilitate the transmission of impulses through nerves in the body.

Psychoneuroimmunology A branch of science that strives to show the connections among psychology, neuroendocrinology, and immunology.

Receptors Sites on cell surfaces that serve as points of attachment for various types of messenger molecules.

Self-Regulation Theory A person's ability to learn cognitive processing of information to bring involuntary body responses under voluntary control.

Traumatic stress response (TSR) When the normal stress response is altered as a result of overwhelming and/or ongoing stress.

■ THEORY AND RESEARCH

Developments in science and concomitant advances in technology continue to reveal human beings in new ways. The mechanistic view of the body–mind has given way to a holistic view.

The habit of looking at persons as their component parts while ignoring interactions and contexts is misleading and might be limiting in its usefulness to help a person achieve optimal health of mind, body, and spirit. As we free our scientific imagination and increase our knowledge of laws such as the concept of nonlocality and superposition of states in quantum physics, our understanding of living systems will continue to change.[1,2]

New Scientific Understanding of Living Systems

1. Quantum theory
   a. Discoveries in quantum physics negate the old ways of viewing phenomena.
   b. In the past, the properties and behavior of the parts were believed to determine those of the whole;[3] now it is clear that the whole also defines the behavior of the parts.
   c. The realization that systems are integrated wholes that cannot be understood simply by analysis shattered scientific certitude; no longer was it possible to believe that given enough time, effort, and money, all questions would have answers.
   d. All scientific concepts and theories have limitations; scientific explanations do not provide complete and conclusive answers but instead generate other questions.[4]
   e. The more we learn, the more we discover how much we do not know; even one additional piece of data can change the whole configuration.
   f. The world is complex and unified; parts complement one another and participate in the whole. Similarly, all parts of the body work together.
   g. Health and illness are indivisible; both are natural and necessary. Hyperpyrexia (fever) can be seen as a sign of illness as well as a sign of the body's healthy response to a threat.[5]
2. Systems Theory
   a. von Bertalanffy's General Systems Theory established systems thinking as the predominant scientific movement in the first half of the 20th century.[6]
   b. Resultant theories and models of living systems initiated a radical shift in the understanding of human beings; it is now believed that persons and their environments make up an interconnected dynamic system in which a change at any point can effect changes at other points.
   c. The idea that the world is hierarchical, with each level organized separately, has been replaced with a new understanding of relatedness and context.
   d. Human beings are living systems, organizationally closed and structurally open, embedded within the web of life.[7]
      - They are *organizationally closed* because they are self-organizing; that is, they establish their own order and behavior rather than submitting to those imposed by the environment.
      - They are *structurally open* because they engage in a continual exchange of energy and matter with their environment.
   e. A dysfunction in any one system of the body reverberates in the other systems (e.g., hypothyroidism [an endocrine dysfunction] can manifest itself by thinning hair or clinical depression but might, in fact, be secondary to a dysfunction in another organ system).[8]
   f. It is not possible to identify conclusively a single cause of what was formerly named a primary dysfunction.
   g. All body systems participate in the biodance; changes in one system result in changes in the other systems and, in circular fashion, changes in itself.
   h. Feedback, integration, rhythm, and dynamic equilibrium are all part of the biodance.
3. Theory of Relativity
   a. Einstein developed a system of mechanics that acknowledges the relative character of motion, velocity, and mass, as well as the interdependence of matter, time, and space.[3]
   b. The theory is based on the principle that there is no absolute frame of reference independent of the observer; each person views others from his or her own perspective, including his or her particular biases. Scientists can no longer describe their work as finding a piece to a puzzle or as adding a building stone to a firm foundation of knowledge.

c. It has become increasingly apparent that scientific knowledge is a network of concepts and models, none of which is any more fundamental than the other.

d. All things (objects) and events (happenings) in one's life are connected and relative within the whole.

e. The mind and body are inseparably intertwined; whatever happens in one's life is interconnected.

f. Thoughts, feelings, and actions all influence a person's state of health and illness.

4. Principles of Self-Organization

a. The key ideas of current models of self-organizing systems were refined and extended during the 1970s and 1980s, and a unified theory of living systems emerged.[7,8]

b. This unified theory encompassed the creation of structures and modes of behavior in the processes of development, learning, and coevolution.

c. In the past, living systems were viewed from two perspectives:

  ▪ Physical matter (structure): Concerned with quantities, things weighed and measured

  ▪ The configuration of relationships (pattern): Concerned with qualities and is expressed by a map of the configuration of relationships

d. Systems, whether nonliving or living, are configurations of ordered relationships whose attributes are the properties of pattern.

e. Living systems are fundamentally different from nonliving systems:

  ▪ Living systems do not function mechanically and are not explained just by physical principles.

  ▪ The components of living systems are interconnected by internal feedback loops in a nonlinear fashion and are capable of self-organization (autopoiesis).[9] In humans, for example: homeostatic mechanisms maintain body temperature, repair body tissues in response to a wound, preserve integrity of the body; and complex instinctual patterns for protection and reproduction ensure survival of the individual and the species.

f. If the pattern of a living system is destroyed, the system dies even though all the components of the system remain intact.

g. A living system cannot be restored simply by re-creating the pattern. However, a nonliving system, such as a bicycle, will regain function if the parts are reassembled correctly.

h. Living systems do not rest in a steady state of balance as do nonliving systems but rather operate far from equilibrium.[10] Stability in living systems embodies change.

i. Relationships are not linear, but extend in all directions. Bifurcation occurs and generates new feedback loops.[7]

j. Living systems regulate and re-create themselves.

k. Organisms appear to be under the direction of an overall design or purpose and do not just function mechanically.[7] For example, the symptoms experienced by humans represent attempts to gain health and, therefore, are signals of stability, not breakdown. The human immune system recognizes an invading organism as dangerous and quickly reacts to counter the threat. Symptoms are really signs of the inherent organization and adaptability of a living system. We cannot unerringly predict the outcome of these complex relationships among organisms—one person might become sick and die whereas another might be seemingly unaffected and yet infect others with whom he has contact. Even invading organisms, also living systems, learn and adapt. The ability of pathogens to modify themselves and develop resistance to antibiotics is a striking example of the ability of a living system to reorganize.

5. Bell's Theorem

a. Cause-and-effect thinking with its before, after, now, and later sequence is no longer acceptable.

b. According to Bell's Theorem, the whole determines the actions of the parts, and changes occur instantaneously[7,11]

c. Experience teaches us that not all people respond in the same way to the same treatment; even a fleeting thought or a passing feeling can hasten or hinder recovery. Changes do not happen in an orderly stepwise sequence.

d. Healing does not take time, but is dependent on hope and belief beyond time. Beliefs, thoughts, and feelings are all part of the configuration, and each affects the human states of wellness and illness.

e. Miller classifies people as monitors and blunters:[12]
- Monitors need information to reduce their stress.
- Blunters prefer distraction.
- Explaining the details of upcoming surgery to a monitor can be expected to reduce stress and promote healing. Blunters prefer to trust in the skills of the caregiver and do not even want to hear how that will be accomplished.

6. Personality and wellness

a. Researchers have unsuccessfully tried to link specific illnesses with particular personality constellations.

b. Several researchers, however, have uncovered particular personality traits associated with wellness.[11,13,14]

c. Schwartz discovered that persons who with willful, mindful effort attend to symptoms, sensations, and feelings and who believe they can do something about their symptoms can alter their brain chemistry and move toward health.

d. Kabat-Zinn found that healthy attention and meditation helped persons effectively cope with chronic illness and intractable pain.

e. Pennebaker found that persons who admit their feelings to themselves and others have healthier psychological profiles and had fewer illnesses than those who do not.

f. Scientific studies of forgiveness have revealed that whenever people choose to forgive a transgression, areas in the emotional limbic center of the brain are activated.[15] The activity decreases when the person focuses on the unfairness of the situation, but increases when the person imagines forgiving the offender.

g. There is increasing interest in the benefits of positive emotions on the immune system.[16] Altogether, studies suggest that transient positive mood states such as humor and joy are associated with an up-regulation of components of the innate immune system among healthy volunteers and a reduction in allergic responses among allergy sufferers.

h. Even though a direct cause-and-effect relationship between any personality factor and health or illness cannot be determined, the research suggests that developing personality strengths to protect one from the stresses of living seems to bolster one's defense against illness.

7. Information Theory

a. Patterns of communication and patterns of organization in organisms can be viewed analogously.[9]

b. Information Theory, a mathematical model, was developed to define and measure amounts of information transmitted through telegraph and telephone lines; the theory was used to explain how to get a message coded as a signal to determine what to charge customers.

c. A coded message (signal) is essentially a pattern of organization.

d. Information flow (i.e., pattern of communication and pattern of organization) in human beings is able to unify physiologic, psychological, sociological, and spiritual phenomena in a holistic framework.

e. Information flow is the missing piece that makes it possible to transcend the body–mind split because information resides in both the body and the mind; our emotions and feelings are sources of vital information.

f. Emotions-proper are life-regulating phenomena that help maintain our health by making adaptive changes in our body states and form the basis for feelings.[17]

g. The information generated by these processes is designed to be protective and is more complex than reflexes.[18]

8. Santiago Theory of Cognition

a. Derived from the study of neural networks, the Santiago Theory of Cognition is linked to the concept of autopoiesis.[9]

b. Cognition is generally defined as the process of knowing or perceiving; it is associated with the mind, implicitly with the brain and nervous system.

c. The Santiago Theory offers a radical expansion of the traditional concept of cognition; in this new view, cognition involves the whole process of life, including perception, emotion, and behavior.

d. Even the cells that make up the immune system perceive the characteristics of their environment and will, for example, move to the site of a wound and increase in numbers to deal with an invading organism. Despite the absence of a brain, cognition is present; in this event, it can be described as embodied action.[9] Perception and action in these cells are inseparable.

e. Fundamental shifts in our understanding of the human mind help explain how humans receive, generate, and transduce information.

f. New ideas and events evoke body–mind changes; that is, neural pathways and consciousness couple to enable information transduction.[16]

9. Energy Model: Dr. Ginger Bowler showed that everything is energy with a respective frequency.[19] One can list these frequencies on a continuum. In her model, the line (midrange on the continuum) is neutral. Anything above the line is a higher vibrational frequency, which in general, improves health of mind, body, and spirit. Anything below the line is a slower, denser energy frequency that leads to disease and unhealthiness.

Emotions and the Neural Tripwire

1. The traditional view in neuroscience has been that:
   a. Sensory organs transmit signals to the thalamus and
   b. From there to the sensory process areas of the neocortex.
   c. The neocortex translates the signals into perceptions and attaches meanings.[17]
   d. The signals then move to the limbic system, which sends the appropriate response to the body.
2. The discovery of a smaller bundle of neurons that leads directly from the thalamus to the amygdala and in addition to those that connect with the neocortex has changed the traditional view.
   a. Sensory impulses go directly from the sensory organs to the amygdala, allowing for a faster response.

b. The amygdala triggers an emotional response even before the person fully understands what is happening. Taking immediate action, the amygdala sends impulses through the brain to the body.

c. If the stimulus is traumatic, the amygdala responds with extra strength. Key changes take place in the locus ceruleus, which regulates catecholamines; adrenaline and noradrenaline are released.

d. Other limbic structures, such as the hippocampus and the hypothalamus, respond, and the main stress hormones bring about the typical body responses labeled *fight, flight, faint,* or *freeze.*

e. Changes in the brain opioid system that secretes endorphins prepare the person to meet the danger.

f. The neocortex processes the impulse, and a more considered response follows.

g. Emotions are not dispensable, but rather an integral part of the whole; there is a positive benefit to negative emotions. They are a warning that some need is not being met.

3. Figure 31-1, Emotions and the Neural Tripwire, can be found in Chapter 31 of *Holistic Nursing: A Handbook for Practice* (6th edition).

State-Dependent Memory and Recall

1. Feelings are integral to human living; what people learn depends on their mood or feelings at the time of the experience.[20]
2. The emotion-carrying molecules or ligands, which accompany all human activity, bind to cellular receptors and send an informational message to the cell where they can be stored as memories; feelings and actions are intertwined (e.g., people are more likely to help others when they are in a good mood and more likely to hurt others when they are in a bad mood).
3. Likewise, feelings and memories are intertwined; thoughts that occur throughout daily routines are repeated patterns of memories and their associative emotional connections.
4. Memories are accompanied by emotions that, in turn, are influenced and affected by the context in which they were acquired (e.g., a particularly traumatic experience

is stamped in the memory with special strength. Subsequent stimuli in new situations and emotional experiences can attach to and reawaken past memories. These reactivated thoughts and emotions direct and shape our actions in the present).
5. Feelings or mood also plays a major role in body–mind healing.
    a. Recent work with persons suffering from post-traumatic stress disorder (PTSD) revealed that relearning is the route to healing. The following can be used to unfreeze a picture frozen in the amygdala that is capable of triggering the fight, flight, freeze, or faint response provoked by seemingly benign stimuli: writing therapy, bibliotherapy, bodywork, art therapy, traditional talk therapies.[21]

Location of the Brain Centers

1. Brain function can be best understood using the model of a hologram.
    a. A hologram is a specially processed photographic record that provides a three-dimensional image when a light from a laser is beamed through it.
    b. If any part of the hologram should be destroyed, any one of the remaining parts is capable of reconstructing the whole image.
    c. This holographic model is congruent with the new understanding of the way in which information is transmitted, received, and stored (learned).
2. Memories are not stored in any specific part of the brain, but rather in multiple overlapping areas. They can be retrieved in their entirety by a stimulus to more than one area of the brain. Loss of specific memory is related more to the amount of brain damage than to the site of the injury (e.g., the ability to recall what was lost when gunshot wounds injure the brain often returns).
3. The brain has the ability to grow whole new neurons.
4. Paranormal events, including the transpersonal healing associated with shamanism and other approaches to metaphysical healing, involve communicating information in ways that do not conform to the current

understanding of receiving, processing, and sending energy.
5. Phenomena such as phantom limb sensations and auras that extend beyond the corpus challenge traditional perceptions of body image, as well as the understanding of the physical boundaries of the body.
6. Mechanisms of consciousness, such as the ability of the person to reflect on the self or create and retrieve images, cannot be explained simply in terms of the structure and function of current anatomic models.
7. Experience can change brain structure; viewing the brain in a holographic manner reveals its influence on psychophysiologic functioning.
8. Cognitive therapy is an example of an attempt to modify negative irrational thinking that leads to emotional distress.
9. The revolutionary discovery of the neuroplasticity of the brain is opening new worlds of possibility in human development.[13,16,22]

Neuroplasticity

1. It was once believed that the hardware of the brain was fixed and immutable; according to that belief, the brain virtually establishes all its connections, such as the auditory cortex and the visual cortex, in the first years of life. Depictions of the specific areas and functions of the different parts of the brain were commonly accepted. If an area responsible for one function was injured, it was believed no other area of the brain assumed its function (e.g., rehabilitation focused on forgetting what function was lost and strengthening and compensating for whatever function remained intact).
2. Current neurorehabilitation efforts not only compensate for the loss of cognitive abilities, but also are directed to restore those abilities; we acknowledge that the brain can respond to altered sensory inputs and reprogram itself to resume previous functions.
3. Our brain is continuously getting rewired in keeping with the world of digital technology and the information revolution. The human brain changes throughout a person's lifetime.

Epigenetics

1. Our genes are not fixed; we are not simply genetically determined.
2. Our genes are modulated by our inner environment—the emotional, chemical, mental, energetic, and spiritual landscape—as well as our outer environment—the social and ecological systems in which we reside.
3. Genes can be activated or deactivated by the meaning we assign to an experience.
4. We are formed and molded by the thoughts that stimulate the formation of neural pathways that either reinforce old patterns or initiate new ones.
5. The process by which a gene produces a result in the body is well established.[23,24]
   a. Signals pass through the cell membrane to the nucleus, enter the chromosome, and activate a specific strand of DNA.
   b. Each strand of DNA is protected by a protein. The protein serves as a barrier between the information contained in the DNA and the rest of the intracellular environment. As long as the DNA is wrapped by the protein, the DNA lies dormant.
   c. When a signal arrives, the protein around the DNA unwraps and, with the assistance of RNA, the DNA molecule replicates an intermediate template molecule.
   d. At this point, the targeted gene moves into active expression where it creates other actions within the cell by constructing, assembling, or altering products.
   e. What was dormant potential is moved into active expression by a signal that comes from outside the cell and not from the DNA.
6. This process can take 1 second or hours.[23,24]
7. Epigenetic mechanisms program gene expression.[25]
8. Key neuronal genes are fine-tuned by early life experience and govern learning and memory throughout life.
9. Enriched postnatal experience enhances spatial learning, whereas chronic early life stress can result in persistent deficits in the structure and function of hippocampal neurons.
10. Epigenetic mechanisms are an integral part of a multitude of brain functions, including basic neuronal functions and higher-order cognitive processes.[26]
11. Evidence suggests that maternal stress influences programming of integrated physiologic systems in the offspring beginning in pregnancy, suggesting stress effects can be transgenerational.
12. Biological, psychological, and social processes clearly interact throughout life to influence the expression of strengths as well as disorders.

◼ MIND MODULATION

1. Indirect and direct anatomic and biochemical pathways connect the neuroendocrine, nervous, and immune regulatory systems.[27] Communication among these systems is multidirectional with signal molecules and their receptors regulating the cellular outcomes.
2. Feedback loops, up-regulation, and down-regulation of hormones and receptors function to protect the body.

Stress Response

1. The stress response is designed to protect against threats to well-being.[27] Threats can be physical, social, psychosocial, real, and/or simply perceived.
2. Biochemical functions of the major organ systems are modulated by the mind.[28]
3. Thoughts and feelings are transduced into chemicals (i.e., neurotransmitters, neurohormones, and peptides) that circulate throughout the body and convey messages to various systems within the body.
4. The stress response illustrates the way in which various systems cooperate to protect an individual from harm. An example of this response is found in Chapter 31 of *Holistic Nursing: A Handbook for Practice*.
5. Physiologic effects of stress: Increased heart and respiratory rates, tightened muscles, increased metabolic rate, general sense of foreboding, fear, nervousness, irritability, negative mood, elevated blood pressure, dilated pupils, stronger cardiac contractions, increased levels of blood glucose, serum

cholesterol, circulating free fatty acids, and triglycerides.

6. Although these responses prepare a person for short-term stress, they can lead to structure changes and clinical illness if prolonged. The memory of this traumatic experience is stored in the brain and other body cells and has psychological and spiritual effects. The individual might reexperience the stress reaction in future similar events with less intense stress, such as having a friend brush against his arm as they walk toward the car. Indeed, just thinking about this experience can initiate a stress response.

7. Table 31-1, Effects of Sympathetic and Parasympathetic Stimulation, reviews the effects of sympathetic and parasympathetic stimulation. It can be found in Chapter 31 of *Holistic Nursing: A Handbook for Practice*.

8. When the stress has been dealt with or is no longer a threat, the body returns to its normal, homeostatic state.

9. However, when one experiences a threat so traumatic or the threat is so chronic, the normal stress response is altered, resulting in the traumatic stress response (TSR).[29]

10. Severe traumatic threats range from childhood abuse to a near-death automobile accident or the sudden, unexpected death of a child; chronic ongoing threat or stress could be caregiving for an elderly spouse with Alzheimer's disease or unpleasant work conditions.

11. Initiation of the stress response that is short lived does not lead to adverse health results, whereas severe and/or long-term stress can lead to adverse health events.[30]

12. Homeostasis, the body's steady state, is maintained through ongoing changes in response to physical and environmental challenges.

13. Allostasis is the process used to maintain homeostasis and well-being.[31]

14. The general adaptation syndrome, the nonspecific physiologic stress response, is part of allostasis; the number of demands requiring adaptation determines the allostatic load.

15. When an individual experiences overwhelming stress or has inadequate coping skill to deal with the stress, allostatic overload occurs; allostatic overload can lead to structural changes in the body and illness.[29]

16. Long-term effects of stress can negatively influence cardiovascular disease and gastrointestinal problems; lead to depression, drug problems, and accidents; promote lipolysis in the extremities and lipogenesis in the face and back as a result of long-term presence of high levels of cortisol; suppress the inflammatory process; increases the risk of osteoporosis and ulcers; lead to atrophy of immune system organs; cause levels of various reproductive hormones (e.g., progesterone, estrogen, and testosterone), growth and thyroid hormones, and insulin to decline, probably to conserve energy.[32]

17. The stress response is modulated by
   a. Disposition
   b. Personality
   c. Coping skills

18. Psychological stressors stimulate a physiologic response and are referred to as a reactive response; students can have a reactive response when taking an examination.

19. Anticipatory stressors can also elicit the stress response; children who have been abused by a parent might experience a physiologic response when the parent comes near.

20. Perceived stressors begin in the area of the brain that controls cognition and emotions, the cerebral cortex and the limbic system; one person can have a full-blown stress response to a damaged fingernail whereas another person might not have a stress response to the loss of a best friend.

21. Additionally, there are individual differences in hormonal, neuroendocrine, and immunologic responses to stress.[28,32]

22. Three major body systems are involved with the stress response: the nervous, endocrine, and immune systems. These systems work in symphony-like ways to protect the body from harm.

Nervous System

1. The brain is the cognitive center. It is here that memories are stored, ideas generated, and emotions expressed.[14]

2. Emotions that affect the body originate in the brain; the brain, then, has a powerful influence over the body and is also the link to emotions and the immune system.

3. The interconnectedness of the central nervous system (CNS) means that frontal

cortex thoughts and images are in intimate communication with the emotion-related limbic center.

4. As the biochemicals transduced from thoughts and ideas circulate through the limbic-hypothalamic system, memory cells from past experiences affect their structure.

5. The hypothalamus, the central control center, coordinates the biochemical cascade, integrating neuroendocrine functions by secreting both releasing and inhibiting hormones, as well as stimulating the sympathetic nervous system (SNS).[33]

6. The SNS branch of the autonomic nervous system (ANS) is connected to the limbic system, has fibers extending into the adrenal medulla, and includes a pathway of nerves to the thymus, lymph nodes, spleen, and bone marrow; hence, the connections are not only biochemical, but also anatomic.

7. The SNS with preganglionic fibers that terminate in the adrenal medulla stimulate the secretion of epinephrine (80%) and norepinephrine (20%) that begin the physiologic stress response and result in increased heart and respiratory rates, elevated blood pressure, and increased blood to skeletal muscle.

8. The effects of epinephrine occur within seconds.[34,35]

9. Integration of the stress response occurs in the CNS.

10. Communication is dependent on neuronal pathways among the cerebral cortex, the limbic system, the thalamus, the hypothalamus, the pituitary gland, and the reticular activating system (RAS).[32 34]

11. The focus of the cerebral cortex is on cognition, focused attention, and vigilance.

12. The limbic system is the emotional center focused on feelings such as rage, anger, and fear. This system elicits an endocrine response indirectly via stimulation of neural pathways for sensory information and stimulates a central response by direct stimulation of the locus coeruleus (LC).

13. The thalamus is the relay station. In the thalamus sensory data are sorted and distributed.

14. The hypothalamus is the coordinator of the endocrine system and the ANS.

15. The RAS is the modulator of ANS activity, skeletal muscle tone, and mental alertness.

16. The LC, located in the brain stem, has afferent pathways connecting the hypothalamus, hippocampus, limbic systems, and cerebral cortex; it is rich with norepinephrine-producing cells, integrating the ANS response.

17. The entire process is not only complex but also not completely clear.[27] Understanding the psychophysiologic stress response as it affects the nervous system helps to clarify how different holistic therapies work.

18. It is possible to interrupt feelings of anxiety by using a relaxation technique to calm the self or a cognitive restructuring technique to change thought patterns. For example, when patients learn to use relaxation, imagery, music therapy, or certain types of meditation training, their sympathetic response to stress decreases and the calming effect of the parasympathetic system takes over, leading to body–mind healing.

19. Biofeedback can reduce arousal and tension, and it is so effective that it has become a common intervention for a number of conditions induced or exacerbated by uncontrolled stimulation of the stress response.[27] For example, warming the fingers by using biofeedback decreases the discomfort that accompanies Raynaud's disease.

20. Changes in physiology change thoughts and feelings; changes in thoughts and feelings, conversely, change physiology.

Endocrine System

1. The nervous and endocrine systems are so closely connected and interactive that they are referred to as the neuroendocrine system.

2. The specific organs of the endocrine system and the stress response are the pituitary and adrenal glands.

3. Hormones, secreted by the endocrine glands, are the specialized chemical messengers that act to modulate both cellular and systemic responses; they are always present in body fluids, but their concentrations vary. They produce both localized and generalized effects.

4. One hormone can stimulate a variety of effects in different tissues, and a single function can be subject to regulation by more than one hormone.

5. Hormones include amines and amino acids (e.g., norepinephrine, epinephrine,

dopamine), peptides, polypeptides, proteins, and steroids.[36]

6. Each cell has a multitude of receptor molecules that can be modified or altered.

7. Hormones act by binding to their specific receptor on target cell surfaces. For example, treatment with methadone is effective for heroin addicts because the methadone binds to the opioid receptor sites.

8. A decrease in hormone levels can increase the number of receptor sites available. This is *up-regulation*. Conversely, an elevated hormone level leads to a decrease in receptors, or *down-regulation*.[36]

9. Many of the hormones have a negative feedback loop that maintains the *balance* in serum hormonal levels.

10. Stimuli such as circadian rhythms, the environment, and emotional and physical stressors influence the secretion of hypothalamic hormones.

11. The major endocrine hormones in the stress response are:
    a. Epinephrine from the adrenal medulla
    b. Glucocorticoids from the adrenal cortex

12. Other hormones associated with the stress response include pituitary hormones (growth hormone, prolactin, estrogen, and testosterone).

13. Growth hormone (GH) and prolactin are secreted by the anterior pituitary during stress; GH affects metabolism of carbohydrates, protein, and lipids.

14. Estrogen might attenuate the hypothalamic-pituitary-adrenal axis (HPA) effects because women tend to respond more to stressors with a greater HPA stress response.

15. Decreased testosterone levels occur in men during stressful experiences, but more research is needed to understand the significance.

16. The opioids (i.e., endorphins, enkephalins) are synthesized in the pituitary and other parts of the CNS. Opioids have a morphine-like effect with receptors throughout the body. These naturally occurring hormones produce the "runner's high," increase a person's pain threshold, and explain how people can "ignore" their own serious injury to save a loved one.

17. The endorphins are secreted by immune cells during stress, leading to analgesia.[33]

Corticotropin-Releasing Factor

1. Corticotropin-releasing factor (CRF), a peptide and neurotransmitter, is part of the neuroendocrine stress response.

2. CRF is found in the brain stem, hypothalamus, limbic systems, and extrahypothalamic structures. When released from the hypothalamus, CRF leads to pituitary secretion of adrenocorticotropic hormone (ACTH).

3. ACTH induces the secretion of glucocorticoid hormones from the adrenal cortex.

4. Cortisone helps to mediate the stress response and has a number of physiologic outcomes.[27]

5. There is a sympathetic nervous system connection to the blood vessels supplying the immune cells, thereby creating a direct nervous system and immune system pathway.[33]

6. Cortisol produces similar effects as those of epinephrine, but the effects last from minutes to days. To explain, epinephrine is secreted quickly during the alarm stage and cortisol is secreted for the long term during the resistant and exhaustion stages. Cortisol stimulates gluconeogenesis, increasing blood glucose levels and resulting in protein breakdown. This breakdown leads to loss of muscle, negative nitrogen balance, increased gastrointestinal secretion, and suppression of the immune system.[33]

Immune System

1. The immune, endocrine, and nervous systems communicate with hormones, neuropeptides, neurotransmitters, and products of immune cells; this communication is bidirectional.[32]

2. Anatomically, the nervous system has direct connections to immune system organs (thymus, bone marrow, lymph nodes, and spleen); likewise, immune system cells produce messengers that signal the nervous system.[14]

3. There are receptors on the immune system cells for the neurotransmitters such as the opioid peptides, dopamine, catecholamines, and ACTH.[32]

4. The nervous system has direct sympathetic innervation of immune system blood vessels.[33]

5. The SNS pathways of norepinephrine and epinephrine secretion and the hypothalamic-pituitary-adrenal axis with glucocorticoid secretion have direct effects on immune system cells. Glucocorticoids suppress the immune system. For example, cortisol suppresses white blood cells and is even administered to suppress the immune system in people with autoimmune diseases.

6. Recent findings indicate that CNS and ANS neuropeptides and endocrine hormones stimulated by the nervous system directly affect immune system cells. Receptor sites located on the surface of the T and B lymphocytes have the ability to activate, direct, and modify immune function. For example, CRF suppresses monocytic macrophages and T helper lymphocytes. Lymphocytes produce the stress hormone ACTH and the brain peptide endorphin.[32] Endorphins have both enhancing and suppressing effects on immune system cells, depending on their concentration. They can elevate active T cells whereas too many endorphins can suppress the immune system.[14,33] In turn, cytokines, that is, secretions of immune system cells, affect the nervous and endocrine systems.

7. Interventions to reduce the stress response can have a positive effect on the immune system.

8. Interventions that induce the parasympathetic response have healing effects on the body.

9. Because all systems are interconnected, holistic interventions contribute to health and healing by innervating multiple facets of the nervous, endocrine, and immune systems. It is important to remember that there are individual differences in immunologic reactivity, hormonal responses, and autonomic responses to stress as well as healing modalities.[28]

Neuropeptides

1. With their receptors, neuropeptides help further explain body–mind interconnections and the way that emotions are experienced in the body.

2. Circulating throughout the body, neuropeptides are considered the messengers that connect body and mind.

3. The first neuropeptides were discovered in the intestine, which has many receptors; this might help explain those "gut feelings."

4. Neuropeptides can be exchanged and produced by most all body tissues, even inflammatory cells.[37]

5. The limbic system and hippocampus are rich with neuropeptide receptors, containing almost all of them and connecting emotions and learning. The concept of emotions as neuropeptides explains why people have trouble remembering and learning when they are experiencing psychophysiologic stress.

6. Performance, too, is affected. For example, those who experience severe anxiety and panic before speaking in public or performing a concert benefit from relaxation techniques and cognitive restructuring.

7. This ability to alter biochemicals and the consequent effects on memory and learning occur when the unconscious mind is brought into consciousness with hypnosis.

8. Emotions and spirituality cannot be ignored; nurses who attend only to the body are not providing holistic care.

9. Referrals to chaplains or therapists are positive interventions but might leave patients and families feeling uncared for, unattended, unheard, and lonely.

10. Interventions to support and enhance coping offer another opportunity to promote healing and wholeness.[36]

■ CONCLUSION

1. New scientific understandings of living systems, such as principles of self-organization and mind modulation of the body–mind systems, provide a theoretical base for holistic healing interventions.

2. Understanding the physiologic principles that are involved in nursing interventions helps nurses design individualized and appropriate holistic care for clients.

3. Nurses, aware of their own wounds and sensitive to the wounds of clients, are strategically placed to lead clients in facilitating health and healing.

4. Walking the talk is about being authentic and congruent, allowing nurses to relate to patients in authentic and congruent ways.

5. Caring for oneself is essential for nurses to model wholeness. For, if truth be known, nurses who do not care for themselves are unable to provide holistic care for their patients.

6. The process of becoming authentic makes one sensitive to the needs of others. Modeling is, perhaps, the strongest teaching strategy.

7. Clients are becoming much more knowledgeable of complementary interventions.

8. It is essential, therefore, to educate nurses to empower them as well.

9. Knowledge of the communication of the nervous, endocrine, and immune systems is necessary but insufficient for holistic nursing—neither does it explain all aspects of illness.

10. New scientific information invalidates the idea of the dualism of mind and body.

11. Thoughts, emotions, and consciousness do not reside solely in the brain, but are present in various body parts—the brain, the glands, and the immune, enteric, and sexual systems.

12. The research data overwhelmingly document the body–mind interrelationships.

13. There are still many unanswered questions. Does the mind exist after the physical death? Does the soul survive death of the body? Why do some people experience phantom pain after an amputation?

14. Nurses must continue to incorporate wholeness into their own lives while exploring effective ways to deliver holistically oriented care to their clients.

15. The meaning of the illness, the method of giving the diagnosis, the tone of voice and the touch of the nurse, and the relationships to family and friends must all be investigated.

16. To achieve this goal, nurses must be aware of what they focus on and what they choose to ignore.

■ NOTES

1. Leddy, S. K. (2006). *Integrative health promotion conceptual bases for nursing practice*. Sudbury, MA: Jones and Bartlett.

2. Dossey, L. (2004–2005, December–February). The unsolved mystery of healing. *Shift: At the Frontiers of Consciousness*, 24–26.

3. Lindley, D. (2007). *Uncertainty: Einstein, Heisenberg, Bohr, and the struggle for the soul of science*. New York, NY: Doubleday.

4. Haisch, B. (2001). Freeing the scientific imagination. *IONS Noetic Science Review*, 24–29.

5. Boyd, M. A., & Nihart, M. A. (2003). *Psychiatric nursing*. Philadelphia, PA: Lippincott-Raven.

6. von Bertalanffy, L. (1968). *General Systems Theory*. New York, NY: George Braziller.

7. Laszlo, E. (2002). *The systems view of the world. A holistic vision of our time*. Cresskill, NJ: Hampton Press.

8. Prigogine, I. (1997). *The end of certainty*. New York, NY: Free Press.

9. Capra, F. (1996). *The web of life*. New York, NY: Doubleday.

10. Larter, R. (2002, March–May). Life lessons from the newest science. *IONS Noetic Science Review*, 22–27.

11. Kabat-Zinn, J. (2005). *Coming to our senses*. New York, NY: Hyperion.

12. Bartol, G. M. (1998). Creating a healing environment. *Seminars in Perioperative Nursing, 92*(7), 90–95.

13. Rabin, B. (2007). Stress: A system of the whole. In R. Ader (Ed.), *Psychoneuroimmunology* (4th ed., Vol. 1, p. 216). New York, NY: Elsevier.

14. Karren, K. J., Hafen, B. Q., Smith, N. L., & Frandsen, K. J. (2006). *Mind/body health. The effects of attitudes, emotions and relationships* (3rd ed.). New York, NY: Pearson.

15. Simac, V. (2006–2007, December–February). The challenge of forgiveness. *Shift: At the Frontiers of Consciousness*, 13, 29–33.

16. Begley, S. (2006). *Train your mind, change your brain*. New York, NY: Ballantine.

17. Pert, C. B. (1997). *The molecules of emotion: Why you feel the way you feel*. New York, NY: Charles Scribner's Sons.

18. Damasio, A. (2003). *Looking for Spinosa*. New York, NY: Harcourt.

19. Bowler, G. (2000). *Listening and communicating with energy*. Madison, WI: Focus on the Light.

20. Goleman, D. (1995). *Emotional intelligence*. New York, NY: Bantam.

21. Frisch, N. C., & Frisch, L. E. (2011). *Psychiatric mental health nursing* (4th ed.). New York, NY: Delmar.

22. Graham, J. E., Christian, L. M., & Kiecolt-Glaser, J. K. (2007). Close relationships and immunity. In R. Ader (Ed.), *Psychoneuroimmunology* (4th ed., Vol. 1, p. 792). New York, NY: Elsevier.

23. Mark, C. W. (2010). *Spiritual intelligence and the neuroplastic brain*. Bloomington, IN: Authorhouse.

24. Church, D. (2007). *The genie in your genes*. Santa Rosa, CA: Elite Books.

25. McClelland, S., Korosi, A., Cope, J., Ivy, A., & Baram, T. Z. (2011). Emerging roles of epigenetics mechanisms in the enduring effects of early-life

stress and experience on learning and memory. *Neurobiology of Learning and Memory, 96*(1), 79–88.

26. Graff, J., Kim, D., Dobbin, M. M., & Tsai, L. H. (2011). Epigenetic regulation of gene expression in physiological and pathological brain process. *Physiological Reviews, 91*(2), 603–649.

27. Porth, M. C. (2010). *Essentials of pathophysiology: Concepts of altered health states* (4th ed.). Philadelphia, PA: Lippincott Williams & Wilkins.

28. Ader, R. (2005). Integrative summary: On the clinical relevance of psychoneuroimmunology. In K. Vedhara and M. Irwin (Eds.), *Human psychoneuroimmunology*, 344–349. Oxford, England: Oxford University Press.

29. Wilson, K. R., Hansen, D. J., & Li, M. (2010). The traumatic stress response in child maltreatment and resultant neuropsychological effects. *Aggression and Violent Behavior, 16*, 87–97.

30. Piazza, J. R., Almeida, D. M., Dmitrieve, N. O., & Klein, L. C. (2010). Frontiers in the use of biomarkers of health in research on stress and aging. *Journal of Gerontology Series B: Psychological Sciences and Social Sciences, 65B*, 513–525.

31. Emerson, R. J. (2010). Homeostasis and adaptive responses to stressors. In L.-C. Copstead and J. L. Banasik (Eds.), *Pathophysiology* (4th ed., pp. 14–27). St. Louis, MO: Elsevier Saunders.

32. McCance, K. L., Forshee, B. A., & Shelby, J. (2006). Stress and disease. In McCance, K. L. & Huether, S.E. (Eds). (pp. 311–332). *Pathophysiology: The biologic basis for disease in adults and children.* 5th ed St. Louis, MO: Elsevier Mosby.

33. Oakley, L. D. (2005). Stress, adaptation, and coping. In L. C. Copstead and J. L. Banasik (Eds.), pp. 23–45. *Pathophysiology* (3rd ed.). St. Louis, MO: Elsevier Saunders.

34. M. C. Porth, *Essentials of Pathophysiology: Concepts of Altered Health States,* 4th ed. (Philadelphia, PA: Lippincott Williams & Wilkins, 2010).

35. Huether, S. E. (2006). Mechanisms of hormonal regulation. In K. L. McCance and S. E. Huether (Eds.), *Pathophysiology: The biologic basis for disease in adults and children.* (pp. 655–681).St. Louis, MO: Elsevier Mosby.

36. N. P. M. Van der Kleij and J. Bienenstock (2007). "Significance of Sensory Neuropeptides and the Immune Response," in *Psychoneuroimmunology,* (4th ed., pp. 97–129). Vol. 1, ed. R. Ader. New York, NY: Elsevier.

■ STUDY QUESTIONS

Basic Level

1. Which of the following changes in our understanding of our body–mind system can be attributed to Einstein's theory of relativity?

   a. All body–mind events have an identifiable cause and effect.
   b. All things and events connect and are relative to the others.
   c. Symptoms indicate a breakdown in our body–mind system.
   d. All diseases can be broken down and separated into parts to determine the root cause.

2. Which of the following answer choices does not modulate the physiologic stress response?

   a. Age
   b. Disposition
   c. Personality
   d. Coping skills

3. Which of the following systems are involved in the stress response?

   a. Lymphatic, circulatory, and nervous systems
   b. Musculoskeletal, immune, and gastrointestinal systems
   c. Endocrine, immune, and nervous systems
   d. Cardiovascular, respiratory, and endocrine systems

4. What physiologic changes would be expected in a patient experiencing a highly stressful situation?

   a. Low levels of protein with muscle buildup
   b. High levels of serum fatty acids and glucose
   c. High levels of serum albumin and enhanced tissue healing
   d. High levels of hydrochloric acid in the gut

5. Which of the following answer choices best explains the therapeutic benefit of holistic nursing interventions such as imagery, touch, and relaxation with patients who are experiencing chronic pain?

   a. They bring about changes in one part of the system that lead to changes in the whole system.
   b. They exert a placebo effect.
   c. They distract a person from the pain.
   d. These interventions are only effective in patients who believe they will be beneficial.

Advanced Level

6. Which of the following are the major endocrine hormones in the stress response?
   a. Norepinephrine and dopamine
   b. Corticotropin-releasing factor (CRF) and somatostatin
   c. Adrenocorticotropic hormone (ACTH) and prolactin
   d. Epinephrine and glucocorticoids

7. By which mechanism do holistic interventions promote health and healing?
   a. Enhancing parasympathetic dominance, which promotes balance in all the body-mind systems
   b. Up-regulating emotional responses to down-regulate stressful stimuli
   c. Increasing the production of the body's natural endorphins to produce a relaxed state
   d. Creating a feedback loop from the locus ceruleus to the amygdala to promote relaxation

8. Fundamental shifts in our understanding of the human mind have supported the interconnectedness of body, mind, and spirit. Neural pathways and consciousness couple to enable information transduction resulting in transformed physiologic outcomes. This is best described by which theory?
   a. Einstein's Theory of Relativity
   b. Plank's quantum mechanics
   c. Santiago Theory of Cognition
   d. Unified Theory of Living Systems

9. Which of the following is an appropriate nursing intervention for patients that Miller describes as "blunters"?
   a. Review all significant details of the upcoming procedure and ask patients to repeat their understanding of your explanation.
   b. Show a model of the heart and bypass grafts so that patients can understand exactly what will be done in the open heart surgery.
   c. Encourage patients to go online and read all about the upcoming surgery.
   d. Encourage patients to listen to relaxing music as they awake in the postanesthesia care area.

10. Which of the following concepts contributes significant science on how the body–mind reframes and/or desensitizes responses to traumatic events to attain homeostasis?
    a. Consciousness
    b. Allostatic overload
    c. Autopoiesis
    d. Neural trip wires

Chapter 31

Spirituality and Health

Mary Helming

Original Authors: Margaret A. Burkhardt
and Mary Gail Nagai-Jacobson

■ DEFINITIONS

Religion An organized system of beliefs regarding the cause, purpose, and nature of the universe that is shared by a group of people, and the practices, behaviors, worship, and ritual associated with that system. Religion connects persons through shared beliefs, values, and practices, making clear particular belief systems that are different from other belief systems, thus defining differences among groups of persons.

Spirituality The essence of our being. It permeates our living in relationships and infuses our unfolding awareness of who we are, our purpose in being, and our inner resources. Spirituality is active and expressive. It shapes—and is shaped by—our life journey. Spirituality informs the ways we live and experience life, the ways we encounter mystery, and the ways we relate to all aspects of life. Inherent in the human condition, spirituality is expressed and experienced through living our connectedness with the Sacred Source, the self, others, and nature.

■ THEORY AND RESEARCH

1. What is spirituality?
   a. Can spirituality be defined?
      - Most basic, yet least understood aspect of holistic nursing.
      - Intangible in many ways and defies quantification.
      - Mystery and human experience of spirituality cannot be fully defined.
      - Symbols, metaphor, and story more often describe spirituality.[1]
      - From Latin *spiritus*, meaning breath; relates to Greek *pneuma* or breath, which refers to vital spirit or soul.
      - Spirituality is the essence of who we are and how we are in the world and, like breathing, is integral to our human existence.
      - All people are bio-psycho-social-spiritual beings.
      - There are developmental aspects of spirituality; may vary with age.
      - Incorrect common practice of describing spirituality in terms of religious beliefs and practices.
         ◆ Healthcare providers often link spiritual caregiving with determining a patient's religious affiliation and understanding the health-related beliefs, norms, and taboos of that religion.
         ◆ This is incomplete and it is necessary to differentiate spirituality from religion.
      - Spirituality is broader than religion; not everyone is religious, but everyone is spiritual through human nature.
      - Holistic nurses honor the unique ways in which people express, experience, and nurture their spiritual selves.
2. Relationship between spirituality and religion
   a. Nursing and healthcare literature reflect the understanding that spirituality and religion are not synonymous.[2-5]

b. As essence of our being, spirituality is integral to all persons and a manifestation of each person's wholeness and being.

c. Religion is chosen. Spirituality is expressed both within and beyond the context of religion.

d. *Religion* refers to an organized system of beliefs shared by a group of people and the practices related to that system.

- Ritual, worship, prayer, meditation, style of dress, dietary observances are examples of religious practice.
- Culture influences religious and spiritual practices, values, and beliefs.
- Religious practices can assist in development of spirituality, but not necessarily.
- Rites and rituals of religious practice might or might not meet patient's spiritual needs.

e. Spiritual care and interventions must be individualized and reflect the patient's perspectives and worldview, especially when spirituality is not expressed through a particular religion.[6]

3. Understanding spirituality

a. Difficulty expressing spirituality in language.

b. Western cultures: Language used for describing spirit is usually that of science or religion from the Judeo-Christian tradition.

c. Spirituality in nursing and health care tend to reflect Judeo-Christian values and perspectives regarding the Divine, relationships with others and the world, experience of suffering, and prayer.

d. Nurses need to be open to each person's unique expression of spirituality, especially if not of Judeo-Christian background.

e. Western Judeo-Christian-Islamic traditions share beliefs in monotheism, transcendence, and dualism.[7]

- Monotheism: Belief in one God that is above and beyond nature, contrasted with a belief in the existence of many gods (polytheism) or the existence of the sacred in all living things (pantheism) found in Eastern and nature religions.
- Transcendence: To exist above material existence; God is separate from humanity.

- Western traditions: Seek connection with the Divine by focusing *outward* through ritual and prayer.
- Eastern and nature traditions: Focus on *immanence*, the experience of the Divine within each person, looking inward through meditation and spiritual exercises.
- Dualism: Separation of spirit and matter, of science and religion as dominant in Western cultures.
- Monism: Reality is a unified whole, metaphysical tradition of Eastern cultures.

4. Elements of spirituality

a. Increased interest in health and spirituality over recent years.

b. Defining spirituality is like trying to lasso wind: Wind can be felt and its effects seen, but it cannot be contained within concepts or boundaries.

c. Understanding spirituality requires many ways of knowing: cognitive, intuitive, aesthetic, experiential, and deep inner sensing or knowing.

d. Elements of spirituality: Essence of being, a unifying and animating force, the life principle of each person, a sense of meaning and purpose, and a commitment to something greater than the self.[1,3,8-11]

e. Spirituality permeates life, shapes our life journey, and is vital to the process of discovering purpose, meaning, and inner strength.

f. Spirituality helps find one's place in the world and gives sense of trust that what is needed will be given.

g. Sense of inner peace is element of spirituality, ability to remain calm in times of trouble. Felt in heart. "Peace which passeth understanding" in Christianity.

h. Awareness of life beyond the present.

i. Peace is a product of living in relationship with the Sacred Source, others, and all creation in a way that acknowledges and nurtures soul in the midst of all that life brings.

5. Connectedness with the Sacred Source

a. Research demonstrates people express and experience spirituality in relationships with Sacred Source, Nature, others, and the self.[1,4,12]

b. Mystery of the Sacred Source. Various cultures and faith traditions use names: Life Force, Source, God, Allah, Lord, Goddess, Absolute, Higher Power, Spirit, Vishnu, Inner Light, Tao, Great Mystery, the Way, Universal Love, Sacred Source, God, One with No Name.

c. Connection with Sacred Source is at the heart of one's being. Our rational minds cannot conceptualize, describe God adequately.

d. Connect with Sacred Source through prayer, ritual, reconciliation, stillness, readings.

e. Reverence: Appreciation of human limitations and awe of God. Sense of omnipresence of God.

6. Connectedness with nature

a. Spirituality can be experienced through sense of connectedness with nature, environment, universe.

b. Natural order on Earth, connectedness with web of life. Happenings on Earth and environment affect human beings and human beings affect Earth and environment.

c. Sense of awe and feeling connected with all beings and things on Earth is spiritual.

d. Sense of spirituality often felt while walking on a beach, sitting by a favorite tree, viewing a sunset, listening to flowing water, watching a fire, caring for plants, and so forth.

7. Connectedness with others

a. Spirituality experienced through relationships with other human beings: Comfort, support, conflict, and sharing of joys and sorrows. Healing of relationships is an important aspect of spiritual growth.

b. Experience of community and common bond with humanity.

c. Giving and receiving important to connectedness; presence is sharing with another.

d. Lack of connectedness with others can cause spiritual crisis and isolation.

e. Global connectedness with others is increasing because of technology; sense of world community.

f. Structures: Health care, educational institutions, faith-based services, social organizations, informal affiliations, and Internet links all capable of supporting spirituality and connectedness with others.

8. Connectedness with self

a. Being: Is the art of stillness and presence with self, others, the Sacred Source, and nature. Being includes experiencing present moment more deeply.

- Awareness: Experience of living in the moment, present to body-mind-spirit, without judgment.
- Attentiveness to Being allows person to attune to sources of inner strength and deepest knowing.
- Spirituality infuses the ever-unfolding awareness of who one is—of self-becoming.
- Spirituality can be manifested in doing also: assisting others, tending the sick, attending religious services, praying, meditating, teaching religious education, spending time with friends, caring for family, creating sacred space for self and others, and so forth.
- Sacred space: Home for the spirit, providing rest, stillness, nurture. Examples: sunlit space, a garden or workshop, a room for prayer or meditation, family surrounding a loved one in a hospital.

■ SPIRITUALITY AND THE HEALING PROCESS

Body-Mind-Spirit

1. Holistic paradigm: Every human experience has body-mind-spirit components.

2. Words *healing*, *whole*, and *holy* derive from same root: Old Saxon *hal*, meaning whole. Therefore: healing is a spiritual process that attends to the wholeness of a person.

3. Healing requires recognition of the spiritual dimension of each person, including the healer, and awareness that spirituality permeates every encounter.

4. Shared relationship describes common humanity and connectedness between caregiver and the person being healed, manifestation of spirituality.

Spiritual View of Life Issues

1. Core life issues that often challenge the individual to experience heights and depths

of life. Concepts in spirituality include the following:

a. Mystery: Truth beyond understanding and explanation; spirituality helps people survive the unknowing.

b. Love: Love, which is the source of all life, fuels spirituality, prompting each person to live from the heart, the center where the ego is detached from outcomes. Love is nonlocal, transcending place and time. Love includes self-love, divine love, love for others, and love for all life.

c. Suffering: Core mystery in life; can be physical, emotional, mental, and spiritual. People struggle with finding meaning in suffering; suffering can enhance spiritual awareness and can be spiritually transformative. In others, suffering can cause frustration and anger. The nurse's awareness of his/her own response to suffering is essential to allow greater ability to be present in an intentional, healing manner with patients and honor their suffering. Such presence supports a person's spiritual journey toward discovering transcendent meaning of experience.[13]

d. Hope: An expectation of fulfillment, which goes beyond believing or wishing. Hope is future-oriented, yet in the present moment. Hope can be a goal or desire for a future event or outcome, and also the sense that the future is safe. Hope is a significant factor in overcoming illness and in living through difficult situations.[14,15] It helps people deal with fear and uncertainty and enables them to envision positive outcomes.

e. Forgiveness: Forgiveness does not necessarily mean forgetting, condoning, absolving, or sacrificing; rather, it is a process of extending love and compassion to self and others.[16-18] Beliefs about the nature of the Sacred Source influence one's ability to offer and receive forgiveness. Forgiveness is something one does for oneself, not just for others. Self-forgiveness is essential type of forgiveness for healing and spiritual growth to occur.

f. Peace and peacemaking: Inner peace is a way of being that is healing and nurturing. Peace and justice can be inseparable to many. Inner peace can occur in the midst of hardship and difficulties.

g. Grace: Grace can be seen as a gift from the Sacred Source that assists and empowers a person in the midst of difficult and sometime overwhelming circumstances. Grace can be a blessing that comes into one's life unearned, which causes gratitude. Grace can be life-changing and touch one's spirit in a profound way. Although grace might be considered coincidence by some, others sense it is a connection to something deeper in the web of life. An example is: "My CT scan was clear for the third time, something that the doctors didn't expect and that I didn't dare hope for."

h. Prayer: Is the most fundamental, primordial, and important language that humans speak; prayer starts and ends without words. Prayer is a deep human instinct that flows from the core of one's being where the longing for and awareness of one's connectedness with the source of life are blended. Prayer represents a longing for communication with God or Sacred Source. Prayer varies according to religions and individuals. It can be private, public, communal, individual, in song, chant, dance, meditation, walking, or silence. Types of prayer include petition, intercession, confession, lamentation, adoration, invocation, thanksgiving, being, and showing care and concern for others. Prayer is divine, the universe's affirmation that we are not alone.[19]

- Prayer can affect healing.[20-22] Both directed prayer, which focuses on specific outcome, and nondirected prayer, which focuses on greatest good of the organism, can affect healing. Even at a distance, prayer alters processes in a variety of organisms, including plants and people. In his book *Be Careful What You Pray For*, Dossey reminds us that prayer is potent force that is best used thoughtfully, with discernment.[23]

Spiritual and Psychological Dimensions

1. *Psyche* means spirit or soul. Psychology has put matters of soul into theories and

sometimes pathologies. Holistically speaking, spiritual and psychological matters are interconnected and part of body-mind-spirit as integrated whole. Nurses need to search for spiritual concerns and not label them as psychopathology. "Dark night of soul" is term for process of deep searching for spiritual concerns, sometimes through a process of pain and suffering.

2. Western traditions have less awareness of spiritual nature compared with Eastern and indigenous ones.

3. Dossey recognizes Nightingale as a mystic, although some interpreted Nightingale's health concerns after the Crimean War as psychological pathology.[24,25]

4. Nurses need to appreciate the difference between spiritual and psychological domains to assess spiritual cues and spiritual crises more effectively and foster spiritual growth.

■ SPIRITUALITY IN HOLISTIC NURSING

Nurturing the Spirit

1. Attentiveness to one's own spirituality is living in a healing way and is foundational to integrating spirituality into clinical practice.

2. Care of spirit is a professional nursing responsibility and intrinsic part of holistic nursing. Within a holistic perspective, providing spiritual care is an ethical obligation.

3. Nurses need to nurture themselves to have the strength to help heal others.

4. A persistent barrier to incorporating spirituality into clinical practice is fear of imposing particular religious values and beliefs on others. Nurses who integrate spirituality into their care of others recognize that although each person acts out of and is informed by her or his own spiritual perspective, acting from this foundation is not the same as imposing these beliefs and values on another.

Spirituality in Research and Practice

1. Many researchers approach spirituality study through the lens of religious beliefs and practice, but this can be an issue because not all spirituality is expressed through religious traditions.

2. Not all religions indicate the person's true spirituality either.

3. Current spirituality scales are biased toward Judeo-Christian beliefs.

4. Because spirituality is so difficult to describe, such scales might not always capture a person's spirituality.

Listening and Intentional Presence

1. Attentive listening and focused presence are the heart of caring for the spirit, and essential in any approach to spirituality assessment.

2. Use of broad, open-ended questions is helpful, such as "Tell me more about...," "Help me to understand what you need," "I don't understand what you are trying to say," and "What was that like for you?"

3. Nurses can help create sacred space for these discussions, and encourage use of prayer, centering, and meditation to enhance spiritual discussions and be more fully present to others.

4. Intentional, active listening by the nurse allows client, by sharing with an open-hearted and fully present listener, to hear herself or himself with greater clarity and understanding in a safe space.

5. Nurses need awareness of their own discomforts in discussion as well as how external distractions such as environment or time pressures affect their ability to listen. Be aware of body posture communication, verbal and nonverbal cues.

6. Intentional listening and presence foster authenticity in the nursing process.

7. The core of active listening and healing presence lies in intention of nurse who recognizes all as spiritual.

Using Story and Metaphor in Spiritual Care

1. Nurses' own life stories inform and form them.

2. Listening and encouraging people to share their stories can be assessment and intervention.

3. Sharing stories helps people to understand themselves and their world; through the vehicle of story, people reveal experiences

of relationships, emotions, conflicts, and struggles.

4. Stories challenge nurses to understand wholeness of a person and to listen for the meaning of a life.

Using Guides and Instruments to Facilitate Spirituality Assessment

1. Nurses can use the questions of a spiritual assessment guide or tool to open discussion or serve as reference points for discussing spirituality with patients to know and understand them better.

2. Assessing a person's understanding of spirituality and ways of expressing spirituality includes exploring role and influence of important connections to present circumstances; issues related to meaning and purpose; important beliefs, values, and practices; prayer or meditation styles; and desire for connection with religious groups or rituals.

3. See Exhibits 32-3, 32-4, 32-5, 32-6 in *Holistic Nursing: A Handbook for Practice* (6th edition) for examples of several spiritual assessment tools or scales.

4. The Spiritual Assessment Tool is based on a conceptual analysis of spirituality derived from Burkhardt's critical review of the literature.[26] This instrument poses open-ended, reflective questions that assist nurses in developing awareness of spirituality for themselves and others. These questions are meant to be prompts to focus on pertinent spiritual concerns. Similar types of questions are equally appropriate. Some areas might be addressed more fully than others, depending on a particular client's needs. This instrument is meant to be a guide for nurses, to support and enhance their comfort and skills with spirituality assessment, and is not designed as a self-administered survey. To facilitate the healing process in clients/patients, families, significant others, and yourself, the following reflective questions assist in assessing, evaluating, and increasing awareness of the spiritual process in yourself and others. It includes such overall concepts as Meaning and Purpose, Inner Strengths, and Interconnectedness.

5. Howden's Spirituality Assessment Scale (SAS) is a 28-item instrument based on a conceptualization of spirituality as a phenomenon represented by four critical attributes.[27]

6. The Spirituality Scale (SS) was developed by Delaney as a way to holistically assess beliefs, practices, lifestyle choices, intuitions, and rituals that represent the human spiritual dimension.[28]

7. Personal Spiritual Well-Being Assessment (PSWBA) and Spiritual Well-Being Assessment (SWBA) by B. Barker are yet other scales.[29,30]

■ HOLISTIC CARING CONSIDERATIONS

1. Spiritual caregiving requires an understanding of the holistic caring process that is integrative.

2. Holistic nurses recognize spirituality is an important dimension of any health concern, and use nursing diagnoses regarding spirituality appropriately.

Tending to the Spirit

1. Nurses use assessment, diagnosis, planning, and intervening knowing all persons are spiritual beings.

2. Giving clients opportunity to discuss and reflect on spiritual concerns enables them to become more aware of their spirituality and personal spiritual journeys.

3. Awareness of and care for self as a spiritual being is an important aspect of holistic nursing care.

4. Forming spiritual companionship or support groups within work environments can help nurses maintain their spirits in the midst of daily demands on their energies.

5. Regular prayer, centering, mindfulness, meditation, or starting the day with intention assists nurses in maintaining their own wholeness and grounds their practice of intentional presence.

Touching

1. When words cannot be found, touch can be a powerful expression of spirit and instrument of healing.

2. Appropriate touch, hand on shoulder, handclasp can be supportive.

Fostering Connectedness

1. Relationships are a major aspect of spirituality.
2. Nurses can help strengthen meaningful and supportive bonds by encouraging visits and phone calls from family and friends.
3. Visits from pets can be important; photos, memorabilia, guided imagery all can help.
4. Religious, social, and business visitors can be helpful.
5. Connection with environment can be accomplished by visits outdoors, healing nature scenes, scents, flowers, plants, and so forth.
6. Relationship with the sacred can be difficult for agnostics or atheists. Nurses might need to creatively look for means to engage the spiritual side of these patients.

Using Rituals to Nurture the Spirit

1. Rituals serve as reminders to allow sacred time and space in our lives.
2. Achterberg et al. describe three phases of ritual.[31] First phase is the symbolic breaking away from everyday busyness. Second phase is the transition phase, which calls for identification and focus on areas of life that need attention. Third and final phase, referred to as return phase, is reentry into everyday life.
3. One example of a ritual space: Find a quiet place, a healing place, and go there. Examples include corner of your favorite room where you have placed pictures, a candle, or other symbols that signal peace and inner reflection to you; a park, under an old tree, or in a special place, such as a mountain, a coastline, or a forest.

Developing Centering, Mindfulness, and Awareness

1. Spiritual disciplines are those practices that cause people to pause in the midst of their activities and busyness to attend to matters of the spirit or soul.
2. Eastern and indigenous traditions focus on mindfulness and awareness.
3. Judeo-Christian traditions can focus on centering prayer for quietness.
4. Awareness is observing what is going on with oneself or others without judgment, noting feelings, thoughts, and physical sensations.

Praying and Meditating

1. In the clinical setting, both the nurse's and the patient's understanding of prayer will determine the role of prayer.
2. Clarifying patients' understanding of and need for prayer as part of holistic nursing care. Some patients want others to pray with or for them, while others do not believe in prayer.
3. Nurse can encourage quiet time, participation in religious worship or observances.

Ensuring Opportunities for Rest and Leisure

1. Integrate aspects of holistic living and care of the spirit with rest, leisure, and Sabbath time, which enhances growth, creativity, and renewal.[32-34]
2. Leisure is an attitude of the heart that facilitates connection with the inner self and the Sacred Source and opens one to reflect on and envision a life of doing to allow for more Being. Authentic leisure implies an approach to living that allows one to relax into a level of being that deepens self-awareness, nourishes one's wholeness, and enriches connections with Sacred Source and other people.
3. Assisting persons to consider place of rest and leisure in their lives is part of holistic nursing.

■ ARTS AND SPIRITUALITY

1. Artists can include anyone who creates. Can be an expression of spirituality.
2. Literature, poetry, music, pottery, dance, photography, gardens all are aspects of creativity that can express spirituality.

■ NOTES

1. Burkhardt, M. A., & Nagai-Jacobson, M. G. (2002). *Spirituality: Living our connectedness.* Albany, NY: Delmar Thompson Learning.
2. Chiu, L., Emblen, J. D., Van Hofwegen, L., Sawatzky, R., & Meyerhoff, H. (2004). An integrative review of the concept of spirituality in the health sciences. *Western Journal of Nursing Research, 26,* 405–428.

3. McBrien, B. (2006). A concept analysis of spirituality. *British Journal of Nursing, 15*(1), 42–45.

4. Lewis, M., Hankin, S., Reynolds, D., & Ogedeghe, G. (2007). African American spirituality: A process of honoring God, others, and self. *Journal of Holistic Nursing, 25*(1), 16–23.

5. Chung, L. Y. F., Wong, F. K. Y., & Chan, M. F. (2007). Relationship of nurses' spirituality to their understanding and practice of spiritual care. *Journal of Advanced Nursing, 58*(2), 158–170.

6. Mok, E., Wong, F., & Wong, D. (2010). The meaning of spirituality and spiritual care among the Hong Kong Chinese terminally ill. *Journal of Advanced Nursing, 66*(2), 360–370.

7. Engebretson, J. C., & Headley, J. H. (2013). Cultural diversity and care. In B. M. Dossey & L. Keegan (Eds.), *Holistic nursing: A handbook for practice* (6th ed.). Burlington, MA: Jones & Bartlett Learning.

8. Burkhardt, M. A. (1994). Becoming and connecting: elements of spirituality for women. *Holistic Nursing Practice, 8,* 12–21.

9. Lemmer, C. M. (2005). Recognizing and caring for spiritual needs of clients. *Journal of Holistic Nursing, 2*(3), 310–322.

10. Noble, A., & Jones, C. (2010). Getting it right: Oncology nurses' understanding of spirituality. *International Journal of Palliative Nursing, 16*(11), 565–569.

11. Craig, C., Weinert, C., Walton, J., & Derwinksi-Robinson, B. (2006). Spirituality, chronic illness, and rural life. *Journal of Holistic Nursing, 24*(1), 27–35.

12. Tuck, I., Alleyne, R., & Thinganjana, W. (2006). Spirituality and stress management in healthy adults. *Journal of Holistic Nursing, 24*(4), 245–253.

13. Ferrell, B. R., & Coyle, N. (2008). The nature of suffering and the goals of nursing. *Oncology Nursing Forum, 35*(2), 241–247.

14. Johnson, S. (2007). Hope in terminal illness: An evolutionary concept analysis. *International Journal of Palliative Nursing, 13*(9), 451–459.

15. Pipe, T. R., Kelly, A., LeBrun, G., Schmidt, D., Atherton, P., & Robinson, C. (2008). A prospective descriptive study exploring hope, spiritual well-being, and quality of life in hospitalized patients. *MEDSURG Nursing, 17*(4), 247–257.

16. Seaward, B. L. (2005). *Quiet mind, fearless heart: The Taoist path through stress and spirituality.* Hoboken, NJ: Wiley.

17. Grossman, W. (2007). *To be healed by the earth.* New York, NY: Seven Stories Press.

18. Recine, G., Werner, J. S., & Recine, I. (2007). Concept analysis of forgiveness with a multi-cultural emphasis. *Journal of Advanced Nursing, 59*(3), 308–316.

19. Dossey, L. (1996). *Prayer is good medicine.* San Francisco, CA: Harper.

20. Narayanasamy, A., & Narayanasamy, M. (2008). The healing power of prayer and its implications for nursing. *British Journal of Nursing, 17*(6), 394–398.

21. Helming, M. B. (2011). Healing through prayer: A qualitative study. *Holistic Nursing Practice, 25*(1), 33–44.

22. Breslin, M. J., & Lewis, C. A. (2008). Theoretical models of the nature of prayer and health: A review. *Mental Health, Religion & Culture, 11*(1), 9–21.

23. Dossey, L. (1997). *Be careful what you pray for.* San Francisco, CA: HarperCollins.

24. Dossey, B. M. (2000). *Florence Nightingale: Mystic, visionary, healer.* Springhouse, PA: Springhouse.

25. Dossey, B. M. (2010). Florence Nightingale: A 19th-century mystic. *Journal of Holistic Nursing, 28*(1), 10–35.

26. Burkhardt, M. A. (1989). Spirituality: An analysis of the concept. *Holistic Nursing Practice, 3,* 69–77.

27. Howden, J. W. (1992). *Development and psychometric characteristics of the Spirituality Assessment Scale.* Unpublished doctoral dissertation, Texas Woman's University, Denton.

28. Delaney, C. (2005). The Spirituality Scale: Development and psychometric testing of a holistic instrument to assess the human spiritual dimension. *Journal of Holistic Nursing, 23*(2), 145–167.

29. Barker, E. R. (1996, November). *Patient spirituality assessment: A tool that works.* Paper presented at the Uniformed Nurse Practitioners Association Meeting, Seattle, WA.

30. Barker, E. R. (1998). *How to do research, get finished, and not lose your balance.* Presentation at the Nursing Research Symposium, San Diego, CA.

31. Achterberg, J., Dossey, B. M., & Kolkmeier, L. (1994). *Rituals of healing: Using imagery for health and wellness.* New York, NY: Bantam.

32. Mueller, W. (2000). *Sabbath: Restoring the sacred rhythms of rest.* New York, NY: Bantam.

33. Grafanaki, S., Pearson, D., Cini, F., Godula, D., McKenzie, B., Nason, S., & Anderegg, M. (2005). Sources of renewal: A qualitative study on the experience and role of leisure in the life of counselors and psychologists. *Counseling Psychology Quarterly, 18*(1), 31–40.

34. Heintzman, P. (2008). Leisure-spiritual coping: A model for therapeutic recreation and leisure services. *Therapeutic Recreation Journal, 42*(1), 56–73.

STUDY QUESTIONS

Basic Level

1. Which of the following statements best describes spirituality?
   a. Anyone who belongs to a religious faith is a spiritual person.
   b. Spirituality is the essence of who and how we are in the world and is integral to our human existence.
   c. The word *spirituality* comes from the Latin and the Greek, meaning "breath."
   d. Spirituality is difficult to define and not everyone has a spiritual side.

2. The *primary* distinction between religion and spirituality is:
   a. Religion is an organized belief system shared by groups of people.
   b. Spirituality is involved with matters of the spirit, whereas religion involves rituals.
   c. Religion can involve cultural practices, dietary laws, and particular dress codes.
   d. Spirituality is a life choice, whereas people are often raised in a specific religious practice.

3. What is the separation of science and spirit also known as?
   a. Monism
   b. Monotheism
   c. Dualism
   d. Polytheism

4. Spirituality involves a sense of connectedness with which of the following?
   a. Self
   b. Sacred Source
   c. Others
   d. Nature
   e. All of the above

5. Which of the following is one of the best ways for the holistic nurse to assess a patient's sense of spirituality and open communication about spirituality?
   a. Listening with intention
   b. The use of story
   c. Obtaining the patient's religious preference and associated cultural practices
   d. Using a spiritual assessment scale or guide

6. Which of the following is the best example of a holistic nurse creating sacred space for a patient who is in a skilled nursing facility recovering from a stroke?
   a. Asking the family members to bring in photos, memorabilia, and a candle to light for prayers.
   b. Bringing the patient outdoors in warm weather where family members can sit at the front entrance.
   c. Asking a Healing Touch practitioner to work with the patient once a week.
   d. Placing prints of nature scenes, a fragrant plant, and playing soft music near the patient's bedside.

Advanced Level

7. The advanced holistic nurse is aware that demonstrating presence and intentionality with patients most involves which of the following?
   a. The fact that the nurse must be very spiritual himself or herself
   b. Active listening and the intention and attention of the nurse who recognizes all persons as spiritual beings
   c. Praying for or with the patient if the patient so desires it
   d. The nurse needing to focus on his or her own nurturing to enhance spirituality

8. The advanced holistic nurse is asked to pray with a patient. He or she understands that which one of the following is one of the most problematic issues nurses consider in praying with patients?
   a. Fear of imposing his or her own spiritual beliefs and values.
   b. Prayer has a variety of types to select from: silence, spoken, communal, singing, and chanting.
   c. Not every prayer is answered in the way the patient wishes it to be answered.
   d. Some religions see suffering and illness as punishment for sins.

9. A dying patient in hospice care asks a nurse to discuss spiritual issues. The nurse is very uncomfortable discussing death because of a personal tragedy that she has not yet come to terms with. Which of the following statements is most important in guiding the nurse's decision?
   a. Whether the nurse and/or the patient believe in God or a Higher Power is all-important.
   b. If the nurse is uncomfortable in this discussion, he or she should call in the chaplain.
   c. Nursing knowledge of culture, religious traditions, and family backgrounds assists in understanding the meaning of suffering for patients who are dying.
   d. Providing spiritual care is an ethical obligation that, if ignored, deprives patients of their dignity as human beings.

10. Several key concepts in spirituality are essential for the advanced holistic nurse to understand. Which of the following key concepts is correct in its meaning?
    a. Mystery is a future-oriented expectation of fulfillment.
    b. Grace is truth beyond understanding or explanation.
    c. Hope is a blessing that comes into life unexpectedly.
    d. Inner peace is a way of being that is healing and nurturing.

11. The concept of being involves all of the following statements except which one?
    a. Being is the art of stillness and presence with self, others, the Sacred Source, and Nature.
    b. Being includes experiencing the present moment more deeply.
    c. Being involves a sense of spiritual transformation and transcendence.
    d. Being involves awareness of one's own body-mind-spirit, without judgment.

12. The advanced holistic nurse is aware that which of the following concepts related to spirituality is true?
    a. Nurses do not need to nurture themselves spiritually to have the strength to heal others.
    b. Lack of connectedness with the environment can lead to spiritual crisis.
    c. Spirituality involves the search for meaning and purpose in life.
    d. Healing does not necessarily require recognition of the spiritual dimension of each person.

Chapter 32

Energy Healing

Victoria E. Slater

■ DEFINITIONS

Aura An atmosphere; a vague, luminous glow surrounding something. It can be an information-containing electromagnetic field and can be likened to the data contained within a computer.

Capacitor A device that stores electric charge.

Centering An altered state of consciousness that results in the centered person's hands emitting measurable extra-low-frequency magnetic pulses of 0.3–3.0 hertz (Hz), that is, cycles per second.

Chakra An energy center in the subtle, or energetic, body that is described as a whirling vortex of light.

Electromagnetic induction The causing or inducing of voltage, a change in an electric current.

Energy healing The deliberate process of using an external energy field to induce a change in one's own or another's field for the purpose of physical, mental, emotional, and spiritual healing. Energy healing can involve the presence of a caring person.

Entrainment The phenomenon of rhythmic processes synchronizing with each other. Synchronization is recognized in pendulum clocks, planets, music, an organism adjusting to the light/dark cycle, brain waves, social groups, and more.

Intention Purpose, aim, or objective; the choice to act or think in a certain way.

Meridian Microvolt electrical conduits organized in an electrical mesh that permeates the body and precedes development of vessels and organs. In Eastern philosophies, the meridians are said to conduct *chi*, or universal energy.

Resistor Part of an electrical device that resists the flow of charge.

Subtle energies Barely noticeable electrical and magnetic fields of living organisms that might be related to internal electrical and magnetic activity.

Voltage A measurement related to the difference in potential energy between two adjacent areas.

■ INTRODUCTION

Energy healing appears to involve two physics principles: electromagnetic induction and entrainment. If these are shown to be active in energy healing, it would suggest that the body is an electromagnetic organism that responds to electricity, magnetism, and frequencies of light and sound. Likewise, the aura, chakras, and meridians might be or have electrical and magnetic properties.

If the human is an electromagnetic phenomenon, the nurse's presence might be more than theoretical; it might be a very real electrical and magnetic event. Also, laying on of hands modalities of all kinds, such as Healing Touch, Therapeutic Touch, Reiki, and more might be electromagnetic phenomena. Sound healing, flower essences, homeopathy, and aromatherapy might be entrainment, or frequency-influencing, modalities.

The concepts of this chapter are put forth to stimulate thought and, possibly, research.

■ THEORY AND RESEARCH

Energy Healing

1. Many, if not all, cultures have an energy healing practice. The Chinese and Japanese practice *Chi Kung* (qi gong) and the Hawaiians *Huna*. There is the Hindu practice of *prana* and the Native American practices of *shaking hands* and drumming.
2. Energy healing came to nursing through Dolores Krieger[1] and her Therapeutic Touch. Janet Mentgen continued the expansion of energy healing into nursing with Healing Touch.[2] Many nurses have studied various types of energy modalities and have added some of them to their nursing practices.[3]
3. Energy medicine might or might not be the same as energy healing, which can involve *presence*.

Energy Anatomy

1. The aura
   a. Traditional explanations of the aura
      ▪ A golden light surrounding the body.
      ▪ People describe the aura differently and those differences can be the result of what Daniel Benor calls the "window of observation," or the unique limitations of a person's perceptual ability.[4]
      ▪ The aura is believed to be able to be damaged, leading to physical, emotional, and social problems, including those associated with posttraumatic stress disorder (PTSD).
   b. Research in to the aura
      ▪ Auric research is in its infancy.
      ▪ Two types of camera have been invented that show energy moving around the body.
   c. Scientific explanations of the aura: Comparing the aura to an electromagnetic field
      ▪ A traditional electromagnet has an iron core surrounded by an electric current. When the current is turned on an electromagnetic field is formed and the electromagnet is able to do work. This electromagnetic field is easier to discern closer to the core and more difficult to detect farther away.

▪ The human being has an iron core of hemoglobin that is surrounded by the electric currents of neurons and meridians. The result enables the person to do more work than just the biological musculature would allow. The aura is easier to detect closer to the body than farther away.
▪ Both an electromagnetic field and the human aura are capable of carrying information.
   d. Intuitive experiences of the aura
      ▪ Use your hands to sense the space around different individuals, plants, and animals. Sense movement, temperature changes, and distortions such as the field pulling in or bulging out. Compare a healthy person to an ill one, someone who exercises to a couch potato, a man to a woman, and an adult to a child.
2. Chakras
   a. Traditional explanations of chakras
      ▪ There are many explanations of chakras including some that are not recognized as such, including Maslow's Hierarchy of Needs.[5]
      ▪ Chakras are believed to be portals through and by which the individual gathers information and energy from the environment and releases them to the environment.
      ▪ Chakras are lined up like keys on a piano, each working with a higher frequency of sound and light than the one below it.
      ▪ Each chakra has a different job, from survival (the lowest chakra) to responding to the environment (second and third chakras), loving and being loved (fourth or heart chakra), speaking your own truth (fifth or throat chakra), insight (sixth or brow chakra), and access to spiritual mysteries (seventh or crown chakra). Different chakra models assign different jobs to the various chakras, but every model has the lowest chakra dealing with the simplest tasks and the higher chakras with more complex ones.
      ▪ If you think of Maslow's lowest need level, survival, a person's lowest chakra would gather the information of how

safe the surroundings are and release the information that it is either safe or threatening. The problem is interpreting the information the lowest chakra has gathered; that is the task of the higher chakras. Their ability to sift through and interpret what is received is influenced by the person's personal experiences and choices.

- As with Maslow's hierarchy, the work of each chakra, each hierarchy, is dependent upon the work of the lower ones.
- Various chakra models place chakras at different locations in and beyond the body. While most chakra models portray seven major chakras along the center of the body, five along the spine and two in the head, those are not the only ones. There is a chakra associated with every organ; there is one at the sole of each foot and palm of each hand; and there is one with every joint such as each vertebra, the joints of the fingers and toes, and the two joints in the middle ear. Different cultures emphasize some and ignore others.
- Chakras are associated with sounds and colors that move up in frequency as chakras are higher on the body. For example, the root chakra at the base of the spine is seen as red and heard as middle C. Each chakra in turn is the next higher color/sound from red to orange, yellow, green, blue, indigo, and violet and from middle C, to D, E, F, G, A, B.
- Chakras are present and function at birth but mature over a lifetime. Again, various models have this maturation occurring at different ages. Rosalyn Bruyere's intuitive interpretation is one, and another is based on the mathematical model of the Fibonacci sequence. (See the "Websites" section at the end of this chapter.)

b. Research into chakras
- The best known chakra research has been done by Valerie Hunt and Hiroshi Motoyama, both of whom recorded the electrical frequencies and states of chakras.

- Hunt found that they produce regular, high-frequency, wave-like signals from 500 to 20,000 cycles per second, which is higher than any other measured human body frequency.[6]
- Motoyama found that advanced meditators had increased frequency and amplitudes of their chakras compared to nonmeditators. He learned that some people could consciously project energy through their chakras, thus controlling their own energy.[7]
- Newer researchers, such as Curtis, Zeh, Miller, and Rich found that people with more psychological symptoms had more poorly functioning chakras than psychologically healthy people, which is consistent with chakra theory. The research team was unable to determine which came first, the symptoms or change in chakra functioning or even if the two situations are related.[8]

c. Scientific explanations of chakras: Comparing chakras to electrical components
- Chakra processing of frequencies and amplitudes of sound and light is similar to the ability of a television, radio, cell phone, or computer to receive and transmit information. They can only process what they receive and are capable of processing. Remember that each chakra is capable of processing a different frequency than the chakra above and below it.
- Like computer programs, chakras have "hidden files" that can interfere with healthy functioning. Those chakra files are developed during childhood, often before the individual has language, and includes such behaviors as how to respond to violent shouting, to hugs, to abandonment, to love, that is, to the individual's life experiences.
- Televisions, cell phones, and chakras are capable of transmitting information across distances. Electronic devices can transmit that information across long distances; chakras, across short ones.
- Electronic devices and chakras can be damaged by an overload of power.

Both can be repaired—electronic devices through repair or replacement of parts; chakras through energy healing and meditation.

   d. Intuitive experiences of chakras
- Do the chakra exercise on page 762 of *Holistic Nursing: A Handbook for Practice* (6th edition).

3. Meridians
   a. Traditional and not so traditional explanations of meridians
- Meridians are described as a structure involving 12 pairs (12 in each side of the body) of subtle flows of energy that might be electricity plus the information carried on the current.
- Meridians carry information slowly but completely as a gestalt.
- Meridians might bring energy and information to each cell. This needs to be studied.

   b. Research into meridians
- Gerber, in *Vibrational Medicine*, describes the meridian system as a continuous mesh that precedes the early development of any of organs. Imagine a mesh. Now imagine the organs of the body developing within the mesh, with a meridian strand snaking into every cell. Research suggests that this image is correct; more research needs to be done.[9]
- Robert Becker, in *The Body Electric*, found that meridians are smaller than a single human hair, about 0.5–1.5 microns in diameter, and have a current that has been measured at less than one-billionth of an ampere.[10] (That is very, very, very small and might be small enough to flow into a single cell without damaging it.)
- Meridians have acupoints that act like boosters. Those acupoints are located at just the right distances apart to boost an electric current of such a miniscule voltage.
- Meridians appear to act like biological fiber-optic light cables. This means that, like all fiber-optics, they are able to carry light and information.
- Meridians appear to be electromagnetic, which means that nearby electrical and magnetics fields can influence them.
- Meridians also appear to conduct sound waves, suggesting that they bring sound throughout the body.
- Meridian techniques, such as acupuncture, bring the body into balance. For example, the same needle placement is used for hyper- and hypothyroidism.

   c. Scientific explanations of meridians: Comparing meridians to electric currents
- If meridians carry electric currents, as research suggests, then a nearby electrical, magnetic, and/or electromagnetic field affects them. That impact can lead to a voltage surge (imagine boosting the speed of the flow of current) or can damage the mesh, if the nearby field is too powerful for the tiny meridians. (Such damage can be part of post-traumatic stress disorder symptoms.)
- Imagine a human or animal being constructed of a continuous mesh that might equate to a structure of thousands of tiny electric currents. Some flow up, some down, some diagonally. The currents flowing up negate those flowing downward, but there is an overall type of steady state of power within the mesh and the individual.
- This suggests that each person produces an electromagnetic field. Each person electrically and magnetically influences the person/people next to them. This might be the physics behind *presence*.
- Because meridians might carry information and sound, they might help bring information from the external environment into the body, acting as a fundamental information gathering and processing system.

   d. Intuitive experiences of meridians
- Become still within. Pay attention to the subtle flows within your body. Focus on your skin. Sense the flow of the 12 meridians on each side of your body. Most of them seem to flow from feet to head. Can you notice this flow?

- Shake hands with someone or touch another in some way. All of the meridians, all 12 pairs, terminate in the hands; this suggests that our hands gather lots of information that then flows up the arms and into the body. Set a timer and in about 15 minutes or so, become quiet and let your body reveal the gestalt that you learned about the person you touched. Could this be part of the reason for shaking hands with a stranger?

4. Summary of energy anatomy
   a. The three-part aura, chakra, meridian system gathers, processes, stores, and transmits information, much as computers do.
   b. Chakras, with their frequency-processing function, give you multiple pieces of information (bits and bytes) quickly.
   c. Meridians, with their continuous flow of information from the environment, provide you with the complete picture, the gestalt, but too slowly to act on in an emergency. As complex organisms, we need both the quick responsiveness of the chakras and the gestalt of the meridians.
   d. The aura stores information in addition to being an electromagnetic field that might act as a shield.

Laying On of Hands Modalities, the Healer, Electromagnetic Induction, and Presence

1. Laying on of hands and the healer
   a. Several researchers (Zimmerman,[11] Waechter and Sergio,[12] and Moga and Bengston[13]) have found that prepared laying on of hands practitioners emit a pulsed electromagnetic wave from their hands. This wave pulsed from 0.3 to 30 Hz (the upper limit of the measuring device) but concentrated in the 7- to 9-Hz range.
   b. Practitioners prepared in different ways. Therapeutic Touch practitioners learned to center, or enter a meditative state. Bengston and his students created 20 positive images and just scrolled through this memory while doing the work. Both groups might have entered an altered state of consciousness, one meditative and the other a different type of altered state of consciousness while focusing primarily on positive images.[14]
   c. Bengston suggested that individuals who believe that their healing approach will work might get in the way of the results by anticipating healing. He suggested that having no expectations might be a more healing attitude.

2. Electromagnetic induction
   a. A physicist would tell you that the phrase "energy healing" or "energy medicine" is incorrect; the word *energy* is not used properly. A more accurate description might be "electromagnetic induction healing" or "applied electromagnetic induction."
   b. Electromagnetic induction occurs naturally; it is a product of the changing flow of electrons (a current) that creates a magnetic field surrounding the electric current. The magnetic field influences a nearby electric current, causing a "voltage surge" in the electric current, or a speeding up of the flow of electrons. The boost in the electric current causes a stronger magnetic field that causes even greater voltage surges in surrounding electric currents.
   c. When a system is designed where there are many parallel electric currents, each current's magnetic field influences the nearby currents, creating a succession of voltage surges.
   d. This is called "an induced" current, or electromagnetic induction, where one electric current and its magnetic field induces a current/field in nearby currents/fields.
   e. This is useful because you can take one long electrical wire, curl it around something such as an iron core (remember electromagnets?), and you have a series of parallel electric currents/parallel magnetic fields each inducing a voltage surge in the ones near it. It is an exceedingly efficient way to generate power from a relatively small input.
   f. Imagine the meridian mesh. It can be seen as a series of parallel electric

currents with their magnetic fields each inducing a voltage surge in the nearby ones. The result might be to create more power for the individual than would be available from the meridians alone.

g. A changing electric current is one of the requirements to induce a current. Engineers can change the direction of the flow; humans and animals can change the current with our thoughts. Research needs to be done on this.

h. Another source of that change might found in the discovery that healers and tai chi students build up a charge in their bodies and release it. Such a release would cause a voltage surge in the nearby person.

3. Presence

a. Presence might be an electromagnetic induction event. One human electromagnet next to another human electromagnet can induce a voltage surge in each other. The person who is able to enter an altered state of consciousness through stillness imagining positive results might produce a healing electromagnetic moment.

b. If so, the presence of a sham healer in energy healing research can be expected to be healing. Moreover, the presence of any person other than the participant in any research can be expected to have an effect on the outcome of the study.

Other Forms of Energy Healing

1. Homeopathy

a. Homeopaths prepare remedies from natural substances, such as plants, animals, mother's milk, gems, and snake and spider venom, essentially anything and potentially everything.

b. The theory behind homeopathy is that "like cures like." If a remedy causes the symptoms, homeopaths believe it can be used to cure the symptom and the underlying problem.

c. There is some evidence that the means of preparing a homeopathic remedy changes the magnetic field of the preparation.

2. Flower essences

a. Flower essences, also, can be created from natural and synthetic substances.

b. The substance is placed in or near water. The theory is that the essence of the substance is transferred to the water, which is then stabilized with alcohol, vinegar, or salt.

c. This essence might be the electromagnetic frequency of the substance. You can imagine that the frequency of a rose differs from that of a cactus or any other plant. If the frequency changed, the rose would no longer be a rose but something else.

3. Aromatherapy, or essential oils

a. Aromatherapy is a misnomer. It is not the aroma that is the active factor, but the biology, chemistry, and energy of the oil extracted from a plant.

b. To a nurse, the biology and chemistry of the plant's oil is understandable; they can be antifungal, antibiotic, antiviral, soothing, irritating, and so forth.

c. The energy of the oil is more subtle. For example, the oil of evergreen trees act as if they "unzip" memories within the person (think of a zipped computer file in which a lot of data are stored very compactly). When used with skillful counseling, such essential oils can help a person gain access to painful and hidden memories and release them.

4. Sound

a. Drumming and chanting might be the best known forms of sound healing to Westerners.

b. Research has shown that drumming improves mood scores in nursing students and lowers turnover in long-term care workers.

c. More recently, tuning forks are being used to insert a particular sequence of sounds into the recipient's field.

d. Music can be designed or used to change the habitual state of a person's energy field.

e. Sound can work as an environmental stimulus that might or might not be healing. The notes can be healing, but excessive volume and any percussive effects can damage the aura, the meridians, and the sound-sensitive chakras.

5. Light
   a. Sunlight was used to treat tuberculosis patients until effective medications were discovered.
   b. People with Seasonal Affective Disorder Syndrome (SADS) are fully aware of the effect of the presence and absence of sunlight on their mood and ability to be productive.
   c. The eyes, pineal glands, and acupoints all appear to be light sensitive and/or to allow light to enter the body.
   d. Sitting in the sun for a short time daily might be needed for a healthy being.

6. Color therapies
   a. Different colors each have different frequencies. Exposing yourself to or thinking about different colors can have a subtle effect on the body.
   b. One self-care method might be to vividly imagine being filled with the colors of the rainbow in turn, from red to orange, yellow, green, blue, indigo, and violet (ROYGBIV).
   c. Intuitive experiences of aromas, flower essences, sound, light, and color.
   d. Do the intuitive exercises on page 769 of *Holistic Nursing: A Handbook for Practice* (6th edition).

7. Entrainment
   a. Entrainment is a common phenomenon seen in two pendulum clocks in which the pendulums are swinging at different rates and patterns. Over a short time, they will begin to beat in unison. They have entrained with each other.
   b. In entrainment, one of the pendulums had to slow down, one speed up, or both change and meet somewhere in between their two initial patterns.
   c. Humans entrain with each other.
   d. Social entrainment is when cyclical processes in a group begin to be synchronized. A well-known example is when the menstrual cycles of the women of a tribe or family synchronize, when they all have their menses at the same time.
   e. Interactional synchrony is how skilled and empathic listeners naturally adjust their posture and natural speech rhythms to match the person with whom they are speaking.
   f. Laying on of hands modalities may involve both electromagnetic and entrainment processes.
      - People's rhythms include rate of respiration, heartbeat, brain wave patterns, and, more elusively, the electromagnetic pulsing natural to the individual. For entrainment to occur between two people or within a group one person must speed up or slow down his or her rhythm while the others remain static, or they all must change to meet somewhere in the middle of their habitual rhythms.
      - In social entrainment, this shift is unconscious; in interactional synchrony, it might be conscious.
      - This might be part of the impact of presence; the nurse who is conscious of herself and her impact naturally uses interactional synchrony and might also unconsciously create a calming *presence* that the patient/client entrains to.
      - In energy healing, entrainment is often conscious; the various forms of energy healing teach practitioners a way to do this.
      - This is part of how energy healing and presence might work—the provider maintains a particular state and the client shifts his rhythm to more closely mimic the provider's.
      - Aromatherapy, flower essences, homeopathy, light, sound, and music can work because of entrainment.
      - The natural substances used to create essential oils, flower essences, and homeopathy do not change; the recipient must shift to match their rhythms. Why the same plant such as a rose that is prepared differently for a flower essence, an essential oil, or homeopathically works differently in all three cases is unknown, but part of the active mechanism might be entrainment.

- Light, sound, and music are more varied, but to get a clue as to how your rhythms respond to them, stand outside in the sunlight, on a gloomy day, and at night. How do you change?
- Similarly, how does your body and mood shift with the changes in the noise around you? Do you respond differently to a quiet day on the nursing unit than you do when the vacuum cleaner is running?
- How about your responses to music? You entrain to these, or try to, because they are unlikely to change to meet your pattern.
- Wilken and Wilken suggest that we don't like a particular type or selection of music because it is ugly but because it activates a blockage within us. As we expose ourselves to the music (as we choose to entrain to it), we will find ourselves enjoying it more and might find that an old emotional pattern has been released.[15]

Summary of the Holistic Nurse, Entrainment, Electromagnetic Induction, and Presence

1. The holistic nurse who is with a patient might be using interactional synchrony, entrainment, and electromagnetic induction simultaneously. Perhaps this is one description of an expert nurse.

Intention

1. Lynne McTaggart's book *The Intention Experiment* teaches us that how a space is used seems to be imprinted on the space. Something that occurs in that same space repeatedly becomes easier. If that activity is moved to a different room, your usual results might change. This has been shown to be a problem when research is moved to a different lab.[16] The space seems to have memory.

2. This suggests that to maximize healing, rooms should be dedicated to healing activities with no other activities occurring within them. This would indicate that a healing room in your home should not double as an office or guest room.

3. This also suggests that the pain, death, and grief that occur in hospitals, nursing homes, and even your own home might be imprinted on the space. It is useful to occasionally energetically clean your personal and work spaces, especially if a physically or emotionally painful event has occurred there. This might be one effect of spring cleaning.

4. There are many ways to energetically clean a room, but the easiest is to ask the Holy to clean it for you and to fill it with light, love, joy, peace, and so forth.

■ RESEARCH IMPLICATIONS

Electromagnetic Induction

1. Researching energy healing, a phenomenon that might be based on principles of physics rather than biology, is not easy. In 40 years of research, we might have learned more about how not to research these modalities than how to.

2. As Diane Wardel has clearly stated, you cannot use the biology gold standard research design of experiment-control to study laying on of hands modalities. Because the presence of a person changes the phenomenon, you cannot test these modalities using a sham provider.[17]

3. Expert laying on of hands providers have different results from novices, which is to be expected, but sometimes the novice has better results. The supposition is that the expert wants the treatments to work and, thus, gets in the way; the novice doesn't care, so is more open and fluid.

4. Results of laying on of hands modalities seem to be cumulative, beginning with attitudinal changes, emotional changes, and finally physical ones. Thus, if a person complains of pain, his attitude toward something in his life will change before the pain mitigates. This sequence makes it difficult to study the short-term effects of the treatments and get a good picture of what is really happening.

5. Electromagnetic induction might be one reason for the types of results common with laying on of hands modalities. The presence of a nearby human electromagnet might make enough of a change in the electrical flow of the chakras, meridian, the

currents flowing across the connective tissue and other electrical currents in the body to influence gradual and gentle changes that become healing. These changes need to be measured, if they exist.

Entrainment

1. The entrainment modalities are even more difficult to study than are laying on of hands.
2. In Western allopathic medicine, prescriptions are given because of how the drug works, not because of a person's specific characteristics. The entrainment modalities such as homeopathy, flower essences, aromatherapy, light, sound, and music are specific to the individual and can work differently for different people. Before we are able to predict their results accurately, we first need to know more about how they work.

Directions for Future Research: A Few Possible Studies

1. Is there an electromagnetic induction effect between humans? How small is the voltage range of this effect? Is it what Becker discovered—less than a billionth of an ampere?
2. If there is an electromagnetic induction effect between humans, how does this differ between the expert and the novice laying on of hands healer?
3. What is the electromagnetic effect of presence?
4. What are the long-term effects of electromagnetic and entrainment modalities?
5. How do the different laying on of hands modalities differ electromagnetically?
6. Do the electromagnetic and entrainment techniques support a person better before or after an allopathic treatment?
7. How healthy are providers and long-time users of these techniques compared to the nonusing population?

■ HOLISTIC CARING PROCESS

1. The holistic nurse assessing any individual brings unique skills to the assessment. This includes the nurse's experience with energy healing. You can only determine that an individual might benefit from one of the energy therapies if you have experienced and studied it, and even then the results are specific to the recipient.
2. The holistic nurses' identifications of the patient/client's patterns, challenges, and needs, the outcome identification, the therapeutic plan of care, and implementation of the particular modality do not differ from any other nursing intervention except that the nurses who have studied energy healing modalities can add these to their assessments and plans.
3. The aspect of energy healing that involves all nurses is presence. If presence is an electromagnetic induction phenomenon, the nurse can be an actual instrument of healing, perhaps as much or more so than the medical intervention the person is receiving. A nurse who brings a healing presence to the patient can have a different effect on that individual than one who does not.
4. An example of an institutional healing presence culture is the Heart Hospital in Albuquerque, New Mexico. The nurse and staff are not directly taught to walk slowly, not rush, speak in a friendly and cheerful manner, and not scare the patient, but they do. The nursing culture teaches the physicians, medical students, orderlies, and other staff how to be a healing presence to the patients and even to the other staff. Compare this example to your experiences where you work. Also, compare the healing presence you, as a holistic nurse, now bring to your working environment to what you brought earlier in your career. How have you changed on your holistic nursing journey?

■ WEBSITES

1. National Center for Complementary and Alternative Medicine, "What Is Complementary and Alternative Medicine?" http://nccam.nih.gov/health/whatiscam/
2. To learn more about electromagnetic induction:
   a. http://www.youtube.com/watch?v=BKXw2OjuPpY
   b. http://www.youtube.com/watch?feature=endscreen&v=gfJG4M4wi1o&NR=1

3. Platonic Realms, "The Fibonacci Sequence." http://www.mathacademy.com/pr/prime /articles/fibonac/index.asp.

4. M. Clayton, R. Sager, and U. Will. (2004). In time with the music: The concept of entrainment and its significance for ethnomusicology. *ESEM CounterPoint, 1*, 1–82. http://ethnomusicology.osu.edu/EMW /Will/InTimeWithTheMusic.pdf

■ NOTES

1. Krieger, D. (1979). *The Therapeutic Touch*. New York, NY: Prentice Hall.

2. Hover-Kramer, D., Mentgen, J., & Scandrett-Hibdon, S. (2001). Healing touch: A guide book for practitioners (2nd ed). Independence, Ky: Cengage Learning.

3. Brennan, B. A. (1987). *Hands of light: A guide to healing through the human energy field*. New York, NY: Bantam.

4. Benor, D. J. (1992). Intuitive diagnosis. *Subtle Energies, 3*(2), 41–64.

5. Maslow, A. H. (1954). *Motivation and Personality*. New York, NY: Harper.

6. Hunt, V. V. (1995). *Infinite Mind: The Science of Human Vibrations* (pp 19–21). Malibu, CA: Malibu Publishing.

7. Motoyama, H. (2009). *Karma and Reincarnation, the Key to Spiritual Evolution and Enlightenment* (pp. 125–134). Encinitas, CA: CIHS Press.

8. Curtis, R., Zeh, D., Miller, M., & Rich, S. C. (2004). Examining the validity of a computerized chakra measuring instrument: A pilot study. *Subtle Energies and Energy Medicine, 15*(3), 209–223.

9. Gerber, R. (2000). *Vibrational medicine for the 21st century: The complete guide to energy healing and spiritual transformation*. New York, NY: HarperCollins.

10. Becker, R., & Selden, G. (1985). *The body electric: Electromagnetism and the foundation of life*. New York, NY: William Morrow/Quill.

11. Zimmerman, J. (1990). Laying-on-of-hands healing and therapeutic touch: A testable theory. *BEMI Currents: Journal of the Bio-Electro-Magnetics Institute, 2*, 8–17.

12. Waechter, R. L., & Sergio, L. (2002). Manipulation of the electromagnetic spectrum via fields projected from human hands: A qi energy connection? *Subtle Energies and Energy Medicine, 13*(3).

13. Moga, M. M., & Bengston, W. F. (2010). Anomalous magnetic field activity during a bioenergy healing experiment. *Journal of Scientific Exploration, 24*(3), 397–410.

14. Bengston, W. F. (2010). Breakthrough: Clues to healing with intention. *EdgeScience Magazine, 2*, 5–9.

15. Wilken, A., & Wilken, J. (2005). Our sonic pathways. *Subtle Energies and Energy Medicine, 16*(3).

16. McTaggart, L. (2007). *The intention experiment: Using your thoughts to change your life and the world*. New York, NY: Free Press.

17. D. Wardell, personal conversation, June 2010.

■ STUDY QUESTIONS

Basic Level

1. Which phenomenon provides more power than is provided by just the initial source of power?
   a. Electricity
   b. Magnetism
   c. Electromagnetic induction
   d. Entrainment

2. Which of the following carries information that you receive as a gestalt?
   a. Aura
   b. Chakras
   c. Meridians
   d. Neurons

3. Which of the following is organized to process different frequencies of sound and light?
   a. Aura
   b. Chakras
   c. Meridians
   d. Neurons

4. A patient/client wants to talk about her fears about an impending surgery. You know that the physician has done a good job of explaining it. What is one approach you might use as a holistic nurse to comfort the patient/client?
   a. Explain the surgery and discover whether the individual really understands it.
   b. Ask the patient/client to explain what she knows to you.
   c. Find out what scares the patient/client.
   d. Listen to the person and be present.

5. You have just begun working in a new clinic and the music being played drives you nuts. What can you do to help yourself?
   a. Ask that no music be played.
   b. Ask that different types of music be played throughout the day.
   c. Decide to put up with it even though it is so irritating.
   d. Realize that as you get used to it, it will become less irritating.

Advanced Level

6. You are cleaning and bandaging a wound. What could you do to increase the electromagnetic induction that might lead to increased healing?
    a. Place a heat lamp over the area around the wound after you clean and bandage it.
    b. Become calm and peaceful as you are working and talking with the patient.
    c. Ask the patient to listen to his favorite music after you finish.
    d. Place a cell phone, iPad, or computer over the wound for a few seconds.

7. Construction has begun next to your unit and the noise is intermittent but loud. You are aware of the problem of the patients entraining to the noise. What might you do to mitigate the entrainment?
    a. Ignore the noise; there is nothing you can do.
    b. Give the patients and family members ear plugs.
    c. Turn up the TV or radio.
    d. Move everyone as far away from the noise as possible.

8. Your son has fallen and hurt his knee. How can you apply electromagnetic induction to the wound?

    a. Kiss the "boo-boo."
    b. Tell him he is a big boy and you are proud of him.
    c. Give him his favorite cookie to distract him.
    d. Panic briefly.

9. You are having an argument with someone you love. How can you use entrainment to help bring a truce/peace between you?
    a. Match his or her mood and actions. If the person yells, you yell.
    b. Pay attention to yourself and think loving thoughts.
    c. Leave the room so that that there is no one for him or her to fight with.
    d. Verbally agree with everything he or she says while silently disagreeing.

10. You have just had three patients die in the same room, one right after another. What can you do to remove the energy of death?
    a. Ask housekeeping to clean the walls as well as the bed and floor.
    b. Place flowers in the room between patients.
    c. Make sure the next patient in the room is not terminal.
    d. Stay in the room while you ask the Holy to clean it.

Chapter 33

Holistic Nursing Research

Rothlyn P. Zahourek

■ DEFINITIONS

Bias Having preconceived ideas and expectations about a research study's outcome. Can be overt or more subtle as a hope or expectation.

Bracketing Characteristic of qualitative research. The researcher outlines in writing his or her philosophies, biases, or concerns and expectations about the research project process and/or outcome.

Credibility A term used in qualitative research that accounts for the researcher's trustworthiness in demonstrating the process of data collection and interpretation of results.

Hawthorne effect When people know they are being observed in a study, their behavior is affected simply by being observed.

Healing Both a process and result; defined by the individual as perception of shift or meaningful change. The central concept in holistic nursing research.

Healing relationship The quality and characteristics of interactions between healer and the one being healed (healee) that facilitate healing, including empathy, care, love, warmth, trust, confidence, honesty, courtesy, respect, and communication, as well as compassion, presence, intent, and intentionality.

Heisenberg's Uncertainty Principle The principle that observation of phenomena or objects changes the nature of what is studied.

Integral The appreciation for the interactions and interrelationships of the many parts within the whole of a system.

Meta-analysis A statistical technique that combines the results of many studies related to one topic to establish an overall estimate of the therapeutic effectiveness of an intervention.

Mixed methods research A type of research that combines paradigms, philosophies, and methods on a specific topic to grasp a more complete representation of reality and/or confirm the credibility of the research findings; also might be referred to as triangulation.

Placebo A medically inert medication, preparation, treatment, technique, or ritual that has no intended effects on the person and no actual therapeutic value. The fact that the placebo is inert is now in question based on the impact of suggestion and intention.

Praxis The bringing together of practice and research. It is a synthesizing and reflective process in which theory is dynamic and practice reflects research and theory in a unified whole.

Qualitative research A systematic, subjective research approach that describes life experiences and searches for how participants find meaning in their experiences; based on philosophical, psychological, and sociological theory; focuses on understanding the whole, which is consistent with the philosophy of holistic nursing.

Quantitative research A systematic, formal, reductionistic, objective approach in which numerical data are used to obtain and interpret information about the world. It embodies the principles of the scientific method and describes variables, examines relationships among variables, determines cause-and-effect interactions between variables, and predicts future responses.

Reductionism The approach of breaking down phenomena to their smallest possible parts; also called positivism and equated with the linear, logical nature of the scientific method.

Reliability Generally associated with quantitative research and the ability of a scale or a tool to consistently measure a phenomenon when used repeatedly.

Research A diligent, systematic inquiry or investigation to validate and refine existing knowledge and generate new knowledge.

Systematic review A specific form of review of research studies that yields more convincing evidence. Several methods exist; these are invaluable in discovering what has already been discovered about a particular phenomenon.

Translational research Taking basic bench highly reductionist (molecular or cellular) research and translating that into clinical application. It generates new research questions that are fed back to the bench. More broadly, translating any research into practice.

Unitary The recognition that parts cannot be separated from the whole because the whole is greater than, and different from, the parts; contention that separating phenomenon into parts undermines the understanding of the whole.

Validity Generally associated with quantitative research; internal and external; relates to the interpretation of data; meaningful, appropriate, and useful results are required for validity. Internal validity is related to the controls placed on the research design and process and ensures that the effects of the independent variable are causing the results in the dependent variable. External validity ensures that the results are generalizable to other populations, settings, and times and depends on internal validity.

■ THEORY AND RESEARCH

What Is Holistic Nursing Research?

1. How do we understand and connect science and spirit?
2. How do we explore the healing relationship and healing itself?
3. What is different about holistic nursing research (HNR)?
4. HNR must occur within a framework of theory and practice that accepts holism as its base.
   a. Integral definition of holism
   b. Unitary definition of holism

Worldviews and Ways of Knowing and Nursing Theory

1. Historically, nursing research and theory generation have been based on Carper's classical work. She proposed a system of *four ways of knowing*:[1]
   a. Empirical: Objective, logical, and positivistic science
   b. Ethical: Obligations, what should be done in a given situation; what is acceptable practice; requires openness to differences in philosophical positions[2]
   c. Personal: Self-knowledge; determined by ability to self-actualize; comfort with ambiguity; commitment to patience and self-care
   d. Aesthetic: Artful knowledge; abstract; defies formal description and measurement; understanding of subjective experiences; creative pattern
2. Fawcett developed a classic paradigmatic system that describes three frameworks of increasing degrees of abstractness:[3]
   a. Particulate–deterministic: Reductionist, concrete
   b. Interactive–integrative: Reality is multidimensional and contextual; reciprocal relationships
   c. Unitary–transformative: Human beings are unitary, evolving, self-organizing fields, and defined by pattern; highly abstract[3]

3. Nurse theorists Watson, Newman, Parse, and Rogers are associated with the unitary–transformative paradigm. Enzman-Hagedorn and Zahourek developed an integrated model that combines Carper's and Fawcett's paradigms with specific research approaches for holistic nursing research.[4]
4. Dossey's integral nursing model is another. Mariano provides a slightly different framework described as four "attributes of scholarship": wide awake, reflective, caring, and humorous.[5]
5. Other frameworks and bodies of knowledge that influence HNR: Knowing-unknowing, healing concepts and research, observer effect, consciousness and energy.

■ IMPACT OF THE NCCAM 2011 STRATEGIC PLAN

NCCAM Strategic Plan: Goals and Objectives

1. Goals
   a. Advance the science and practice of symptom management.
   b. Develop effective, practical, personalized strategies for promoting health and well-being.
   c. Enable better evidence-based decision making regarding complementary and alternative medicine (CAM) use and its integration into health care and health promotion.
2. Strategic objectives
   a. Advance the research on mind–body interactions practices and disciplines.
   b. Advance research on CAM natural products.
   c. Increase understanding of real-world patterns and outcomes of CAM use and its integration into health care and health promotion.
   d. Improve the capacity of the field to carry out rigorous research.
   e. Develop and disseminate objective, evidence-based information on CAM interventions.
3. Types of evidence
   a. Basic science: Investigates biological effects and mechanisms of action; it clarifies hypotheses and answers the question, "How does it work?"
   b. Translational research: Might identify markers of biological effect; develops and validates measures of outcome; develops algorithms and preliminary clinical efficacy; estimates sample size for future studies. Answers the question, "Can it be studied in people?"
   c. Efficacy studies: Highly controlled studies to determine specific effects of an intervention. Answers the question, "What are the specific effects?"
   d. Effectiveness and outcome studies: What is the usefulness and safety of the intervention in general populations and healthcare settings? Answers the question, "Does it work in the real world?"

■ EXAMPLES OF THE CURRENT STATUS OF HOLISTIC NURSING RESEARCH

1. Research using randomized controlled trials to evaluate mindfulness-based stress reduction for solid organ transplant patients[6]
2. A quasi-experimental pre–post intervention design evaluating the effect of live music on patients' experience of pain, anxiety, and muscle tension[7]
3. Mixed method study on garden walking for depressed elders[8]
4. A qualitative historical study on the nature of the caring relationships in Florence Nightingale's writing[9]
5. A descriptive hermeneutic phenomenologic investigation of the transformational and extraordinary experiences of nurse healers[10]
6. A phenomenologic study of eco-spirituality exploring the experience of environmental meditation in patients with cardiovascular disease[11]

■ HOLISTIC RESEARCH METHODS AND ENHANCING HOLISTIC NURSING

1. Quantitative research
   a. Descriptive research, which describes phenomena
   b. Correlational research, which examines relationships between and among variables
   c. Quasi-experimental research, which explains relationships, examines causal

relationships, and clarifies the reasons for events

d. Experimental research, the randomized controlled trial (RCT), which examines cause-and-effect relationships between variables[12]

e. Critique of quantitative research:
   - Distinctive features of unique individuals can be lost in aggregate means, standard deviations, and various statistical analyses.[13]
   - Many complementary therapies are not testable under blinded and sham conditions, and the choice of an appropriate control condition is not always clear.[14]
   - In highly controlled research, it is difficult to include the individualistic whole human being response to variables.

2. Qualitative research
   a. Appropriate when little information is known about a phenomenon or when phenomena are difficult to measure.[15]
   b. Systematically describes and promotes understanding of human experiences such as health, healing, energy, intention, caring, comfort, and meaning.
   c. The context of this approach is meaning of observed patterns.
   d. Critique: Not as easily replicable, more subjective.
   e. Methods include the following:
      - Phenomenology: Focuses on experience as the whole person lives it
      - Hermeneutics: Seeks to understand meaning and the individual's sociocultural experiences
      - Ethnography: Describes a culture and the people within the culture
      - Grounded theory: Uncovers psychosocial problems and how people manage
      - Historical research: Describes or analyzes past events to better understand the present[12]
      - Narrative and aesthetic forms of inquiry

■ ENHANCING HOLISTIC RESEARCH

1. Mixed methods: Avoids paradigmatic wars but can be very positivistic rather than holistic; increases reliability and validity

2. Synthesis, systematic reviews, and meta-analyses: Highest levels of evidence

3. Additional methods: Aesthetic and transpersonal
   a. Increase understanding of real-world patterns and outcomes of CAM use and its integration into health care and health promotion
   b. Improve the capacity of the field to carry out rigorous research
   c. Develop and disseminate objective, evidence-based information on CAM interventions

4. Confounds for holistic nursing research
   a. The passage of time; the impact of many interventions is not observable or measurable immediately and can develop over time
   b. The qualitative interpretation and meaning of an experience that might not be measured physiologically
   c. Other intervening life experiences
   d. Environmental impacts (e.g., natural and human-made disasters)
   e. Cultural influences (e.g., an Hispanic as opposed to Chinese interpretation of an experience)
   f. Personality temperament influences
   g. Standardization of method (e.g., can Therapeutic Touch be standardized?), variation in method, approach, and skill used by individual practitioners
   h. Sensitivity and reliability of tools and instruments to measure change
   i. Placebo and expectation effect (valuable in one's personal experience of being healed, but a problem in conducting controlled research)
   j. The Heisenberg principle and the Hawthorne effect
   k. The impact of the interpersonal relationship and the intentions of healer and healee

How Is Holistic Nursing Research Different?

1. The shift in emphasis to understanding the healing relationship through a holistic (unitary or integral) model.
2. Certain phenomena related to holistic research are not accessible to reductionist

scientific investigation because they cannot be objectively measured.

3. The individual who experiences certain effects in a holistic nursing relationship might be unable to conceptualize, express, translate, or communicate these effects to another.

4. As we accumulate a database that includes various approaches and methodologies our body of supportive evidence grows.

5. Holistic nursing research not only evaluates the effects of alternative and complementary modalities but also puts that evaluation into the context of a whole. What do we consider the "whole"? What worldview do we use to understand holism? Holistic nursing research is different because it simply is based in a holistic paradigm.

Please refer to Tables 34-1 and 34-2 in *Holistic Nursing: A Handbook for Practice, Sixth Edition,* for more explanations.

■ NOTES

1. Carper, B. (1978). Fundamental patterns of knowing in nursing. *Advances in Nursing Science, 1*(13), 13–23.

2. Porter, S. (2010). Fundamental patterns of knowing in nursing; the challenge of evidence-based practice. *Advances in Nursing Science, 33*(1), 3–14.

3. Fawcett, J. (1993). *Analysis and evaluation of nursing theories.* Philadelphia, PA: F. A. Davis.

4. Enzman-Hagedorn, M., & Zahourek, R. P. (2007). Research paradigms and methods for investigating holistic nursing concerns nursing. *Nursing Clinics of North America, 42*(2), 335–353.

5. Mariano, C. (2006). The many faces of scholarship. *Beginnings, 26*(5), 3.

6. Gross, C. R., Kreitzer, M. J., Thomas, W., Reilly-Spong, M., Cramer-Bornemann, M., Nyman, J. A.,...Ibrahim, H. N. (2010). Mindfulness-based stress reduction for solid organ transplant recipients: A randomized controlled trial. *Alternative Therapies in Health and Medicine, 12*(4), 30–38.

7. Sand-Jecklin, K., & Emerson, H. (2010). The impact of a live therapeutic music intervention on patients' experience of pain, anxiety and muscle tension. *Holistic Nursing Practice, 24*(1), 7–15.

8. McCaffrey, R., Hansen, C., & McCaffrey, W. (2010). Garden walking for depression: A research report. *Holistic Nursing Practice, 24*(5), 252–259.

9. Wagner, D., & Whaite, B. (2010). An exploration of the nature of caring relationships in the writings of Florence Nightingale. *Journal of Holistic Nursing, 28*(4), 225–234.

10. Hemsley, M., Glass, N., & Watson, J. (2006). Taking the eagle's view: Using Watson's conceptual model to investigate the extraordinary and transformative experiences of nurse healers. *Holistic Nursing Practice, 20*(2), 85–94.

11. Delaney, C., & Barrere, C. (2009). Ecospirituality: The experience of environmental meditation in patients with cardiovascular disease. *Holistic Nursing Practice, 23*(6), 361–369.

12. Polit, D. F., Beck, C. T., & Hungler, B. P. (2001). *Essentials of nursing research: Methods, appraisal, and utilization* (5th ed.). Philadelphia, PA: Lippincott.

13. Lukoff, D., et al. (1998). The case study as a scientific method for researching alternative therapies. *Alternative Therapies in Health and Medicine, 4*(2), 44–52.

14. Margolin, A., et al. (1998). Investigating alternative medicine therapies in randomized controlled trials. *Journal of the American Medical Association, 280*(18), 1626–1628.

15. Sandelowski, M. (1993). Rigor or rigor mortis: The problem of rigor in qualitative research revisited. *Advances in Nursing Science, 16*(2), 1–8.

■ STUDY QUESTIONS

Basic Level

1. **For which of the following reasons is holistic nursing research different?**
   a. Deals with a CAM approach
   b. Uses a nursing theory
   c. Uses a holistic framework in planning, conducting, or interpreting the research and the results
   d. Is easily applied by nursing administration

2. **Which of the following is a resource for nurses and clients on holistic nursing research?**
   a. The AHNA website research section
   b. The NCCAAM website
   c. The Carlat reports
   d. The *American Journal of Nursing*

3. **Which of the following is a confounding aspect of holistic nursing research?**
   a. The amount of time it takes for the result of many interventions to become evident
   b. The Heisenberg effect
   c. The placebo effect
   d. All of the above

4. What is the influence of being studied and a confound for many research studies called?
   a. The placebo effect
   b. The Heisenberg effect
   c. The Hawthorn effect
   d. The randomized control effect

5. Examples of qualitative research include all of the following except which one?
   a. Phenomenology
   b. Grounded theory
   c. Ethnography
   d. Survey

6. When evidence from a randomized controlled trial is applied in a clinical study and evaluated what is it called?
   a. Basic science
   b. Translational research
   c. Survey
   d. Efficacy studies

7. A study that looks at the relationship of parts to the whole uses which framework?
   a. Unitary framework
   b. Integral framework
   c. Particulate framework
   d. Deterministic framework

Advanced Level

8. What must the holistic nurse do when interpreting a holistic nursing research study?
   a. The nurse must see statistically significant results.
   b. The nurse must see that the results are applicable in HN practice.
   c. The nurse must be sure the study is based in a holistic framework.
   d. All of the above

9. A patient asks you about the evidence for *Ginkgo biloba*. You inform her that the best evidence comes from where?
   a. A completed meta-analysis
   b. A report in the *New York Times*
   c. A qualitative study
   d. A systematic review of studies

10. A holistic nurse researcher is interested in studying the effect of aromatherapy on pain. Which is the most comprehensive study that yields the most convincing evidence?
    a. Quantitative double-blind study with two groups: one that received aromatherapy and the other that was a control group and did not receive the therapy
    b. A mixed method study with comparison groups and a narrative qualitative component
    c. A phenomenological study of the experience of pain and relief
    d. A review of literature on pain and aromatherapy

11. What do holistic nurse researchers do to control for confounding effects?
    a. Acknowledge the effect from the start
    b. Conduct more longitudinal studies
    c. Accept that statistical significance might not be the same as clinical significance
    d. All of the above

Chapter 34

Evidence-Based Practice

Cynthia C. Barrere and Carol M. Baldwin

Original Authors: Alyce A. Schultz, Bernadette Mazurek Melnyk,
Carol M. Baldwin, and Jo Rycroft-Malone

■ DEFINITIONS

Comparative effectiveness research (CER)
The conduct and synthesis of research that compares the benefits and harms of various interventions and strategies for preventing, diagnosing, treating, and monitoring health conditions in real-world settings. The purpose of this research is to improve health outcomes by developing and disseminating evidence-based information to patients, clinicians, and other decision makers about which interventions are most effective for which patients under specific circumstances.

Evidence-based practice (EBP) The conscientious use of the best available evidence combined with the clinician's expertise and judgment and the patient's preferences and values to arrive at the best decision that leads to high-quality outcomes.

PICOT A standardized format for asking the searchable, answerable question: population of interest (P); the intervention or issue of interest (I); the comparison intervention, if relevant (C); the outcome (O); and time frame (T), if relevant.

■ THEORY AND RESEARCH

Holistic Nursing and Evidence-Based Practice

1. The science and art of holistic nursing honor an individual's subjective experience about health, health beliefs, and values and develop therapeutic partnerships with individuals, families, and communities that are grounded in nursing knowledge, theories, research expertise, intuition, and creativity.[1]

2. Evidence-based practice (EBP) is the conscientious use of the best available evidence combined with the clinician's expertise and judgment and the patient's preferences and values to arrive at the best decision that leads to high-quality outcomes.[2,3]

3. Figure 35-1, Evidence-Based Practice Conceptual Framework, can be found in *Holistic Nursing: A Handbook for Practice* (6th edition).

Historical Underpinnings of Current Evidence-Based Practice

1. Knowledge translation or the use of research evidence to improve clinical outcomes is not a 21st-century phenomenon.

2. Florence Nightingale, as a nurse in the Crimean War (1853–1856), found that washing hands between patients along with other public health measures reduced morbidity and mortality among the soldiers.[4]

3. Recognized as the first nurse to conduct and use research, Nightingale showed that the quality of care can be improved through sanitary conditions, careful data collection, and critical thinking.[5]

4. More than 150 years later, Nightingale's insight into the need for research laid the groundwork for evidence-based practice in holistic nursing.[6]

Nursing Research into Evidence-Based Practice

1. Research skills and knowledge have become a requirement for the professional nurse; concern for use of research findings in practice and strategies to increase research utilization is a top priority.
2. It is also evident that much of nursing care is based on best practice and the methodology for and emphasis on quality improvement continue to increase; therefore, additional forms of evidence are used as the basis for practice.
3. Sackett and colleagues coined the term *evidence-based medicine* in the early 1990s to add credibility to internal quality improvement data and common practices that were providing good patient outcomes.[7] *Evidence-based practice* is the term used to describe practices by all healthcare professionals.
4. From the mid-1990s to the present, a number of new quality improvement and evidence-based practice models and frameworks have been developed.

■ CONCEPTUAL MODELS FOR EVIDENCE-BASED PRACTICE

The DiCenso Model

1. The DiCenso Model of EBP,[8] adapted from Haynes,[9] promotes the use of research findings within the context of an evidence-based decision-making framework.[10]
2. The individual clinician integrates the best research evidence with the patient's clinical status, preferences, action, and circumstances; available healthcare resources; and clinical expertise to decide on the interventions or type of care to be delivered.

The Clinical Scholar Model and Program

1. Clinical scholars are agents of change.
2. The Clinical Scholar Model is inductive, decentralized, and predicated on "building a community" of clinical scholars to serve as mentors anywhere patient care is provided.[11]
3. The clinical scholar is always questioning whether a procedure needs to be performed at all and, if so, whether there is a more efficient and effective way of providing the same care.

4. The Clinical Scholar Program, based on the Clinical Scholar Model, is a series of six interdisciplinary all-day workshops, generally presented one month apart. The goals of the program are as follows:
   a. Promote a culture of EBP and clinical scholarship through a program of interdisciplinary clinical research and EBP at the bedside, extending work that has already been initiated in a clinical setting.
   b. Prepare a cadre of direct care providers as clinical scholars to implement change and evaluate practice based on evidence.

Promoting Action on Research Implementation in Health Services (PARIHS) Model

1. The PARIHS framework was developed to represent the complexities involved in implementing evidence into practice.[12,13]
2. The successful implementation (SI) of evidence into practice is a function (f) of the nature and type of evidence (E), the qualities of the context (C) in which the evidence is to be implemented, and the way the process is facilitated (F); therefore, SI = $f(E,C,F)$.
3. It provides a practical and conceptual heuristic to guide implementation and practice improvement activity, which takes multiple factors into account and acknowledges the dynamism in implementation processes.
4. This conceptual and theoretical framework has been used for research and evaluation, the basis for tool development, modeling research utilization, and evaluating the facilitation of interventions.[13]

Advancing Research and Clinical Practice Through Close Collaboration (ARCC) Model for Systemwide Implementation and Sustainability of EBP

1. The ARCC Model includes multiple strategies for advancing EBP within healthcare organizations.
2. The key element for implementing and sustaining system-wide EBP in the model is a cadre of EBP mentors who facilitate clinician and organizational culture change to EBP.[10]
3. Within the conceptual framework of the ARCC Model, the first step to systemwide

implementation is the assessment of an organization's strengths and limitations in advancing EBP.

4. Once strengths and limitations are identified, a key implementation strategy in the ARCC Model, the development of a cadre of EBP mentors (such as an advanced practice nurse), is initiated.

5. Goals of the ARCC Model include the following:
   a. Promoting EBP among advanced practice and staff nurses as well as transdisciplinary clinicians.
   b. Establishing a cadre of EBP mentors to facilitate systemwide implementation of EBP in healthcare organizations.
   c. Disseminating and facilitating use of the best evidence from well-designed clinical studies.
   d. Designing and conducting studies to evaluate the effectiveness of the ARCC Model on the process and outcomes of clinical care.
   e. Conducting studies to evaluate the effectiveness of the EBP implementation strategies.[3,14]

CHALLENGES TO AND STRENGTHS OF EVIDENCE-BASED CARE

1. Barriers to providing care based on the latest evidence include lack of searching skills, inability to critically appraise studies, insufficient institutional support, as well as negative attitudes toward research.[15-17]

2. Nurses who incorporate EBP into their care report that it gives them a voice, allows them to reclaim their authentic selves as real nurses, and supports them as patient advocates to improve the quality of care.[18]

3. Holistic nurses need a sound understanding of strategies to reduce barriers when implementing EBP to nurture the holistic caring process based on evidence that can empirically support the science and art of holistic nursing.[19]

MAGNET RECOGNITION AND EVIDENCE-BASED PRACTICE

1. The Magnet Recognition Program, developed in the early 1990s by the American Nurses Credentialing Center (ANCC),

added impetus to the EBP movement, particularly in nursing.[20]

2. The expectation for nurses in Magnet facilities is to generate new knowledge through the conduct of research.[20]

3. There is the expectation that nurses at all levels of practice will apply research-based evidence and utilize practice-based evidence as appropriate.

4. Practice-based evidence is defined in the Magnet Program as interventions that have been shown effective in improving outcomes but have not been scientifically validated.[21]

APPLYING EBP TO THE HOLISTIC CARING PROCESS STEP BY STEP:

1. The seven-step EBP process requires that the holistic nurse:
   a. Cultivate a spirit of inquiry.
   b. Determine a clinical issue of interest and formulate a searchable, answerable question (PICOT).
   c. Perform an efficient, focused search to find an answer to the clinical question (akin to an abbreviated literature search).
   d. Assess the article(s) using rapid critical appraisal techniques.
   e. Apply the valid and reliable evidence.
   f. Evaluate the outcomes of the implementation of evidence.
   g. Disseminate the outcomes of the EBP decision or change.[10,22-25]

2. *Clinical Scenario: Music for Reducing Dyspnea and Anxiety in Patients with COPD*[26] provides a detailed example of the application of EBP. This scenario can be found in Chapter 35 of *Holistic Nursing: A Handbook for Practice*.

3. Both qualitative and quantitative methods were used to enrich the project outcomes.

4. The qualitative information provided by the participants gives insight into their lived experiences with dyspnea and reinforces the idea that holistic nurses need to be considerate regarding clients' music preferences and the potential effects on dyspnea, such as assisting patients to achieve their goals.

5. The quantitative findings were both statistically and clinically significant. Hence, moving from critical appraisal of the evidence to action, the holistic nurse decides

to incorporate music therapy into care of patients with COPD, emphasizing the music is to be selected by the clients.

■ EBP AND HOLISTIC NURSING PRACTICE, EDUCATION, AND SCHOLARSHIP

1. On average, it takes 17 years to translate research findings into clinical practice.[27]
2. Leading professional and healthcare organizations and policymakers have placed a major emphasis on accelerating EBP in the educational, practice, and research settings.
3. In the landmark document *Crossing the Quality Chasm*, the Institute of Medicine (IOM) emphasizes that one of the 10 "rules for health care" is evidence-based decision making.[28]
4. The five core competencies for educational programs for healthcare professionals deemed essential by the IOM's Health Professions Educational Summit include employing EBP.[29]
5. EBP must be the foundation of practice, education, and research.
6. Holistic nursing requires valid evidence-based practice that is conducted to assist clinicians at the point of care to have the latest and best information upon which to base their care.[14,30]

■ GLOBAL HEALTH, HOLISTIC CULTURE CARE, AND EBP

1. The teaching, implementation, and application of EBP are shared concerns globally.[31]
2. To guide all nurses toward understanding the implications and applications of EBP internationally, the peer-reviewed journal *Worldviews on Evidence-Based Nursing: Linking Evidence to Action* is an information resource for nurses worldwide that is published on a quarterly basis under the auspices of STTI.
3. The Joanna Briggs Institute collaborates internationally with more than 60 entities around the world, including in Singapore, Canada, China, and the United States, to promote and support the synthesis, transfer, and utilization of evidence through identifying feasible, appropriate,

meaningful, and effective healthcare practices to assist in the improvement of healthcare outcomes globally.[32]

■ EBP AND COMPARATIVE EFFECTIVENESS RESEARCH

1. It is important for holistic nurses to know the advances in moving evidence forward to inform national and global health policy and to support informed consumer choices.[33,34]
2. Initiated by the National Institutes of Health and the Institute of Medicine in 2009, the purpose of Comparative Effectiveness Research (CER) is to improve health outcomes by developing and disseminating evidence-based information to patients, clinicians, and other decision makers about which interventions are most effective for which patients under specific circumstances at individual and population levels.[34–36]
3. Characteristics of CER studies include:
   a. Studies directly inform clinical or health policy decisions.
   b. Studies compare at least two alternatives, each with the potential to be best practices.
   c. Results are generated at population and subgroup levels.
   d. Outcome measures are important to patients.
   e. Methods and data sources (qualitative and/or quantitative) are appropriate for the decision of interest.
   f. Studies are conducted in real-world settings.
4. Interventions can include medications, procedures, medical and assistive devices and technologies, diagnostic testing, holistic practices, behavioral change, and delivery system strategies.
5. A focus of CER is to implement practice- and cost-effective interventions to improve health outcomes in large patient populations.

■ NOTES

1. American Holistic Nurses Association. (n.d.). What is holistic nursing? Retrieved from http://www.ahna.org/AboutUs/WhatisHolisticNursing/tabid/1165/Default.aspx

2. Melnyk, B., & Fineout-Overholt, E. (2006). Consumer preferences and values as an integral key to evidence-based practice. *Nursing Administration Quarterly, 30,* 123–127.

3. Fineout-Overholt, E., Melnyk, B. M., & Schultz, A. (2005). Transforming healthcare from the inside out: Advancing evidence-based practice in the 21st century. *Journal of Professional Nursing, 21,* 335–344.

4. Dossey, B. M. (2010). *Florence Nightingale: Mystic, visionary, healer.* (Commemorative ed.). Philadelphia, PA: F. A. Davis.

5. Stringer, H. (2010). The evolution of evidence-based practice. *Nursing Spectrum & NurseWeek, Commemorating Nightingale's Legacy,* 70–72.

6. Nightingale, F. (1969). *Notes on nursing: What it is, and what it is not.* Mineola, NY: Dover. (Original work published 1860)

7. Sackett, D. L., DiCenso, A., Guyatt, G., & Ciliska, D. (2000). *Evidence-based medicine: How to practice and teach EBM.* New York, NY: Churchill Livingstone.

8. DiCenso, A., Guyatt, G., & Ciliska, D. (2005). *Evidence-based nursing. A guide to clinical practice.* St. Louis, MO: Mosby.

9. Haynes, R. B., Devereaux, P. J., & Guyatt, G. H. (2002). Clinical expertise in the era of evidence-based medicine and patient choice. *ACP Journal Club, 136,* A11–A14.

10. Melnyk, B., & Fineout-Overholt, E. (2011). *Evidence-based practice in nursing and healthcare: A guide to best practice.* Philadelphia, PA: Lippincott Williams & Wilkins.

11. Schultz, A. A. (2005, February). Advancing evidence into practice: Clinical scholars at the bedside [Electronic version]. *Excellence in Nursing Knowledge.*

12. Rycroft-Malone, J., Harvey, G., Seers, K., Kitson, A., McCormack, B., & Titchen, A. (2004). An exploration of the factors that influence the implementation of evidence into practice. *Journal of Clinical Nursing, 13,* 913–924.

13. Rycroft-Malone, J. (2010). Promoting Action on Research Implementation in Health Services (PARIHS). In J. Rycroft-Malone & T. Bucknall (Eds.), *Models and frameworks for implementing evidence-based practice: Linking evidence to action.* Oxford, England: Wiley Blackwell/STTI.

14. Melnyk, B., & Fineout-Overholt, E. (2002). Putting research into practice. *Reflections on Nursing Leadership, 28,* 22–25.

15. Melnyk, B. (2002). Strategies for overcoming barriers in implementing evidence-based practice. *Pediatric Nursing, 28,* 159–161.

16. Pravikoff, D. S., Pierce, S. T., & Tanner, A. (2005). American Academy of Nursing Publication Advisory Committee Evidence-Based Practice Readiness Study supported by Academy Nursing Informatics Expert Panel. *Nursing Outlook, 53,* 49–50.

17. Baldwin, C. M., Melnyk, B., Fineout-Overholt, E., Cometto, M. C., & Avila, G. (2009, February 20). *Individual and institutional barriers to implementing EBP in clinical practice: A comparison of pan American and U.S. nurses.* Paper presented at the 10th Annual National/International EBP Conference, Phoenix, AZ. (2/19-20/09). *Received best EBP Implementation podium presentation award.*

18. Strout, T. (2005). Curiosity and reflective thinking: Renewal of the spirit. *Online Journal of Excellence in Nursing Knowledge, 2,* 39.

19. Melnyk, B. (2006). Calling all educators to teach and model evidence-based practice in academic settings. *Worldviews on Evidence-Based Nursing, 3,* 93–94.

20. Reigle, B. S., Stevens, K. R., Belcher, J. V., Huth, M. M., McGuire, E., Mals, D., & Volz, T. (2008). Evidence-based practice and the road to Magnet status. *Journal of Nursing Administration, 38,* 97–102.

21. American Nurses Credentialing Center. (2008). *Magnet Recognition Program, application manual.* Silver Spring, MD: Author.

22. Baldwin, C. M., & Fineout-Overholt, E. (2005). Evidence-based practice as holistic nursing research. *Beginnings, 25,* 16.

23. Melnyk, B. (2003). Finding and appraising systematic reviews of clinical interventions: Critical skills for evidence-based practice. *Pediatric Nursing, 29,* 147–149.

24. Melnyk, B., & Fineout-Overholt, E. (2002). Key steps in implementing evidence-based practice: Asking compelling, searchable questions and searching for the best evidence. *Pediatric Nursing, 28,* 161–162, 266.

25. Melnyk, B., & Fineout-Overholt, E. (2005). Rapid critical appraisal of randomized controlled trials (RCTs): An essential skill for evidence-based practice (EBP). *Pediatric Nursing, 31,* 50–52.

26. McBride, S., Graydon, J., Sidani, S., & Hall, L. (1999). The therapeutic use of music for dyspnea and anxiety in patients with COPD who live at home. *Journal of Holistic Nursing, 17,* 229–250.

27. Balas, E. A., & Boren, S. A. (2000). Managing clinical knowledge for healthcare improvements. In V. Schattauer (Ed.), *IMIA yearbook of medical informatics* (pp. 65–70). Chicago, IL: American Health Information.

28. Committee on Quality of Health Care in America, Institute of Medicine. (2001). *Crossing the quality chasm: A new health system for the 21st century.* Washington, DC: National Academy Press.

29. Greiner, A., & Knebel, E. (Eds.). (2003). *Health professions education: A bridge to quality.* Washington, DC: National Academy Press.

30. Krueger, J. C. (1978). Utilization of nursing research. The planning process. *Journal of Nursing Administration, 8,* 6–9.

31. Sigma Theta Tau International Honor Society in Nursing. (n.d.). *Global development*. Retrieved from http://www.nursingsociety.org/aboutus/Position Papers/Documents/policy_development.doc

32. Joanna Briggs Institute. (n.d.). Home page. Retrieved from http://www.joannabriggs.edu.au/

33. Bauer, J. G., & Chiappelli, F. (2011). Transforming scientific evidence into better consumer choices. *Bioinformation, 7,* 297-299.

34. Chalkidou, K., Tunis, S., Lopert, R., Rochaix, L., Sawicki, P. T., Nasser, M., & Xerri, B. (2009). Comparative effectiveness research and evidence-based health policy: Experience from four countries. *Milbank Quarterly, 87,* 339-367.

35. Iglehart, J. K. (2009). Prioritizing comparative effectiveness research. IOM recommendations. *New England Journal of Medicine, 361,* 325-228.

36. Nabel, E. (2009). *Role of the NIH in comparative effectiveness research.* Paper presented at the National CER Summit, Washington, DC. Retrieved from http://www.ehcca.com/presentations/comp effective1/nabel_1.pdf

■ STUDY QUESTIONS

Basic Level

1. To arrive at the best decision that leads to high-quality outcomes, evidenced-based practice is advocated. Evidence-based practice is the conscientious use of which of the following?
   a. Findings from clinical experimental studies that are randomized control trial designs
   b. The best available evidence, clinicians' expertise and judgment, and the patient's preferences and values
   c. Quality improvement surveys and questionnaires, clinicians' expertise and judgment, and the patient's preferences and values
   d. Well-designed qualitative research studies combined with quantitative research endeavors and the patient's preferences and values

2. The purpose of comparative effectiveness research is to improve health outcomes by developing and disseminating evidence-based information to patients, clinicians, and other decision makers about which of the following?
   a. Which holistic interventions are the most effective for all patients under specific circumstances

   b. Which CAM interventions are the most effective for the general population under stress
   c. Which interventions are most effective for a limited patient population under limited circumstances
   d. Which interventions are most effective for which patients under specific circumstances

3. PICOT is a standardized format for asking the searchable, answerable question. What do the letters stand for?
   a. Population, invention, comparison, outcome, and time frame
   b. People, intervention, comparison, outcome, and time frame
   c. Population, intervention, condition, outcome, and time frame
   d. Population, intervention, comparison, outcome, and time frame

4. How do Magnet programs define practice-based evidence?
   a. Interventions that have been shown effective in improving outcomes but have not been scientifically validated
   b. Interventions that have been shown effective in improving outcomes and have also been scientifically validated
   c. Practice outcomes that have been demonstrated effective and are ready for replication
   d. Practice outcomes that have not yet been demonstrated effective and that need further investigation

5. Barriers to providing care based on the latest evidence are not only national issues but also global challenges in nursing as well. What are these barriers?
   a. Nurses' lack of skills in searching the literature, inability to critically appraise studies, insufficient institutional support, yet positive attitudes toward research
   b. Nurses' lack of skills in searching the literature, inability to critically appraise studies, insufficient institutional support, and negative attitudes toward research
   c. Nurses' strength in ability to search the literature, inability to critically appraise studies, insufficient institutional

support, and negative attitudes toward research

d. Nurses' strength in ability to search the literature, ability to critically appraise studies, insufficient institutional support, and negative attitudes toward research

Advanced Level

6. Robert Spencer, a home hospice nurse, is reviewing the literature about Healing Touch and its effectiveness in relieving pain. He finds a case study reported in the literature about a clinical situation in which Therapeutic Touch was used successfully to relieve one patient's pain. Robert knows that case study reports are ranked lower in the hierarchy of evidence for intervention questions because of their lack of objectivity. Which of the following questions should Robert include in his critical appraisal of this report?

   a. Is this case study appealing in the way it is written to describe the situation?
   b. Does the case study provide valid comparative results?
   c. What are the case study patient's values and expectations?
   d. How do the case study results compare with results of published research?

7. Sean Walden, RN, works on a surgical unit in which he led an EBP team to improve postoperative pain management. Sean and his team have used reliable and valid measures to evaluate the practice change. Which of the following answer choices would be an appropriate next step for Sean and his team to make?

   a. Submit an abstract about the EBP project.
   b. Recheck the outcomes to be sure they are accurate.
   c. Critically appraise the evidence again.
   d. Ask another clinical question.

8. Kristen Noonan, RN, works on a medical inpatient unit of a Magnet hospital. Evidence-based practice is an important aspect of her nursing role. Which one of the following situations would likely spur Kristen to initiate an evidence-based project?

   a. The nurse manager returns from a conference and shares a new fall prevention protocol with the nursing staff.
   b. Kristen identifies there has been an increase in the number of patient falls during the past 3 months.
   c. The vice president of nursing informs staff that the hospital will need to conform to a newly adopted state guideline for the use of restraints.
   d. ANA guidelines for the use of restraints are revised and circulated to all schools of nursing.

9. Romana Sanchez is an advanced practice nurse who provides assessments and consultation for residents in a residential elder care facility. The facility supervisor requests a consult in regard to the results of a 12-month audit that indicated a total of 52 falls during that period. One of the suggestions the advance practice nurse includes is a critical review of the literature. Which type review will likely provide the best evidence for the examination of patient fall prevention measures?

   a. A systematic review
   b. A review of randomized controlled trials
   c. A review of phenomenologic studies
   d. A review of mixed methods studies

10. Tracey Shustan, RN, is asked by her nurse manager to serve on a committee charged with developing an evidence-based practice protocol for one of the unit's routine nursing procedures. As the committee begins to explore the issue, it becomes clear that little research has been conducted on this procedure. Tracey knows that when the body of research is limited, she needs to use other venues of information such as which of the following?

    a. Case studies
    b. Expert opinions
    c. Computer-assisted instructional programs
    d. There are no other sources; only research findings can be utilized for evidence-based practice.

Chapter 35

Teaching Future Holistic Nurses: Integration of Holistic and Quality Safety Education for Nurses (QSEN) Concepts

Cynthia C. Barrere

■ DEFINITIONS

Holistic nursing learning activities Learning activities in which students are encouraged to reflect on ways to interface nontraditional healing therapies with traditional medical therapies to help patients heal in mind, body, and spirit.

Quality safety education for nurses (QSEN) A project in which the overall goal is to meet the challenge of preparing future nurses who will have the knowledge, skills, and attitudes (KSAs) necessary to continuously improve the quality and safety of the healthcare systems within which they work.[1]

■ THEORY AND RESEARCH

1. The realization of the importance of holistic nursing as essential to effective nursing practice is increasing as demonstrated by the recognition of holistic nursing as a specialty by the American Nurses Association (ANA)[2] and the merging of the American Holistic Nurses Association and ANA scope and standards of practice. Despite this evidence supporting the need for nurses to provide high-quality, whole-person caring, room for improvement exists.[3]
2. Schools of nursing are encouraged to integrate holistic concepts and quality improvement into content in undergraduate curriculums.
   a. The revised 2008 *Essentials of Baccalaureate Education for Professional Nursing Practice* advocates the preparation of the baccalaureate graduate to practice from a holistic caring framework.[4]
   b. A National Nursing Advisory Board and the American Association of Colleges of Nursing, funded by the Robert Wood Johnson Foundation, developed six quality and safety education for nurses competencies: patient-focused care, teamwork–collaboration, informatics, safety, quality improvement, and evidence-based practice.[5,6]
   c. The Institute of Medicine (IOM) in its most recent 2010 report echoes the sentiments regarding new graduate nurse preparation.[3]
3. Holistic caring and QSEN competencies both emphasize compassionate and respectful care in a safe, healing environment. Students need to learn holistic nursing and quality safety as fundamental to practice.

■ PATIENT-FOCUSED CARE

1. QSEN highlights patient-focused care as one of the essential competencies for nursing and defines it as the "recognition of the patient or designee as the source of control and full partner in providing compassionate and coordinated care based on respect for a patient's preferences, values, and needs."[7]
2. Holistic nursing subscribes to a similar definition: "Patient-focused and family focused care actively involves patients and family members or significant others, as the patient desires, in the care process. This type of care provides services based on patient's needs."[8p503]
3. These definitions complement one another by demonstrating the blending of Eastern and Western schools of thought and

emphasizing the importance of patient empowerment to facilitate healing.

4. Nursing students at Quinnipiac University begin their initial junior clinical rotation at a long-term care or rehabilitation facility.

5. The course includes a reflective assignment that teaches students the power of caring as they learn how small acts of kindness lead to meaningful nurse–patient connections that are equally as important and, at times, more healing than medications or treatments.

6. A student nurse who learns how to use the whole self as an instrument of healing will likely be more sensitive to cues from others and make a profound healing difference in the lives of others.

7. An example of a successful reflective teaching/learning student activity can be found in Chapter 36 of *Holistic Nursing: A Handbook for Practice* (6th edition) in an exercise called Healing Others.

■ INFORMATICS

1. Nursing informatics is a more recently recognized competency for nursing that supports safe, patient-centered care.[9,10]
   a. Inclusion of informatics in an undergraduate nursing curriculum teaches students how to evaluate the quality of health-related websites and search electronic scientific databases.[11]
   b. The QSEN definition of informatics is "use information and technology to communicate, manage knowledge, mitigate error, and support decision making."[7]

2. Complementary and alternative modalities (CAM) therapies are often available in healthcare facilities.
   a. Nurses need to be knowledgeable of the more common CAM interventions and be able to locate information on modalities less often used.
   b. Nurses need to support or refute the use of a selected modality based on the evidence.
   c. Nursing students exposed to selected healthcare library resources and websites will gain comfort in accessing appropriate resources.

3. A description of an effective teaching/learning student activity can be found in Chapter 36 of *Holistic Nursing: A Handbook*

for Practice in an exercise called Complementary and Alternative Modalities and Older Individuals.

■ TEAMWORK–COLLABORATION

1. Teamwork and collaboration among interprofessionals are necessary for high-quality patient care, yet are challenging to achieve.[12,13]
   a. The QSEN definition of teamwork–collaboration is "function effectively within nursing and inter-professional teams, fostering open communication, mutual respect, and shared decision-making to achieve quality patient care."[7]
   b. From a holistic perspective, relationship-centered philosophies such as practitioner-to-practitioner relationships are a priority to enhance the creation of healing environments.[14]

2. Interprofessional education during preprofessional licensure education programs has been identified as one way to improve communication, collaboration, and trust after graduation.
   a. Nursing students find clinical simulation, a teaching/learning strategy in which students interact with a high-fidelity mannequin, an effective way to practice "performing in the moment" as they demonstrate psychomotor skills, therapeutic nurse–patient interaction, clinical reasoning, and caring.[15]
   b. Clinical simulation offers a wonderful opportunity for the practical application of teamwork and collaboration as well.
   c. Real-life clinical simulation scenarios provide nursing students and physician assistant (PA) students with actual opportunities to communicate and collaborate in much the same way they will work together in the future.
   d. Running a code is one common example where students have a chance to use teamwork as expected to occur in practice.
   e. A particularly instructive teaching moment often occurs spontaneously. Planned spontaneity to teach nursing and students from other health professions to work together on behalf of a patient can be built into a simulation scenario. Exhibit 36-1 in *Holistic Nursing:*

A Handbook for Practice provides an example of an interprofessional teamwork/collaboration clinical simulation scenario.

QUALITY IMPROVEMENT

1. Engaging nurses in quality improvement processes is critical to delivering excellent patient care.[16]
   a. In QSEN, the definition of quality improvement is "use data to monitor the outcomes of care processes and use improvement methods to design and test changes to continuously improve the quality and safety of health care systems."[7]
   b. A comparable definition from a holistic perspective is the use of reflective practice in the holistic caring process.[17,18] After the nurse reflects on the information, the nurse can make practice changes as necessary. An individual nurse can apply reflective techniques by thinking back to a specific patient situation to contemplate whether interventions were effective or ineffective and to consider how she or he might do things differently in the future. A group of nurses can also use reflective techniques by considering ways to improve care for a group of patients on an inpatient unit or in the community.
   c. Quality improvement (QI) and reflective practice dovetail with evidence-based practice when nurses examine ways to "do things better" by evaluating data and current research that leads to more effective nursing interventions.
2. Many nursing schools are enhancing QI content in undergraduate nursing curriculums to better prepare new nurses in practice for active participation in QI activities.[19]
3. A description of a clinical student teaching/learning activity can be found in Chapter 36 of *Holistic Nursing: A Handbook for Practice* in an exercise on quality improvement and reflective practice.

EVIDENCE-BASED PRACTICE

1. Nurses must embrace evidence-based practice (EBP) as the underpinning for nursing interventions to provide optimal patient care.[20]

2. The QSEN definition for EBP is "integrate best current evidence with clinical expertise and patient/family preferences and values for delivery of optimal health care."[7]
3. Holistic standards concur with this interpretation: "The conscientious use of the best available evidence combined with the clinician's expertise and judgment and the patient's preferences and values to arrive at the best decision that leads to quality outcomes."[21p34]
4. Creative teaching and learning activities for nursing students about EBP are intended to foster attitudes of understanding and appreciation of the importance of examining the literature and other appropriate information when making clinical decisions.[22]
5. EBP teaching/learning activities threaded through a number of nursing courses illustrate the strength of the evidence for the topic under discussion in classes.
6. To draw on students' prior knowledge and skills of reviewing the literature, a senior capstone evidence-based project can be assigned to teams of students in clinical as students examine the evidence behind procedures on their respective units. Intensive librarian support can be available for assistance with literature reviews.
7. An exemplar of a senior-level EBP teaching/learning activity can be found in Chapter 36 of *Holistic Nursing: A Handbook for Practice* in an exercise about team evidence-based practice projects.

SAFETY

1. Management commitment to a patient safety culture is crucial in keeping patients safe while healing takes place.[23]
2. QSEN defines the safety competency as that which "minimizes risk of harm to patients and providers through both system effectiveness and individual performance."[7]
3. Holistic healing occurs in many ways. The concept of safety is included in discussion of healing environments: "With both attention and intention, the environment can become one in which the client can feel safe and explore the dimensions of self in the healing moment."[24p730]
4. The literature documents that there are opportunities for improvement in patient safety curriculums in schools of nursing.[6,25]

5. A myriad of holistic patient safety teaching/learning activities is available on the QSEN website. These activities are highlighted for use in the classroom, lab, or clinical settings.[1]

6. An illustration of a safety teaching/learning activity can be found in Chapter 36 of *Holistic Nursing: Handbook for Practice* in an exercise called No Prescription Needed: Take Ma Huang and Call Me in the Morning.

7. Holistic quality and safety initiatives are a vital part of clinical nursing practice. Nursing students who graduate from schools in which holistic quality and safety learning activities are integrated throughout the curriculum are better prepared to join in improvement projects or suggest topics for improvement to enhance patient caring and healing.

■ NOTES

1. Quality and Safety Education for Nurses Institute. (n.d.). About QSEN. Retrieved from http://www.qsen.org

2. Mariano, C. (2006, December 14). Holistic nursing achieves ANA specialty status [Press release]. Retrieved from http://www.ahna.org/Home/NewsRoom/MostRecentPressReleases/mostyrecentpressreleases/tabid/2165/Default.aspx

3. Institute of Medicine. (2010). *The future of nursing: Leading change, advancing health.* Washington, DC: National Academies Press. Retrieved from http://www.iom.edu/Reports/2010/The-Future-of-Nursing-Leading-Change-Advancing-Health.aspx

4. American Association of Colleges of Nursing. (2008). *The essentials of baccalaureate education for professional nursing practice.* Washington, DC: Author.

5. Brady, D. S. (2011). Using quality safety education for nurses (QSEN) as a pedagogical structure for course redesign and content. *International Journal of Nursing Education Scholarship, 8,* 1–18.

6. Chenot, T. M., & Daniel, L. G. (2010). Frameworks for patient safety in the nursing curriculum. *Journal of Nursing Education, 49,* 559–568.

7. Quality and Safety Education for Nurses Institute. (n.d.). Competencies. Retrieved from http://qsen.org/competencies/

8. Moore, N., & Hanson, J. (2009). Relationship-centered care and healing initiative in a community hospital. In B. M. Dossey & L. Keegan (Eds.), *Holistic nursing: A handbook for practice* (5th ed., p. 503). Sudbury, MA: Jones and Bartlett.

9. Kleib, M., Sales, A. E., Liama, I., Andrea-Baylon, M., & Beaith, A. (2010). Continuing education in informatics among registered nurses in the United States in 2000. *Journal of Nursing Continuing Education, 41,* 329–336.

10. Murphy, J. (2010). Nursing informatics: The intersection of nursing, computer, and information services. *Nursing Economics, 28,* 204–207.

11. Jette, S., Tribble, D. S., Gagnon, J., & Mathieu, L. (2010). Nursing students' perceptions of their resources toward the development of competencies in nursing informatics. *Nurse Education Today, 30,* 742–746.

12. Rose, L. (2011). Interprofessional collaboration in the ICU: How to define? *Nursing in Critical Care, 16,* 5–10.

13. Miller, K.-L., Reeves, S., Zwarenstein, M., Beales, J. D., Kenaszchuk, C., & Conn, L. G. (2008). Nursing emotion work and interprofessional collaboration in general internal medicine wards: A qualitative study. *Journal of Advanced Nursing, 64,* 332–343.

14. Gaboury, I., Lapierre, M., Boon, H., & Moher, D. (2011). Interprofessional collaboration within integrated healthcare clinics through the lens of the relationship-centered care model. *Journal of Interprofessional Care, 25,* 124–130.

15. Cordeau, M. A. (2010). The lived experience of clinical simulation of novice nursing students. *International Journal for Human Caring, 14,* 8–14.

16. Albanese, M. P., Evans, D. A., Schantz, C. A., Bowen, M., Disbot, M., Moffa, J. S.,...Polomano, R. C. (2010). Engaging clinical nurses in quality and performance improvement activities. *Nursing Administration Quarterly, 34,* 226–245.

17. Beam, R. J., O'Brien, R. A., & Neal, M. (2010). Reflective practice enhances public health nurse implementation of nurse–family partnership. *Public Health Nursing, 27,* 131–139.

18. Lange, F. (2009). Nursing management of subarachnoid haemorrhage: A reflective case study. *British Journal of Neuroscience Nursing, 5,* 463–470.

19. Sullivan, D. T., Hirst, D., & Cronenwett, L. (2009). Assessing quality and safety competencies of graduating pre-licensure nursing students. *Nursing Outlook, 57,* 323–332.

20. Makic, M. B. F., VonRueden, K. T., Rauen, C. A., & Chadwick, J. (2011). Evidence-based practice habits: Putting more sacred cows out to pasture. *Critical Care Nurse, 31,* 38–61.

21. Melnyk, B. M., & Baldwin, C. M. (2009). Evidence-based practice. In B. M. Dossey & L. Keegan (Eds.), *Holistic nursing: A handbook for practice* (5th ed., p. 34). Sudbury, MA: Jones and Bartlett.

22. Smith-Strøm, H., & Nortvedt, M. W. (2008). Evaluation of evidence-based methods used to teach nursing students to critically appraise evidence. *Journal of Nursing Education, 47,* 372–375.

23. Feng, X. Q., Acord, L., Cheng, Y. J., Zeng, J. H., & Song, J. P. (2011). The relationship between

management safety commitment and patient safety culture. *International Nursing Review, 58,* 249–254.

24. McKivergin, M. (2009). The nurse as an instrument of healing. In B. M. Dossey & L. Keegan (Eds.), *Holistic nursing: A handbook for practice* (5th ed., p. 730). Sudbury, MA: Jones and Bartlett.

25. Smith, E. L., Cronenwett, L., & Sherwood, G. (2007). Current assessments of quality and safety education in nursing. *Nursing Outlook, 55,* 132–137.

STUDY QUESTIONS

Basic Level

1. Which of the following answer choices characterizes holistic caring and quality and safety education for nurses (QSEN)?
   a. Distinct caring concepts and not related to one another
   b. Distinct caring concepts and provide an evidence base for practice
   c. Closely aligned and complement one another
   d. Closely aligned yet can cause confusion

2. How is teaching nursing students about the quality improvement process best accomplished?
   a. Engaging them in a quality improvement project in their clinical area in which they need to assist with data collection
   b. Presenting a lecture on quality improvement and administering a test to validate what they learned
   c. Assigning them an article on quality improvement and giving them a quiz the next time they come to class
   d. Having students observe data collection, but not allowing them to participate in the process

3. What is evidence-based practice?
   a. The fundamental base for both holistic care interventions and quality care interventions
   b. The underpinning for quality care, but not necessary for providing holistic care
   c. Useful for holistic nursing practice, but not essential for quality care
   d. Rarely helpful when practicing holistic nursing

4. An instructor in an undergraduate nursing program wants to emphasize the incorporation of informatics in nursing practice in a teaching/learning activity that demonstrates holistic concepts and QSEN concepts. Which of the following teaching/learning activities would best demonstrate both concepts?
   a. Assign the students to work in groups of three to write a poem about healing.
   b. Discuss hospital infection rates and ask students to write an outline of the central line dressing change procedure.
   c. Using the electronic medical record in lab, have students document how they empowered a patient in preparation for discharge.
   d. Ask students to collaborate with the dietician on their clinical unit to develop a teaching plan for their assigned patient.

5. To maintain a culture of holistic safety, during medication reconciliation for patients taking enteric-coated medications prior to discharge from the hospital, which statement by the nurse is important to review?
   a. "Swallow this medication whole, do not chew it."
   b. "Avoid taking this medication with water."
   c. "Lie down after taking this medication."
   d. "This medication is likely to irritate your stomach."

Advanced Level

6. The patient has been informed by his clinician that he has type 2 diabetes and needs to begin oral diabetic medications and lose 100 pounds. When the nurse enters the patient's room a few minutes after the clinician leaves, the patient is visibly upset, stating that he cannot lose weight, that he has tried many times before and nothing works. Which of the following actions by the nurse best demonstrates the holistic patient-focused care needed at this time?
   a. Contacting the dietician to teach the patient healthy food choices
   b. Reassuring the patient that his clinician knows best
   c. Teaching the patient about his oral diabetic medications
   d. Being present with the patient as he expresses his feelings and concerns

7. Mr. Finch, an 80-year-old patient, is transferred to a rehabilitation unit after hospitalization for a total joint replacement a week ago. He has type 2 diabetes managed with diet and oral medication. Which of the following demonstrates a collaborative intervention?
   a. The nurse reviews the medical record admission orders, history, and plan of care.
   b. The dietician makes an appointment to interview Mr. Finch about his knowledge of diabetic meal planning later in the afternoon.
   c. The nurse and physical therapist both plan to work with Mr. Finch.
   d. The nurse and physical therapist assist Mr. Finch to safely get out of bed to the chair.

8. A 20-year-old Hispanic male patient is admitted for uncontrolled diabetes resulting from nonadherence to his meal plan and insulin regimen plan at home. A nurse is planning a session with the patient to review this issue and reinforce information as needed to help him maintain glucose levels within normal limits. Prior to the session, which holistic patient-focused care intervention is likely to assist in helping this patient better adhere to an effective treatment regimen?
   a. Provide instructions in the patient's language.
   b. Make sure written materials are in large font.
   c. Give instructions to a family member instead.
   d. Provide the information to the patient's girlfriend.

9. Mrs. Collins, a 75-year-old patient with pancreatic cancer, was just informed by her oncologist that her cancer advanced, there are no more treatment options, and a referral to the hospice program is suggested. Maria, her nurse, is with Mrs. Collins when the oncologist informs her of this news. Knowing that Mrs. Collins is upset, Maria remains with her a while. What response might Maria use that demonstrates holistic patient-focused care when Mrs. Collins asks: "Why is this happening?"
   a. Explain why the cancer advanced in her body using terms Mrs. Collins can understand.
   b. Respond with: "I don't know. I wish I had the answer for you," and remain present with her.
   c. Say: "This is difficult for me to discuss. Let's talk about something more pleasant."
   d. State: "I am not sure, but I know how you feel." Then proceed to share with Mrs. Collins how she felt when her aunt passed away.

10. A nurse working on a medical unit observes that the number of patient falls has increased over the past 3 months. She is concerned about the holistic patient safety culture on her unit. What would be an appropriate next step this nurse might take?
    a. Insist that the nurses and patient care technicians make hourly rounds on all of the patients.
    b. Be sure that patients identified as high risk for falls have a notation about this status in the health record.
    c. Review the health records of the patients who fell over the past 3 months to discern any patterns regarding their falls.
    d. Speak with the patients currently identified as high risk for falls on the unit and elicit the fall prevention measures they are taking.

Chapter 36

The Nurse as an Instrument of Healing

Deborah McElligott

◼ DEFINITIONS

Healing A positive, subjective, unpredictable process involving transformation to a new sense of wholeness, spiritual transcendence, and reinterpretation of life.[1] Healing involves the process of the right relationships forming on any or all levels of the human experience—a goal of holistic nursing.[2]

Health The actualization of inherent and acquired human potential through goal-directed behavior, competent self-care, and satisfying relationships with others, while adjustments are made as needed to maintain structural integrity and harmony with relevant environments; a process of being and becoming an integrated and whole person.[3]

Health promotion Described by Pender as the effort or activity to increase well-being and actualize human health potential.

Inner wisdom The innate inner knowledge or knowing that one can access through meditation, mindfulness, and other methods that connect to the subconscious.

Intuition Sudden insight or knowing without the perceived use of logic or analysis. Often called a right brain activity, intuition can be enhanced through the senses and is often used to guide integrative treatments including energy work.[4]

Self-care The practice of engaging in health-related activities, using health-promoting, desired behaviors to adopt a healthier lifestyle and enhance wellness; activities individuals initiate and perform to maintain life, health, and well-being.

Self-care plan A plan developed with a goal of actualizing behaviors and actions to promote one's health, wellness, and healing.

Transpersonal caring A caring presence where the nurse acknowledges and appreciates the total body, mind, and spirit connection between each interaction with self and others. The relationships occur on sacred ground, and both the nurse and client become part of something larger than themselves. This is the embodiment of the nurse as an instrument of healing.[5]

◼ THEORY AND RESEARCH

1. The American Holistic Nurses Association (AHNA) supports self-care, grounded in nursing theory, in its evidence-based *Scope and Standards of Practice*.[6]
   a. According to the AHNA, self-care translates into the knowledge, skills, presence, and attitude of holistic nurses, involving a lifelong process of education, practice, and self work.
   b. To become an instrument of healing, the nurse identifies at-risk patterns; recognizes the individual capacity to heal; creates a conscious awareness and understanding of his or her purpose, meaning, and connection with a greater being/force; develops an understanding that crisis creates opportunity as he or she continually evolves.

2. Although thousands of years of anecdotal data support many modalities, research is evolving to support practices such as energy work, acupuncture, imagery, and body work that can be used in assessment, treatment, and promotion of self-care and wellness.

3. Healing paradigms supporting self-care include whole medical systems, both ancient and modern. These systems focus on balancing, healing, partnering with, and coaching to reach the person's potential. Examples of such systems include:
   a. Traditional systems such as traditional Chinese medicine (TCM), Ayurvedic medicine, and Shamanism.
   b. Modern systems such as homeopathy, naturopathy, chiropractic, and functional medicine.

■ INTERNATIONAL AND NATIONAL TRENDS

1. International agendas
   a. Partnership of the United Nations with the World Health Organization formed the Eight Millennium Development Goals, focusing on global health problems and an aim to improve well-being by 2015 in eight different areas.[7]
   b. Millennium Goals are to eradicate extreme poverty and hunger, achieve universal primary education, promote gender equality and empower women, reduce child mortality, improve mental health, combat HIV/AIDS, ensure environmental sustainability, develop global partnerships.

2. National agendas
   a. Since 1979, one goal of the U.S. Surgeon General's office has been to develop a healthy and fit nation.[8]
   b. National Prevention and Health Promotion Strategy: A document addressing the need for healthy foods, clean air and water, and safe worksites in the United States.
   c. Healthy People 2020 offers a vision of a society where everyone lives long, healthy lives. Goals of Healthy People 2020 include:
      ■ To "promote quality of life, healthy development and healthy behaviors across all life stages."

■ To focus on quality of life (QOL), conceptualized as well-being, and described as thriving and flourishing;
■ Assessment of QOL may occur through happiness and life satisfaction tools.
■ Recommendations for the National agenda include areas of self-care: healthy behaviors, healthy physical environment, healthy social environment, positive mental health, responsible sexual behavior, and avoidance of tobacco use; a focus on nutrition, physical activity, and stress management across the life span of the population, from childhood to senior years.[9]

■ NURSING THEORY

1. Grand nursing theories such as Roger's Science of Unitary Human Beings, Watson's Theory of Human Science and Human Care, Dossey's Theory of Integral Nursing, and Orem's Self-Care Deficit Nursing Theory individually and collectively support the concept of self-care and the caring process. They support the nurse as an instrument of healing as they:
   a. Direct and define assessment on both physical and energetic levels, supporting the concept of being as opposed to doing.
   b. Support the concepts of reflection, presence, therapeutic relationships, holistic communication, and healing environments.
   c. Support nursing education and research to honor therapeutic presence, intuition, caring science, and the integral role of the nurse.
   d. Support an individual's goals based on the situation, culture, beliefs, and capabilities.
   e. Support the concept of coaching, involving holding the space for an individual's inner wisdom to unfold and guide the development of a personal wellness plan.
   f. Align with other disciplines to support integrative practice grounded in research.

2. Midrange theories such as the Health Promotion Model (HPM) combine perspectives

from nursing and behavioral sciences, integrating factors that can influence health behaviors.[10] In the Health Promotion Model:

a. Nurses identify interpersonal influences, interventions for health behavior change, and individual needs in tailoring the path to reach the necessary and desired changes.

b. This model guides data collection, processing, nursing activities, and possible client outcomes.

c. The motivation for behavior is wellness, not fear.

d. The goal is to expand health potential, not prevent disease.

e. Health is influenced by multidimensional factors.

d. Health is viewed as greater than the absence of disease.

e. The client is an active partner, expressing a unique health potential, assessing competencies, using goal-directed behavior, self-care, satisfying relationships, spiritual wellness, and harmony/balance within the self and with the environment.

f. Health is often viewed as one end of a continuum and a fluid balance of the body, mind, and spirit within and with the environment.

g. A focus on health involves treating minor symptoms, adjusting lifestyle as needed, and discovering the cause, which prevents further imbalances.

■ CONCEPTS RELATED TO SELF-CARE

1. Concept of health
   a. Health can be defined from various perspectives: the absence of illness; the capacity to adapt; the ability to fulfill a role; the ability to incorporate the importance of wholeness, peacefulness, and meaningfulness.[11]
   b. Pender describes health as the actualization of inherent and acquired human potential through goal-directed behavior, competent self-care, and satisfying relationships with others, while adjusting to maintain integrity and harmony with relevant environments.[3]

c. Optimal health is viewed as a dynamic balance of all aspects of the whole person—physical, emotional, social, and spiritual.

2. Concept of health promotion
   a. Health promotion, the effort or activity adopted to achieve health, is centered on self-care and can be applied to an individual or family, community, or society.
   b. Health promotion includes behavior motivated by the desire to increase well-being, a value for growth in positive directions, a desire for balance, and to regulate personal behaviors.
   c. A focus on health can lead to improved health because risks are assessed and interventions are suggested to change perceptions, decrease barriers, gather support, and improve health-promoting behaviors.
   d. Evaluating, addressing, and incorporating health-promoting behaviors into daily activities creates a lifestyle representing self-care or self-management of health promotion.
   e. Measurements of health promotion include the Health-Promoting Lifestyle Profile Tool (HPLPII), which identifies six behaviors or subscales to measure: interpersonal relations, nutrition, health responsibility, physical activity, stress management, and spiritual growth.[12]

3. Concept of self-care
   a. Self-care directly relates to health promotion and self-responsibility.
   b. Orem describes self-care as the "practice of activities that individuals initiate and perform on their own behalf in maintaining life, health and well-being."[13]
   c. Self-care involves deliberate action (one maintains health and recognizes and treats symptoms).
   d. Self-care is a learned behavior, naturally culturally specific and necessitating individualization of recommendations for activities.
   e. Self-care is dynamic in nature—traditionally focused on body, mind, and spirit, seeking to rebalance the system when imbalances occur.
   f. Statistics highlight the number of chronic diseases that can be prevented,

modified, or eradicated by healthier lifestyles.

g. Self-care can be motivated by suffering, discord, or imbalances in the person's system, such as a newly diagnosed disease or disorder.

h. Self-care can be operationalized through the examination of health-promoting behaviors as listed on various wellness instruments such as the HPLP II or the Integrative Health and Wellness Assessment (IHWA) tool.[4]

i. Educational efforts to support self-care include overall health assessment, goal setting, skill building, experiential activity, demonstration, and opportunities for feedback.

j. Coaching is expanding as one method of enhancing self-care and supports the individual as a partner in wellness efforts.

k. Self-care plans are often used to list specific, measurable, achievable goals for both the short and long term.

l. Self-care goals are based on the individual's inner knowledge, current assessment, and priorities.

4. Concept of healing: Aspects of healing, the goal of nursing care, have been widely discussed.

a. Healing can be defined as a positive, subjective, unpredictable process involving a transformation to a new sense of wholeness, spiritual transcendence, and reinterpretation of life.[1]

b. Quinn sums up healing as the development of a right relationship.[2]

c. Concept analysis can be used to understand healing. This includes the examination of the antecedents, mediators, attributes, and consequences of healing.

d. Antecedents are factors that occur before healing is initiated. One antecedent is suffering, a relentless threat or a severe state of distress that can occur on many levels including physical, emotional, spiritual, and social. Suffering is a subjective experience; an individual's perception of suffering warrants attention no matter how it appears to others—if it is perceived, we honor it as real.[14]

e. Mediators in healing can be internal or external and can involve traits of the patient or traits of the environment and the nurse.. These traits influence the degree to which the individual accepts and participates in the transpersonal caring process. The nurse, through transpersonal caring, becomes the healing environment as a caring moment is created, and both the nurse and the patient are changed.

f. Attributes of healing include subjective, positive process, transformation to wholeness, a spiritual transcendence, and reinterpretation of life.

g. Consequences of healing include feelings of serenity, a sense of interconnectedness, gratitude, new meaning, purpose, and peace.

h. To assist in the healing process, nurses can partner with clients to enhance self-responsibility and self-care, motivation and skill development.

i. Clients can be supported through modeling, memory, and perspective. Modeling brings intention, education, and reassurance to the relationship; memory identifies internal resources; perspective models acceptance and supports change.[15]

j. The role of the nurse varies, moving from one of support to becoming a bystander as the person gains a new relational system. The patient is not passive and control of the healing is not in the nurse's hands.

■ SELF-CARE IN NURSES

1. The need for self-care in nurses is recognized because there are more than 15 million nurses globally. Nurses form the largest group of employees in hospitals, yet the profession is projected to have a shortage of more than a million by 2020.

2. Nightingale highlighted the need for self-care in nurses. In fact, Nightingale's legacy:

a. Emphasizes the need for nurses to focus on self-care.

b. Emphasizes the need for the care and support of other nurses (the *esprit de corps*).

c. Emphasizes the need for care of the environment.

d. Discusses the need for environments to support healing.

e. Highlights spiritual self-care in letters directing nurses to develop a sacred space for reflection, gain support from a Being greater than themselves, and to see that reflection in each and every person.[16]

3. Research studies have identified the need for self-care in nursing, citing the following:

a. Nurses often neglect their own care with study results on nurses' actual health status and health-promoting behaviors ranging from good general overall health ratings to overall poor health-promoting behaviors on standardized tools.[17]

b. Poor behaviors include poor diet, lack of physical activity, obesity, stress, and compassion fatigue.

c. Poor health-promoting behaviors are linked to stress, illness, increased health-care costs, obesity, job turnover, errors, and poor-quality care.

d. From a business perspective, promoting health in nurses and their work environment can decrease the cost of turnover, disability, and employer health care and improve quality of care.[18]

4. Process of self-care

a. The core value of self-care includes self-reflection and self-assessment.

b. Assessment includes the identification of patterns that put one at risk for disease and imbalances. Both internal and external risks can exist including toxic living or working environments; using tobacco, unnecessary drugs, and alcohol; working long hours; experiencing stress; lack of sleep; lack of physical activity; poor eating habits—undereating/overeating.

c. The nurse must recognize and believe in his or her own innate healing ability, realizing the power of emotions, thoughts, and practices to influence the body-mind-spirit.

d. Reflective practices that enhance self-care are developed and incorporated into a daily lifestyle with a goal of reaching the greatest potential of one's health.

e. Self-evaluation is ongoing and identifies areas of strength as well as those needing further development.

5. Nursing presence

6. To provide meaningful care nurses must be able to be present and resonate positive feelings such as love and appreciation. Because nursing is a calling and healing is the essence of nursing, healing and self-care must be a central core of every nurse's life. This necessitates nursing knowledge, skills, and caring and includes the following:

a. Consciousness toward one's purpose—a powerful component of self-care, guiding one from daily to lifelong living

b. Development of meaning in one's life (directly related to connection to a force greater than oneself)

c. Viewing change as part of the joy of living, where opportunity can arise from crisis

d. Enhancing the skills of reflection, presence, therapeutic relationship, and communication

e. Developing a lifestyle building resilience through meditative practices, healthy nutrition, exercise, supportive relationships, and ongoing assessment

f. Self-compassion skills: balancing compassion ("opening the heart to suffering") with equanimity ("the state of being nonpartial")[19]

■ SELF-CARE IN THE WORKPLACE

1. Nurses can align their institutional values with the core values of the American Holistic Nurses Association and use nursing theory to guide and evaluate holistic programs focusing on self-care and health promotion.

2. Nurses can partner with national agendas and harness data, such as one Institute of Medicine (IOM) report— poor communication and lack of teamwork contributes to workplace errors—for support.[20]

3. Nurses can lead the opportunity to create workplace goals to increase well-being and actualize human health potential for staff through the use of processes such as nurse coaching.

a. The nurse coaching process involves six steps (may occur simultaneously): establish relationship & readiness for change; identify opportunities and issues; assist client to establish goals; structure the coaching interaction; empower client to reach goals; assist client to determine the level of goal achievement. [4]

4. Nurses can assist in self-assessment through:
   a. Identifications of perceived barriers to health promotion, including stressors, both individual and group. Examples include excessive work demands, injustices, unsafe work environments, lack of time, lack of education regarding healing strategies, and lack of social support.[18]
   b. Identification of the benefits of health promotion activities.
   c. Identification of situational influences on health behaviors.

5. Because obstacles to self-care can be unique to different areas of nursing, generic recommendations for workplace wellness might include the following:
   a. Individual and team assessment using wellness tools and the development of individual/team/unit wellness goals
   b. Development of group wellness plans and opportunities
   c. Identification of themes that cross units and services that might require institutional changes or programs (onsite gym, meditation room, walking path, wellness clinic)

6. Recommendations for successful worksite programs include the following:
   a. The use of appreciative inquiry (a positive approach to transformative change with focus on clients' strengths) to assist with change
   b. Decreasing perceived barriers to health promotion
   c. Providing convenient time and location for interventions
   d. Encouraging a holistic approach to wellness
   e. Considering employee preferences
   f. Strengthening social and peer support
   g. Supporting structured periods/places to support mindfulness and reflective practice
   h. Creating healing environments
   i. Offering healthy choices for onsite food

7. Effects of supporting self-care in the workplace:
   a. Increased health-promoting behaviors and health benefits
   b. Increased quality of life
   c. Decreased health expenditures
   d. Increase in work team productivity
   e. Increased quality of care

■ SELF-CARE USING THE HOLISTIC CARING PROCESS

1. A focus on self-care does not need to be an independent, lonely process.

2. As clients are partnering with holistic nurses and other integrative practitioners to improve self-care they are often involved in the transpersonal caring process. Transpersonal caring involves moving toward a higher sense of self and harmony with the body, mind, and soul. In transpersonal caring relationships, the nurse has a moral commitment to human dignity, the intent and will to affirm the subjective significance of others, the ability to detect feelings, and the ability to feel a union with another and the nurse's own history.[5]

3. Numerous self-care practices enhance whole-person healing and can include the following:
   a. Healthy nutrition, regular exercise, reflective/meditative practices, relaxation, spirituality, music, art, energy healing, bodywork, imagery, affirmations, aromatherapy, journaling, storytelling, yoga, tai chi
   b. The development of a therapeutic relationship with a practitioner who can assist one in holistic assessment and treatments, as needed, involving whole-person healing

4. The holistic caring process includes the following:
   a. Holistic assessment is ongoing and nourished by the centering of the practitioner, development of the relationship with the client, and the deep listening of the story, which includes the assessment of a readiness to change.
   b. Nursing diagnosis becomes the analysis or interpretation of the information by both the client and practitioner. Incorporation of both Western and traditional assessment methods and patterns can be used to determine areas of focus.
   c. Identification of patterns/challenges/needs allows the person to assess strengths and prior success as well as

identify support systems and potential threats to a successful self-care plan.

d. Outcome identification or goals are driven by the self but can be fostered by the discussion with the holistic nurse and the development of a self-care plan that is clear, action-oriented, realistic, and time-lined.

e. The implementation of the therapeutic care plan involves the actual behaviors by both the client and the nurse as determined by the plan.

f. Evaluation is primarily done by the individual and involves his or her perception of self-care goals attained, as well as next steps.[4]

COACHING THE CORE VALUE OF SELF-CARE FOR PATIENTS AND COMMUNITY

1. Whether coaching the individual or group, the nurse can use the six-step process, described by Hess, to enhance self-care:[21]
   a. Establish relationship and assess client readiness for change.
   b. Identify opportunities and issues.
   c. Assist client to establish goals according to his or her priorities.
   d. Structure the interaction.
   e. Empower client to reach goals.
   f. Assist client to evaluate goals.
2. Nursing actions include the following:
   a. Centering and holding the space for the client, creating a safe space
   b. Asking the right questions
   c. Considering health literacy and cultural diversity
   d. Focusing on positive individual traits
   e. Fostering realistic, measurable, and sustainable goals
3. Partner with individuals and communities to develop self-care programs.
   a. Identify at-risk populations and support the need with research, needs assessments for your area of interest.
   b. Identify interested groups, seeking community, including faith-based community, support.
   c. Align with local healthcare institutions or governmental programs.
   d. Use coaching skills to assess, inspire, and maintain change.

e. Identify champions to align with to present at community events.
f. Write short articles for local papers.
g. Use the power of technology, Internet, and websites.

4. Use holistic principles and concepts such as improving one "part of the whole" enhances other "parts," just as caring for one family member in some way affects the whole family.
5. Possible talking points for the community—use simple assessment questions such as:
   a. For body/physical wellness: How is/are your...sleep, nutrition, exercise (aerobic, strength, flexibility), habits, physical exams/screenings, home and work environments?
   b. For mind/emotional wellness: Have you ever tried...affirmations, appreciative inquiry, breath work, meditation, being creative, use of imagination, learning something new, cognitive therapy, self-reflection, journaling, humor, relaxation, open communication, or stress management?
   c. For spirit/social wellness: How are your relationships with family and friends? Do you give and feel love and appreciation? What gives your life meaning? Do you feel connected to something greater as well as to others? Can you forgive? Do you use your intuition, laughter, play? Do you have a sense of community?

SUPPORTING THE CORE VALUE OF SELF-CARE FOR THE ENVIRONMENT

1. As holistic nurses practice self-care, attention to the environment is a natural progression.
2. Research highlights several concerns when caring for the environment and self including the following:
   a. Chemical pollutants, radiation, noise, pollution
   b. The effects of technology (for example, cell phone usage), and the relationships to health and illness
   c. Ways to conserve and protect our planet and natural resources, including water and energy

3. Strategies for healing environments can include the following:
   a. Soothing sounds and nature scenes
   b. Aromatherapy—ensuring cautions, indications, and contraindications are reviewed
   c. The creation of a sacred space in one's home and workplace
   d. Go-Green efforts such as recycling, buying organic when possible, avoiding foods with added chemicals and artificial coloring, prudent energy use, and partnering with community activists to increase safeguarding of the environment

■ CONCLUSION

1. Nursing care begins with self-care, a practice underutilized in the nursing workforce.
2. The core values of holistic nursing provide a structure to support self-care and a mandate to practice.
3. As nurses focus on self-care and model caring behaviors in the workplace, patient care can be enhanced.
4. A lifelong practice of reflection, self-awareness, and self-care supports the nurse in the role of an instrument of healing.

■ NOTES

1. McElligott, D. (2010). Healing: From concept to nursing practice. *Journal of Holistic Nursing, 28*(4), 251–259.
2. Quinn, J. F. (2000). The self as healer: Reflections from a nurse's journey. *AACN Clinical Issues, 11*(1), 17–26.
3. Pender, N., Murdaugh, C., & Parsons, M. (2006). *Health promotion in nursing practice* (5th ed.). Upper Saddle River, NJ: Prentice Hall.
4. Dossey, B. M., Keegan, L., & Guzzetta, C. (2009). *Holistic nursing: A handbook for practice* (5th ed.). Sudbury, MA: Jones and Bartlett.
5. Watson, J. (2005). *Caring science as sacred science*. Philadelphia, PA: F. A. Davis.
6. American Holistic Nurses Association, American Nurses Association. (2007). *Holistic nursing: Scope and standards of practice*. Silver Spring, MD: Nursebooks.org.
7. World Health Organization. (n.d.). Millennium Developmental Goals (MDGs). Retrieved from http://www.who.int/topics/millennium_development_goals/about/en/index.html
8. U.S. Department of Health and Human Services. (2010, January). *The surgeon general's vision for a healthy and fit nation*. Rockville, MD: U.S. Department of Health and Human Services, Office of the Surgeon General.
9. Institute of Medicine. (2011). *Leading health indicators for Healthy People 2020; letter report*. Washington, DC: National Academy Press.
10. Peterson, S., & Bredow, T. (2004). *Middle range theories: Application to nursing research*. Philadelphia, PA: Lippincott Williams & Wilkin.
11. Smith, J. (1981). The idea of health: A philosophical inquiry. *Advanced Nursing Science, 3*(3), 43–50.
12. Walker, S. N., & Hill-Polrecky, D. (1996). Psychometric evaluation of the Health Promoting Lifestyle Profile II. In *Proceedings of the 1996 scientific session of the American Nurse Association's Council of Nurse Researchers*. Washington, DC: American Nurses Foundation.
13. Orem, D. (2001). *Nursing: Concepts of practice* (6th ed.). St. Louis, MO: Mosby.
14. Egnew, T. (2009). Suffering, meaning and healing: Challenges of contemporary medicine. *Annals of Family Medicine, 7*(2), 170–175.
15. Bolles, S., & Maley, M. (2004). Designing relational models of collaborative integrative medicine that support healing processes. *Journal of Alternative and Complementary Medicine, 10*, S61–S69.
16. Dossey, B. M., Selanders, L., Beck, D. M., & Attewell, A. (2005). *Florence Nightingale today: Healing leadership global action*. Silver Spring, MD: American Nurses Association.
17. McElligott, D., Siemers, S., & Thomas, L. (2009). Nursing wellness: Is there a healthy nurse in the house? *Applied Nursing Research, 22*(3), 211–215.
18. McElligott, D., Capitulo, K., Morris, D., & Click, E. (2010). The effect of a holistic intervention on the health promoting behaviors of registered nurses (CNE activity). *Journal of Holistic Nursing, 28*(3), 174–186.
19. Halifax, J. (2009). *Being with dying*. Boston, MA: Shambhala.
20. Institute of Medicine. (2003). *Keeping patients safe: Transforming the work environment of nurses*. Retrieved from http://www.iom.edu/Reports/2003/Keeping-Patients-Safe-Transforming-the-Work-Environment-of-Nurses.aspx
21. Hess, D., Bark, L. A., & Southard, M. E. (2012). Holistic nurse coaching. Retrieved from http://www.ahncc.org/images/HessWhite_Paper_Holistic_Nurse_Coaching.pdf

■ STUDY QUESTIONS

Basic Level

1. Which of the following answer choices has a focus on the following agenda: to eradicate extreme poverty and hunger, achieve universal primary education, promote gender equality and empower women, reduce child mortality, improve mental health, combat HIV/AIDS, and ensure environmental sustainability?
   a. National Health Care Agenda
   b. IOM report
   c. WHO Millennium Goals
   d. Healthy People 2020

2. The effort or activity adopted to achieve health centered on self-care that can be applied to an individual, family, or community is best described as which of the following?
   a. Healing
   b. Counseling
   c. Health promotion
   d. Self-assessment

3. Which of the following answer choices characterizes the Health Promotion Model as a midrange theory?
   a. It is motivated by disease and illness.
   b. It is used only for self-care in nurses and healthcare workers.
   c. It is focused on expanding health potential.
   d. It cannot be measured.

4. Which of the following supports the need for self-care in healthcare workers?
   a. Union contracts
   b. State law
   c. IOM report
   d. National healthcare workers legislation

5. A positive, subjective, unpredictable process involving a transformation to a new sense of wholeness, spiritual transcendence, and a reinterpretation of life can be described as which of the following?
   a. Healing
   b. Health promotion
   c. Wellness
   d. Self-care

Advanced Level

6. Which of the following best describes an example of nursing presence?
   a. The nurse sitting facing the patient
   b. The use of eye-to-eye contact
   c. The use of an interpreter to assist with communication when a patient has another primary language
   d. The nurse centering prior to walking into a patient's room

7. What are the benefits in the workplace of improved self-care?
   a. Increased quality of life, increased work team productivity, and increased quality of care
   b. Increased number of nurses and improved healthcare benefits
   c. No need for managers
   d. The attraction of predominantly younger nurses with better education

8. What are common nursing workplace stressors identified in the literature?
   a. Salary, hospital regulations
   b. Traffic, parking
   c. Need for continuing education, working holidays
   d. Lack of time, work demands

9. Transpersonal human caring relates to self-care because it involves which of the following?
   a. Six stages of assessment
   b. A primary focus on the needs of others
   c. An acknowledgment and appreciation of the total body, mind, and spirit connection between each interaction with self and others
   d. A focus on the individual journey of the person without regard to the environment surrounding him or her

10. When nursing actions include centering and holding the space for the client, asking the right questions, a focus on positive individual traits, and fostering realistic, measurable, and sustainable goals, they are reflecting which of the following?
    a. Self-care
    b. Nurse coaching
    c. Appreciative inquiry
    d. Self-assessment

Reflections

Pause for a moment...*While studying for HN-BC, HNB-BC, or AHN-BC certification, remember to pause periodically, take some deep breaths, and reflect on your efforts to succeed. We suggest that you read a reflection after each chapter to mindfully relax, renew and refocus...then continue on with your review.*

I am studying the *AHNA Core Curriculum for Holistic Nursing* to enhance my ability to enunciate the knowledge base for holistic nursing.

I am studying the *AHNA Core Curriculum for Holistic Nursing* to accomplish by personal goal of successfully completing the HN-BC, HNB-BC, or AHN-BC holistic nursing certification exam at the appropriate basic or advanced level for me.

I am proud of the goal that I have set for myself to earn the distinction of excellence in the area of holistic nursing.

I will study in a quiet environment, I will commit to a study plan with specific times and dates, and I will assemble all the materials that I need to study: this *Core Curriculum* and other references suggested by AHNCC located at www.ahncc.org .

I know the content areas where I am strong and those where I need more study time.

I can visualize complete success in the holistic nursing certification process (HN-BC, HNB-BC, or AHN-BC)

I give myself positive affirmations and feedback.

I become aware of my breathing...my inbreath and outbreath are balanced...as I stay with my breathing, I find a deeper place of inner peace.

I watch my belly rise and fall with the rhythm of my relaxed breathing. This balanced breathing helps me in my work and life.

I am using my distraction techniques: anytime that worry or fear comes into my mind, I will let go of the anxiety; if a thought of failure comes to my mind, I take a deep breath and with the next exhalation, I let that worry flow out.

I am eating nourishing food and will do so before the HN-BC, HNB-BC, or AHN-BC examination Complex carbohydrate foods will provide me with the most energy. I am avoiding excessive use of caffeine or sugar and will continue to do so before the examination.

I am relaxed and at ease and will arrive at the HN-BC, HNB-BC, or AHN-BC examination in this same relaxed state—this will enhance my success.

Answer Key

Chapter 1

Basic Level

1. Correct answer: B
2. Correct answer: D
3. Correct answer: D
4. Correct answer: B
5. Correct answer: A

Advanced Level

6. Correct answer: B
7. Correct answer: C
8. Correct answer: D
9. Correct answer: C
10. Correct answer: B

Chapter 2

Basic Level

1. Correct answer: B
2. Correct answer: C
3. Correct answer: B
4. Correct answer: A
5. Correct answer: A

Advanced Level

6. Correct answer: C
7. Correct answer: B
8. Correct answer: A
9. Correct answer: D
10. Correct answer: A

Chapter 3

Basic Level

1. Correct answer: D
2. Correct answer: B
3. Correct answer: B
4. Correct answer: B

Advanced Level

5. Correct answer: C
6. Correct answer: A
7. Correct answer: C
8. Correct answer: B

Chapter 4

Basic Level

1. Correct answer: C
2. Correct answer: D
3. Correct answer: D
4. Correct answer: A
5. Correct answer: A
6. Correct answer: B
7. Correct answer: C
8. Correct answer: A
9. Correct answer: B
10. Correct answer: D

Chapter 5

Basic Level

1. Correct answer: A
2. Correct answer: C
3. Correct answer: D
4. Correct answer: D
5. Correct answer: A

Advanced Level

6. Correct answer: D
7. Correct answer: A
8. Correct answer: C
9. Correct answer: D
10. Correct answer: B

Chapter 6
Basic Level
1. Correct answer: B
2. Correct answer: C
3. Correct answer: A
4. Correct answer: C
5. Correct answer: B

Advanced Level
6. Correct answer: D
7. Correct answer: A
8. Correct answer: C
9. Correct answer: D
10. Correct answer: B

Chapter 7
Basic Level
1. Correct answer: B
2. Correct answer: E
3. Correct answer: B
4. Correct answer: D
5. Correct answer: C

Advanced Level
6. Correct answer: B
7. Correct answer: D
8. Correct answer: A
9. Correct answer: C
10. Correct answer: D

Chapter 8
Basic Level
1. Correct answer: D
2. Correct answer: B
3. Correct answer: A
4. Correct answer: A
5. Correct answer: D

Advanced Level
6. Correct answer: C
7. Correct answer: D
8. Correct answer: A
9. Correct answer: B
10. Correct answer: A

Chapter 9
Basic Level
1. Correct answer: B
2. Correct answer: A
3. Correct answer: D
4. Correct answer: C
5. Correct answer: C

Advanced Level
6. Correct answer: A
7. Correct answer: C
8. Correct answer: B
9. Correct answer: D
10. Correct answer: C

Chapter 10
Basic Level
1. Correct answer: B
2. Correct answer: C
3. Correct answer: B
4. Correct answer: B
5. Correct answer: C
6. Correct answer: D

Advanced Level
7. Correct answer: C
8. Correct answer: D
9. Correct answer: A
10. Correct answer: C
11. Correct answer: B

Chapter 11
Basic Level
1. Correct answer: D
2. Correct answer: B
3. Correct answer: B
4. Correct answer: D
5. Correct answer: D

Advanced Level
6. Correct answer: C
7. Correct answer: B
8. Correct answer: A
9. Correct answer: A
10. Correct answer: A

Chapter 12
Basic Level
1. Correct answer: C
2. Correct answer: B
3. Correct answer: A
4. Correct answer: A
5. Correct answer: D

Advanced Level
6. Correct answer: A
7. Correct answer: B
8. Correct answer: A
9. Correct answer: C
10. Correct answer: B
11. Correct answer: C
12. Correct answer: D

Chapter 13
Basic Level
1. Correct answer: D
2. Correct answer: B
3. Correct answer: D
4. Correct answer: C
5. Correct answer: B

Advanced Level
6. Correct answer: B
7. Correct answer: B
8. Correct answer: D
9. Correct answer: C
10. Correct answer: A

Chapter 14
Basic Level
1. Correct answer: D
2. Correct answer: D
3. Correct answer: D
4. Correct answer: D
5. Correct answer: A
6. Correct answer: D

Advanced Level
7. Correct answer: D
8. Correct answer: C
9. Correct answer: C
10. Correct answer: D

Chapter 15
Basic Level
1. Correct answer: D
2. Correct answer: C
3. Correct answer: A
4. Correct answer: B
5. Correct answer: D

Advanced Level
6. Correct answer: C
7. Correct answer: B
8. Correct answer: D
9. Correct answer: C
10. Correct answer: A

Chapter 16
Basic Level
1. Correct answer: B
2. Correct answer: D
3. Correct answer: C
4. Correct answer: D
5. Correct answer: B
6. Correct answer: C
7. Correct answer: A

Advanced Level
8. Correct answer: B
9. Correct answer: D
10. Correct answer: A
11. Correct answer: D
12. Correct answer: B
13. Correct answer: B

Chapter 17
Basic Level
1. Correct answer: C
2. Correct answer: A,B,D
3. Correct answer: A,C,D
4. Correct answer: D
5. Correct answer: A

Advanced Level
6. Correct answer: A, B,C
7. Correct answer: C
8. Correct answer: A, B, C, D
9. Correct answer: A, B, D
10. Correct answer: A, B, C

Chapter 18
Basic Level
1. Correct answer: D
2. Correct answer: C
3. Correct answer: C
4. Correct answer: D
5. Correct answer: B
6. Correct answer: B
7. Correct answer: C

Advanced Level
8. Correct answer: C
9. Correct answer: B
10. Correct answer: C

Chapter 19
Basic Level
1. Correct answer: B
2. Correct answer: D
3. Correct answer: C
4. Correct answer: B
5. Correct answer: B

Advanced Level
6. Correct answer: C
7. Correct answer: C
8. Correct answer: A
9. Correct answer: C
10. Correct answer: C

Chapter 20

Basic Level

1. Correct answer: D
2. Correct answer: A
3. Correct answer: B
4. Correct answer: B
5. Correct answer: C

Advanced Level

6. Correct answer: A
7. Correct answer: C
8. Correct answer: A
9. Correct answer: B
10. Correct answer: C

Chapter 21

Basic Level

1. Correct answer: B
2. Correct answer: D
3. Correct answer: C
4. Correct answer: B
5. Correct answer: B

Advanced Level

6. Correct answer: B
7. Correct answer: A
8. Correct answer: C
9. Correct answer: A
10. Correct answer: C

Chapter 22

Basic Level

1. Correct answer: A
2. Correct answer: C
3. Correct answer: D
4. Correct answer: A
5. Correct answer: C
6. Correct answer: B
7. Correct answer: D
8. Correct answer: A

Advanced Level

9. Correct answer: C
10. Correct answer: D
11. Correct answer: B
12. Correct answer: D
13. Correct answer: B
14. Correct answer: D
15. Correct answer: B

Chapter 23

Basic Level

1. Correct answer: B
2. Correct answer: D
3. Correct answer: C
4. Correct answer: A
5. Correct answer: D

Advanced Level

6. Correct answer: C
7. Correct answer: A
8. Correct answer: B
9. Correct answer: A
10. Correct answer: D

Chapter 24

Basic Level

1. Correct answer: C
2. Correct answer: A
3. Correct answer: A
4. Correct answer: D
5. Correct answer: B

Advanced Level

6. Correct answer: C
7. Correct answer: A
8. Correct answer: C
9. Correct answer: A
10. Correct answer: B

Chapter 25

Basic Level

1. Correct answer: B
2. Correct answer: B
3. Correct answer: C
4. Correct answer: C
5. Correct answer: C

Advanced Level

6. Correct answer: B
7. Correct answer: C
8. Correct answer: A
9. Correct answer: A
10. Correct answer: C

Chapter 26

Basic Level

1. Correct answer: D
2. Correct answer: C
3. Correct answer: A
4. Correct answer: B
5. Correct answer: C

Advanced Level

6. Correct answer: D
7. Correct answer: A
8. Correct answer: A
9. Correct answer: B
10. Correct answer: A

Chapter 27

Basic Level

1. Correct answer: B
2. Correct answer: B
3. Correct answer: A
4. Correct answer: D
5. Correct answer: C
6. Correct answer: D

Advanced Level

7. Correct answer: C
8. Correct answer: B
9. Correct answer: B
10. Correct answer: D
11. Correct answer: C

Chapter 28

Basic Level

1. Correct answer: D
2. Correct answer: D
3. Correct answer: C
4. Correct answer: D
5. Correct answer: D

Advanced Level

6. Correct answer: C
7. Correct answer: A
8. Correct answer: B
9. Correct answer: A
10. Correct answer: A

Chapter 29

Basic Level

1. Correct answer: C
2. Correct answer: B
3. Correct answer: D
4. Correct answer: A
5. Correct answer: A

Advanced Level

6. Correct answer: D
7. Correct answer: D
8. Correct answer: C
9. Correct answer: B
10. Correct answer: C

Chapter 30

Basic Level

1. Correct answer: B
2. Correct answer: A
3. Correct answer: C
4. Correct answer: B
5. Correct answer: A

Advanced Level

6. Correct answer: D
7. Correct answer: A
8. Correct answer: C
9. Correct answer: D
10. Correct answer: C

Chapter 31

Basic Level

1. Correct answer: B
2. Correct answer: A
3. Correct answer: C
4. Correct answer: E
5. Correct answer: D
6. Correct answer: D

Advanced Level

7. Correct answer: B
8. Correct answer: A
9. Correct answer: D
10. Correct answer: D
11. Correct answer: C
12. Correct answer: C

Chapter 32

Basic Level

1. Correct answer: C
2. Correct answer: C
3. Correct answer: B
4. Correct answer: D
5. Correct answer: D

Advanced Level

6. Correct answer: A
7. Correct answer: D
8. Correct answer: A
9. Correct answer: B
10. Correct answer: D

Chapter 33
Basic Level

1. Correct answer: C
2. Correct answer: A
3. Correct answer: D
4. Correct answer: B
5. Correct answer: D
6. Correct answer: B
7. Correct answer: A

Advanced Level

8. Correct answer: D
9. Correct answer: A
10. Correct answer: B
11. Correct answer: D

Chapter 34
Basic Level

1. Correct answer: B
2. Correct answer: C
3. Correct answer: D
4. Correct answer: A
5. Correct answer: B

Advanced Level

6. Correct answer: D
7. Correct answer: A
8. Correct answer: B
9. Correct answer: A
10. Correct answer: B

Chapter 35
Basic Level

1. Correct answer: C
2. Correct answer: A
3. Correct answer: A
4. Correct answer: C
5. Correct answer: A

Advanced Level

6. Correct answer: D
7. Correct answer: D
8. Correct answer: A
9. Correct answer: B
10. Correct answer: C

Chapter 36
Basic Level

1. Correct answer: C
2. Correct answer: C
3. Correct answer: C
4. Correct answer: C
5. Correct answer: A

Advanced Level

6. Correct answer: D
7. Correct answer: A
8. Correct answer: D
9. Correct answer: C
10. Correct answer: B

Index